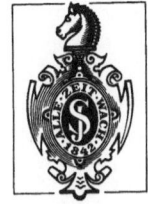

Experimental Lung Cancer

Carcinogenesis and Bioassays

International Symposium
Held at the Battelle Seattle Research Center
Seattle, WA, USA, June 23-26, 1974

Edited by
Eberhard Karbe and James F. Park

With 312 Figures and 144 Tables

Springer-Verlag Berlin Heidelberg GmbH 1974

The Symposium was sponsored by
The Battelle Memorial Institute
The Battelle Institute Life Science Program
The Division of Biomedical and Environmental Research (AEC, USA)
Deutsche Forschungsgemeinschaft, W. Germany

The program was planned with the cooperation of the Carcinogenesis Program
of the National Cancer Institute (NIH, USA)

Dr. Eberhard Karbe
Chief, Toxicology, Physiology and Experimental Medicine Division,
Battelle-Institut e.V., Frankfurt, W. Germany
Privatdozent, Veterinary Pathology, University of Zurich, Zurich, Switzerland

Dr. James F. Park
Associate Manager, Biology Department, Battelle Pacific Northwest Laboratories,
Richland, Wash., USA

ISBN 978-3-642-61941-0   ISBN 978-3-642-61939-7 (eBook)
DOI 10.1007/978-3-642-61939-7

Preface

These are the proceedings of the international symposium on "Experimental Respiratory Carcinogenesis and Bioassays", held from 23 to 26 June 1974 at the Battelle Seattle Research Center, Seattle, Wash., USA.

Human lung cancer is already very common in industrialized countries, and its incidence is increasing. This increase involves mainly epidermoid and small-cell carcinoma. Evidence is accumulating that these tumors are associated with such exogenic factors as automobile exhaust, asbestos, chemicals, cigarette smoke, and radionuclides. These proceedings are concerned with finding the most suitable experimental designs for investigating the genesis of these particular types of tumor, and with the development of specific bioassays to test suspected carcinogens.

Spontaneous epidermoid and small-cell carcinomas are extremely rare in the respiratory organs of animals, and it has proved rather difficult until recently to produce them experimentally. Epidermoid carcinomas are now readily obtained by using methods of intratracheal instillation of carcinogens with particulate materials such as that described by SAFFIOTTI and co-workers, which is the technique most frequently mentioned in these proceedings. While the experimental production of small-cell carcinomas has remained difficult, it is described by two authors in this volume.

The development of an animal model for studying respiratory carcinogenesis or to test suspected respiratory carcinogens must allow for both exogenous factors associated with the material and methods of exposure and factors endogenous to the animal, e.g. particular sensitivity to chemical carcinogens, detailed knowledge of genetic make-up, resistance to respiratory inflammation and CO toxicity, dimensions of the respiratory tract and life span. Special attention has been focused on the correlation between aryl hydrocarbon hydroxylase activity and sensitivity to the carcinogenic effect of polycyclic aromatic hydrocarbons. The induction of a malignant tumor in a simian primate by a polycyclic aromatic hydrocarbon is reported here for the first time.

Inhalation experiments with carcinogens carry a high risk of human exposure, and because of this hazard special precautionary measures have to be taken. The sophisticated equipment required is available in only a few laboratories; we are fortunate that these proceedings include several reports on experiments in this field. Further studies are necessary to improve the exposure design, especially as regards bioassays concerned with the deposition and dosimetry of inhaled particulate matter. Other methods of applying carcinogens to the target tissue, e.g. instillation, injection or implantation, are discussed.

In vitro systems offer unique possibilities for investigating carcinogenesis under defined conditions, and the experiments reported here
indicate that organ cultures are particularly suitable for studying
carcinogenesis at the cellular or molecular level. This approach does
not replace animal experiments; instead, it opens us new avenues in
the study of respiratory carcinogenesis. A topic of very particular
interest is the role of synergistic effects in carcinogenesis. It has
been appreciated during the presentation of papers and in discussions
that superadditive effects may be produced by combinations of carcinogens, or co-carcinogens, and that promoters may be involved in respiratory carcinogenesis. The potentiating effects of components of combustion products were discussed, and the need to identify additional
active principles in polluted air was recognized. The deposition pattern and clearance rate of carcinogens are affected by particle size
and may significantly influence carcinogenesis.

Cigarette smoke, being a major causative factor of human lung cancer,
received a great deal of attention. The best animal model to test the
carcinogenic activity of inhaled cigarette smoke appears at present
to be the Syrian hamster, which develops epidermoid carcinomas in the
larynx. The disadvantages of this model are a low tumor yield (below
2o%) and the fact that the induced respiratory tract tumor is located
only in the larynx.

Another special topic was the effect of inhaled alpha-emitting radionuclides on the incidence of lung cancer, as observed in uranium
miners. Various uranium-mine air contaminants are being tested in
rodents and dogs, and it has been demonstrated that radon daughters
alone can cause lung cancer. Pulmonary deposition of other alpha-
emitting radionuclides (^{239}Pu, ^{238}Pu, ^{244}Cm, ^{241}Am, and ^{210}Po) increases the incidence of pulmonary cancer in rodents. The chemical
form of the isotopes influences distribution of the radiation dose
in the lung; a rather uniformly distributed dose will induce cancer
more readily than a heterogeneously distributed dose from particulate
matter. Alpha-emitting radionuclides induce primarily epithelial tumors
in the lung. At the radiation dose levels studied to date, dogs that
inhaled beta-emitting radionuclides (^{144}Ce and ^{90}Sr) developed mainly
hemangiosarcomas, i.e. tumors of endothelial origin.

The results of animal experiments on the process of carcinogenesis
and the testing of suspected carcinogens depend on interpretation of
the histopathologic lesions. Because of its key role, the histology
of precancerous and cancerous lesions was discussed in detail during
a three-hour slide session; this discussion is not included in these
proceedings.

We were fortunate in that many outstanding scientists in the field of
experimental lung cancer attended the symposium and contributed to
these proceedings. In particular, we would like to thank Dr. UMBERTO
SAFFIOTTI for introducing the symposium, Drs. WALTER DONTENWILL,
SIDNEY LASKIN, PAUL NETTESHEIM, and MICHAEL SPORN for introducing and
chairing the sessions, and Dr. SWEND NIELSEN for organizing and chairing the slide session. These scientists helped to plan the symposium
and made a significant contribution to its success. A wealth of scientific information was given in 58 papers by authors from various countries, presenting the state of the art in the field of experimental
lung cancer at an international level. The 1o3 participants came from
France, Germany, Great Britain, Japan, Switzerland, and the United
States of America.

We are also greatful to numerous people for their technical assistance in assuring the smooth running of the symposium and the rapid publication of these proceedings. In this respect we would like to acknowledge the efforts of SHIRLEY LAKE, who helped to organize the symposium, and ELLEN BRANDT, who helped to edit these proceedings, both in Seattle. Last but not least, we extend thanks, not only for their help, but also for their great patience, to our secretaries, INGEBORG SCHIECHEL in Frankfurt and JUDITH HARRISON in Richland.

Finally, we thank the publisher for publishing these proceedings less than six months after the symposium took place.

September 1974   Eberhard Karbe
                                        Battelle-Institut e.V.
                                        Frankfurt, W.Germany

                                        James F. Park
                                        Battelle Pacific Northwest
                                        Laboratories
                                        Richland, Wash., USA

Contents

X

SESSION V

In vitro Bioassays of Respiratory Carcinogens. Chairman: M.B.
SPORN

Keynote Address: Progress in Respiratory Carcinogenesis

Umberto Saffiotti

National Cancer Institute, National Institutes of Health, Bethesda, MD, USA

I wish to thank the Symposium Chairmen for giving me the privilege of opening the proceedings of this conference on respiratory carcinogenesis, which stimulates great anticipation for much new information and for the discussion of many exciting developments in this field.

Many of us, reunited here today, have been directly involved in the development of research in respiratory carcinogenesis for many years. It is therefore a pleasure for us to meet with old friends for a renewed exchange of scientific news in such delightful surroundings. This pleasure is enhanced by the presence of several colleagues who have more recently entered this field and who will bring to us new ideas and new perspectives.

Progress in respiratory carcinogenesis has been remarkable in the last 10 to 15 years and its momentum is increasing. Only a few, rather isolated laboratories were active in this field until the early 1960s, when new animal models were developed. These models allowed a good experimental reproduction of the main type of respiratory neoplasia, i.e., bronchogenic carcinoma, and made it feasible to approach the experimental study of the complex factors and mechanisms involved in the pathogenesis of respiratory tract cancers.

As is witnessed by the present symposium, a broader and more articulated effort has now developed, with a great deal of collaboration and joint efforts by different research groups.

In the last decade, a series of conferences have provided the framework for an assessment of the state of our knowledge on respiratory carcinogenesis. In June 1965, a conference on "Lung Tumors in Animals" was organized by Professor SEVERI at the University of Perugia (SEVERI, 1966). It provided the first comprehensive review of our field and a demonstration of the new methods of induction of bronchogenic carcinomas. I had the opportunity to review the field again at the International Symposium on Carcinogenesis and Carcinogen Testing organized in Boston in 1967 by Dr. HOMBURGER (SAFFIOTTI, 1969).

Two other conferences were jointly sponsored by the National Cancer Institute and by the Atomic Energy Commission, organized by the Biology Division of the Oak Ridge National Laboratory, and held in Gatlinburg, Tennessee. One of these conferences, devoted to "Inhalation Carcinogenesis" and related methods, was held in October 1969 (HANNA et al., 1970); the other, devoted to the "Morphology of Experimental Respiratory Carcinogenesis", took place in May 1970 (NETTESHEIM et al., 1970). The present symposium comes, after an interval of 4 years, at an opportune time to review a great deal of progress with emphasis on new bioassay methods.

Lung cancer is still a growing threat to our society, its death toll still increasing in most countries.

In 1969, at the first Gatlinburg Conference, I noted that the projected mortality from lung cancer for that year in the United States was 60,000 deaths, which meant 165 deaths per day or one every 8 1/2 minutes. The lung cancer mortality now projected for 1974 in the United States is 75,000 deaths (National Cancer Institute Fact Book, 1974) which means that we have now 205 deaths per day from lung cancer or one every 7 minutes. The current projections are reported in Table 1.

Table 1. Estimated cancer deaths and new cases of respiratory cancers for the United States, 1974

Cancer Site	Estimated Deaths			Estimated New Cases		
	Total	Male	Female	Total	Male	Female
Lung	75,400	59,900	15,500	83,000	67,000	16,000
Larynx	3,200	2,800	400	9,500	8,300	1,200
Other and Unspecified	1,300	800	500	2,700	1,700	1,000
Total Respiratory System	79,900	63,500	16,400	95,200	77,000	18,200

Many considerations and research methods that apply to lung cancer also apply to cancer of the larynx (SAFFIOTTI and KAUFMAN, in press). The greatest single factor in a tragedy of such immense proportions as those implicit in the figures in Table 1 has been well identified: it is cigarette smoking, a habit that could well be avoided, thus preventing such disastrous consequences.

A number of other environmental exposures to chemical and physical carcinogens have also been found to be causally linked to respiratory cancers in man. Exposures to some of these hazards, such as asbestos or radiation from radon and radon daughters, act synergistically with the exposure to cigarette smoke, producing a multiplicative rather than a simply additive effect.

Undoubtedly, our society is presently subject to a very high level of respiratory cancer risk from tobacco smoke and from other environmental factors. Does this mean that our society accepts such a risk? I do not believe so. Our society is actually showing more and more clearly that it does not want to accept such a risk. Our being here today and our own work are proofs of the refusal of our society to accept such a risk passively. In the United States, the Federal Government through its several agencies, as well as universities and research institutes, private agencies, industry, and public interest groups are contributing to a major effort aimed at the prevention of lung cancer.

The Carcinogenesis Program of the National Cancer Institute has been a focal point of much of this work, and I would like to share with you some of the concepts that have been the basis for our development of a program on the pathogenesis of lung cancer and its prevention.

Recognizing the complexity and multiplicity of the causative factors and of the host control mechanisms, we addressed our program to several levels of investigation. The development of more specific animal models was followed by histogenesis studies, by the bioassay of new environmental agents, and by the study of their dose-response relationships and possible synergism. The role of cofactors, such as particulate materials or intercurrent infections, was also investigated in the animal models.

A major effort was devoted in our NCI laboratories to the development of methods for the biochemical analysis of the target tissues, namely the epithelia of the tracheobronchial tract, and to the elucidation of morphological-biochemical correlations in the early stages of the specific carcinogenic response.

It became possible for us to establish in 1970 a Lung Cancer Unit, which later became the Lung Cancer Branch in the Carcinogenesis Program. This Branch, and the corresponding Lung Cancer Segment for collaborative research, are directed by Dr. Michael B. SPORN and have the collaboration of Drs. David G. KAUFMAN, Curtis C. HARRIS, Luigi DE-LUCA, Carl SMITH, and a few others.

Recent key developments have been the establishment of methodologies for the analysis of the target epithelia *in vitro*, using organ cultures, and the combination of *in vivo* and *in vitro* techniques of exposure to carcinogens, inhibitors, and markers to obtain a dynamic analysis of steps involved in the pathogenesis of respiratory cancers. The microsomal enzyme systems responsible for carcinogen activation at the target site are being studied in this context, since it becomes necessary to define this important parameter of susceptibility in precise measurable terms as they relate to the cells of origin of respiratory cancers.

Another approach has been devoted to developing inhibitory mechanisms for those cellular control factors which regulate cellular differentiation and carcinogenesis, such as those dependent on vitamin A. Dr. SPORN will discuss these developments in detail in Session V.

Using the methods of biochemical analysis of the target cells, the binding of carcinogens to the respiratory epithelial cells and to their DNA has been demonstrated and quantitated. Its dependence on both the microsomal enzyme system and on vitamin A have been shown (KAUFMAN et al., 1972 and 1973; HARRIS et al., 1973; GENTA et al., 1974).

Finally, and perhaps most importantly, we have continued to relate the experimental systems to the problem of carcinogenesis in man. High-risk groups have been identified and followed up, particularly asbestos workers and uranium miners. The frequently long duration of a preneoplastic stage in the bronchial epithelium, such as carcinoma *in situ* before invasive cancer sets in, gives us hope that if we succeed in developing effective means for a pharmacologic intervention in anticarcinogenesis, this could be successfully applied to selected high-risk populations to prevent or markedly delay the onset of malignancy. The need for direct experimental study of the human respiratory epithelium is now being met by the application of the previously developed *in vitro* methods directly to the human bronchial epithelium in organ cultures. Dr. TRUMP will give the first report of these studies in Session V. A program on tobacco carcinogenesis and on the identification of less hazardous cigarettes was supported by the Carcinogenesis Program until October 1973, when it was established as a separate Program on Smoking and Health within the National Cancer Institute.

I could not begin to do justice in such a short time to all the investigators who have greatly contributed to the development of our program on lung carcinogenesis. Suffice it to say that the program of this symposium is a representative sample of the state of this work and of its international nature.

Major new trends have clearly appeared in the 4 to 5 years since the Gatlinburg meetings and are going to be discussed in this symposium. Methods will be reported from several laboratories for the induction of respiratory neoplasia by direct inhalation of tobacco smoke, localized in the larynx. Several conditions will be demonstrated in which different factors or cofactors combine to produce respiratory cancers, in some instances by a clearly synergistic mechanism reminiscent of the effects observed in man. Combined effects will be illustrated for chemical carcinogens in association with other chemicals, with physical factors such as particulated materials and radiation, and with viral infections. Many of these systems also represent new bioassay methods, such as the implantation in the lung of wax pellets with tobacco smoke condensate, which was proposed by STANTON. Advances in radiation carcinogenesis will also be discussed. Histopathology of the induced lesions will be discussed in detail; particular interest will be given to the suggested induction of tumors similar to small-cell undifferentiated carcinomas presented by BLAIR and by GRICIUTE.

Finally, this symposium will devote a major portion of its program to the new developments based on *in vitro* methodologies, which represent not only the focusing of our research tools on the fundamental cellular and molecular mechanisms that control respiratory carcinogenesis, but also the development of powerful new bioassay methods that can be addressed both to the identification of carcinogens or anticarcinogens at the cellular level and to the measurement of individual susceptibility of the target tissues in animals and in man.

I am delighted to share with you these exciting developments and I wish you all a successful meeting.

References

GENTA, V.M., KAUFMAN, D.G., HARRIS, C.C., SMITH, J.M., SPORN, M.B., SAFFIOTTI, U.: Vitamin A deficiency enhances binding of benzo(a)-pyrene to tracheal epithelial DNA. Nature, 247, 48-49 (1974).

HANNA, M.G., Jr., NETTESHEIM, P., GILBERT, J.R. (Eds): Inhalation Carcinogenesis. AEC Symposium Series no. 18 (Conf. 691001), 524 pp. Oak Ridge, Tennessee: U.S. Atomic Energy Commission, Division of Technical Information Extension, 1970.

HARRIS, C.C., KAUFMAN, D.G., SPORN, M.B., BOREN, H., JACKSON, F., SMITH, J.M., PAULEY, J., DEDICK, P., SAFFIOTTI, U.: Localization of benzo(a)pyrene-^{3}H and alterations in nuclear chromatin caused by benzo(a)pyrene-ferric oxide in the hamster respiratory epithelium. Cancer Res., 33, 2842-2848 (1973).

KAUFMAN, D.G., BAKER, M.S., HARRIS, C.C., SMITH, J.M., BOREN, H., SPORN, M.B., SAFFIOTTI, U.: Coordinated biochemical and morphologic examination of hamster tracheal epithelium. J. nat. Cancer Inst., 49, 783-792 (1972).

KAUFMAN, D.G., GENTA, V.M., HARRIS, C.C., SMITH, J.M., SPORN, M.B., SAFFIOTTI, U.: Binding of ^{3}H-labeled benzo(a)pyrene to DNA in hamster tracheal epithelial cells. Cancer Res., 33, 2837-2841 (1973).

National Cancer Institute Fact Book 1974. U.S. Department of Health, Education and Welfare. Publication No. (NIH) 74-512, 46 pp. Washington, D.C.: U.S. Government Printing Office 1974.

NETTESHEIM, P., HANNA, M.G., Jr., DEATHERAGE, J.W., Jr. (Eds): Mor-
phology of Experimental Respiratory Carcinogenesis. AEC Symposium
Series no. 21 (Conf. 700501), 483 pp. Oak Ridge, Tennessee: U.S.
Atomic Energy Commission, Division of Technical Information Exten-
sion, 1970.
SAFFIOTTI, U.: Experimental Respiratory Tract Carcinogenesis. In:
Progr. Exp. Tumor Res., Vol. 11, pp. 302-333 (F. Homburger, ed.).
New York, Basel: Karger 1969.
The Laryngoscope, in press.
SEVERI, L. (ed.): Lung Tumours in Animals. Proc. 3rd Quadrennial
Internat. Conf. on Cancer, 970 pp. Perugia. Italy: Division of Cancer
Research, University of Perugia 1966.

Session I Methods in Experimental Respiratory Carcinogenesis and Bioassays

Chairman: Sidney Laskin

New York University Medical Center, New York, NY, USA

Models in Chemical Respiratory Carcinogenesis*

Sidney Laskin and Arthur Sellakumar

New York University Medical Center, Department of Environmental Medicine, New York, NY 10016, USA

The first landmark conference on respiratory carcinogenesis was that held in Perugia, Italy in 1965 (SEVERI, 1966). It is of interest to note that at this conference, much of the discussion is related to the search for appropriate techniques and the search for an ideal animal model. FRANCIS ROE outlined specifications for the ideal model (ROE, 1966). These specifications can be summarized as follows:

1. Realistic exposure (inhalation)
2. Small species in large numbers
3. Short lifespan
4. Low incidence of spontaneous lung cancer
5. No interference by other respiratory disease
6. Anatomical similarity to man
7. Similar histologic types and sites.

ROE also made the point of relationships of cancer to background disease, pre-existing scars, and other clinical problems which may be related to the etiology of lung cancer. It is recognized that human lung cancer is a disease with multiple etiology, which is interrelated with a variety of factors and co-factors which, in turn, may be dependent upon the anatomical and physiological mechanisms involved. The present state of our knowledge finds the animal that most closely meets the requirements of the ideal model to be the common laboratory rat. Squamous cell carcinoma of bronchogenic origin has been clearly demonstrated in a variety of more recent studies. In over 20 years, our experience with the Sprague-Dawley strain has never demonstrated this cancer to arise spontaneously. This is in agreement with the findings of other laboratories. A note of caution, however, must be considered with the use of SPF animals. A recent study by PREJEAN et al. (1973) does indeed show a low but real spontaneous incidence of this type of cancer.

The problem at stake is multiple - man is exposed to complex mixtures and the identification of carcinogens in such mixtures are best accomplished with the rat model. In order to elucidate mechanisms and to distinguish between true carcinogens, co-carcinogens, and other factors, a variety of other models may be of particular value. Noteworthy among these is the hamster intratracheal model of SAFFIOTTI et al. (1965).

Table 1 briefly outlines the variety of factors which must be considered in the selection of a model. Many of these factors will be demonstrated in the studies reported at this session. A constant underlying factor is the genetic background of the individual animal. Al-

---

*Excluding radioactive materials and tobacco products which will be considered in other sessions.

8

Table 1. Factors in the model

1. Animal	2. Compound
species strain anatomy and respiratory physiology metabolic pathways immunologic mechanisms endocrine responses	physical and chemical state metabolic intermediates mode of action secondary toxic reactions
3. Combined actions	4. Interrelationship with disease
vehicle co-carcinogenesis promotion	pre-existing disease virus interactions

though a large body of information exists for the laboratory mouse, there is a definite need for the development of genetic information for other species.

The materials dispersed in the atmosphere are primarily in 2 forms; particulates or aerosols which include dusts, fumes, mists, smokes, and gases and vapors. Particulates vary greatly in particle size, shape, and uniformity of dispersion. Gases and vapors, on the other hand, usually are dispersed in molecular form and are more uniformly distributed. The action of gases and vapors is directly proportional to their concentration in the atmosphere. Generally, the region of deposition in the respiratory system is related to the solubility of the gas; most soluble gases are largely deposited in the upper respiratory passages, less soluble and insoluble gases will penetrate to the alveolar region.

Factors determining injury from inhaled particulates are summarized in Table 2. The division of a solid into small particles and their subsequent dispersion into the atmosphere results in 2 important changes. Tremendous increases occur in both the surface area and total space occupied. The effect of these changes is to intensify the chemical and physical activity of the material. These properties show in increased rates of reactions involving oxidation, solubility, evaporation, adsorption, and electrical activity. Changes in these properties may also cause subsequent changes in other physical properties. Thus the adsorption of a gas film on a particle surface may interfere with its chemical reactions and also with physical phenomena, such as wetting.

The physiological effect of air-borne particles is also intimately associated with their physical and chemical properties. Since these properties are related to particle size, the significance of particle size to the inhalation problem is considerable. In general, small particles may be expected to be more active than large ones. Moreover the effective sizes depend upon the amount of a given size retained by the animal.

Problems relating to the deposition and clearance of particulate matter have been reviewed (Air Quality Criteria for Particulate Matter, 1970). Toxic action of particulates may be due to one or more of 3 mechanisms (Air Quality Criteria for Particulate Matter, 1970):

1. The particle may be intrinsically toxic due to its inherent chemical and/or physical characteristics.

2.   The particle may interfere with one or more of the clearance mechanisms in the respiratory tract.

3.   The particle may act as a carrier of an adsorbed toxic substance.

Almost 6 decades have passed since the first description of chemical carcinogenesis by YAMAGIWA and ICHIKAWA (1915). During this time various investigators have tried numerous techniques; the majority of which resulted in failure. It is only within the last 20 years that successful techniques have been developed. The most notable of these are: intratracheal intubation, implant techniques, systemic administration, inhalation exposures.

In this brief review, successful techniques considered will be largely those resulting in histologic types of lung cancer similar to that seen in man. These include squamous cell carcinoma, adenocarcinoma, small or oat cell carcinoma, and undifferentiated carcinoma. It must be recognized that classification and description of histopathologic types is still a controversial area. For the purposes of this review, each author's definitions or descriptions have been accepted as stated.

Table 2.   Factors determining injury from inhaled particulates

---

1.   Quantity of particulate inhaled

a)   Concentration in the atmosphere
b)   Particle size distribution
c)   Duration of the exposure
d)   Respiratory rate and volume

2.   Quantity of particulate retained

a)   Physiochemical properties of the particulate
b)   Anatomical structure
c)   Clearance mechanisms

3.   Site of action

a)   Particle size and other physical properties define region of deposition
b)   Physical and chemical nature, solubility, etc. determine the site and specific response

---

Intratracheal Intubation Studies

Table 3 shows selected references for intratracheal studies. Although one of the early negative findings was that reported by SANNIE (1935) where benzo(a)pyrene (BP) is given in olive oil to rats, NISKANEN (1949), using a similar technique with dibenz(a,h)anthracene (DBA) was successful in inducing squamous cell carcinoma. The first to show that bronchogenic carcinoma could be induced in hamsters was DELLA PORTA et al. (1958) using 7,12-dimethylbenz(a,h)anthracene (DMBA).

Many of the early intratracheal studies were complicated by tissue destruction and inflammatory responses which may be important factors in the pathogenesis of these experimentally induced tumors. The introduction of the BP + ferric oxide technique of SAFFIOTTI represents a major advance with the induction of a high incidence of tumors without the presence of marked irritation and inflammation. The role of the so-called 'inert dust' such as iron oxide may relate to the clearance and/or penetration of the carcinogen. However, recent studies by MONTESANO et al. (1970) suggest that iron oxide may act similarly

Table 3. Selected references for intratracheal intubation studies (positive findings)

Dibenz(a,h)anthracene in olive oil	Rats	1949, NISKANEN (1949)
7,12-Dimethylbenz-(a)anthracene	Hamsters	1958, DELLA PORTA et al. (1958)
Diethylnitrosamine	Hamsters	1962, DONTENWILL et al. (1964)
Benzo(a)pyrene in tween-60	Hamsters	1962, HERROLD and DUNHAM (1962)
7,12-Dimethylbenz-(a)anthracene in mineral oil	Hamsters	1965, GROSS et al. (1965)
Benzo(a)pyrene in mineral oil	Hamsters	1965, GROSS et al. (1965)
Chrysotile + benzo(a)pyrene	Hamsters	1965, MILLER et al. (1965)
Benzo(a)pyrene + ferric oxide	Hamsters	1965, SAFFIOTTI et al. (1965)
N-nitroso-N-methylurea	Hamsters	1970, HERROLD (1970)
Methylcholanthrene	Hamsters	1970, LASKIN et al. (1970)
Benzo(a)pyrene + india ink	Rats	1970, SHABAD and PYLEV (1970)
Chrysotile + benzo(a)pyrene in tween-60	Hamsters	1970, SMITH et al. (1966)
Methylcholanthrene	Mice	1971, NETTESHEIM et al. (1971)
Methylcholanthrene	Rats	1972, SCHREIBER et al. (1972)
Benzo(a)pyrene	Hamsters	1972, FERON (1972)
Chrysotile + benzo(a)pyrene	Rats	1972, PYLEV (1972)
7H-Dibenzo(c,g)-carbazole + ferric oxide	Hamsters	1972, SELLAKUMAR and SHUBIK (1972)
Chrysotile + benzo(a)pyrene	Rats	1972, VÔSAMÄE (1972)
7,12-Dimethylbenz-(a)anthracene	Rats	1973, BLAIR et al. (1973)

to a tumor promoting agent. It is of interest to note, in examining Table 3, that the majority of the positive compounds are in combination with other materials or vehicles which may have co-carcinogenic or promoting effects. Recent studies have shown that with modifications of technique and selection of more appropriate strains of animals, pure carcinogens could indeed result in positive findings. Of particular interest is the use of methylcholanthrene (MCH) in hamsters by LASKIN et al. (1970), in mice by NETTESHEIM et al. (1971), and in rats by SCHREIBER et al. (1972). FERON (1972) has also been able to produce carcinomas in hamsters with high concentrations of BP.

Implant Techniques

Implant techniques (Table 4) have been highly successful and have
proven useful as a screening procedure. ANDERVONT (1937) was the first
to use this technique successfully to produce squamous cell carcinoma
in animals. His technique involved passing thread impregnated with
DBA through the intact chest wall of mice. Modifications of this technique have been described by KUSCHNER et al. (1957) which resulted in
induction of bronchogenic carcinoma in rats and mice with MCH and DBA.

Table 4. Selected references for implant techniques

Thread implants			
1,2,5,6 Dibenzan-thracene	Mice	1937,	ANDERVONT (1937)
Methylcholanthrene	Rats	1957,	KUSCHNER et al. (1957)
Dibenzanthracene	Rats	1957,	KUSCHNER et al. (1957)
Methylcholanthrene	Rats	1963,	BROWN (1963)
Intrabronchial pellet implants			
Benzo(a)pyrene	Rats, hamsters	1970,	LASKIN et al. (1970)
Methylcholanthrene	Rats, hamsters	1970,	LASKIN et al. (1970)
Calcium chromate	Rats	1970,	LASKIN et al. (1970)
Lung pellet implant			
Methylcholanthrene	Rats	1972,	STANTON and BLACKWELL (1961)
Intrapleural implant[a]			
Asbestos	Rats	1972,	STANTON and WRENCH (1972)
Fiberglass	Rats	1972,	STANTON and WRENCH (1972)

[a]All other techniques - squamous cell carcinoma; this technique -
mesothelioma.

The intrabronchial pellet implant technique (LASKIN et al., 1970) was
developed in our laboratory to provide selective exposure of a well-
defined area of the bronchial mucosa. This technique, although highly
artificial, has aided in the development of dose-response relationships
and the evaluation of serial pathogenesis in rats and hamsters.

The technique of STANTON and BLACKWELL (1961) represents a blind introduction of materials in a beeswax carrier pellet. In a more recent
technique which utilizes an intrapleural implant, STANTON and WRENCH
(1972) have successfully induced mesotheliomas with both asbestos
and fiberglass particles.

Systemic Administration

The development of studies with nitrosamines by MAGEE and BARNES in
the fifties (MAGEE and BARNES, 1967) introduced a new concept to the
study of respiratory tract carcinogenesis. Here was a class of chemicals which could be introduced by a variety of systemic routes which
led to lung cancer. Table 5 shows some of the variety of successful
studies performed with nitrosamines and related compounds. MOHR (1970)
has recently reviewed extensive studies by the German workers.

Table 5. Selected references for systemic administration[a]

Dimethylnitrosamine	Rats	Subcutaneous	1962, DRUCKREY and PREUSSMANN (1962)
4-Nitroquinoline-N-oxide	Rats	Subcutaneous	1962, MORI (1962)
Diethylnitrosamine	Hamsters	Subcutaneous	1964, DONTENWILL (1964)
Diethylnitrosamine	Rabbit	Oral	1965, RAPP et al. (1971)
Nitrosoheptamethylene-imine	Rats	Oral	1969, LIJINSKY et al. (1969)
Diethylnitrosamine	Hamsters	Subcutaneous	1970, MONTESANO et al. (1970)
Dibutylnitrosamine	Hamsters	Subcutaneous and oral	1971, ALTHOFF et al. (1971)
Di-N-propylnitrosamine	Hamsters	Subcutaneous	1974, POUR et al. (1974)

[a]Predominantly adenocarcinomas except for nitrosoheptamethyleneimine
which is predominantly squamous cell carcinoma.

Diethylnitrosamine (DEN) is the compound which has been extensively
studied. Although primarily a liver carcinogen in rats, it is a significant respiratory tract carcinogen in hamsters regardless of the
route of administration. Dose-response relationships after subcutaneous
injection of DEN were investigated by MONTESANO and SAFFIOTTI (1968).

The nitrosamines are of particular importance since human exposure
occurs in certain chemical industries. They may also pose general
health problems in that they can occur in foods, tobacco smoke, and
may be formed *in vivo* from nitrites and secondary amines. The role of
nitrosamines as possible co-factors with polycyclic hydrocarbons may
become an important area for study. Synergistic effects with DEN plus
BP and ferric oxide and with ferric oxide alone have already been reported by MONTESANO et al. (1970).

Inhalation

SAFFIOTTI, at the first Gatlingburg Conference (SAFFIOTTI, 1970), considered experimental inhalation exposures as the ultimate tool for the
study of respiratory tract carcinogenesis. Although inhalation studies
were described as early as 1865 (EULENBERG, 1865), it is only with the
development of modern technology that adequate definition, control,
and reproducibility of experimental conditions could be attained. This
technology has recently been described in a review by DREW and LASKIN
(1973). The literature of the last 90 years contains results of literal-
ly hundreds of studies which are predominantly negative with respect
to the problem of inhalation carcinogenesis. The major reason for
failure in these studies were that exposures were poorly defined or
controlled and most represented acute or limited periods of exposure.
Chronic or lifespan studies have been rare until the last 20 years.

In the recent literature on chronic studies, a variety of materials
examined showed negative findings. These range from the vanadium pentoxide studies of SJÖBERG to the more recent studies of NETTESHEIM et
al. with ozonized gasoline plus influenza virus (Table 6).

A variety of studies with mice showed only increases in adenoma incidences as shown in Table 7. This appears to be a characteristic
responce in the mouse and its spontaneous incidence is well documented

Table 6. Selected references for inhalation studies (negative findings)

Vanadium pentoxide	Rabbits	1951, SJÖBERG (1951)
Asbestos	Mice, dogs, monkeys, guinea pigs	1951-64, various authors SMITH et al. (1966)
Silica dust	Rats	1957, SCHEPERS et al. (1957)
Chrome compounds	Mice, rats, rabbits, guinea pigs	1959, BAETJER et al. (1959)
Glass dust	Rats, guinea pigs	1960, GROSS et al. (1960)
Asphalt	Guinea pigs, mice	1960, HUEPER and PAYNE (1960)
Nickel dust	Rats, hamsters	1962, HUEPER and PAYNE (1962)
Titanium dioxide	Rats	1963, CHRISTIE et al. (1963)
Asphalt	Mice	1964, SIMMERS (1964)
Ozonized gasoline + influenza virus	Mice	1970, NETTESHEIM et al. (1970)

to be related to genetic factors. Its relationship, however, to human carcinogenesis is not yet understood. ROE argues that agents which produce such lesions in mice, when adequately tested, usually do indeed induce cancer in other sites or tissues (ROE, 1966). He states, therefore, that this model may well be an extremely sensitive bioassay system for detecting carcinogenicity.

Inhalation studies with mice where adenocarcinomas are the most advanced finding are not as prominent in the literature (Table 8).

Adenocarcinomas, though found occasionally in rats and hamsters, are not the most advanced finding for these species. In the recent literature, a wide variety of materials have resulted in findings of squamous cell carcinomas (Table 9). It is of interest to note that ozonized gasoline, which by itself resulted only in adenocarcinomas, when combined with influenza virus produced squamous cell carcinoma. This tumor has also been demonstrated in mice with coal tar by HORTON et al. (1963) and more recently with MCH by NETTESHEIM (1971).

The majority of the successful studies shown in Table 9 were predominantly performed with rats. These were largely combined-action studies or utilized materials which had strong action as respiratory irritants.

The studies of GROSS et al. (1967) and REEVES et al. 1971) clearly confirm the carcinogenicity of asbestos. It must be recognized, however, that this material contains trace metals and that asbestos may be an effective adsorber of BP. Also GROSS's experiments have been criticized since his grinding procedures significantly increased quantities of chromium in the final dust.

A variety of industrial materials have quite recently been implicated as potential human carcinogens. These are reported in the studies of VIOLA (1970) and LASKIN et al. (1971, 1972, 1973). Of particular interest is bis(chloromethyl)ether (BCME). The studies of LEONG with mice (LEONG et al., 1971) yielded only increased incidences of adenomas with BCME whereas those reported by LASKIN et al. (1971) with rats resulted in significant numbers of squamous cell carcinomas in addi-

Table 7. Inhalation studies

1. Increase in adenoma incidence		
Tarred road dust	Mice	1934, CAMPBELL (1934)
Gasoline + tetra ethyl lead	Mice	1936, CAMPBELL (1936)
Chimney soot	Mice	1938, SEELIG and BENIGNUS (1938)
Street dust	Mice	1942, MCDONALD and WOODHOUSE (1942)
Ozonized gasoline	Mice	1956, KOTIN and FALK (1956)
Coal tar fractions + phenolics	Mice	1967, TYE and STEMMER (1967)
Bis(chloromethyl)ether	Mice	1971, LEONG et al. (1971)

Table 8. Inhalation studies

2. Adenocarcinoma		
Ozonized gasoline	Mice	1956, KOTIN and FALK (1956)
3-Nitro-3-hexane	Mice	1963, DEICHMAN et al. (1963)
Ozonized gasoline	Mice	1970, NETTESHEIM et al. (1970)
Calcium chromate (dust)	Mice	1971, NETTESHEIM et al. (1971)

Table 9. Inhalation studies

3. Squamous cell carcinomas		
Nickel carbonyl	Rats	1959-65, SUNDERMAN et al. (1959, 1961, 1963, 1965)
Diethylnitrosamine	Hamsters	1962, DONTENWILL et al. (1962)
Ozonized gasoline + influenza virus	Mice	1963, KOTIN and WISELEY (1963)
Coal tar	Mice	1963, HORTON et al. (1963)
Asbestos (chrysotile)	Rats	1967, GROSS et al. (1967)
Sulfur dioxide + benzo(a)pyrene	Rats	1970, LASKIN et al. (1970)
Vinyl chloride	Rats	1970, VIOLA (1970)
Crocidolite	Rats	1971, REEVES et al. (1971)
Bis(chloromethyl)ether	Rats	1971, LASKIN et al. (1971)
Polyurethane	Rats	1972, LASKIN et al. (1972)
Calcium chromate	Rats	1973, LASKIN et al. (1973)

tion to a high incidence of esthesioneuroepitheliomas. The extremely
low levels used (O.l ppm) suggested a very serious new industrial
hazard. Subsequent to the original publication, a number of epidemiologic studies have confirmed this material as a human carcinogen
(FISHBEIN, 1972; Occupational safety and health letter, 1972; SAKABE,
1973; THEISS et al., 1973).

Inhalation of BP in combination with exposures to sulfur dioxide has
resulted in the production of squamous cell carcinomas in rats (LASKIN

et al., 1970). These findings are of particular interest since both
materials have been implicated in community air pollution problems and
since these represent the first duplication of human lung cancer in
animals by inhalation exposures to polycyclic hydrocarbons. The industrial coke oven problem may also relate directly to this type of
exposure. Both BP and sulfur dioxide are present in coke oven emissions
and may interact in humans as they do in rats (Criteria for a Recommended
Standard, 1973).

In current studies at our laboratory, hamsters intubated with carcinogen
are being exposed to sulfur dioxide atmospheres. BP, which has previously shown negative results by intubation only, in combination with
sulfur dioxide exposures has resulted in the appearance of squamous
cell carcinomas. This combination of techniques may provide another
useful model for respiratory tract carcinogenesis.

We now have at our disposal a series of animal models for respiratory
carcinogenesis which closely simulate the disease in man. These model
systems have begun to be useful for the identification of environmental
carcinogenic agents and co-factors which may be involved. If inhalation
is accepted as the ultimate model, then studies in recent years tend
to suggest that the rat may be the species of choice most closely
resembling man.

Acknowledgements

The authors wish to acknowledge the technical help of ANNAMARIE VERDE
and DOROTHY NATALIZIO in the preparation of this review.

This review was prepared under the support of Contract Number NO1-CP-
33260 from the United States Public Health Service, National Cancer
Institute and is part of a center program supported by the National
Institutes of Environmental Health Sciences, Grant No. ES00260.

References

Air Quality Criteria for Particulate Matter. Chap. 9. U.S. Department
    H.E.W. National Air Pollution Control Administration Publication
    No. AP-49, 1970.
Air Quality Criteria for Particulate Matter, p. 141, U.S. Department
    H.E.W. National Air Pollution Control Administration Publication
    No. AP-49, 1970.
ALTHOFF, J., KRÜGER, F.W., MOHR, W., SCHMÄHL, D.: Dibutylnitrosamine
    carcinogenesis in Syrian golden and Chinese hamsters. Proc. Soc.
    exp. Biol. (N.Y.) 136, 168-173 (1971).
ANDERVONT, H.B.: Pulmonary Tumors in Mice. IV. Lung tumors induced
    by subcutaneous injection of 1,2,5,6-Dibenzanthracene in different
    media and by direct contact with lung tissues. Publ. Hlth Rep.
    (Wash.) 52, 1584-1589 (1937).
BAETJER, A.M., LOWNEY, J.F., STEFFEE, H., BUDACZ, U.: Effect of
    chromium on incidence of lung tumors in mice and rats. AMA Arch.
    Ind. Health 20, 124-135 (1959).
BLAIR, W.H., OTERO, N., RAO, H.: Development of lung neoplasms in rats
    treated with 7,12-Dimethyl-benz(a)anthracene. In: Proc. Amer. Ass.
    Cancer Res., 64th annual meeting, Atlantic City, N.J., Apr. 11-13,
    1973.
BROWN, C.E.: Carcinoma of the rat lung from intrapleural methyl-
    cholanthrene. Arch. Path. (Chicago) 76, 347-353 (1963).

CAMPBELL, J.A.: Cancer of the skin and increase in incidence of primary tumors of lung in mice exposed to dust obtained from tarred roads. Brit. J. exp. Path. 15, 287-294 (1934).

CAMPBELL, J.A.: The effect of exhaust gases from internal combustion engines and of tobacco smoke upon mice with special reference to incidence of tumors of the lung. Brit. J. exp. Path. 17, 146-158 (1936).

CHRISTIE, H., MACKAY, R.J., FISHER, A.M.: Pulmonary effects of inhalation of titanium dioxide by rats. Amer. industr. Hyg. Ass. J. 24, 42-46 (1963).

Criteria for a Recommended Standard. Occupational Exposure to Coke Oven Emissions. U.S. Dept. H.E.W., HSM 73-11016, 1973.

DEICHMANN, W.B., MACDONALD, W.E., ANDERSON, W.A.D., BERNAL, E.: Adenocarcinoma in the lungs of mice exposed to vapors of 3-Nitro-3-Hexane. Toxicol. and App. Pharmacol. 5, 445-456 (1963).

DELLA PORTA, G., KOLB, L., SHUBIK, P.: Induction of tracheobronchial carcinomas in the Syrian golden hamster. Cancer Res. 18, 592-597 (1958).

DONTENWILL, W.: Experimentelle Untersuchungen zur Genese der Lungencarcinomas. Arzneimittel-Forsch. 14, 774-780 (1964).

DONTENWILL, W., MOHR, U., ZAGEL, M.: Über die unterschiedliche Lungencarcinogene Wirkung des Diäthylnitrosamin bei Hamster und Ratte. Z. Krebsforsch. 64, 499-502 (1962).

DREW, R.T., LASKIN, S.: Environmental inhalation chambers. In: Methods in animal experimentation (W.I. Gay, ed.), Vol. 4, pp. 1-41. New York, London: Academic Press, 1973.

DRUCKREY, H., PREUSSMANN, R.: Erzeugung von Lungenkrebs durch subcutane Injection von N, N-Diamylnitrosamin an Ratten. Naturwissenschaften 49, 111-112 (1962).

EULENBERG, H.: Die Lehre von den schädlichen und giftigen Gasen. Braunschweig: Vieweg 1865.

FERON, V.J.: Respiratory tract tumors in hamsters after intratracheal instillations of benzo(a)pyrene along and with furfural. Cancer Res. 32, 28-36 (1972).

FIGUEROA, W.G., RASZKOWSKI, R., WEISS, W.: Lung cancer in chloromethyl methyl ether workers. New Engl. J. Med. 288, 1096-1097 (1973).

FISHBEIN, G.W.: Occupational Health and Safety Letter, Vol. 2, Nr. 6, March 22, 1972.

GROSS, P., de TREVILLE, R.T.P., TOLKER, E.B., KASCHAK M., BABYAK, M.A.: Experimental asbestosis. The development of lung cancer in rats with pulmonary deposits of chrysotile asbestos dust. Arch. Environ. Health 15, 343-355 (1967).

GROSS, P., TOLKER, E., BABYAK, M.A., KASCHAK, M.: Experimental lung cancer in hamsters. Arch. Environ. Health 11, 59-65 (1965).

GROSS, P., WESTRICK, M.L., MCNERNEY, J.M.: Glass Dust: A Study of Its Biologic Effects. AMA Arch. Ind. Health 21, 10-23 (1960).

HERROLD, K.M.: Upper respiratory tract tumors induced in Syrian hamsters by N-methyl-N-nitroso-urea. Int. J. Cancer 6, 217-222 (1970).

HERROLD, K.M., DUNHAM, L.J.: Induction of carcinoma and papilloma of the tracheobronchial mucosa in the Syrian hamster by intratracheal instillations of benzo(a)pyrene. J.N.C.I. 28, 467-491 (1962).

HORTON, A.W., TYE, R., STEMMER, R.L.: Experimental carcinogenesis of the lung. Inhalation of gaseous formaldehyde or an aerosol of coal tar by C3H mice. J.N.C.I. 30, 31-43 (1963).

HUEPER, W.C., PAYNE, W.W.: Carcinogenic studies on petroleum asphalt, cooling oil and coal tar. Arch. Path. (Chicago) 70, 372-384 (1960).

HUEPER, W.C., PAYNE, W.W.: Experimental studies in metal carcinogenesis. Arch. Environ. Health 5, 445-462 (1962).

KOTIN, P., FALK, H.L.: Experimental induction of pulmonary tumors in strain A mice following their exposure to an atmosphere of ozonized gasoline. Cancer 9, 910-917 (1956).

KOTIN, P., WISELEY, D.V.: Production of lung cancer in mice by inhalation exposure to influenza virus and aerosols of hydrocarbons. Prog. exp. Tumor Res. 3, 186-215 (1963).

KUSCHNER, M., LASKIN, S., CRISTOFANO, E., NELSON, N.: Experimental carcinoma of the lung. In: Proc. 3rd Nat. Cancer Conf., pp. 485-495. Philadelphia: Lippincott 1957.

LASKIN, S., CAPPIELLO, V.P., ISOLA, D., KUSCHNER, M.: Chronic inhalation exposures with calcium chromate aerosols. A.I.H.A. Ind. Health Conf., Abstract No. 164, p. 175. Boston, Mass., May, 1973.

LASKIN, S., DREW, R.T., CAPPIELLO, V.P., KUSCHNER, M.: Inhalation studies with freshly generated polyurethane foam dust. In: Assessment of Airborne Particles (T.T. Mercer, P.E. Morrow, W. Stober, eds), pp. 382-404. Springfield, Illinois: Charles C. Thomas 1972.

LASKIN, S., KUSCHNER, M., DREW, R.T.: Studies in pulmonary carcinogenesis. In: Inhalation Carcinogenesis (M.G. Hanna, Jr., P. Nettesheim, J.R. Gilbert, eds). AEC Symposium Series no. 18, pp. 321-351. Oak Ridge, Tennessee: U.S. Atomic Energy Commission, Division of Technical Inf. 1970.

LASKIN, S., KUSCHNER, M., DREW, R.T., CAPPIELLO, V.P., NELSON, N.: Tumors of the respiratory tract induced by inhalation of bis(chloromethyl) ether. Arch. Environ. Health 23, 135-136 (1971).

LEONG, B.K.J., MACFARLAND, N.H., RUSE, W.H.: Induction of lung adenomas by chronic inhalation of bis(chloromethyl) ether. Arch. Environ. Health 22, 663-666 (1971).

LIJINSKY, W., TOMATIS, L., WENYON, C.E.: Lung tumors in rats treated with N-nitrosoheptamethyleneimine and N-nitrosooctamethyleneimine. Proc. Soc. exp. Biol. (N.Y.) 130, 945-949 (1969).

MAGEE, P.N., BARNES, J.M.: Carcinogenic nitroso compounds. In: Advances in Cancer Research (A. Haddow, S. Weinhouse, eds), Vol. 10, pp. 163-246. New York, London: Academic Press 1967.

MCDONALD, S., JR., WOODHOUSE, D.L.: On the nature of mouse lung adenomata, with special reference to the effects of atmospheric dust on the incidence of these tumors. J. Path. Bact. 54, 1-12 (1942).

MILLER, L., SMITH, W.E., BERLINER, S.W.: Tests for effect of asbestos on benzo(a)pyrene carcinogenesis in the respiratory tract. Ann. N.Y. Acad. Sci. 132, 489-500 (1965).

MOHR, U.: Effects of diethylnitrosamine in the respiratory system of Syrian golden hamsters. In: Morphology of experimental respiratory carcinogenesis (P. Nettesheim, M.G. Hanna, Jr., J.W. Deatherage, Jr., eds). AEC Symp. Series no. 21, pp. 255-265. Oak Ridge, Tennessee: U.S. Atomic Energy Commission, Division of Technical Inf. 1970.

MONTESANO, R., SAFFIOTTI, U.: Carcinogenic response of the respiratory tract of Syrian golden hamsters to different doses of diethylnitrosamine. Cancer Res. 28, 2197-2210 (1968).

MONTESANO, R., SAFFIOTTI, U., SHUBIK, P.: The role of topical and systemic factors in experimental respiratory carcinogenesis. In: Inhalation Carcinogenesis (M.G. Hanna, Jr., P. Nettesheim, J.R. Gilbert, eds). AEC Symposium Series no. 18, 353-371. Oak Ridge, Tennessee: U.S. Atomic Energy Commission, Division of Technical Inf. 1970.

MORI, K.: Induction of pulmonary tumors in rats by subcutaneous injection of 4-nitroquinoline-1-oxide. Gann 53, 303-308 (1962).

NETTESHEIM, P., HANNA, M.G., JR., DOHERTY, D.G., NEWELL, R.F., HELLMAN, A.: Effects of chronic exposure to artificial smog and chromium oxide dust on the incidence of lung tumors in mice. In: Inhalation Carcinogenesis (M.G. Hanna, Jr., P. Nettesheim, J.R. Gilbert, eds). AEC Symposium Series no. 18, pp. 305-320. Oak Ridge, Tennessee: U.S. Atomic Energy Commission, Division of Technical Inf. 1970.

NETTESHEIM, P., HANNA, M.G., JR., DOHERTY, D.G., NEWELL, P.F., HELL-
    MAN, A.: Effect of calcium chromate dust, influenza virus and 100R
    whole-body X-radiation on lung tumor incidence in mice. J.N.C.I. 47,
    1129-1144 (1971).
NISKANEN, K.O.: Observation on metaplasia of bronchial epithelium
    and its relation to carcinoma of the lung; pathoanatomical and ex-
    perimental researches. Acta path. microbiol. scand., Suppl. 80,
    1-80 (1949).
Occupational safety and health letter (G. Fishbein, ed.), 2 (6).
    1 March 22, 1972.
POUR, P., CARDESA, A., ALTHOFF, J., MOHR, U.: Tumorigenesis in the
    nasal olfactory region of Syrian golden hamsters as a result of
    Di-n-propylnitrosamine and related compounds. Cancer Res. 34,
    16-26 (1974).
PREJEAN, J.D., PECKHAM, J.C., CASEY, A.E., GRISWOLD, D.P., WEISBURGER,
    E.K., WEISBURGER, J.H.: Spontaneous tumors in Sprague-Dawley rats
    and Swiss mice. Cancer Res. 33, 2768-2773 (1973).
PYLEV, L.N.: Morphological lesions in rat lungs induced by intra-
    tracheal injection of chrysotile asbestos alone and with benzo(a)
    pyrene. Vop. Onkol. 18, 40-45 (1972).
RAPP, H.J., CARLETON, J.H., CHRISLER, C., NADEL, E.M.: Induction of
    malignant tumors in the rabbit by oral administration of diethylnitro-
    samine. J.N.C.I. 34, 453-511 (1971).
REEVES, A.L., PURO, H.E., SMITH, R.G., VORWALD, A.J.: Experimental
    asbestos carcinogenesis. Environ. Res. 4, 496-511 (1971).
REEVES, A.L., VORWALD, A.J.: Beryllium carcinogenesis II. Pulmonary
    deposition and clearance of inhaled beryllium sulfate in the rat.
    Cancer Res. 27, 446-451 (1967).
ROE, F.J.C.: The relevance and value of studies of lung tumors in
    laboratory animals in research on cancer of the human lung. In:
    Lung tumors in animals. Proc. 3rd Quad. Conf. on Cancer, U. Perugia,
    June 1965 (L. Severi, ed.), pp. 101-126. Perugia: Division of Cancer
    Research 1966.
SAFFIOTTI, U.: Experimental respiratory tract carcinogenesis and its
    relation to inhalation exposures. In: Inhalation Carcinogenesis
    (M.G. Hanna, Jr., P. Nettesheim, J.R. Gilbert, eds). AEC Symposium
    Series no. 18, pp. 27-54. Oak Ridge, Tennessee: U.S. Atomic Energy
    Commission, Division of Technical Inf. 1970.
SAFFIOTTI, U., CEFIS, F., KOLB, L.H., SHUBIK, P.: Experimental studies
    of the conditions of exposure to carcinogens for lung cancer induc-
    tion. J. Air Pollution Control Ass. 15, 23-25 (1965).
SAKABE, H.: Lung cancer due to exposure to bis(chloromethyl) ether.
    Ind. Health 11, 145-148 (1973).
SANNIE, C., OBERLING, C., GUERIN, M., GUERIN, P.: Les modalités de
    action cancérigène du 1,2-benzopyrène. C.R. Soc. Biol. (Paris) 120,
    1196-1198 (1935).
SCHEPERS, G.W.H.: Neoplasia experimentally proceeded by beryllium
    compounds. In: Progress in Experimental Tumor Research (F. Homber-
    ger, ed.), Vol. 2, pp. 203-245. New York: Hafner Publ. Co., Inc.,
    1961.
SCHEPERS, G.W.H.: Biological action of beryllium. Reaction of the
    monkey to inhaled aerosols. Ind. Med. Surg. 33, 1-16 (1964).
SCHEPERS, G.W.H., DURKEN, T.M., DELAHANT, A.B., CREEDON, F.T., REDLIN,
    A.J.: The biological action of Degussa submicron amorphous silica
    dust (Dow Corning Silica). AMA Arch. Ind. Health 16, 125-146 (1957).
SCHREIBER, H., NETTESHEIM, P., MARTIN, D.H.: Rapid development of
    bronchiolo-alveolar squamous cell tumors in rats after intratracheal
    injection of 3-methylcholanthrene. J.N.C.I. 49, 541-554 (1972).
SEELIG, M.G., BENIGNUS, E.L.: Lung tumor development in a resistant
    strain of mice subjected to inhalation of soot. Amer. J. Cancer 34,
    391-398 (1938).

SELLAKUMAR, A.R., SHUBIK, P.: Carcinogenicity of 7H-Dibenzo(c,g)
carbazole in the respiratory tract of hamsters. J.N.C.I. $\underline{48}$,
1641-1646 (1972).

SEVERI, L.: Lung tumors in animals. Proceedings of the Thırd
Quadrennial Conference on Cancer, University of Perugia, June, 1965.
Perugia: Division of Cancer Research, 1966.

SHABAD, L.M., PYLEV, L.N.: Morphological lesions in rat lungs in-
duced by polycyclic hydrocarbons. In: Morphology of Experimental
Respiratory Carcinogenesis (P. Nettesheim, M.G. Hanna, Jr., J.W.
Deatherage, Jr., eds). AEC Symposium Series no. 21, pp. 227-242.
Oak Ridge, Tennessee: U.S. Atomic Energy Commission, Division of
Technical Inf. 1970.

SIMMERS, M.H.: Petroleum asphalt inhalation by mice. Effects of
aerosols and smoke on the tracheobronchial tree and lungs. Arch.
Environ. Health $\underline{9}$, 727-734 (1964).

SJÖBERG, S.: Health hazards in the production and handling of
vanadium pentoxide. Arch. industr. Hyg. $\underline{3}$, 631-646 (1951).

SMITH, W.E., MILLER, L., ELSASSER, R.E., HUBERT, D.D.: Test for
carcinogenicity of asbestos. Ann. N.Y. Acad. Sci. $\underline{132}$, 456-488
(1966).

STANTON, M.F., BLACKWELL, R.: Induction of epidermoid carcinoma
of the lungs of rats. A 'new' method based upon deposition of methylcholanthrene in areas of pulmonary infarction. J.N.C.I. $\underline{27}$, 375-407
(1961).

STANTON, M.F., WRENCH, C.: Mechanism of mesothelioma induction with
asbestos and fibrous glass. J.N.C.I. $\underline{48}$, 797-821 (1972).

SUNDERMAN, F.W., JR.: Studies of nickel carcinogenesis: Alterations
of ribonucleic acid following inhalation of nickel carbonyl. Amer.
J. clin. Path. $\underline{39}$, 549-561 (1963).

SUNDERMAN, F.W., DONNELLY, A.J.: Studies of nickel carcinogenesis.
Metastasizing pulmonary tumors in rats induced by the inhalation
of nickel carbonyl. Amer. J. Path. $\underline{6}$, 1027-1041 (1965).

SUNDERMAN, F.W., DONNELLY, A.J., WEST, B., KINCAID, J.F.: Nickel
poisoning IX. Carcinogenesis in rats exposed to nickel carbonyl.
Arch. industr. Hlth $\underline{20}$, 36-41 (1959).

SUNDERMAN, F.W., SUNDERMAN, F.W., JR.: Nickel poisoning XI. Implica-
tion of nickel as a pulmonary carcinogen in tobacco smoke. Amer.
J. clin. Path. $\underline{35}$, 203-209 (1961).

THEISS, A.M., HEY, W., ZELLER, H.: Zur Toxikologie von Dichlordi-
methyläther-Verdacht auf kanzerogene Wirkung auch beim Menschen.
Zbl. Arbeitsmed. $\underline{23}$, 97-102 (1973).

RYE, R., STEMMER, K.L.: Experimental carcinogenesis of the lung II:
Influence of phenol in the production of carcinoma. J.N.C.I. $\underline{39}$,
175-186 (1967).

VIOLA, P.L.: Cancerogenic effect of vinyl chloride. In: Program
of Tenth International Cancer Congress. Vol. 29, p. 20, Houston,
Texas, 1970 (Abs.).

VÔSAMÄE, A. In: International Agency for Research on Cancer, Annual
Report 1971, p. 46, Lyon, 1972.

YAMAGIWA, K., ICHIKAWA, K.: Experimentelle Studie über die Pathogenese
der Epithelialgeschwülste. Mitt. med. Fak. Tokyo $\underline{15}$, 295-344 (1915).

The Role of the Host in the Development of *in vivo* Models for Carcinogenesis Studies*

Carrie E. Whitmire, Charles F. Demoise, and Richard E. Kouri

Department of Experimental Oncology, Viral-Chemical Carcinogenesis Section, Bethesda, MD 20014, USA

ABSTRACT

The development of cancer depends upon the integrated response of the host to the carcinogen and to the initial transformation event. Genetic factors determine the host's potential to respond to chemical and viral carcinogens, while endogenous and exogenous environmental factors influence the realization of the genetic potential. In chemical carcinogenesis, inducibility (the capacity to metabolize polycyclic aromatic hydrocarbons (PAH) to the ultimate carcinogen) has been demonstrated to be under genetic control; however, tumors will occur to a lesser degree and after a longer delay when large doses of PAH are administered to noninducible mice. Aryl hydrocarbon hydroxylase induction by noncarcinogenic materials may also influence the effects of PAH carcinogens.

In viral carcinogenesis, evidence points to genetic transmission of the RNA oncogenic viruses with expression of the viral genome under host control. Host control over RNA tumor viruses may be demonstrated by the existence of epigenetic, xenotropic, and pantropic viruses; permissive, restrictive, producer, and nonproducer cell lines; and the presence of viral group specific antigen, infectious virus, and/ or neoplasia in the host.

The development of cancer from the initial transformed cells (chemical and/or viral induced) is dependent on the host response which is influenced by numerous factors. Immunosurveillance is probably the first line of defense against these transformed cells. Genetic control of immunocompetence is evidenced by the variety of responses to various antigenetic stimuli in genotypically different strains of mice. Immunosuppressive effects of carcinogens, drugs, infections, etc., appear to make possible the initial act of establishing clones of transformed cells by overriding the immunocompetence of the host. Other factors related to diet, aging, stress, etc., effect the host control over the carcinogenic event and may be related to the increased susceptibility to carcinogens and/or the increase in the incidence of "spontaneous" tumors.

In our laboratory, we have undertaken studies to provide the best possible mouse model system for studying respiratory carcinogenesis. These studies with inbred mice have included the determination of relative susceptibility to various carcinogens, AHH inducibility, type C

*This work was supported by the Council for Tobacco Research and by Contract NO1-CP 43240 within the Virus Cancer Program of the National Cancer Institute, National Institutes of Health, U.S. Public Health Service.

RNA viral expression, immunocompetence when challenged by various antigens, and the immunosuppressive effects of various chemical carcinogens. We plan to further evaluate our model systems with regard to environmental stress factors, cocarcinogenesis, and viral infections. In this way, we hope to establish the integrated host response to the events occurring in respiratory carcinogenesis.

Introduction

The ultimate solution of the cancer problem is dependent not only on the determination of the causes of cancer but also on the mechanisms whereby the host regulates the prevention and surveillance of the carcinogenic event(s) and the ultimate growth of the cancer. We must now ask what are the differences between susceptible and resistant hosts to the causes of cancer. Cancer, as a disease entity, differs in many respects from infectious diseases, in that there is a greater host-parasite involvement. Evidence points to cancer being an epigenetic disease (i.e., its development is dependent on an innate genetic resistance predisposed to gradual failure of control surveillance mechanisms). However, this is not the entire picture, since the response of the host to carcinogenic and subsequent events is an integrated response dependent on the interactions of both genetically controlled mechanisms and internal as well as external environmental factors.

A prerequisite to the etiological studies of any disease is the development of an appropriate animal model system. With the resolution of this problem, rapid progress in treatment and prevention can generally be made. Perhaps the greatest problem in carcinogenesis research has been the lack of a classical experimental animal model system. MEKLER (1973) has suggested that certain fundamental laws of biology pertinent to carcinogenesis have either escaped the attention of researchers or have not yet been discovered. The great strides which have been made in the study of host factors believed relevant to cancer have led us to the conclusion that we must better understand the role of the host in carcinogenesis before we can judiciously select the best animal model.

What species of laboratory animals provides us with the most information regarding those host surveillance mechanisms that may play a role in carcinogenesis? At this time, one would have to agree that there is more available information for various inbred strains of mice. For this reason, we suggest the mouse is still our best hope for selecting one or more model systems where inbreeding can provide the characterization of genetic factors related to carcinogenic susceptibility. There is probably no greater justification for using rats, rabbits, or for that matter, primates to demonstrate the carcinogenic potential of most chemicals. There are other justifications for the use of mice. Much of our knowledge regarding oncogenic viruses comes from mouse studies and has only recently been expanded to other species. In many ways, because of the broad knowledge of mouse genetics, we can come closer in mice to mimicking the situation that exists in man than in any other animal. Mice are easy to handle and require less space than most other animals; therefore, statistically significant results can be obtained by the use of large populations. Their relatively short life span of 2 to 3 years also makes them ideal subjects for lifetime studies. Their extraneous virus flora have been relatively well characterized and can be controlled by quarantine procedure. Their "spontaneous" tumor incidences have also been characterized.

There are of course various disadvantages, as is true with any model
system. For respiratory carcinogenesis studies, mice have the disadvantage of being obligate nose breathers and this may present a different picture from that seen in man. Rats and mice have 4 nasal
glands (vs 1 in man) which discharge fluids upon breathing noxious
chemical or physical irritants. Mice also have more goblet cells per
surface area of the respiratory epithelium (WYNDER and HOFFMANN, 1969).
The organs and blood supply in mice are also small, thus presenting
the disadvantage that only a limited number of studies can be undertaken with any one animal.

For the past 10 years, our laboratory has been actively defining certain parameters of viral-chemical carcinogenesis. Fortunately, other
laboratories have pursued other aspects of genetically controlled surveillance mechanisms, which play important roles in cancer. It is our
purpose in this paper to look at the integrated host (i.e., the inbred
mouse) in an attempt to pull together many of the factors we feel play
a role in the selection of the best possible animal model system for
respiratory carcinogenesis. Our discussion of the mouse model system
presents several aspects of host control over susceptibility:

- Susceptibility to chemical carcinogens
- Chemical carcinogen metabolism
- Viral etiology of cancer
- Tumor immunology
- Other genetic controls of neoplastic development
- Cells at risk to carcinogens and DNA repair

Chemical Carcinogenesis Susceptibility

During the past 7 years we have concentrated primarily on the characterization of various genotypically different mouse strains as to
their susceptibility to 3-methylcholanthrene (MCA), 7,12-dimethyl-
benz(a)anthracene (DMBA), and benzo(a)pyrene (BaP) when given subcutaneously to female mice 4 weeks of age (WHITMIRE et al., 1971;
WHITMIRE and SALERNO, 1972; KOURI et al., 1973b). These studies were
based on an 8 month observation period, since most tumors occur during
the first 5 to 6 months. The doses selected were relatively small,
since our primary aim was to determine relative susceptibility in a
reasonable period of time with as few adverse effects on the host as
possible. The basis for comparison has been the cumulative tumor incidence, latency period (SHIMKIN and ANDERVONT, 1940), carcinogenic
index (CI), (% cumulative tumors divided by the average days latency
X 100)(IBALL, 1939), and tumor inducing dose in 50% of the animals
in the defined observation period (TuD$_{50}$), (REED and MUENCH, 1938).
We studied those mouse strains (inbred and random bred) most frequently used in cancer research. We have found correlation of the extensive
literature difficult due to the numerous variables that inevitably
exist between laboratories. Our results from studies carried out over
an extended period using the same techniques, carcinogen dose, vehicle,
and mice of comparable age and sex are presented in Table 1. Table 2
gives some of the host genetic factors for these inbred strains as a
ready reference for later discussions.

These earlier studies with MCA have demonstrated a wide variation in
the tumor incidence as well as average latency period among the genotypically different strains. Although the most susceptible strains
generally develop tumors in the least amount of time, this is not

necessarily the case. For this reason the carcinogenic index (CI) has been utilized as a valuable index in rating the relative susceptibility of the various mouse strains (IBALL, 1939; WHITMIRE and SALERNO, 1972a). Probably the most outstanding examples of variation between tumor incidence and latency are the C3H/fMai and the C3H/HeJ, whose average latency is 14 weeks in each incidence but which produce 93% and 62% tumors respectively. Another example is that of the C3H/HeJ mice (14 weeks latency), which produce only 62% tumors, and the C57BR/cdJ strain, which produce 67% tumors with a relatively long average latency (22 weeks). These studies demonstrate that, although NIH Swiss, Ha/ICR, CFW, and CF-1 random bred strains have been used extensively in carcinogenesis studies, they are not as susceptible as a number of inbred strains. To define the relative susceptibility to MCA carcinogenesis still further, several dose levels were used and we found the C3H/fMai mouse strain to be consistently more susceptible than the other strains tested (Table 3). These studies also demonstrate a difference in mice of the same strain obtained from different sources. This is one variable in carcinogenesis studies of which most investigators are not aware and undoubtedly accounts for some of the variations in reported findings from one laboratory to another. The C57BL/6 mice from 3 sources act as entirely different strains (WHITMIRE and SALERNO, 1972a).

Table 1. Subcutaneous chemical carcinogenous characterization of variou mouse strains with 150µg MCA

MOUSE STRAIN	TUMOR INCIDENCE Tu/T	%	AV. TU. LATENCY (WKS)	C.I.[a]	AHH[b] INDUCI-BILITY	gs-1 ANTIGEN INCIDENCE P/T[c]	%	INFECTIOUS TYPE-C VIRUS
INBRED								
C3H/f Mai	51/55	93	13	102	9	16/23	70	±
C57BL/6 Cum	18/20	90	17	76	10	3/26	12	−
C58/J	20/23	87	16	76	10	10/10	100	+++
C57BL/10ScSnJ	22/27	81	18	64	12	0/14	0	−
BALB/cCr (Mai)	35/49	71	19	53	8	5/23	22	±
C57BR/cdJ	18/27	67	22	44	7	2/18	11	−
C3H/HeN	33/53	62	14	63	10	13/24	50	+
SWR/J	11/22	50	23	33	1	6/10	60	−
129/J	14/30	47	27	25	1	0/15	0	−
C57L/J	13/28	46	20	33	6	0/13	0	−
AKR/J	20/51	39	26	21	1	9/9	100	+++
SJL/J	13/35	37	22	24	1	11/15	73	++
DBA/2J	5/35	14	28	7	1	12/12	100	+
DBA/1J	6/53	11	27	6	1	4/8	50	+
RANDOM BRED								
SWISS-WEBSTER (N)	26/35	74	17	62	1	13/25	52	−
Ha/ICR (RPMI)	46/63	73	19	55	1	14/23	61	++
CFW	21/29	72	17	61	1	9/13	69	+
CF-1	37/66	56	23	33	1	15/15	100	++
SNELL/Mai	9/25	36	24	14	1	11/15	73	+

[a]CARCINOGENIC INDEX = $\dfrac{\text{\% TUMORS}}{\text{AV. DAYS LATENCY}} \times 100$

[b]AHH INDUCIBILITY = $\dfrac{\text{AHH LEVELS FROM MCA-TREATED MICE}}{\text{AHH LEVELS FROM TRIOCTANOIN TREATED MICE}}$
HEPATIC AHH LEVELS WERE DETERMINED 24 HOURS AFTER IP ADMINISTRATION OF 80 µg MCA/g BODY WEIGHT OR 0.05 ml TRIOCTANOIN. CONSTITUTIVE AHH LEVELS WERE SIMILAR FOR EVERY STRAIN TESTED

[c]$\dfrac{P}{T} = \dfrac{\text{NUMBER OF POSITIVE SAMPLES BY CF TEST}}{\text{TOTAL SAMPLES TESTED}}$

Table 2. Genes influencing AHH inducibility, tumor virus histocompatibility, and immunological responses

MOUSE STRAIN	GENE DESIGNATION[a]						IMMUNOLOGICAL RESPONSES[b]									
							H-2 ASSOCIATED				NON H-2 ASSOCIATED					
							Ir-1 GENES				Ir-Ig GENES		Ir-3 GENES			
							SYNTHETIC POLYPEPTIDE COPOLYMERS (,)-A-L			GAT$_{10}$	BALB/c MYELOMA PROTEIN		POLYPEPTIDES (,)-Prol-L		SC[c]	
	Ah	Fv-1	Fv-2	H-2	Ir-1	Ir-3	(T,G)	(H,G)	(Phe,G)		IgG	IgA	(H,G)	(T,G)	A	C
C3H/f	b	n	s	k	a	H9	L	H	H	H	L	H	H	H	H	
C57BL/6	b	b	r	b	b	H9	H	L	H	H	H	L	H	M	M	
C58	b	n	r	k	a	H9	L	H	H	H	L	H				
C57BL/10ScSn	b	b	r	b	b	H9	H	L	H	H	H	L				
BALB/c	b	b	s	d	a	H9	Mv	Mv	H	H	L	L				
C57BR/cd	b	n	r	k	a	H9	L	H	H	H	L	H				
C3H/He	b	n	s	k	a	H9	L	H	H	H	L	H				
SWR	d	n	s	q	c	H9	L	L	H		L	L	H	L	H	H
129	d	n	s	b	a	H9	H	L	H	H	H	L	H	H	H	H
C57L	b	n	r	b	a	H9	H	L	H	H	H	L				
AKR	d	n	s	k	d	H-	L	H	H	H	H	L	H	L	H	M
SJL	d	n	s	s	b	H9	L	L	L	neg	H	H	H	H	H	M
DBA/2	d	n	s	d	c	H9	Mv	Mv	H	H	L	L	H	L	H	M
DBA/1	d	n	s	q	c	H9	L	L	H	H	L	L	L	L	H	L

a STATTS, 1972

b McDEVITT AND LANDY, 1972

L = LOW
M = MEDIUM
Mv = MEDIUM VARIABLE
H = HIGH

c STREPTOCOCCAL CARBOHYDRATE ANTIGENS

Table 3. Comparison of tumor incidence, mean latency, CI, and TuD$_{50}$ in various strains of mice treated subcutaneously with various doses of MCA at 4 weeks of age

AHH INDUCIBLE

MOUSE STRAIN	9.38 µg				37.5 µg				150.0 µg				TuD$_{50}$
	TUMOR INCIDENCE Tu/T	%	MEAN LAT (WKS)	CI	TUMOR INCIDENCE Tu/T	%	MEAN LAT (WKS)	CI	TUMOR INCIDENCE Tu/T	%	MEAN LAT (WKS)	CI	µg MCA
C3H/fMai	9/28	32	23	20	24/29	83	18	68	27/30	90	13	96	21
C3H/AnfCum	9/29	31	21	21	16/29	55	17	46	25/29	86	14	89	57
C57BL/6Cum	10/28	36	21	21	14/27	52	23	32	26/27	96	17	83	26
C57BL/6Mai	—	—	—	—	12/30	40	21	28	20/27	74	19	50	61
C57BL/6J	—	—	—	—	14/29	48	20	34	16/27	59	20	44	64
BALB/cCR (Mai)	3/30	10	27	7	17/28	61	20	45	23/28	82	16	71	34
BALB/cSPF (Mai)	—	—	—	—	20/30	67	17	57	26/31	84	12	98	>38
C57BL/10ScSn	—	—	—	—	12/30	40	23	25	22/27	81	18	64	41

AHH NON-INDUCIBLE

MOUSE STRAIN	150.0 µg				300.0 µg				500.0 µg				TuD$_{50}$
	TUMOR INCIDENCE Tu/T	%	MEAN LAT (WKS)	CI	TUMOR INCIDENCE Tu/T	%	MEAN LAT (WKS)	CI	TUMOR INCIDENCE Tu/T	%	MEAN LAT (WKS)	CI	µg MCA
129/J	14/30	47	27	25	16/28	57	21	39	20/28	71	22	46	203
DBA/2J	10/24	42	25	24	14/24	58	22	38	21/24	88	21	59	212
DBA/1J	4/27	15	25	9	13/24	62	25	35	10/19	53	23	33	238

The susceptibility of an animal to one carcinogen does not insure its responsiveness to another carcinogen. Therefore, studies were undertaken with DMBA and BaP in selected strains. As seen in Table 4, the C3H/fMai strain is highly susceptible to all 3 carcinogens, while the other strains are relatively insensitive to tumor induction with BaP and show varying sensitivity to DMBA. In all instances, the latency periods were longer with DMBA and BaP than with MCA. Although all polycyclic aromatic hydrocarbons are believed to be metabolized by the AHH enzyme system, there is evidence that their metabolism pathways are slightly different (NEBERT et al., 1973), which may account for genetic differences in the strains tested.

Chemical Carcinogen Metabolism

In order for polycyclic aromatic hydrocarbons (PAH) to exert cell transformation, mutagenicity, and tumor induction, they must be metabolized to water soluble active forms (e.g., the epoxide), (MARQUARDT and HEIDELBERGER, 1972; HUBERMAN et al., 1972) by the microsomal bound, mixed function oxidases of which aryl hydrocarbon hydroxylase (AHH) enzymes are a major system found in the tissues of man (KELLERMANN et al., 1973) and animals (GELBOIN, 1967). Constitutive enzyme levels are normally detectable without induction; however, the inducibility of AHH is associated with the carcinogenic effects of PAH (SELKIRK et al., 1971). The AHH system is inducible by a variety of endogenous chemicals (corticorsteroid hormones and bilirubin), as well as exogenous chemicals (barbiturates, insecticides, and PAH); therefore, these enzymes obviously may function as a two-edged sword. Our studies with various strains of mice have demonstrated a direct correlation between inducibility of AHH activity and 150µg MCA subcutaneous carcinogenesis (KOURI et al., 1973b). The results are summarized in Table 1. If, however, one gives higher doses of MCA (Table 3) to noninducible mice, the incidence of tumors can be increased, while the latency period remains at 5 to 6 months and the CI index below 60. The TuD_{50} dose is 3 to 11 times that of the inducible mice.

The role of AHH appears highly specific for each PAH. Thus, the metabolism of MCA, DMBA, and BaP does not necessarily follow the same pathways indicated by subcutaneous and skin carcinogenesis studies (KINOSHITA and GELBOIN, 1972; KOURI et al., 1973b; NEBERT et al., 1973). These differences in the carcinogenic effects (Table 4) indicate that the C3H/f mouse was the only strain capable of handling all 3 carcinogens equally well. It would appear that these variations in the AHH system could be clarified by studying congenetic crosses between the C3H/f strain and another strain giving low levels of tumor induction with BaP and DMBA and might help explain important etiological differences in chemical carcinogenesis.

The inducibility of the AHH system by various chemicals has been shown to be under host regulation. Susceptibility to MCA induction segregates as a single autosomal dominant gene in crosses involving the C57BL/6 (B6) and DBA/2 (D2) strains of mice (THOMAS et al., 1972; NEBERT et al., 1972b; GIELEN et al., 1972b). The B6 is the prototype inducible strain and its allele Ah^b designates the dominant gene. The D2 strain is the prototype strain for the recessive Ah^d allele. We utilized this mouse genetic system to extend our observations on the relationship between AHH inducible and sensitivity to MCA tumorigenesis (KOURI et al., 1973a, 1974c). The results in Table 5 demonstrate that inducible animals were approximately 10 times more sensitive to MCA carcino-

Table 4. Tumor incidence, mean latency, and CI in various strains of mice (females) inoculated subcutaneously with 150μg MCA, DMBA and BaP

MOUSE STRAIN	150 μg MCA				150 μg DMBA				150 μg BaP			
	Tu/T	%	MEAN LAT (WK)	CI	Tu/T	%	MEAN LAT (WK)	CI	Tu/T	%	MEAN LAT (WK)	CI
C3H/fMai	51/55	93	13.2	100	24/25*	96	17.5	78	20/24*	83	18.3	65
B10.BR/J	26/28	93	16.3	83	16/29	55	21.0	37	3/25	12	21.7	8
C57BL/6Cum	18/20	90	16.5	78	5/17	29	22.4	19	2/24	8	19.0	7
C57BL/10ScSn	22/27	81	18.1	64	10/24	42	22.8	26	4/29	14	24.0	8
129/J	14/30	47	27.0	25	11/33	33	26.5	18				
Snell/Mai	9/25	36	23.6	24	8/23	35	24.0	29	3/29	10	22.0	6

*THESE ANIMALS WERE MALES

genesis than noninducible animals when comparing the CI values. In
every case where a tumor was observed on a noninducible animal, it
occurred late in the observation period after tumor development had
ceased in the inducible animals. It is assumed that some metabolism
of this carcinogen took place at a much slower rate (possibly by the
constitutive levels of AHH enzymes), leading to cell transformation
and tumor induction.

The significance of AHH induction in the transformation of tissue
culture cell lines by PAH carcinogens has been demonstrated (KOURI
et al., 1974b). Only those cell lines potentially sensitive to chemically induced transformation possessed the particular type of metabolism
involving the AHH inducible enzymes. The carcinogenic effect of a hydrocarbon is probably determined by the amounts activated to the carcinogenic form. The low levels of these enzymes in many tissue culture
cell lines are probably a factor in the inability to obtain chemically induced transformation.

Enhancement and interference in the metabolism of chemicals by the
AHH system can occur. CONNEY (1974) has demonstrated that oral treatment with MCA, DMBA, and BaP enhanced the metabolism of intravenously (IV) administered radioactive BaP in rats, while phenobarbital
(which stimulates AHH induction) did not enhance MCA, BaP, or DMBA
metabolism. Chronic administration of BaP stimulates the metabolism
of radioaction BaP. These observations are of interest since treatment of rodents with AHH inducers provides protection for the carcinogenic effects of BaP, DMBA, N-2-fluorenylacetamide, 4-dimethylamino-
stibene, urethane, aflatoxin, diethylnitrosamine, and aminoazo dyes
(CONNEY, 1974). THAMAVIT et al. (1974) have also reported that treatment with 3 carcinogens at one time decreases their carcinogenesis
in rats and was believed due to an interference phenomena. WEBER et

Table 5. Relationship of hepatic inducibility and
subcutaneous tumor induction with 150μg MCA in
C57BL/6 x DBA/1, F1, and F2 mice

MOUSE STRAINS	AHH INDUCIBLE		AHH NON-INDUCIBLE	
	TUMOR INCIDENCE		TUMOR INCIDENCE	
	Tu/T	%	Tu/T	%
AHH NONSEGREGATING:				
B6 (Ah^b/Ah^b)	23/29	79		
D2 (Ah^d/Ah^d)			2/30	7
F1 (Ah^b/Ah^d)	54/90	60		
F1 x B6 (Ah^b/Ah^d and Ah^b/Ah^b)	81/94	86		·
TOTALS:	158/213	74	2/30	7
AHH SEGREGATING:				
F1 x D2 (Ah^b/Ah^d and Ah^d/Ah^d)	15/24	75	5/34	15
F2 (Ah^b/Ah^b Ah^b/Ah^d Ah^d/Ah^d)	23/25	92	2/21	10 ·
TOTALS:	38/45	84	7/55	13
TUMOR TOTALS:	196/258	77	8/85	11
AV. DAYS TUMOR LATENCY:	131		195	
CARCINOGENIC INDEX:	59		6	

al. (1974) recently reported that nicotine reduced the metabolism
of benzopyrene in tobacco smoke thus demonstrating interference between chemicals metabolized by the same enzyme system.

Not all known carcinogens belong to the group of chemicals known as
PAH and their metabolism proceeds along different pathways. They have
not been studied as extensively as the PAH group and the relationship
to genetic patterns of susceptibility to carcinogenesis has not been
determined. The dimethylase associated with the metabolism of the
dimethylnitrosamines (DMN) may bear a mirror-image relationship to
the AHH system, since high levels of induced AHH may act as potent
repressors of DMN-dimethylase activity (VENKATESAN et al., 1971).
This suggests that DMN may be a more potent carcinogen in AHH noninducible animals. We are undertaking studies in AHH inducible and
noninducible animals to test this hypothesis.

Virus Etiology of Cancer

Although a number of tumor viruses have been isolated from a variety
of animal species since ROUS (1911) first discovered the avian sarcoma
virus, the concept of viral etiology of cancer has been untenable for
many scientists. The development of inbred mouse strains produced high
and low incidence leukemia strains and ultimately led to the demonstration that RNA tumor viruses could be transmitted both horizontally and
vertically (GROSS, 1944, 1950, 1970). Transmission can take place by
congenital infection of the germ cells or via the placenta or milk;
however, the usual mode of spread appears to be by genetic inheritance
from one generation of animals or cells to the next as DNA copies of
viral RNA integrated into the genetic material of the cells (WEISS,
1973; BUFFET et al., 1969; HILGERS et al., 1972).

Two concepts have been proposed for the origin of RNA tumor viruses:
the oncogene hypothesis of HUEBNER and TODARO (1969)(TODARO and HUEB-
NER, 1972) and the protovirus hypothesis of TEMIN (1971, 1972). The
oncogene theory suggests that viral genetic material is present in
normal cells expressed as infectious virus or as noninfectious viral
subunits (as viral group specific (gs) antigen) and that a noninfectious portion of the viral genome (the oncogene) is responsible for
cellular transformation and cancer. The protovirus hypothesis differs
from the oncogene hypothesis by suggesting that infectious viral genetic information is transferred by transcription and reverse transcription and, in combination with mutation or recombination events, produces neoplastic transformation.

Regardless of the hypothesis for the origin of the RNA tumor viruses,
there are certain cellular controls which govern their expression.
These controls will vary somewhat between endogenous and exogenous
viruses; therefore, it is pertinent that some of the properties of
each be considered. Endogenous viruses are transmitted vertically,
either as viral genome or as infectious virus by congenital means.
Multiple copies of the virogene are present in the DNA of all somatic
and germ cells of all animals in a species. The type of viral expression is under cellular control and may be present as gs antigen,
defective virus, or complete virus capable of growth under proper
conditions with the production of reverse transcriptase (RT). Clonal
lines established from these tissues will either spontaneously release virus or induce virus release after varying intervals of cultivation, depending on the original viral expression and the strength

or degree of cellular control. Induction can also be accomplished with
5'-iododeoxyuridine (IudR) or 5-bromodeoxyuridine (BudR). Complete
virogene is known to be present in chickens, Chinese and Syrian hamsters, mice, rats, cats, pigs, and baboons and has been demonstrated
by single cell clones with release of infectious virus. These cells
with endogenous virogene are generally resistant to exogenous infection by the homologous endogenous virus. The expression of endogenous virus is influenced by the genetic properties of the virus and
the cell as well as exogenous factors, such as radiation, chemical
carcinogens, etc. Exogenous viruses differ from endogenous viruses
in that they are spread horizontally as infectious virus (with evidence of RT) from animal to animal or cell to cell.

The characterization of the mouse type C viruses has recently been reviewed by SARMA and GAZDAR (1974). The type C RNA viruses from mice
can be divided into 2 groups. The sarcoma viruses (MSV) produce solid
tumors *in vivo* and transformed or cytopathogenic foci *in vitro*. These
have been isolated rarely from laboratory adopted stocks of mouse
leukemia viruses (MuLV), (HARVEY, 1964; MOLONEY, 1966; KIRSTEN and
MAYER, 1971) or from several spontaneously occurring mouse sarcoma
(FINKEL et al., 1966; GAZDAR et al., 1972). MSV can transform cells
and release virus or they can fail to release virus, as seen in the
nonproducer cell lines where the viral genome is integrated into the
genetic material of the host cell. In such cases the viral genome can
be rescued by superinfection with MuLV, which provides the envelope
for the defective MSV. The mouse leukemia viruses (MuLV) are noncyto-
pathogenic *in vitro* when propagated in permissive cells. *In vivo*, some
produce leukemia while others fail to produce evidence of any neoplastic potential under the test conditions. They have been isolated
from spontaneous and chemically induced solid tumors.

Recently, it has been shown that 2 classes of murine, RNA, type C
viruses exist, based on their ability to replicate in mouse tissue.
Those which will not replicate in mouse tissue but require rabbit,
human, cat, etc., tissue are called xenotropic viruses (X-tropic),
(LEVY, 1973) or S-tropic (SHERR et al., 1974). These viruses have
typical murine type C antigenic markers but differ distinctly by
nucleic acid hydridization from the N-tropic MuLV (BENVENISTE et al.,
1974). The significance of the X-tropic viruses has not been determined at this time although they are apparently widespread. Their
presence in the mouse with the apparent inability to propagate at
least *in vitro* in mouse tissues presents an interesting type of genetic
control that requires additional study. The implications of such
viruses in humans provide a possible explanation to our inability to
propagate a human cancer virus. MuLV, which replicate preferentially
in mouse tissues, have been classified as ecotropic viruses (LEVY,
1974), and make up the group of murine viruses for which considerably more information is available. It is these viruses that will be
discussed in this paper.

Vertical transmission of virogene information bypasses the host controls associated with infectious viral (but not necessarily oncogene)
expression. Such host controls over infectious virus are common to
vertically and horizontally transmitted infectious virus expression.
Evidence of viral genetic information in the absence of infectious
virus has been demonstrated by several systems. Virus-like molecule
sequences were reported by HAREL et al. (1967) in the DNA of uninfected murine cells. CHASE and PIKO (1973) and VERNON et al. (1973) observed C-type particles, and gs antigen (HUEBNER et al., 1970a) has
been demonstrated in embryonic tissues of mice. The Gross$_{IX}$ MuLV
associated antigen was demonstrated by STOCKERT et al. (1971). Spon-

taneous and induced appearance of MuLV from clones of nonproducer cell lines has been demonstrated by TODARO (1972), AARONSON et al. (1969, 1971).

Based on our present technology for detecting type C RNA viral expression there appear to be 4 categories of mouse strains: 1. the C57L mouse expresses no viral antigen or infectious virus; 2. the NIH Swiss mouse has only the gs-1 antigen and no G_{IX} antigen, and the 129 strain expresses some gs-1 and G_{IX} antigen (neither of these 2 mice has infectious ecotropic MuLV, although type C particles have been observed in NIH Swiss mice); 3. certain mice have a low incidence of early ecotropic MuLV expression as gs-1 antigen that gradually increases and is accompanied by low levels of infectious MuLV expression as seen in the BALB/c mouse (PETERS et al., 1972a); and 4. a high level of infectious virus is detected early in life, accompanied by a high incidence of leukemia as demonstrated in AKR, C58, and C3H/Fi.

Several genes have been associated with endogenous virus expression; however, their roles have not been fully evaluated and may be related more to the expression of neoplasia than the virus per se. The TL antigen, determined by the Tla locus, may represent a viral genome since it appears only on leukemic cells and thymocytes of certain strains (BOYSE and OLD, 1969). The G_{IX} antigen is found on thymocytes and lymphocytes, but all murine leukemic cells are not G_{IX}^{+} (STOCKERT et al., 1971). TAYLOR et al. (1971) described 2 independent genes (no designation made) for gs antigen expression in the AKR mouse and postulated one locus for gs antigen expression and another for infectious virus in the AKR X C57BL/6 F2 cross. It is possible these 2 genes may be the same as the V_1 and V_2 loci for complete virus production in the AKR mouse described by ROWE (1972). These V-loci and the Ind locus (STEPHENSON and AARONSON, 1972a, 1972b) predispose cells to virus induction by IudR and BudR (ROWE et al., 1971). TAYLOR et al. (1973) also described the Mlv-1 allele in the C57BL/10 and DBA/2 strains as a determinate of gs antigen expression. Another gene (Fv-2) has been characterized for host control over propagation of the spleen focus-forming virus (SFFV) component of Friend virus complex. The susceptibility phenotype (Fv-2^s) is dominate and the Fv-2^r denotes absolute resistance. This linkage is unrelated to the H-2 linkage and has no direct influence on the lymphatic leukemia virus of Friend (MCDEVITT and LANDY, 1972).

Interferon has been shown to be a potent antiviral agent and its production has been shown to be under host control (deMAEYER and deMAEYER-GINGNARD, 1969). This control is apparently related to the host response to various interferon inducers (BARON, personal communication, 1974) therefore demonstrating another variation in host control of infectious virus expression.

The best defined of the host cellular control genes for MuLV is that governing the replication of infectious virus. This spreading factor influences the ability of endogenous as well as exogenous ecotropic viruses to express themselves as infectious virus. The Fv-1 locus controls the host range permissiveness of mouse cells for the replication of MuLV (PINCUS et al., 1971a, 1971b). HARTLEY et al. (1970) demonstrated 3 groups of MuLV based on their ability to grow more efficiently in NIH Swiss (N) cells (Fv-1^n) or BALB/c (B) cells (Fv-1^b) and designated this predilection of the viruses as "N- and B-tropic" and NB-tropic" for those viruses that grow equally well in both types of cells. The tropism of the various mouse strains and their embryonic tissue culture cells have been classified as N-type or B-type. In the case of the MSV, the tropism is dependent on the tropism of the helper virus. Mice strains that develop early leukemia belong to the $Fv-1^n$ group (AKR, C58, C3H/Fi). These mice also carry the V_1 and V_2 alleles for high incidence activation of the endogenous MuLV. See Table 6 for summary of host genes associated with RNA type C viral expression control.

These type C viruses and the various host control mechanisms have been shown to play a role in the incidence of "spontaneous" (PETERS et al., 1972b) and virally induced neoplasia (LILLY and PINCUS, 1973; ROWE, 1972). They have been postulated to be switched on by chemical carcinogens (HUEBNER et al., 1970b, 1972; MEIER and MYERS, 1973); however, their significance in chemical carcinogenesis is still open to speculation. If one does undertake induced viral-chemical carcinogenesis studies, one must be cognizant of the susceptibility of the mouse strain not only to the chemical carcinogen used but also to the virus selected for these studies. It is also necessary to recognize the importance of endogenous viruses and the ensuing natural incidence of early or late development of leukemia when selecting inbred strains and congeneic strains for carcinogenesis studies related to the interaction of spontaneous and induced neoplasia (WHITMIRE et al., 1972b, 1972c, 1973a; SALERNO et al., 1973).

To determine the occurrence and concomitants of viral expression during MCA carcinogenesis in the various mouse strains, we have followed the incidence of gs antigen and infectious virus in the induced tumors (WHITMIRE et al., 1971, 1973b; WHITMIRE and SALERNO, 1972a). These results are summarized in Table 1. There is no significant correlation between susceptibility to MCA and the presence of viral expression as gs antigen or infectious virus. Other studies have confirmed this finding with DMBA and BaP (KOURI et al., 1973b). The gs antigen expression in chemically induced tumors follows the same pattern as that of the spleens of normal animals (MYERS et al., 1970) and could be related to the degree of expression that increases with age, as observed in the BALB/c mouse (WHITMIRE et al., 1973b).

Tumor Immunology

The significance of the host's ability to respond immunologically to the events of carcinogenesis was recognized early, yet today not all the ramifications of tumor immunology are understood. Further advances in technology and more knowledge regarding the integrated nature of host defense mechanisms might shed some light on this complex area. There exists the dichotomy between the healthy immune stimulus that provides for elimination of the initial transformed cells or the holding action in the host-parasite relationship, and the unhealthy condition where the immunological response enhances tumor growth. A point in cancer research has been reached when we must use the available knowledge regarding immunological competence for the selection of our animal models. It is my purpose to review some of these factors to be defined or at least recognized as existing in the animal models selected for the study of viral, chemical, and viral-chemical carcinogenesis. Sweeping conclusions regarding carcinogenic events can no longer be made in model systems without considering the integrated host reactions.

The metabolism of chemical carcinogens and factors related to viral etiology have already been considered; however, it will be necessary to consider the immunological response involved in those 2 facets that

Table 6. Genes influencing ecotropic mouse tumor virus expression (TOOZE, 1973)

ALLELE	PHENOTYPE	EXPRESSION	EXAMPLE STRAIN	REFERENCE
Tla	TL ANTIGEN	+	A, C58	BOYSE & OLD (1969)
		−	AKR, C57BL/6	
NOT DESIGNATED	gs ANTIGEN	+	AKR	TAYLOR, MEIER, MYERS (1971)
		−	C57L	
NOT DESIGNATED	INFECTIOUS MuLV	+	AKR	TAYLOR, MEIER, MYERS (1971)
		−	C57L	
V_1	N-TROPIC MuLV INDUCTION	V_1	AKR, C58, C3H/Fi	ROWE (1972)
		v_1		
V_2	N-TROPIC MuLV INDUCTION	V_2	AKR, C58, C3H/Fi	ROWE & HARTLEY (1972)
		v_2		
Ind	N-TROPIC MuLV INDUCTION	+	BALB/c NIH-SWISS	STEPHENSON & AARONSON (1972b)
		−		
Fv-1	TISSUE TROPISM FOR VIRAL REPLICATION	n	AKR, C58	ROWE & HARTLEY (1972) STEPHENSON & AARONSON (1972a)
		b	C57BL/6, BALB/c	
		nb	NZB	
H-2	EARLY LEUKEMIA LATE LEUKEMIA	k	AKR	BOYSE, OLD, STOCKERT (1972)
		b	AKR/H-2^b	
G_{IX}	G_{IX} ANTIGEN	+	129	BOYSE, OLD, STOCKERT (1972)
		−	C57L	
Mlv-1	gs ANTIGEN	a	C57BL/10, DBA/2	TAYLOR, MEIER, HUEBNER (1973)
		b		

allow the initial carcinogenic event to establish itself. Immunosuppressive effects of virus (SHEARER et al., 1973) and chemical carcinogens (STJERNSWÄRD, 1965; REES and SYMES, 1973; MATSUOKA et al., 1972; PARMIANI et al., 1971; BALL et al., 1966; BALL, 1970) undoubtedly play a significant part in the initial carcinogenic event. We are currently addressing ourselves to defining the immunosuppressive effects of various chemical carcinogens given intratracheally for the induction of lung cancer in several strains of mice (DEMOISE et al., 1974). Just as NETTESHEIM and HAMMONS (1971) have shown differences in susceptibility to lung carcinogenesis by MCA, STUTMAN (1969) indicates differences in the immunosuppressive effects in genotypically different strains. Based on our studies with MCA we would anticipate that both differences in tumor induction and immunosuppression may be correlated with the AHH inducibility of the various mouse strains (KOURI et al., 1973b).

The possible mechanisms whereby chemical carcinogens bring about carcinogenic events may be dependent not only on the transforming events but also on immunodepression, that allows these transformed cells to bypass the immunological defense mechanisms of the host. Immunosuppression by chemical carcinogens may, in fact, not be a single event, but cumulative, recurring events that allow frequent bypassing of host defense mechanisms and consequently slow interrupted but progressive growth of tumor cells.

The term "immunologic surveillance" coined by THOMAS (1959) and further expounded by BURNET (1970a, 1970b) denotes the idea of "seeking out and destroying" transformed cells by immunological means. This idea may not be totally correct, because rather than destruction, a "holding action" (LAPPE, 1971, 1972) may develop until such time as events in the integrated host's defense provide a favorable climate for the growth of the transformed cells (HESTON, 1963). This "sneaking through" event of some transformed cells that ultimately leads to the development of cancer is more of apparent scientific basis than it initially appeared. "Sneak through" has been thought to occur due to the location of the transformed cells in sites not exposed, or exposed less frequently to concomitant immunity. This unequal exposure to immune mechanisms is also believed to play a role in the site of metastites (VAAGE et al., 1971).

Another factor allowing "sneak through" of initial transformed cells is the low antigenic profile of some tumor cells as well as the low antigen load presented by only a few cells. For tumor cells to escape immune surveillance there must first be a barrier to escape. Nonimmunogenic or low immunogenic tumors may not be capable of surveillance by immunological means. One must then define what we mean by "nonimmunogenic". Is it that these tumor cells are so like normal cells that they cannot be recognized as foreign by the host? Self-non-self discrimination is not fully understood and is intertwined with immunological tolerance, immunological paralysis, and immunological recognition. Is it that the host is tolerant to these cells since they contain certain embryonic antigens or endogenous viral genome antigens? Or, is it that the host is not capable of recognizing these antigens due to genetic variations within the species? This is where the inbred laboratory animals help us understand the role of genetic determinants in the immune process and, ultimately, to understand the events of neoplastic initiation and developments. Genetic variation in the immunological response can definitely influence neoplasia. Many of the differences in specific immunological responses have been linked to the histocompatibility gene in the mouse, rat, and guinea pig. Viral susceptibility has also been closely associated with the H-2 locus and such variations in susceptibility may be shown to be related, at least

in part, to inability to produce an immunological response in susceptible mice. These immune responses are under the control of individual dominant autosomal genes. Differences in response are not
usually all or none but are concerned with quality and/or specificity
of the antibody response.

The Ir-1 locus is closely linked to the H-2 gene in mice. Evidence
indicates responsiveness to the various peptides (L-tyrosine and
L-glutamic acid [T,G], L-phenylalanine and L-glutamic acid [P,G], and
L-histidine and L-glutamic acid [H,G] built on multichain poly-DL-
alanine) are under the control of different Ir-1 alleles (MCDEVITT,
1968). All of these polypeptides are antigenic in some strain of mice,
but not necessarily in any one strain. They will not cross-immunize
although antibody will cross react extensively. The Ir-1 gene functions
at the T-cell level and controls cellular immune functions in the
recognition of antigens, thus low responders are those who have reduced numbers of detectable precursor cells or cells with lower affinity for the specific immunogens. Low responder animals can, however,
recognize these polypeptide antigenic determinants and produce large
amounts of antibody when these hapten polypeptides are coupled with
an immunogenic protein carrier. This shows one means of bypassing
genetic defects (MCDEVITT, 1968).

The Ir-1 genes appear to have at least 2 or 3 separate loci. The Ir-
IgA gene controls the immune response of mice to allotypic and idio-
typic determinants on the IgA myeloma proteins derived from BALB/c
mice. The Ir-IgG gene is linked to different H-2 specificities than
the Ir-IgA and controls the immune response to γG (γ2a) of the same
antigen (LIEBERMAN and HUMPHREY, 1971, 1972).

Various immunological responses have been shown to be non-H-2 linked.
In immune responses to the (T,G) or (Phe-G)-Prol--L portion of multichain synthetic polypeptides, the response is controlled by the dominant, autosomal, Ir-3 gene (MOZES et al., 1973). The SJL mouse is the
prototype for the high responders and the DBA/1 for the low responders.
These responses are expressions of B cell activity and demonstrate
antibodies can be made to 2 determinants on the same antigen under
the control of 2 genes. Other non-H-2 linked gene controls of immune
responses are reviewed by MCDEVITT and LANDY (1972), demonstrating
dependence on the recognition of the antigenic determinant.

Antibody response to streptococcal polysaccharides differs dramatical-
ly with some strains, producing more to the group A than the group C
carbohydrates, whereas in others, the reverse is true. These responses
can give rise to a rather homogenous or a wide variation in the heterogeneity of the immune responses. B cell dependent responses to Sal-
monella lipopolysaccharides have also shown differences in mouse strain
response and are dependent on recognition of the antigen (PAULI, 1972).

Having reviewed some of these various aspects of immunogenetic responses,
one finds that new scientific discoveries are being made at a rate and
volume beyond our ability to assimilate, evaluate, and make use of them
as building blocks for rational progress. Unequal progress in the research prevents total integration of this knowledge into the understanding of host-parasite relationships. These studies with natural
and synthetic antigens have demonstrated immunogenetic differences
in responses which can not at this time be correlated with the viral
and tumor specific membrane antigens. Recent advances in characterizing
the amino acid sequences in the tumor virus (OROSZLAN et al., 1970;
NOWINSKI et al., 1972) and the mouse myeloma protein (FRANCIS et al.,
1974), the isolation of the viral envelope glycoproteins (KENNEL et

al., 1973), and studies with carcinoembryonic antigens (TOMITA et al.,
1974) will lead to a greater understanding of their immunogenetic
potential. Each host responds to some of these antigens but probably
not to all of the exposed antigenic configurations making up the tumor
cell membranes and soluble antigens. The immunological reactions
summarized in Table 2 for the various mouse strains in our carcinogenic studies amplify the subtle difference in their responses to
various defined immunogens. Those differences in the capabilities of
the host to mount an adequate response to produce a "killer" or
"holding" effect influence the capabilities of these genotypic strains
to allow "sneaking through" events to occur for the establishment of
the initial carcinogenic event as a pathologic entity and also to influence the process of metastasis and the blocking phenomenon (HELL-
STRÖM and HELLSTRÖM, 1970) that accompanies rapid growth and terminal
events of the neoplastic process. The genetic capabilities of the
host to respond may be one of the important factors governing the
variation in latency period of tumor development in the animal models
as demonstrated in Table 1.

We have elected to characterize the susceptibility of a mouse strain
not only by the tumor incidence and latency but also by the carcinogenic index (IBALL, 1939), which equates susceptibility to latency
and incidence of tumor induction. It is obvious that certain strains
have longer latency periods than others yet produce comparable numbers
of tumors. We cannot say at this time whether this represents an inability to respond to certain tumor antigens allowing "sneak through"
events to occur or whether these inbred strains actually are capable
of mounting a high level of response leading to the blocking phenomena
and insuring rapid tumor growth. HALPERN (1973) developed high and low
responder lines of Swiss mice to various unrelated antigens. These 2
lines were clearly separated for their humoral responsiveness but showed similar cell mediated reactions. When allogenic Sarcoma 180 implants
were made, the high responders allowed the tumor to grow and 90% of
the animals were killed, while in the low responders, all tumors re-
gressed. The high responders synthesized high levels of antibody believed to have allowed the tumors to grow due to the blocking reaction,
while the low responders produced only enough antibody to provide for
effective cellular immunity. If the type C viral antigens play a significant role in chemical carcinogenesis, it may well be that of providing antigenic components in the tumor cell surface which may make
them more antigenic as postulated by BARBIERI et al. (1971) and GREEN-
BERGER and AARONSON (1973). On the other hand, a tolerance to these
antigens may exist or these endogenous viral antigens may act rapidly to overload the system leading to the blocking phenomena. It is
difficult to speculate regarding the wide divergence in antigenicity
of chemically induced tumors. It could be assumed, however, that
either the individual mice have a wide variation in capability to
respond or that the antigenicity of the various chemically induced
tumors varies significantly accounting for variations in the immunological response. Such variations in capability to respond would influence the time required for the blocking type phenomena to develop,
thereby influencing the rate of tumor development on an individual
animal basis (BARTLETT, 1972). The latter of the 2 hypotheses seems
most likely since we are dealing with inbred strains, although we
have noted a wide variation between individual mice in the mixed
lymphocyte studies. We need to define molecular serology of antigens,
antibodies, and antigen-antibody complexes in order to study the
mechanisms of immune interaction in the mouse model system where the
science of immunogenetics is well advanced. Various sensitive serological procedures, such as the radioimmune assay, are available for
analyzing the specific antigenic components of the tumor antigens.

Using such studies, we should be able to develop better diagnostic
tools and, consequently, a knowledge of the potential usefulness of
immunotherapy or immunological preventive procedures without producing an adverse stimulatory effect to those clones of transformed cells
maintained in a "holding" state by host control mechanisms.

Other Genetic Controls of Neoplastic Developments

Many known genes have been associated with the occurrence of various
forms of neoplasms; however, in many instances this relationship
appears to have no connection with cancer development (HESTON, 1972).
Early experiments in cancer research were concerned mainly with the
inheritance of susceptibility to spontaneous neoplasia. The development of the inbred strains and the use of congenic strains have allowed
for more specific genetic analysis of host susceptibility to carcinogenesis. In most cases, it has been shown that carcinogenesis is dependent on multiple genetic and environmental factors. We will review
only a few of the genetic linkages reported to influence cancer development.

HESTON (1963) reported linkage between pulmonary tumors and 8 specific
genes (hr, A^Y, vt, sh-2, wa-2, Fu, ah, and f), while LITTLE (1934),
BITTNER (1945), and HESTON and DERINGER (1948) demonstrated linkage
of mammary tumors with lethal yellow, brown, and agouti genes. STRONG
(1945) linked gastric tumors with the brown gene while MACDOWELL (1945)
and LAW (1952) demonstrated leukemia linked with dilute and flexed-
tail genes. Although these associations have been made, their correlation with specific biochemical or physiological pathways has not
been made. The H-2 histocompatibility loci has been associated with
susceptibility or resistance to leukemia, the $H-2^k$ being considered
susceptible while $H-2^b$ denotes resistance (LILLY, 1966). How the H-2
locus influences viral leukemia is not known but may represent influences discussed earlier in viral and immunological factor in the
development of cancer.

MEIER et al. (1969) have described the genetic control of susceptibility or resistance to viral leukemogenesis by the hairless locus (hr).
Hairless is an autosomal recessive mutation maintained in strain HRS/J.
The incidence of leukemia is nearly 50% greater in the hairless (hr/hr)
mouse than the haired mouse (hr/+) and occurs 6 months earlier. An
N-tropic MuLV was isolated from both the hr/hr and hr/+ mice. The
latency of neoplastic expression would appear to be related to an
immunodeficiency factor rather than infectious virus expression
(HEINIGER et al., 1974).

YAMAMOTO et al. (1973) propose that malignancy is induced by carcinogens by producing chromosomal changes resulting in a change in the
balance between expression (E) and suppression (S) genes. E exists
in normal cells but is neutralized by S, and malignancy occurs only
when E increases or S decreases. Their studies with hamster cells
injected with polyoma virus or treated with dimethylnitrosamine
identified the location of the E and S chromosomes. These studies
have been confirmed using Ara-C treatment of hamster cells (BENEDICT
et al., 1974).

Cells at Risk to Carcinogens and DNA Repair Synthesis

In addition to the previously discussed genetic factors that provide
varying degrees of protection against the initial carcinogenic event,
there is an additional factor we wish to discuss: the cells at risk
to carcinogenesis. Many factors influence this population of cells,
as dose of carcinogens, chronic exposure, site of exposure, aging
processes, hormonal influences, stress factors that induce hormonal
changes, diet that influences protein metabolism, and promoters such
as dust, asbestos, physical, microbiological and chemical irritants,
etc. The list is long and cannot be fully exploited here. If, however,
one examines this list closely, it is found these factors have one
thing in common. They all influence some function of DNA repair.
PIERCE (1970) points out that tumors arise only in those tissues
capable of mitotic activity. Chemical carcinogens transform only
those cells which are entering mitosis which makes up only 0.03% to
0.13% of the body's cells at any one time (MEKLER, 1973). The cells
at risk are few and far between unless there are intervening factors
that stimulate unscheduled DNA repair. STICH and SAN (1973) indicate
a link exists between the oncogenicity of a compound and its capability to provoke DNA repair synthesis. This, however, is not the entire
picture, since cocarcinogenic effects do occur requiring both inducers and promoters. Cancer research has made use of this process
for years in the form of croton oil in back painting carcinogenesis
experiments. This has been carried over into lung carcinogenesis with
the use of ferric oxide with BaP (SAFFIOTTI et al., 1968, 1972) and
carbon dust or aluminum oxide with BaP (HENRY and KAUFMAN, 1973).
STANTON and BLACKWELL (1961) and BLENKINSOPP (1968) stimulated repair
and regeneration of pulmonary epithelium by pulmonary infarction.
Chronic respiratory infections also promote regeneration of lung
tissue and may play a role in carcinogenesis.

The various factors involving DNA repair have not been fully defined.
HEINIGER et al. (1972) determined the overall DNA-turnover in 19 inbred strains and F1 hybrid mice. The range of DNA turnover observed
suggested polygenic control (H-1, H-3, and H-4) of the steady state.
The mouse strains with the shorter turnover time were C57BR/cdJ,
DBA/2, SWR/J, and BALB/c. The intermediate turnover rate was represented
by C57BL/10, C57BL/6, AKR, C57L, SJL, C58, and C3H/He, while DBA/1
has the longest turnover rate, which was almost 3 times that of
C57BR/cdJ. The DNA turnover rate showed no correlation with spontaneous
tumorigenesis.

Significant differences in ulcer formation in mice has been observed
(LILLY and DURAN-REYNALS, personal communication; NEBERT et al., 1972).
The form of host control appears to be primarily that of cells at risk.
Much of the body receiving the greatest assault from carcinogenic
agents is extracorporeal and has special defense mechanisms. The skin
is made up of stratified layers of epithelial cells, with those involved in mitosis being the least exposed to toxic substances. In the
respiratory and alimentary systems there is a high degree of vascularization and lymphatic involvement and secretatory activity which tends
to produce rapid detoxification and also provides a high level of
immunological protection decreasing the incidence of carcinogenic
"sneak-through" events occurring. The ciliary action of the respiratory
tract also provides for elimination of particulate irritants that induce cellular division.

In the experimental animal models, most chemically induced tumors have
had their origin in cells other than the epithilial cells. However,

in lung carcinogenesis, our primary concern is with the induction of squamous cell carcinomas. Alveoli are lined with squamous cells and are suspected to be the site of lung tumors. It is proposed that the use of ferric oxide or other particulate matter or chemicals that will induce mitotic activity increases the cells at risk and may in reality be only an exaggeration of what takes place in nature. Cigarette smoke carcinogenesis may be related to the cocarcinogenesis effects of weak carcinogens and particulate matter requiring extended chronic exposure. We have found that filtered cigarette smoke fails to induce AHH activity in the lungs of mice while unfiltered smoke induced for extended periods (KOURI et al., 1974). The particulate matter appears to play several roles, the trapping of AHH inducers and as promoters for weak carcinogen by increasing cellular proliferation. For these reasons it would appear the use of those agents that bring about unscheduled DNA synthesis are warranted in experimental models. Although we have considered primarily the influence of DNA synthesis on chemical carcinogenesis, this process is also important in triggering the hypothesized depression of repressors of tumor virus genome, protovirus, or oncogenes that may play an integrated role in the host as the etiological agents of cancer, be they viral, chemical or viral-chemical.

Summary and Application in Experimental Pulmonary Carcinogenesis Studies

The selection of animal models for cancer research must be based on the understanding and subsequent characterization of those host regulatory systems that define the differences between susceptible and resistant hosts. We have reviewed such host factors that appear to play decisive roles in carcinogenesis in the inbred mouse as an animal model. Differences in susceptibility to subcutaneous carcinogens with MCA, DMBA, and BaP have been demonstrated between various genotypically different strains of mice. Susceptibility to PAH carcinogens has been shown to be directly related to the inducibility of hepatic AHH, although differences in relative susceptibility to MCA, DMBA, and BaP were demonstrated in AHH inducible strains.

The host control of the type C RNA virus expression was reviewed. Although the frequency of occurrence of "spontaneous" neoplasia has been demonstrated to be related to infectious virus expression in mice, no direct influence of gs antigen or infectious virus expression on chemical carcinogenesis can be demonstrated. Various parameters of immunogenetics were discussed in relationship to the emergence of the initial transformed cells and the ultimate development of cancer. The immunosuppressive effects of carcinogens may play a role in the establishment of transformed cells and their growth. Differences in tumor latency are believed to be related to genetic differences in ability to recognize and respond to the various tumor cell antigens. The full impact of immunogenetics might be further understood when tumor cell antigens are more fully characterized.

We must consider not only the integrated host response but also the cells at risk to chemical carcinogens. Since DNA repair and mitotic activity may increase susceptibility to transformation, this aspect of susceptibility was discussed.

Based on our findings with subcutaneous chemical carcinogens in inbred mice, we have selected several strains for lung carcinogenesis studies. The effects of intratracheal inoculation of chemical carcinogens on AHH induction in the lungs (KOURI et al., these proceedings) and host immunocompetence (DEMOISE et al., these proceedings) will be correlated with respiratory tumor induction. Studies are also in progress using ferric oxide in combination with chemical carcinogens in hopes of increasing the cells at risk and inducing higher incidences of squamous cell carcinomas. The use of wax pellet carcinogen implants (STANTON and BLACKWELL, 1961) is also being evaluated as a means of inducing lung cancers in mice. By examining these various parameters and methods of tumor induction, we will evaluate the inbred mouse as a model system for lung carcinogens.

Acknowledgements

We wish to thank Dr. RONALD A. SALERNO, Dr. LOUISE S. RABSTEIN, Dr. IVETTE M. GARCIA, Dr. VIRGINIA M. MEROLD, Dr. MINA L. VERNON and our technician staff for their assistance through the years represented by these studies. We also wish to thank Dr. JOHN H. KREISHER and Dr. ROBERT J. HUEBNER for their assistance in this program supported by The Council for Tobacco Research - U.S.A. and by Contract No. NO1-CP-43240 within the Virus Cancer Program of the National Cancer Institute.

References

AARONSON, S.W., HARTLEY, J.W., TODARO, G.J.: Mouse leukemia virus: "Spontaneous" release by mouse embryo cells after long-term *in vitro* cultivation. Proc. nat. Acad. Sci. (Wash.) 64, 87-94 (1969).

AARONSON, S.A., TODARO, G.J., SCOLNICK, E.M.: Induction of murine C-type viruses from clonal lines of virus-free BALB/3T3 cells. Science 174, 157-159 (1971).

BALL, J.K.: Immunosuppression and carcinogenesis contrasting effects with 7,12-dimethylbenz(a)anthracene benz(a)pyrene and 3-methylcholanthrene. J. nat. Cancer Inst. 44, 1-10 (1970).

BALL, J.K., SINCLAIR, N.R., MCCARTER, J.A.: Prolonged immunosuppression and tumor induction by a chemical carcinogen injected at birth. Science 152, 650-651 (1966).

BARBIERI, D., BELEHRADEK, J., BARSKI, G.: Decrease in tumor-producing capacity of mouse cell lines following infection with mouse leukemia viruses. Int. J. Cancer 7, 364-371 (1971).

BARON, S.: Personal communication, 1974.

BARTLETT, G.L.: Effect of host immunity on the antigenic strength of primary tumors. J. nat. Cancer Inst. 49, 493-504 (1972).

BENEDICT, W.F., RUCKER, N., MARK, C., KOURI, R.E.: Correlation between the balance of specific chromosomes and the expression of malignancy in hamster cells. In preparation (1974).

BENVENISTE, R.E., LIEBER, M.M., TODARO, G.J.: A distinct class of inducible murine type C viruses which replicate in the rabbit SIRC cell line. Proc. nat. Acad. Sci. (Wash.) 71, 602-606 (1974).

BITTNER, J.J.: Inciting influences in the etiology of mammary cancer in mice. AAA Research Conference on Cancer, 63-96 (1945).

BLENKINSOPP, W.K.: Relationship of injury to chemical carcinogenesis in the lungs of rats. J. nat. Cancer Inst. 40, 651-661 (1968).

BOYSE, E.A., OLD, L.J.: Some aspects of normal and abnormal cell surface genetics. Ann. Rev. Genetics 3, 269-290 (1969).

BOYSE, E.A., OLD, L.J., STOCKERT, E.: The relation of linkage group IX to leukemogenesis in the mouse. In: RNA Viruses and Host Genome in Oncogenesis (P. Emmolot, P. Bentvelzen, eds), pp. 171-185. Amsterdam: North-Holland Publ. Co. 1972.

BUFFET, R.F., GRACE, G.T., DIBERANDINO, L.A., MIRAND, E.A.: Vertical transmission of murine leukemia virus. Cancer Res. 29, 588-595 (1969).

BURNET, F.M.: Immunological Surveillance. New York: Pergamon Press 1970a.

BURNET, F.M.: The concept of immunological surveillance. Prog. exp. Tumor Res. 13, 1-27 (1970b).

CHASE, D.G., PIKO, L.: Expression of A- and C-type particles in early mouse embryos. J. nat. Cancer Inst. 51, 1971-1975 (1973).

CONNEY, A.H.: Factors influencing benzo(a)pyrene metabolism in animals and man. In: World Symposium on Model Studies in Carcinogenesis (J. DiPaolo, P. Ts'O, eds). Cleveland: Chemical Rubber Co. (in press) 1974.

DEMAEYER, E., DEMAEYER-GUIGNARD, J.: Gene with quantitative effect on circulating interferon induced by Newcastle disease virus. J. Virol. 3, 506-512 (1969).

DEMOISE, C.F., KOURI, R.E., WHITMIRE, C.E.: Cell-mediated immunity after intratracheal exposure to 3-methylcholanthrene, and its relationship to tumor transplant growth in C3H/f Mai mice. In: These Proceedings.

FINKEL, M.P., BISKIS, B.O., JINKINS, P.B.: Virus induction of osteosarcomas in mice. Science 151, 698-701 (1966).

FRANCIS, S.H., GRALAM, R., LESLIE, Q., HOOD, L., EISEN, H.N.: Amino-acid sequence of the variable region of the heavy (alpha) chain of a mouse myeloma protein with anti-hapten activity. Proc. nat. Acad. Sci. (Wash.) 71, 1123-1127 (1974).

GAZDAR, A.F., CHOPRA, H.C., SARMA, P.S.: Properties of a murine sarcoma virus isolated from a tumor arising in an NZW/NZB F$_1$ hybrid mouse. I. Isolation and pathology of tumors induced in rodents. Int. J. Cancer 9, 219-233 (1972).

GELBOIN, H.V.: Carcinogens, enzyme induction, and gene action. Advanc. Cancer Res. 10, 1-81 (1967).

GIELEN, J.E., GOUJON, R.M., NEBERT, D.W.: Genetic regulation of aryl hydrocarbon hydroxylase induction. II. Simple mendelian expression in mouse tissues *in vivo*. J. biol. Chem. 247, 1125-1137 (1972).

GREENBERGER, J.S., AARONSON, S.A.: *In vivo* inoculation of RNA C-type viruses inducing regression of experimental solid tumors. J. nat. Cancer Inst. 15, 1935-1938 (1973).

GROSS, L.: Is cancer a communicable disease? Cancer Res. 4, 293-303 (1944).

GROSS, L.: "Spontaneous" leukemia developing in C3H mice following inoculation in infancy, with AK leukemic extracts or AK embryos. Proc. Soc. exp. Biol. (N.Y.) 76, 27-32 (1950).

GROSS, L.: Oncogenic Viruses. New York: Pergamon Press, Oxford 1970.

HALPERN, B.: Paradoxes in immunology. In: Mechanism in Allergy (L. Goodfriend, A.H. Sehon, R.P. Orange, eds), pp. 527-542. New York: Marcel Dekker, Inc. 1973.

HAREL, L., HAREL, J., HUPPERT, J.: Partial homology between RNA from Rauscher mouse leukemia virus and cellular DNA. Biochem. Biophys. Res. Commun. 28, 44-49 (1967).

HARTLEY, J.W., ROWE, W.P., HUEBNER, R.J.: Host range restrictions of murine leukemia viruses in mouse embryo cell cultures. J. Virol. 5, 221-225 (1970).

HARVEY, J.J.: An unidentified virus which causes the rapid production of tumors in mice. Nature (Lond.) 204, 1104-1105 (1964).

HEINIGER, H.J., CHEN, H.W., MEIER, H., TAYLOR, B., COMMERFORD, L.S.: Studies on the genetic control of cell proliferation: I. Clearance of DNA-bound radioactivity in 19 inbred strains and hybrid mice. Life Sci. 11, 87-96 (1972).

HEINIGER, H.J., MEIER, H., KALISS, N., CHERRY, M., CHEN, H.W., STONER, R.D.: Hereditary immunodeficiency and leukemogenesis in HRS/J mice. Cancer Res. 34, 201-211 (1974).

HELLSTRÖM, K.F., HELLSTRÖM, I.: Immunological enhancement as studied by cell culture technique. Ann. Rev. Microbiol. 24, 373-398 (1970).

HENRY, M.C., KAUFMAN, D.G.: Clearance of benzo(a)pyrene from hamster lungs after administration on coated particles. J. nat. Cancer Inst. 51, 1961-1964 (1973).

HESTON, W.E.: Genetics of neoplasia. In: Methodology in Mammalian Genetics (W.J. Burdette, ed.), pp. 247-268. San Francisco: Holden-Day, Inc. 1963.

HESTON, W.E.: Genetic Factors in Tumorigenesis. In: RNA Viruses and Host Genome in Oncogenesis (P. Emmolot, P. Bentvelzen, eds), pp. 13-24. Amsterdam: North-Holland Publ. Co. 1972

HESTON, W.E., DERINGER, M.K.: Relationship between the agouti gene and mammary tumor development in mice. Acta Univ. Internat. Centre de Cancer 6, 262-263 (1948).

HILGERS, J., BEYA, M., GEERING, G., BOYSE, E.A., OLD, J.J.: Evidence for mendelian inheritance. In: RNA Viruses and Host Genome in Oncogenesis (P. Emmolot, P. Bentvelzen, eds), pp. 187-192. Amsterdam: North-Holland Publ. Co. 1972.

HUBERMAN, E., KUROKI, T., MARQUARDT, H., SELKIRK, J.K., HEIDELBERGER, C., GROVER, P.L., SIMS, P.: Transformation of hamster embryo cells by epoxides and other derivatives of polycyclic hydrocarbons. Cancer Res. 32, 1291-1396 (1972).

HUEBNER, R.J., FREEMAN, A.E., WHITMIRE, C.E., PRICE, P.J., RHIM, J.S., KELLOFF, G.J., GILDEN, R.V., MEIER, H.: Endogenous and exogenous RNA tumor virus genomes in chemical carcinogenesis. In: Environment and Cancer, pp. 318-345. Baltimore, Maryland: The Williams and Wilkins Co. 1972.

HUEBNER, R.J., KELLOFF, G.J., SARMA, P.S., LANE, W.T., TURNER, H.C., GILDEN, R.V., OROSZLAN, S., MEIER, H., MYERS, D.D., PETERS, R.L.: Group-specific antigen expression during embryogenesis of the genome of the C-type RNA tumor virus: Implications for ontogenesis and oncogenesis. Proc. nat. Acad. Sci. (Wash.) 67, 366-376 (1970a).

HUEBNER, R.J., TODARO, G.J.: Oncogenes of RNA tumor viruses as determinants of cancer. Proc. nat. Acad. Sci. (Wash.) 64, 1087-1094 (1969).

HUEBNER, R.J., TODARO, G.J., SARMA, P., HARTLEY, J.W., FREEMAN, A.E., PETERS, R.L., WHITMIRE, C.E., MEIER, H., GILDEN, R.V.: "Switched off" vertically transmitted C-type RNA tumor viruses as determinants of spontaneous and induced cancer: A new hypothesis of viral carcinogenesis. In: International Symposium of the Centre National de Recherce Scientifique, Defectiveness, Rescue and Stimulation of Oncogenic Viruses, Vol. 183, pp. 33-57, Paris 1970b.

IBALL, J.: The relative potency of carcinogenic compounds. Amer. J. Cancer 35, 188-190 (1939).

KELLERMANN, G., LUYTEN-KELLERMANN, M., SHAW, C.R.: Metabolism of polycyclic aromatic hydrocarbons in cultured human leukocytes under genetic control. Humangenetik 20, 257-263 (1973).

KENNEL, S.J., DEL VILLANO, B.C., LEVY, R.L., LERNER, R.A.: Properties of an oncornavirus glycoprotein: Evidence for its presence on the surface of virions and infected cells. Virology 55, 464-475 (1973).

KINOSHITA, N., GELBOIN, H.V.: Aryl hydrocarbon hydroxylase and polycyclic hydrocarbon tumorigenesis: Effect of the enzyme inhibitor 7,8-benzoflavone on tumorigenesis and macro-molecule binding. Proc. nat. Acad. Sci. (Wash.) 69, 824-828 (1972).

KIRSTEN, W.H., MAYER, L.A.: Morphologic responses to a murine erythroblastosis virus. J. nat. Cancer Inst. 39, 311-335 (1971).

KOURI, R.E., DEMOISE, C.F., WHITMIRE, C.E.: The significance of the aryl hydrocarbon hydroxylase enzyme systems in the selection of model systems for respiratory carcinogenesis. These Proceedings.

KOURI, R.E., KIEFER, R., ZIMMERMAN, E.M.: Hydrocarbon metabolizing activity of various mammalian cells in culture. *In Vitro*. (In press) 1974b.

KOURI, R.E., RATRIE, H., WHITMIRE, C.E.: Evidence of a genetic re-
    lationship between susceptibility to 3-methylcholanthrene-induced
    subcutaneous tumors and inducibility of aryl hydrocarbon hydroxylase.
    J. nat. Cancer Inst. 51, 197-200 (1973a).
KOURI, R.E., RATRIE, H., WHITMIRE, C.E.: Genetic control of suscepti-
    bility to 3-methylcholanthrene-induced subcutaneous sarcomas. Int.
    J. Cancer 13, 714-720 (1974c).
KOURI, R.E., SALERNO, R.A., WHITMIRE, C.E.: Relationships between
    aryl hydrocarbon hydroxylase inducibility and sensitivity to
    chemically induced subcutaneous sarcomas in various strains of mice.
    J. nat. Cancer Inst. 50, 363-368 (1973b).
LAPPE, M.A.: Failure of long-term immunological control of 3-methyl-
    cholanthrene-induced skin tumors in the autochthonous host. J.
    Reticuloendothel. Soc. 10, 120-130 (1971).
LAPPE, M.A.: Possible significance of immune recognition of pre-
    neoplastic and neoplastic cell surfaces. In: Conference on Immuno-
    logy of Carcinogenesis, DHEW Publication No. (NIH) 72-334. Nat.
    Cancer Inst. Monogr. 35, 49-55 (1972).
LAW, L.W.: The flexed-tail anemia gene (f) and induced leukemia in
    mice. J. nat. Cancer Inst. 12, 1119-1126 (1952).
LEVY, J.A.: Xenotropic viruses: Murine leukemia viruses associated
    with NIH Swiss, NZB and other mouse strains. Science 182, 1151-1153
    (1973).
LEVY, J.A.: Autoimmunity and neoplasia: The possible role of C-type
    virus. Amer. J. clin. Pathol. (in press) 1974.
LIEBERMAN, R., HUMPHREY, W.: Association of H-2 types with genetic
    control of immune responsiveness to IgA allotypes in the mouse.
    Proc. nat. Acad. Sci. (Wash.) 68, 2510-2513 (1971).
LIEBERMAN, R., HUMPHREY, W.: Association of H-2 types with genetic
    control of immune responsiveness to I_GG (γ2a) allotypes in the
    mouse. J. exp. Med. 136, 1222-1230 (1972).
LILLY, F.: The histocompatibility 2 locus and susceptibility to tumor
    induction. J. nat. Cancer Inst. 22, 631-641 (1966).
LILLY, F., PINCUS, T.: Genetic control of murine viral leukemogenesis.
    In: Advances in Cancer Research (G. Klein, S. Weinhouse, A. Haddow,
    eds), Vol. 17, pp. 231-277. New York, London: Academic Press 1973.
LITTLE, C.C.: The relation of coat color to the spontaneous incidence
    of mammary tumors in mice. J. exp. Med. 59, 229-250 (1934).
MACDOWELL, E.C., POTTER, J.S., TAYLOR, M.J.: Mouse leukemia. XII.
    The role of genes in spontaneous cases. Cancer Res. 5, 65-83 (1945).
MARQUARDT, H., HEIDELBERGER, C.: Influence of "feeder cells" and in-
    ducers and inhibitors of microsomal enzymes on hydrocarbon induced
    malignant transformation of cells derived from mouse prostate. Cancer
    Res. 32, 721-752 (1972).
MATSOUKA, Y., SENOH, H., KAWAMOTO, T., KOHMO, T., HAMOAKA, T., KITAGAWA,
    M.: Failure of immunological memory in DMBA-treated mice. Nature
    New Biol. 238, 273-274 (1972).
MCDEVITT, H.O.: Genetic control of the antibody response. III. Quali-
    tative and quantitative characterization of the antibody response
    to [(T,G)-A--L] in CBA and C57 mice. J. Immunol. 100, 482-492 (1968).
MCDEVITT, H.O., LANDY, M.: Genetic Control of Immune Responsiveness.
    New York, London: Academic Press 1972.
MEIER, H., MYERS, D.D.: Chemical co-carcinogenesis: differential
    action of various compounds, derepression of endogenous C-type RNA
    genomes, and influence of different genotypes of mice. In: Unifying
    Concept of Leukemia (Dutcher, ed.), Bibl. haemat., Vol. 39, pp.
    551-573. Basel: Karger 1973.
MEIER, H., MYERS, D.D., HUEBNER, R.J.: Genetic control by the hr-locus
    of susceptibility and resistance to leukemia. Proc. nat. Acad. Sci.
    (Wash.) 63, 759-766 (1969).
MEKLER, L.B.: Chemical carcinogenesis. A new approach to the molecular
    and cellular mechanisms. Oncology 28, 68-82 (1973).

MOLONEY, J.B.: A virus induced rhabdomyosarcoma of mice. In: Conference on Murine Leukemia. Nat. Cancer Inst. Monograph. 22, 139-142 (1966).

MOZES, E., SHEARER, G.M., SELA, M., BRAUN, W.: Genetic control of immune responses to synthetic polypeptides in mice: Cellular analysis of the phenotypic correction of the Ir-3 gene defect by polyadenylic-polyuridiylic acid. J. Immunol. 111, 439-447 (1973).

MYERS, D.D., MEIER, H., HUEBNER, R.J.: Prevalence of murine leukemia virus group specific antigen in inbred strains on mice. Life Sci. 9, 1071-1080 (1970).

NEBERT, D.W., BENEDICT, W.F., BIELEN, J.E.: Aryl hydrocarbon hydroxylase, epoxide hydrase, and 7,12-dimethylbenz(a)anthracene-produced skin tumorigenesis in the mouse. Molecular Pharm. 8, 374-379 (1972a).

NEBERT, D.W., BENEDICT, W.F., KOURI, R.E.: Aromatic hydrocarbon-produced tumorigenesis and the genetic differences in aryl hydrocarbon hydroxylase induction. In: World Symposium on Model Studies in Chemical Carcinogenesis (J. DiPaolo, P. Ts'o, eds.). Cleveland: Chemical Rubber Co. (in press) 1973.

NEBERT, D.W., GOUJON, F.M., GIELEN, J.E.: Aryl hydrocarbon hydroxylase induction by polycyclic hydrocarbons: Simple autosomal dominant trait in the mouse. Nature New Biol. 236, 107-110 (1972b).

NETTESHEIM, P., HAMMONS, A.S.: Induction of squamous cell carcinoma in the respiratory tract of mice. J. nat. Cancer Inst. 47, 697-701 (1971).

NOWINSKI, R.C., FLEISSNER, E., SARKER, N.H., AOKI, T.: Chromatographic separation and antigenic analysis of proteins of the onconaviruses. J. Virol. 9, 359-366 (1972).

OROSZLAN, S., FISHER, C.L., STANLEY, T.B., GILDEN, R.V.: Proteins of the murine C-type RNA tumor viruses. I. Isolation of a group-specific antigen by isoelectric focusing. J. gen. Virol. 8, 1-10 (1970).

PARMIANI, G., COLNAGHI, M.I., DELLA PORTA, G.: Immunodepression during urethan and N-nitrosomethylurea leukemogenesis in mice. Brit. J. Cancer 25, 354-365 (1971).

PAULI, R.D.: Genetics of the immune response. I. Differences in the specificity of antibodies to lipopolysaccharides among different strains of mice. J. Immunol. 109, 394-400 (1972).

PETERS, R.L., HARTLEY, J.W., SPAHN, G.J., RABSTEIN, L.S., WHITMIRE, C.E., TURNER, H.C., HUEBNER, R.J.: Prevalence of the group-specific (gs) antigen and infectious virus expressions of the murine C-type RNA viruses during the life span of BALB/cCr mice. Int. J. Cancer 10, 283-289 (1972a).

PETERS, R.L., RABSTEIN, L.S., SPAHN, G.J., MADISON, R.M., HUEBNER, R.J.: Indicence of spontaneous neoplasms in breeding and retired breeder BALB/cCr mice throughout the natural life span. Int. J. Cancer 10, 273-282 (1972b).

PIERCE, G.B.: Differentiation of normal and malignant cells. Fed. Proc. 29, 1248 (1970).

PINCUS, T., HARTLEY, J.W., ROWE, W.P.: A major genetic locus affecting resistance to infection with murine leukemia viruses. I. Tissue culture studies of naturally occurring viruses. J. exp. Med. 133, 1219-1233 (1971a).

PINCUS, T., ROWE, W.P., LILLY, F.: A major genetic locus affecting resistance to infection with murine leukemia viruses. II. Apparent identity to a major locus described for resistance to Friend murine leukemia virus. J. exp. Med. 133, 1234-1241 (1971b).

REED, L.Z., MUENCH, H.A.: A simple method of estimating fifty percent endpoints. Amer. J. Hyg. 27, 493-497 (1938).

REES, J.A., SYMES, M.O.: Immunodepression as a factor during 3-methylcholanthrene carcinogenesis and subsequent tumour growth in mice. Int. J. Cancer 11, 202-211 (1973).

ROUS, P.: A sarcoma of the fowl transmissable by an agent separable from the tumor cells. J. exp. Med. 13, 397-411 (1911).

ROWE, W.P.: Studies of genetic transmission of murine leukemia virus by AKR mice. I. Crosses with Fv-1^n strains of mice. J. exp. Med. 136, 1272-1285 (1972).

ROWE, W.P., HARTLEY, J.W.: Studies of genetic transmission of murine leukemia virus by AKR mice. II. Crosses with Fv-1^b strains of mice. J. exp. Med. 136, 1286-1301 (1972).

ROWE, W.P., HARTLEY, J.W., LANDER, M.R., PUGH, W.E., TEICH, N.: Non-infectious AKR mouse embryo cell lines in which each cell has the capacity to be activated to produce infectious murine leukemia virus. Virology 46, 866-876 (1971).

SAFFIOTTI, U., CEFIS, F., KOLB, L.H.: A method for the experimental induction of bronchogenic carcinoma. Cancer Res. 28, 104-124 (1968).

SAFFIOTTI, U., MONTESANO, R., SELLAKUMAR, A.R., CEFIS, F., KAUFMAN, D.G.: Respiratory tract carcinogenesis in hamsters induced by different numbers of administrations of benzo(a)pyrene and ferric oxide. Cancer Res. 32, 1073-1081 (1972).

SALERNO, R.A., RAMM, G.M., WHITMIRE, C.E.: Chemical induction of sub-cutaneous tumors in BALB/c and Swiss mice infected with wild type-C RNA viruses derived from BALB/c tissues. Cancer Res. 33, 69-77 (1973).

SARMA, P., GAZDAR, A.F.: Recent progress in studies of mouse type-C viruses. Current Topics in Microbiology and Immunology (in press).

SELKIRK, J.K., HUBERMAN, E., HEIDELBERGER, C.: An epoxide is an inter-mediate in the microsomal metabolism of the chemical carcinogen, dibenz(a,h)anthracene. Biochem. Biophys. Res. Commun. 43, 1010-1016 (1971).

SHEARER, G.M., MOZES, E., HARAN-GHERA, N., BENTWICH, Z.: Cellular analysis of immunosuppression to synthetic polypeptide immunogens induced by a murine leukemia virus. J. Immunol. 110, 736-741 (1973).

SHERR, C.J., LIEBER, M.M., TODARO, G.J.: Mixed splenocyte cultures and graft versus host reactions selectively induce an "S-tropic" murine type C virus. Cell 1, 55-58 (1974).

SHIMKIN, M.B., ANDERVONT, H.B.: Comparative carcinogenicity of three carcinogenic hydrocarbons. J. nat. Cancer Inst. 1, 57-62 (1940).

STAATS, J.: Standardized nomenclature for inbred strains of mice: Fifth listing. Cancer Res. 32, 1609-1646 (1972).

STANTON, M.F., BLACKWELL, R.: Induction of epidermoid carcinoma in lungs of rats: A "new" method based upon deposition of methyl-cholanthrene in areas of pulmonary infarction. J. nat. Cancer Inst. 27, 375-407 (1961).

STEPHENSON, J.R., AARONSON, S.A.: Genetic factors influencing C-type RNA virus. J. exp. Med. 136, 175-184 (1972a).

STEPHENSON, J.R., AARONSON, S.A.: A genetic locus for inducibility of C-type virus in BALB/c cells. The effect of a non-linked regula-tory gene on detection of virus after chemical activation. Proc. nat. Acad. Sci. (Wash.) 69, 2798-2801 (1972b).

STITCH, H.F., SAN, R.H.C.: DNA repair synthesis and survival of re-pair deficient human cells exposed to the K-region epoxide of benz (a)anthracene. Proc. Soc. exp. Biol. (N.Y.) 142, 155-158 (1973).

STJERNSWÄRD, J.: Immunodepressive effect of 3-methylcholanthrene. Antibody formation at the cellular level and reaction against weak antigenic homografts. J. nat. Cancer Inst. 35, 885-892 (1965).

STOCKERT, E., OLD, L.J., BOYSE, E.A.: The G_{IX} system. A cell surface alloantigen associated with murine leukemia virus, implications re-garding chromosomal integration of the viral genome. J. exp. Med. 133, 1334-1335 (1971).

STRONG, L.C.: Genetic analysis of the introduction of tumors by methylcholanthrene. IX. Induced and spontaneous adenocarcinomas of the stomach in mice. J. nat. Cancer Inst. 5, 339-362 (1945).

STUTMAN, O.: Carcinogen-induced immune depression: absence in mice resistant to chemical oncogenes. Science 166, 620-621 (1969).

TAYLOR, B.A., MEIER, H., HUEBNER, R.J.: Genetic control of the group-specific antigen of murine leukemia virus. Nature New Biol. 241, 184-186 (1973).

TAYLOR, B.A., MEIER, H., MYERS, D.D.: Host gene control of C-type RNA tumor virus: Inheritance of the group-specific antigen of murine leukemia virus. Proc. nat. Acad. Sci. (Wash.) 68, 3190-3194 (1971).

TEMIN, H.M.: The protovirus hypothesis: Speculations on the significance of RNA-directed DNA synthesis for normal development and for carcinogenesis. J. nat. Cancer Inst. 46, 3-7 (1971).

TEMIN, H.M.: The protovirus hypothesis and cancer. In: RNA Viruses and Host Genome in Oncogenesis (P. Emmelot, P. Bentvelzen, eds), pp. 351-363. Amsterdam: North-Holland Publ. Co. 1972.

THAMAVIT, W., HAISA, Y., ITO, N., BHAMARAPRAVATI, N.: The inhibitory effects of α-benzene hexachloride on 3-methyl-4-dimethylaminoazo-benzene and DL-ethionine carcinogenesis in rats. Cancer Res. 34, 337-340 (1974).

THOMAS, L.: Cellular and Humoral Aspects of Hypersensitive State (H.S. Lawrence, ed.), p. 530. New York: Hoeber-Harper 1959.

THOMAS, P.E., KOURI, R.E., HUTTON, J.J.: The genetics of aryl hydro-carbon hydroxylase induction in mice: A single gene difference between C57BL/6 and DBA/2J. Biochem. Genet. 6, 157-168.

TODARO, G.J.: "Spontaneous" release of type-C viruses from clonal lines of "spontaneously" transformed BALB/3T3 cells. Nature New Biol. 240, 157-160 (1972).

TODARO, G.J., HUEBNER, R.J.: The viral oncogene hypothesis: New evidence. Proc. nat. Acad. Sci. (Wash.) 69, 1009-1015 (1972).

TOMITA, J.T., SAFFORD, J.W., HIRATA, A.A.: Antibody response to different determinant on carcino-embryonic antigen (CEA). Immunol. 26, 291-298 (1974).

TOOZE, J.: The molecular biology of tumor viruses. New York: Cold Spring Harbor Laboratory 1973.

VAAGE, J., CHEN, K., MERRICK, S.: Effect of immune status on the development of artificially induced metastases in different anatomical locations. Cancer Res. 31, 496-500 (1971).

VENKATESAN, N., ARCOS, J.D., ARGUS, M.F.: Induction and repression of microsomal drug-metabolizing enzymes by polycyclic hydrocarbons and phenobarbital. Theoretical models. J. Theor. Biol. 33, 517-537 (1971).

VERNON, M.L., LANE, W.T., HUEBNER, R.J.: Prevalence of type-C particles in visceral tissues of embryonic and new-born mice. J. nat. Cancer Inst. 5, 1171-1175 (1973).

WEBER, R., COON, J.M., TRIOLO, A.J.: Nicotine inhibition of the metabolism of 3,4-benzopyrene, a carcinogen in tobacco smoke. Science 184, 1081-1083 (1974).

WEISS, R.A.: Ecological genetics of RNA tumor viruses and their hosts. In: Analytical and Experimental Epidemiology of Cancer T. Hirayama, ed.). Tokyo: Univ. of Tokyo Press 1973.

WHITMIRE, C.E., SALERNO, R.A.: RNA tumor virus gs antigen and tumor induction by various doses of 3-methylcholanthrene in various strains of mice treated as weanlings. Cancer Res. 32, 1129-1132 (1972a).

WHITMIRE, C.E., SALERNO, R.A.: Influence of preinfection of C57BL/6 mice with Graffi leukemia virus on 3-methylcholanthrene-induced subcutaneous sarcoma. Proc. Soc. exp. Biol. (N.Y.) 144, 674-679 (1973a).

WHITMIRE, C.E., SALERNO, R.A., MEROLD, V.M., RABSTEIN, L.S.: Effect of age at treatment and dose of 3-methylcholanthrene on development of leukemia and sarcoma in AKR mice. J. nat. Cancer Inst. 49, 1411-1415 (1972b).

WHITMIRE, C.E., SALERNO, R.A., RABSTEIN, L.S.: Effects of thymectomy, splenectomy and 3-methylcholanthrene on neoplasia expression, incidence and latency in AKR mice. Proc. Soc. exp. Biol. (N.Y.) 141, 890-894 (1972c).

WHITMIRE, C.E., SALERNO, R.A., RABSTEIN, L.S., HUEBNER, R.J.: RNA tumor virus antigen expression in chemically induced tumors. In: Unifying Concepts of Leukemia (R.M. Dutcher, L. Chiecobianchi, eds), Bibl. haemat., Vol. 39, pp. 574-588. Munich, Paris, New York: Karger 1973b.

WHITMIRE, C.E., SALERNO, R.A., RABSTEIN, L.S., HUEBNER, R.J., TURNER, H.C.: RNA tumor-virus antigen expression in chemically induced tumors. Virus-genome-specified common antigens detected by complement fixation in mouse tumors induced by 3-methylcholanthrene. J. nat. Cancer Inst. 47, 1255-1265 (1971).

WYNDER, E.L., HOFFMANN, D.: Bioassays in tobacco carcinogenesis. In: Progress in Experimental Tumor Research (F. Homburger, ed.), Vol. 11, pp. 164-193. Basel, New York: Karger 1969.

YAMAMOTO, T., RABINOWITZ, Z., SACHS, L.: Identification of the chromosomes that control malignancy. Nature New Biol. 243, 247-250 (1973).

The Significance of Aryl Hydrocarbon Hydroxylase Enzyme Systems in the Selection of Model Systems for Respiratory Carcinogenesis*

Richard E. Kouri, Charles F. Demoise, and Carrie E. Whitmire

Department of Experimental Oncology, Viral-Chemical Carcinogenesis Section, Bethesda, MD 20014, USA

ABSTRACT

Aryl hydrocarbon hydroxylase (AHH) is a multicomponent, microsomal-bound enzyme system which converts a variety of lipid-soluble compounds to water-soluble forms for subsequent elimination from the body. The enzyme system is inducible by a variety of endogenous and exogenous compounds including steroid hormones, barbiturates, insecticides, polycyclic aromatic hydrocarbons (PAH), and whole cigarette smoke. Recent results have demonstrated that inducibility is host-gene regulated, the inducibility of this enzyme correlates with carcinogenic susceptibility to PAH in animal, and bronchogenic squamous cell carcinoma in humans (probably cigarette smoke induced).

This paper illustrates the types of AHH responses observed in pulmonary tissues following treatment of mice of various strains with either PAH or tobacco related chemicals. Following intratracheal instillation of 3-methylcholanthrene, we observed that: a) pulmonary AHH can be induced preferentially at doses < 200 µg (in contrast to higher doses that induce both hepatic and pulmonary tissues), b) kinetic data demonstrate a 6 to 8 fold increase within 24 hours followed by a broad plateau lasting up to 96 hours, and c) induction is host regulated, segregating as a single autosomal dominant gene in crosses between the C57BL/6 (inducible) and DBA/2 (noninducible) strains of mice. Although DBA/2 pulmonary tissue is slightly inducible (in contrast to the noninducibility of hepatic tissue), evidence indicates that this response results from proliferation of constitutive AHH and not true "induction". Exposure to whole smoke from one 1A1 cigarette (10% smoke in a Walton Horizontal Smoking Machine) will preferentially induce pulmonary AHH, and this response is under the same genetic control as that induced by MCA. Exposure to gas phase alone will not induce this response. Use of cigarette smoke condensate fractions (Stedman fractionation) derived from 1A1 tobacco show that after intratracheal instillation, at least 4 fractions are capable of inducing pulmonary AHH. Fractions 3, 4, 12, and 14 (Bi^a, Bi^b, N$_{NM}$, and N$_{MEOH}$) induce at least a 2 fold increase of pulmonary AHH (at a LD_{10-14} dose). It seems as if the enzymatic potential of the lung tissue itself may be a major determinant in the ultimate fate of this organ in any carcinogenic process.

*This research was supported by the Council for Tobacco Research.

A. Introduction

Aryl hydrocarbon hydroxylase (AHH) is the name given to one of the multi-component, mixed-function oxidases that converts a variety of lipid-soluble endogenous and exogenous compounds to water-soluble forms, usually for subsequent elimination from the body (MASON, 1957; CONNEY, 1967). The enzyme system possesses 2 properties which make it particularly amenable for studying its role in chemically induced cancers: 1. the system is inducible**(NEBERT and GELBOIN, 1969) and 2. this inducibility is regulated by a single autosomal dominant gene in crosses involving the C57BL/6 and DBA/2 strains of mice (THOMAS et al., 1972; NEBERT et al., 1972). Recent information suggests that this enzyme system plays a major role in 3-methylcholanthrene-induced carcinogenesis in the aforementioned mouse strains (KOURI et al., 1973a, 1973b, 1974a).

The lung and skin of mice seem to be under a different type of genetic control from that of hepatic tissue, because these organs appear to be slightly inducible in strains in which the liver is completely non-inducible (BURKI et al., 1973; WIEBEL et al., 1973). There are many questions concerning the pulmonary response: Is there really a separate genetic control for lung AHH levels? Do genetically regulated differences in AHH inducibility exist in pulmonary tissue of inbred mice? What is the effect of other exogenous chemicals (e.g., tobacco-related products) on lung AHH? Do these enzymatic responses play a role in the susceptibility of mice to chemically induced lung cancers? In this report, we attempt to answer some of the questions concerning the pulmonary response.

B. Materials

The polycyclic hydrocarbons benzo(a)pyrene (BaP) and 3-methylcholanthrene (MCA) were purchased (Sigma Chemicals, St. Louis, Missouri) and purified by recrystallization from benzene. 7,8-benzoflavone was purchased from Aldrich Chemicals (Cedar Knolls, New Jersey). Sources of mice were Cumberland View Farms (Clinton, Tennessee), the Jackson Laboratory (Bar Harbor, Maine), or Microbiological Associates (Bethesda, Maryland). For intratracheal (IT) instillations, a Bausch and Lomb stereomicroscope, equipped with fiber optic illumination, and Hamilton syringes with 22 gauge by 38 mm (with 1.5 mm feeder balls) needles were used. Fractions of cigarette smoke condensate from 1A1 cigarettes were provided by Dr. A.R. PATEL (Meloy Laboratories, Springfield, Virginia)(PATEL et al., 1974). Fractionation into acidic, basic, and neutral fractions was performed according to the procedures of SWAIN et al. (1969). Only 3 fractions have been analyzed as to chemical content: the B_E fraction contains 310 mg nicotine per g fraction, the WA_E fraction contains 41.9 mg phenols per g fraction, and the N_{NM} fraction contains 13.2 µg BP per g fraction (PATEL et al., 1974). Walton-type horizontal smoking machines were obtained from Process and Instruments (Brooklyn, New York), cigarettes were either the 1A1 or 1R1 type (University of Kentucky, Lexington). Enzyme determinations were made

---

** The term "inducibility", as used in this paper, denotes a relative increase in rates of de novo synthesis or of activation of enzyme activity from preexisting moieties, or in rate of both when compared to rate of breakdown. No particular mechanism is implied.

using an Aminco-Bowman spectrophotofluorometer (American Instrument Company, Silver Spring, Maryland).

C. Methods

Care and feeding of mice were as previously published (WHITMIRE et al., 1971). Animals were always treated between the hours of 9:00 am and 10:00 am to avoid diurnal variations. The intratracheal instillation technique was similar to that described recently by HO and FURST (1973). Solutions consisted of MCA suspended in 0.2% gelatin in sterile saline or the various cigarette smoke condensate fractions dissolved in corn oil. Condensate fractions were used at an arbitrary level that killed 10% of the mice in 14 days (LD_{10-14}). 0.02 ml of solution was instilled. At various times post-treatment, lungs and livers were excized and frozen at $-70^{o}C$ until assayed.

Microsomes were prepared from liver tissues of mice pretreated with MCA according to the methods of KUPFER and LEVIN (1972) and were stored at $-70^{o}C$ for up to 72 hours before being assayed. Calcium-aggregated and "normal" centrifugally prepared microsomes were used with similar results. Samples were diluted with 0.1M tris-HCl buffer (pH 7.4) to a final ratio of 1.0 ml microsome suspension per wet weight tissue.

The assay for AHH was basically that of NEBERT and GELBOIN (1969), as modified by NEBERT and GIELEN (1972) and THOMAS et al. (1.972). A unit of AHH activity is that amount of enzyme causing the fluorescent equivalent of 1.0nMole 3-OHBP per min at $37^{o}C$. For hepatic and pulmonary tissues, activity is given in terms of units/g wet weight tissue, and for microsome preparations in terms of units/mg protein.

Inhibition of BaP metabolism *in vitro* was done according to the procedures of GOUJON et al. (1972) and WIEBEL et al. (1971). Concentrations of the various condensate fractions were made in dimethylsulfoxide (DMSO); included was the known competitive inhibitor of "induced" AHH activity, 7,8-benzoflavone (WIEBEL et al., 1971). 200 µg, 20 µg, and 2 µg of the fractions were added to the complete reaction mixture (minus BaP), incubated with shaking for 1.0 min, and then BaP (20 µg) was added and incubation continued for 20 min.

Mice were exposed to 1, 2, or 3 cigarettes simultaneously (10%, 20%, or 30% smoke) and were also exposed to the smoke of 1 cigarette (10% smoke) for 1.0 hour (about 7 cigarettes). This latter exposure regimen consisted of exposing mice to 1 cigarette followed by a 10 min rest period followed by 1 cigarette, until a total of 7 cigarettes were smoked. In some cases, mice were exposed to cigarette smoke for at least 60 days at 8 cigarettes per day (4 consecutive cigarettes in morning and 4 in afternoon). At various times after exposure, mice were killed by cervical dislocation and the lungs and livers were removed and stored at $-70^{o}C$ until assayed. Control animals consisted of either untreated, sham-smoked, or gas-phase (Cambridge-filtered smoke) treated animals. Mice were exposed in 1 min cycles consisting of a 2 sec puff, 15 sec holding time, and 43 sec purge. In certain experiments, holding time was increased to 28 sec and purge time was 30 sec.

D. Results

I. Pulmonary and Hepatic AHH Responses to IT Instilled MCA

The pulmonary and hepatic AHH levels 24 hours after IT administration
of various dose of MCA into C57BL/6Cum (B6) DBA/2Cum (D2) and B6D2Fl
mice are shown in Table 1. At doses greater than 200 µg, the AHH responses of pulmonary tissues from B6 and B6D2Fl lungs were maximally
induced (about 7 fold) while hepatic tissues were only minimally
effected. The D2 strain was generally much less responsive: pulmonary
tissue was only minimally induced at a dose of 500 µg and hepatic
tissue was never induced, regardless of MCA dose. Kinetics of induction of pulmonary AHH in these 3 strains following IT treatment with
200 µg MCA are shown in Fig. 1. Maximum induction in the B6 and B6D2Fl
strains occurred by 24 hours and remained constant for at least 96 hours.
The D2 strain was observed to respond slowly to MCA and maximal induction occurred 48 hours posttreatment. The maximum observed increase
(inducibility) for the B6 or B6D2Fl strains was about 10 and for the
D2 strain about 6.

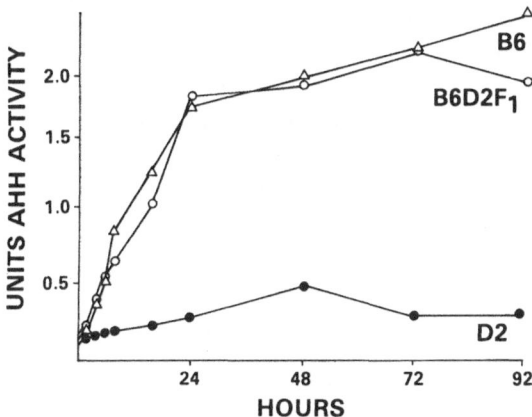

Fig. 1

Responses of 8 other inbred strains to 200 µg MCA given IT are shown
in Table 2. Pulmonary tissues of BALB/cMai C3H/fMai, C57L/J, and
C57BL/6J were observed to be highly induced by 200 µg MCA (4 to 8
fold), while lung tissue from strains AKR/J, SJL/J, DBA/2J, and RF/J
showed no such increase. Hepatic responses were low for all strains
except perhaps for the C57BL/6J and C57L/J, which did express a 1-fold
increase..

II. Genetic Regulation of Pulmonary AHH Induction

The effect of MCA on pulmonary tissue from crosses involving the B6
and D2 strains is shown in Table 3. Animals were classified as inducible or noninducible if, after IT treatment with 200 µg MCA, pulmonary AHH levels were 2.5 ($\pm$ 0.3) units/g tissue (inducible) or 0.3
($\pm$ 0.05) units/g tissue (noninducible). Among 47 backcross animals

Table 1. Effects of intratracheal instillation of various doses of MCA in a 0.2% gelatin solution on pulmonary and hepatic AHH[a] levels

STRAIN AND TISSUE	UNTREATED	GEL	MCA 10 µg	MCA 50 µg	MCA 200 µg	MCA 500 µg
C57BL/6Cum						
LUNG	0.40	0.32	0.89 (2.8)[b]	1.4 (4.4)	2.4 (7.5)	2.4 (7.5)
LIVER	17.50	14.50	13.30 (0.9)	14.51 (1.0)	32.3 (2.2)	33.2 (2.3)
DBA/2Cum						
LUNG	0.30	0.18	––	0.20 (1.1)	0.34 (1.9)	0.56 (3.1)
LIVER	9.80	9.50	––	9.80 (1.0)	10.10 (1.1)	10.20 (1.1)
B6D2F1Cum						
LUNG	0.36	0.26	0.76 (2.9)	1.3 (5.0)	2.0 (7.7)	2.5 (9.6)
LIVER	12.60	10.00	10.30 (1.0)	14.4 (1.4)	18.9 (1.9)	26.5 (2.7)

[a] AHH ACTIVITY GIVEN IN TERMS OF UNITS PER g WET WEIGHT TISSUE. A UNIT IS THAT AMOUNT OF ENZYME CAUSING THE FORMATION OF THE FLUORESCENT EQUIVALENT OF 1.0 nmole 3-OH-BP PER MINUTE AT 37ºC

[b] THE INDUCIBILITY (A RELATIVE INCREASE OF AHH OF TREATED TISSUE COMPARED TO CONTROL TISSUE) IS GIVEN PARENTHETICALLY

Table 2. Effects of intratracheal instillation of 200 µg MCA in 0.2% gelatin on pulmonary and hepatic AHH[a] in various strains of mice

STRAIN	LUNG AHH CONTROL	LUNG AHH MCA	LUNG AHH IND.[b]	LIVER AHH CONTROL	LIVER AHH MCA	LIVER AHH IND.
Balb/cMai	0.71	3.1	4.4	19.2	22.2	1.2
C3H/fMai	0.33	2.5	7.7	7.9	7.3	0.93
C57L/J	0.64	3.4	5.3	13.3	27.4	2.1
C57BL/6J	0.28	2.4	8.0	16.1	32.6	2.0
AKR/J	0.28	0.45	1.6	17.5	15.6	0.89
SJL/J	0.19	0.29	1.5	10.8	11.7	1.1
DBA/2J	0.26	0.36	1.4	8.9	8.5	0.95
RF/J	0.41	0.54	1.3	13.5	13.8	1.0

[a] AHH ACTIVITY GIVEN IN TERMS OF UNITS PER g WET WEIGHT TISSUES. A UNIT IS THAT AMOUNT OF ENZYME CAUSING THE FORMATION OF THE FLUORESCENT EQUIVALENT OF 1.0 nmole OF 3-OH-BP PER MINUTE AT 37ºC

[b] IND. = INDUCIBILITY; RELATIVE INCREASE OF AHH OF TREATED TISSUE COMPARED TO CONTROL TISSUE

tested, 24 were inducible (51%), and among 42-F2 animals tested, 29 were inducible (69%). These numbers were not statistically different from the 50% and 75% ratios that would be expected if a single auto-somal dominant gene were regulating this inducibility.

Table 3. Genetic regulation of pulmonary AHH in crosses involving the C57BL/6Cum and DBA/2Cum strains of mice[a]

STRAIN	NUMBER OF MICE TREATED	NUMBER OF MICE INDUCIBLE	%
B6	50	50	100
D2	50	0	0
B6D2F1	50	50	100
B6D2F1 x D2	47	24	51
B6D2F2	42	29	69

[a]MICE WERE TREATED WITH 200 μg MCA/.02 ml-0.2% GELATIN SOLUTION
INTRATRACHEALLY, AND 24 HOURS LATER, THE PULMONARY AHH WAS
ASSAYED. A MOUSE WAS CONSIDERED INDUCIBLE IF, AFTER MCA TREAT-
MENT, PULMONARY AHH WAS 2.5 (± 0.3) UNITS/g TISSUE AND CONSIDERED
NONINDUCIBLE IF PULMONARY AHH WAS 0.30 (± 0.05) UNITS/g TISSUE.
THE SEX OF THE PROGENY PLAYED NO ROLE IN THIS SEGREGATION
PATTERN

III. Effect of Tobacco Related Products on Pulmonary AHH Levels

1. Effect of Cigarette Smoke. The pulmonary AHH response of B6 mice
exposed to the smoke of one-1A1 cigarette (10% smoke) is shown in
Table 4. The lung tissue responded rapidly and selectively to the
whole smoke. Peak activity occurred approximately 6 hours posttreatment and remained induced for 24 hours. The intervention of a Cambridge-
type filter completely abrogated this induction profile. The use of
2 or 3 cigarettes smoked simultaneously (20% or 30% smoke) gave induction results similar to the use of 1 cigarette (data not shown). Exposure to 1 cigarette-at-a-time for a total of 7 cigarettes (with a
10 min rest between cigarettes) induced pulmonary AHH activity in B6
and C3H/fMai mice, but had only a small effect on D2 mice (Table 5).
This smoking schedule resulted in maximal exposure with minimal death
if nonpretreated animals were used. Using this schedule, the maximal
induction was similar to that induced by 1 cigarette (Table 4): about
2.5 fold in 6 hours. Similar results were also noted using the 1R1
cigarette, i.e., maximal induction occurred within 6 hours after exposure and induction was about 2.5 times that of the sham control or
gas-phase treated animals. Similar results were also noted if the
holding time was increased from 15 to 28 sec. The 28 sec holding time
should allow for maximum deposition of particulate material onto lung
tissue (STOCKLEY, Oak Ridge National Laboratory, personal communication,
1974).

Mice could be adapted to higher smoke exposures by pretreatment with
only 1 or 2 cigarettes per day for 1 week. By slowly increasing the
number of cigarettes (given 1-at-a-time) per day, at 1 month, both
D2 and C3H/fMai mice would accept 16 cigarettes per day, 8 consecutive
cigarettes in the morning and 8 consecutive in the afternoon. Although
slightly more toxic initially, mice would still accept 16-1R1 cigarettes per day using this same schedule. The AHH responses of various
tissues of these 2 strains after exposure to 8 cigarettes per day
(4 in the morning and 4 in the afternoon) for at least 60 days are
demonstrated in Table 6. The chronic high level of smoke seemed to
induce only pulmonary tissue; liver, kidney, and small intestinal
tissue was unaffected. The data with the intestines was difficult to
assess because of the wide mouse-to-mouse variations observed (>200%).
Pulmonary tissue from C3H/fMai mice was induced for the whole 18 hours
observation period, while the induction of D2 lung tissue seemed to

54

Table 4. Effect of exposure to one 1A1 cigarette (10% smoke) on pulmonary AHH levels of C57BL/6Cum mice[a]

| HR. AFTER SMOKE | AHH ACTIVITY (UNITS[b]/g TISSUE) | | |
	WITH FILTER	WITHOUT FILTER	INDUCIBILITY
1.5	0.25	0.24	1.0
3.5	0.21	0.43	1.8
6.5	0.31	0.86	3.6
9.0	0.25	0.53	2.2
12.0	0.25	0.58	2.4
27.0	0.27	0.55	2.3
50.0	0.27	0.38	1.6
74.0	0.27	0.38	1.6
CONTROL	0.24	0.24	

[a]MICE WERE EXPOSED IN A WALTON-TYPE HORIZONTAL SMOKING MACHINE ACCORDING TO THE FOLLOWING 1 MIN CYCLE: 2 SEC PUFF, 15 SEC HOLDING TIME AND 45 SEC PURGE

[b]UNIT IS THAT AMOUNT OF ENZYME CAUSING THE FLUORESCENT EQUIVALENT OF 1 nmole 3-OH-BP/min AT 37°C

Table 5. Effect of 7 consecutive cigarettes[a] on pulmonary AHH activity in various strains of mice

| STRAIN | CONTROL | HOURS[b] POST TREATMENT | | | |
| | | 6 | | 24 | |
		SMOKED	INDUCIBILITY	SMOKED	INDUCIBILITY
C57BL/6Cum	0.20[c]	0.50	2.5	0.45	2.3
DBA/2J	0.25	0.34	1.4	0.32	1.4
C3H/fMai	0.34	0.88	2.6	0.65	1.9

[a]ANIMALS WERE EXPOSED TO CIGARETTE SMOKE USING THE REGIMEN OF ONE CIGARETTE FOLLOWED BY A 10 MIN REST PERIOD FOLLOWED BY ONE CIGARETTE, UNTIL A TOTAL OF SEVEN CIGARETTES WERE SMOKED

[b]HOURS AFTER EXPOSURE TO LAST OF SEVEN (7) 1A1 CIGARETTES

[c]DATA GIVEN IN TERMS OF UNITS AHH ACTIVITY PER g TISSUE. A UNIT IS THAT AMOUNT OF ENZYME CAUSING THE FORMATION OF THE FLUORESCENT EQUIVALENT OF 1 nmole 3-OH-BP PER MIN AT 37°C

have a shorter lifetime and was at background level by 18 hours post-treatment. Responses to the 1R1 cigarettes was similar to that observed for the 1A1 cigarettes.

2. Effect of Cigarette Smoke Condensate Fractions. Fractions of 1A1 cigarette smoke condensate were observed to induce and to inhibit the pulmonary AHH activity of B6 mice 24 hours after IT instillation (Table 7). Fractions B_Ia, B_Ib, N_{MEOH}, and N_{NM} were considered good inducers. The starting material, reconstituted material, B_E, WA_E, WA_I, and N_{CH} were considered weak inducers. Fractions B_W, SA_I, SA_E, and SA_W were actually weak inhibitors of pulmonary AHH activity.

Particular fractions also seemed to have the capability of inhibiting BaP metabolism *in vitro* (Table 8). Data is presented by computing the

Table 6. Effect of smoking[a] on AHH responses of various tissues of 2 inbred strains of mice

| | | HOURS POST TREATMENT | | | | | | | | |
| | | 3 | | | 6 | | | 18 | | |
STRAIN	TISSUE	CONTROL	SMOKED	IND.[b]	CONTROL	SMOKED	IND.[b]	CONTROL	SMOKED	IND.[b]
C3H	LUNG	0.34	1.01	3.1	0.48	0.95	2.0	0.23	0.51	2.2
	LIVER	9.90	10.31	1.1	8.00	9.40	1.2	11.00	13.70	1.2
	KIDNEY	0.06	0.06	1.0	0.07	0.06	0.9	0.06	0.07	1.1
	INTESTINE	1.10	0.63	0.6	0.28	0.30	1.1	0.25	0.35	1.4
D2	LUNG	0.36	0.82	2.3	0.35	1.00	2.9	0.30	0.30	1.0
	LIVER	8.00	10.50	1.3	10.90	9.50	0.9	13.50	14.00	1.0
	KIDNEY	0.08	0.07	0.9	0.06	0.06	1.0	0.07	0.07	1.0
	INTESTINE	0.28	0.99	3.5	0.07	0.08	1.1	0.09	0.07	0.8

[a]ANIMALS WERE PRESMOKED FOR AT LEAST 60 DAYS BY EXPOSURE TO FOUR (4) CONSECUTIVE CIGARETTES GIVEN IN THE MORNING AND FOUR (4) CONSECUTIVE CIGARETTES GIVEN IN THE AFTERNOON. INDICATED TIMES ARE HOURS AFTER EXPOSURE TO LAST OF THE 4 CONSECUTIVE CIGARETTES. CONTROL ANIMALS WERE UNTREATED

[b]IND. = INDUCIBILITY

Table 7. Effect of fractions of the 1A1 cigarette-smoke-condensate on pulmonary AHH activity of C57BL/6Cum mice[a]

FRACTION NO.[b]	FRACTION	µg	UNITS/g TISSUE[c]	INDUCIBILITY
1	STARTING MATERIAL	2000	.22	1.7
2	RECONSTITUTED	500	.24	1.8
3	$B_I a$	1000	.47	3.6
4	$B_I b$	1000	.32	2.5
5	B_E	50	.19	1.5
6	B_W	500	.07	0.5
7	WA_I	1000	.21	1.6
8	WA_E	500	.24	1.1
9	SA_I	500	.07	0.5
10	SA_E	500	.04	0.3
11	SA_W	2000	.05	0.4
12	N_{MEOH}	2000	.32	2.5
13	N_{CH}	500	.15	1.2
14	N_{NM}	500	.43	3.3
CONTROL	CORN OIL	—	.13	1.0

[a]24 HOURS AFTER IT INSTILLATION OF FRACTION, OR CORN OIL VEHICLE

[b]ARRANGED ACCORDING TO SWAIN et al (1969)

[c]A UNIT OF AHH ACTIVITY IS THAT AMOUNT OF ENZYME CAUSING THE FLUORESCENT EQUIVALENT OF 1 nmole 3-OH-BP/min AT 37ºC

Table 8. *In vitro* effect of cigarette smoke condensate fractions on BaP metabolism in hepatic microsomes[a] from MCA treated B6 mice

FRACTION		[X]/[BaP] TO GIVE 50% INHIBITION[b]
1	STARTING MATERIAL	5.0
2	RECONSTITUTED	5.2
3	$B_I a$	0.8
4	$B_I b$	0.5
5	B_E	3.0
6	B_W	>10.
7	WA_I	5.0
8	WA_E	2.0
9	SA_I	>10.
10	SA_E	>10.
11	SA_W	>10.
12	N_{MEOH}	3.0
13	N_{CH}	ND
14	N_{NM}	1.0
—	7, 8-BENZOFLAVONE	1.0

[a]SOURCE OF MICROSOMES WAS HEPATIC TISSUE FROM MICE PRETREATED 24 HOURS PREVIOUS TO SACRIFICED WITH 80 µg MCA/g BODY WEIGHT GIVEN INTRAPERITONEALLY. SPECIFIC ACTIVITY OF MICROSOMES WAS 0.595 units/mg PROTEIN AND DMSO TREATED CONTROL MICROSOMES WAS 0.583 units/mg PROTEIN

[b]200, 20 and 2 µg OF THE VARIOUS FRACTIONS WERE ADDED TO THE COMPLETE REACTION MIXTURE (EXCEPT BaP), INCUBATED WITH SHAKING AT 37ºC FOR 1.0 MIN., AND THEN BaP (20 µg) WAS ADDED AND INCUBATION CONTINUED FOR 20 MIN. DATA GIVEN IN TERMS OF CONCENTRATION OF BaP REQUIRED TO INHIBIT THE FORMATION OF 3-OH-BP BY 50%

concentration of the material over the concentration of BaP necessary to inhibit enzyme activity by 50% (GOUJON et al., 1973). Using a microsomal preparation from MCA-induced livers, fractions B_Ib, B_Ia, and N_{NM} inhibited BaP metabolism at least as effectively as the known competitive inhibitor of induced AHH, 7,8-benzoflavone. The starting material, reconstituted material, B_E, WA_I, WA_E, N_{MEOH}, and N_{CH} fractions were weak inhibitors, while the B_W, SA_I, SA_E, and SA_W fractions had no effect on BaP metabolism.

E. Discussion

There are major strain-to-strain variations in the AHH levels of inbred strains of mice (THOMAS et al., 1972). Similar variations in AHH activity (or inducibility) also exist in the human system (KELLERMANN et al., 1973a). These variations are under host genetic control in both mice and man, segregating as either a dominant, codominant, or recessive gene in mice, depending on strains employed (ROBINSON et al., 1974), and a single codominant gene in man (KELLERMANN et al., 1973b). Recent information suggests that sensitivity or susceptibility to chemically induced cancers is correlated with the AHH responsiveness of that individual. Individual mice or strains of mice which are AHH inducible are much more sensitive to MCA induced tumors than their noninducible counterparts (KOURI et al., 1973a, 1973b, 1974a); and, in man, individuals with high AHH inducibilities seem much more sensitive to cigarette smoke associated bronchogenic squamous cell carcinomas (KELLERMANN et al., 1973c). In the mouse, hepatic tissue has been used to determine the AHH inducibility of individuals. A valid question would be, does the liver activate (or inactivate) carcinogens for other tissues, or can other organs determine their own sensitivity to chemical carcinogens? Results presented here suggest that at least one other organ, the lung, can be a major determinant in its own ultimate susceptibility to chemically induced cancers.

Using the intratracheal route (to limit the enzymatic response to pulmonary tissue alone) and the B6 and D2 inbred strains of mice whose hepatic AHH responses have been extensively studied, we show in this report: 1. MCA given in a 0.2% gelatin solution induces pulmonary AHH, and this induction is dose dependent; 2. a dose of 200 μg MCA maximally induces pulmonary AHH, but has very limited effect on hepatic AHH levels; 3. pulmonary AHH can be induced in D2 mice by IT administration of MCA, but hepatic AHH levels are never induced; 4. although pulmonary AHH is induced in D2 mice, the levels are very low, with about a 5 fold difference between D2 and B6 pulmonary tissues; and 5. this strain difference is under the same genetic control as that of hepatic tissue, e.g., the highly responsive B6 strain differs from the D2 strain by a single autosomal dominant gene controlling this heightened responsiveness. Results with other inbred strains of mice agree with this contention: strains that are nonresponsive to MCA in their hepatic tissues (THOMAS et al., 1972) are low responders in their lung tissue to IT instilled MCA and vice versa.

These results may seem inconsistent in that the pulmonary tissue of both B6 and D2 mice are induced by IT administration of MCA, agreeing with the results of WIEBEL et al. (1973) and BURKI et al. (1973), yet there seem to be basic differences between these 2 "induction" processes because the responses can be discriminated genetically (Table 3). Recent results from our laboratory (KOURI et al., 1974b) suggest that there is, in fact, a difference between the "induction" of pulmonary tissues of the B6 and D2 strains. Use of the competitive

inhibitor of induced AHH, 7,8-benzoflavone, and direct quantification
of the CO-binding cytochromes from B6 and D2 lung tissue demonstrate
that real differences exist between the enzymes in MCA treated B6 and
D2 pulmonary tissue. Available data are consistent with the hypothesis
that MCA treatment of B6 lung tissue induces the genetically mediated
AHH enzyme system associated with the P-448 cytochrome (SLADEK and
MANNERING, 1966), and treatment of D2 lung tissue causes the nonspecific proliferation of enzymes that are very similar to the constitutive,
or P-450 mediated (GILLETTE et al., 1972), enzymes. Thus, pulmonary
AHH is similar, yet different, from hepatic AHH. Similar, in that AHH
inducibility seems to be genetically regulated by the same locus, yet
different, because there seems to be an organ specific response to
MCA in even "noninducible" animals. This response may represent an
adaptive response to the environment, since the lungs are constantly
exposed to air and dust particles containing polycyclic aromatic hydrocarbons, insecticides, and other aromatic chemicals. This interpretation is in accord with the fact that skin is also slightly inducible
in noninducible animals (WIEBEL et al., 1973).

These same strains of mice also respond by increased levels of pulmonary AHH to either whole cigarette smoke (Tables 4, 5, and 6) or
particular fractions of condensates derived from this smoke (Table 7).
Data are consistent with the observations of WELCH et al. (1971) and
MARCOTTE and WITSCHI (1972), who showed that pulmonary AHH can be induced in rats exposed to regular or marijuana cigarettes. The lung
seems to possess definite saturation levels for induction via cigarette smoke, for, regardless of schedule, only a 2 to 3 fold induction is observed. Exposure to 1, 2, or 3 cigarettes consecutively,
or preexposure for up to 60 days with 8 cigarettes per day, yields
quantitatively similar results. The AHH inducible C3H/fMai and B6
strains seem more responsive than the nonresponsive D2 strain (Table 5).
However, after chronic exposure, both the C3H/fMai and D2 pulmonary
tissues were induced (Table 6). Chronic exposure does not induce AHH
levels in the liver, kidney, or intestines. Whether the pulmonary
response of chronically smoked D2 mice represents true "induction"
(e.g., utilizing the P-448 cytochrome) is presently being evaluated.

Results with the cigarette smoke condensate fractions (Table 7) demonstrate that the components of cigarette smoke that induce (or inhibit) pulmonary AHH can be discriminated. The relatively low inducing potential of whole cigarette smoke may reflect the presence of
these inducing and inhibiting components. The BaP containing fraction,
N_{NM}, is observed to be an effective inducer of pulmonary AHH and also
an effective inhibitor of BaP metabolism in $vitro$. The chemical content of the potent $B_I a$ and $B_I b$ fractions is currently being determined. The phenol- or nicotine-containing fractions (WA_E and B_E) are
observed to have little effect on AHH. The severe toxicity observed
with the B_E fraction, however, may conceal any interaction between
nicotine and AHH. Data in Table 8 nicely corroborate these IT results. Using a partially purified microsomal preparation of hepatic
AHH, it was observed that certain fractions (e.g., $B_I a$, $B_I b$, and
N_{NM}) are at least as inhibitory of BaP metabolism as 7,8-benzoflavone.
Thus, there seems to be a correlation between ability to induce pulmonary AHH and ability to inhibit BaP metabolism in $vitro$. The most
likely explanation is that these fractions contain compounds struc-
turally similar to BaP; thus, they are capable of both inducing AHH
and inhibiting BaP metabolism (competitively?) in $vitro$. The use of
IT instillation of chemicals concomitant with tests for inhibition of
BaP metabolism in $vitro$ seems to produce rapid and reproducible tests
for the detection of compounds that can potentially serve as inducers
or substrates for the AHH system. Moreover, preliminary results from

the laboratory of AMES (U. of California, Berkeley) using these same
smoke condensate fractions suggest that certain of these fractions
(especially, B_Ia, B_Ib, WA_I, and neutral fractions) contain potent
mutagenic activity (KIER et al., submitted, 1974). The relative car-
cinogenecity, and cocarcinogenecity, of these fractions are presently
being tested both *in vivo* and *in vitro*.

Published results and preliminary results from our laboratory indicate
pulmonary AHH may play a major role in lung cancer susceptibility.
NETTESHEIM and HAMMONS (1971) reported conditions for induction of
squamous cell carcinoma in inbred strains of mice. These authors
utilized the (C57BL X C3H/f) F_1 and the DBA/2 strains of mice and
500 μg MCA (in 0.2% gelatin) given at weekly intervals for 4 to 6
weeks. The AHH inducible F_1 strain (KOURI, unpublished observation)
was observed to be much more sensitive to MCA induced squamous cell
carcinomas than the AHH "noninducible" DBA/2 strain. Very preliminary
results from our laboratory involving IT administration of MCA into
parent, F_1, backcross, and F2 animals (involving the B6 and D2 strains)
indicate that AHH inducible mice seem to be more susceptible to MCA
induced squamous cell carcinoma. Both results are compatible with the
idea that the increased susceptibility to chemically induced carcinomas
of AHH inducible animals reflects this heightened ability to metabolize chemical carcinogens.

F. Summary

The effects of exogenous factors on lung tissue of inbred strains of
mice seem to be largely determined by the enzymatic activity of lung
tissue itself. The major enzymatic activity studied in this paper was
the inducible enzyme complex, AHH. It was shown that conditions could
be developed so that pulmonary AHH levels were singularly effected.
IT instillation of MCA (≤200 μg), exposure to whole cigarette smoke,
and IT instillation of fractions of cigarette smoke condensate were
shown preferentially to induce pulmonary AHH activity, and, in the
case of MCA, this response was under host genetic control, segregating as a single autosomal dominant gene in crosses involving the B6
and D2 strains of mice. The small increase in D2 lung tissue following MCA treatment was attributed to nonspecific proliferation of
enzymes similar to constitutive AHH, rather than a specific increase
of the new P-448-mediated enzymes.

Exposure to whole cigarette smoke from either the 1A1 or 1R1 cigarette,
using various exposure schedules, resulted in quantitatively similar
increases in pulmonary AHH activity. Pretreatment for 60 days with
8 cigarettes per day did not increase this AHH response. Interposition
of a Cambridge filter abrogated this enzyme response. Particular fractions derived from the smoke condensate of the 1A1 cigarette were observed preferentially to induce pulmonary AHH in B6 mice. These same
fractions (e.g., B_Ia, B_Ib, N_{NM}) also were shown to inhibit BaP metabolism *in vitro*.

Results were discussed in view of the possibility that these enzymatic
responses play a major role in the susceptibility of lung tissue to
chemically induced cancers.

60

G. Acknowledgement

The authors thank Mr. THOMAS RUDE for his excellent technical assistance. This work was supported by contracts from The Council for Tobacco Research.

References

BURKI, K., LIEBELT, A.G., BRESNICK, E.: Induction of aryl hydrocarbon hydroxylase in mouse tissues from a high and low cancer strain and their F_1 hybrids. J. nat. Cancer Inst. 50, 369-380 (1973).

CONNEY, A.H.: Pharmacological implications of microsomal enzyme induction. Pharmacol. Rev. 19, 307-366 (1967).

GILLETTE, J.R., DAVIS, D.C., SASAME, H.A.: Cytochrome P-450 and its role in drug metabolism. Ann. Rev. Pharmacol. 12, 57-84 (1972).

GOUJON, F.M., NEBERT, D.W., GIELEN, J.E.: Genetic expression of aryl hydrocarbon hydroxylase induction IV. Interaction of various compounds with different forms of cytochrome P-450 and the effect on benzo(a)pyrene metabolism *in vitro*. Mol. Pharmacol. 8, 667-680 (1972).

HO, W., FURST, A.: Intratracheal instillation method for mouse lungs. Oncology 27, 385-393 (1973).

KELLERMANN, G., CANTRELL, E., SHAW, C.: Variations in extent of aryl hydrocarbon hydroxylase induction in cultured human lymphocytes. Cancer Res. 33, 1654-1656 (1973a).

KELLERMANN, G., LUYTEN-KELLERMANN, M., SHAW, C.R.: Genetic variation in human lymphocytes. Amer. J. hum. Genet. 25, 327-331 (1973b).

KELLERMANN, G., SHAW, C.R., LUYTEN-KELLERMANN, M.: Aryl hydroxylase inducibility and bronchogenic carcinoma. New Engl. J. Med. 289, 934-936 (1973c).

KIER, L., YAMASAKI, E., AMES, B.: Detection of mutagenic activity in cigarette smoke condensates. (In press) 1974.

KOURI, R.E., SALERNO, R.A., WHITMIRE, C.E.: Relationship between aryl hydrocarbon hydroxylase inducibility and sensitivity to chemically induced subcutaneous sarcomas in various strains of mice. J. nat. Cancer Inst. 50, 363-368 (1973a).

KOURI, R.E., RATRIE, H., WHITMIRE, C.E.: Evidence of a genetic relationship between subcutaneous tumors and 3-methylcholanthrene-induced subcutaneous tumors and inducibility of aryl hydrocarbon hydroxylase. J. nat. Cancer Inst. 51, 197-200 (1973b).

KOURI, R.E., RATRIE, H., WHITMIRE, C.E.: Genetic control of susceptibility of 3-methylcholanthrene-induced subcutaneous sarcomas. Int. J. Cancer 13, 714-720 (1974a).

KOURI, R.E., RUDE, T.H., THOMAS, P.E., WHITMIRE, C.E.: Studies on pulmonary aryl hydrocarbon hydroxylase in inbred strains of mice. (In press) 1974b.

KUPFER, D., LEVIN, E.: Monooxygenase drug metabolizing activity in $CaCl_2$-aggregated hepatic microsomes from rat liver. Biochem. Biophys. Res. Commun. 47, 611-618 (1972).

MARCOTTE, J., WITSCHI, H.P.: Induction of pulmonary aryl hydroxylase by marijuana. Res. Commun. Chem. Path. Pharmacol. 4, 561-568 (1972).

MASON, H.S.: Mechanisms of oxygen metabolism. Adv. Enzymol. 19, 79-233 (1957).

NEBERT, D.W., GELBOIN, H.V.: The *in vivo* and *in vitro* induction of aryl hydrocarbon hydroxylase in mammalian cells of different species, tissues, strains and development and hormone states. Arch. Biochem. Biophys. 134, 76-89 (1969).

NEBERT, D.W., GOUJON, F., GIELEN, F.E.: Aryl hydrocarbon hydroxylase induction by polycyclic hydrocarbons: simple autosomal dominant trait in the mouse. Nature New Biol. 236, 107-110 (1972).

NEBERT, D.W., GIELEN, J.E.: Genetic regulation of aryl hydrocarbon hydroxylase in the mouse. Fed. Proc. 31, 1315-1325 (1972).

NETTESHEIM, P., HAMMONS, A.S.: Induction of squamous cell carcinoma of the respiratory tract of mice. J. nat. Cancer Inst. 47, 697-701 (1971).

PATEL, A.R., HAQ, M.Z., INNERARITY, C.L., INNERARITY, L.T., WEISSGRABER, K.: Fractionation studies of smoke condensate samples from Kentucky reference cigarettes. Tobacco Sci. 1974 (in press).

ROBINSON, J.R., CONSIDINE, N., NEBERT, D.W.: Genetic expression of aryl hydrocarbon hydroxylase. Evidence for the involvement of other loci. J. Biol. Chem. 1974 (in press).

SLADEK, N.E., MANNERING, G.J.: Evidence for a new P-450 hemoprotein in hepatic microsomes from methylcholanthrene treated rats. Biochem. Biophys. Res. Commun. 30, 607-612 (1966).

STOCKLEY, J.: Personal communication, 1974.

SWAIN, A.P., COOPER, J.E., STEDMAN, R.L.: Large scale fractionation of cigarette smoke condensate for chemical and biologic investigations. Cancer Res. 29, 579-583 (1969).

THOMAS, P.E., KOURI, R.E., HUTTON, J.J.: The genetics of aryl hydrocarbon hydroxylase induction in mice: A single gene difference between C57BL/6 and DBA/2J. Biochem. Genet. 6, 157-168 (1972).

WELCH, R.M., LOH, A., CONNEY, A.H.: Cigarette smoke: stimulatory effect on metabolism of 3,4-benzpyrene by enzymes in rat lung. Life Sci. 10, 215-221 (1971).

WIEBEL, F.J., LEUTZ, J.C., DIAMOND, L., GELBOIN, H.V.: Aryl hydrocarbon (benzo(a)pyrene) hydroxylase in microsomes from rat tissues: differential inhibition and stimulation by benzoflavones and organic solvents. Arch. Biochem. Biophys. 144, 78-86 (1971).

WIEBEL, F.J., LEUTZ, J.C., GELBOIN, H.V.: Aryl hydrocarbon (benzo(a)pyrene) hydroxylase: inducible in extrahepatic tissues of mouse strains not inducible in liver. Arch. Biochem. Biophys. 154, 191-194 (1973).

WHITMIRE, C.E., SALERNO, R.A., RABSTEIN, L.S., HUEBNER, R.J., TURNER, H.C.: RNA tumor-virus antigen expression in chemically induced tumors. Virus-genome-specified common antigens detected by complement fixation in mouse tumors induced by 3-methylcholanthrene. J. nat. Cancer Inst. 47, 1255-1265 (1971).

Pulmonary Carcinogenesis by Two Aryl Hydrocarbons on Three Mouse Strains

William Ho, Kristina Wilcox, and Arthur Furst

Institute of Chemical Biology, University of San Francisco, San Francisco, CA 94117, USA

ABSTRACT

A current concept that related the susceptibility to polycyclic hydrocarbon carcinogenesis to the inducible aryl hydrocarbon hydroxylase
(AHH) was tested with benzo(a)pyrene (BaP) and 3-methylcholanthrene
(3-MC) in 3 mouse strains. The carcinogens were suspended in a gelatin
solution and instilled intratracheally into the lungs of mice. The
C57BL/6J strain represented highly inducible AHH, the random - bred
NIH-Swiss/Mai represented variable induction, and the DBA/2J strain
represented low induction of AHH. The 3-MC was more carcinogenic and
toxic than BaP to the NIH-Swiss/Mai and C57BL/6J, but had a less toxic
effect on the DBA/2J mice. Papillary adenoma was the predominent neoplasm detected in all the lungs. The NIH-Swiss/Mai mice had the highest
total lung tumor incidence and the C57BL/6J the lowest. The effective
cumulative carcinogenic dose of 3-MC appeared to be 2 mg. All mice
were equally resistant to pulmonary squamous cell carcinoma induction
by both chemicals regardless of their hepatic AHH activities. The 3-MC
induced only a small percentage of this malignancy in the young adults
in the 3 strains, but produced a higher incidence in the mature C57BL/6J
mice. The results of both the carcinogenesis and the lung clearance
rates of the carcinogens in this study suggested 2 possible explana-
tions: a) in the mouse, AHH of the target tissue may be a more reliable indicator than that of the hepatic AHH of susceptibility to
polycyclic hydrocarbon carcinogenesis; b) the AHH system may play a
subordinate role to genetic, physiologic or viral contribution to
tumor formation.

A. Introduction

Polycyclic hydrocarbons containing the phenanthrene nucleus, such as
benzo(a)pyrene (BaP) and 3-methylcholanthrene (3-MC), are capable of
inducing neoplasms. Although BaP is a product of incomplete combustion
of organic matter, 3-MC has never been isolated from natural substances.
FIESER (1936) synthesized 3-MC from cholic and desoxycholic acids,
leading GREENSTEIN (1954) to postulate that it may be a byproduct of
"abnormal" bile salt metabolism.

Respiratory tract squamous cell carcinoma was reported to be induced
in hamsters (SAFFIOTTI et al., 1968) and rats (PYLEV, 1963) with BaP
and in mice (NETTESHEIM and HAMMONS, 1971) and rats (SCHREIBER et al.,
1972) with 3-MC by the intratracheal instillation method. However,
no study has been conducted comparing the effects of these chemicals
on the same animal model in parallel experiments using this inoculation technique.

We compared the carcinogenic action of BaP and 3-MC in mouse lungs, introduced by our previously described intratracheal instillation procedure (HO and FURST, 1973). The purpose was to determine whether a correlation existed between pulmonary tumor incidence, the duration the carcinogen remained in the lung, and the inducible level of hepatic aryl hydrocarbon hydroxylase complex (AHH). There was a correlation between sarcoma induction by subcutaneous injection of 3-MC and the inducibility of hepatic AHH levels in several strains of mice (KOURI et al., 1973).

The 3 mouse strains utilized, selected on the basis of their inducible levels of hepatic AHH, were C57BL/6 (highly inducible), the DBA/2 (noninducible), and random bred NIH-Swiss (variable induction). The time required by the lungs of the respective strains to eliminate the 2 test carcinogens was measured. 2 other conditions investigated in this study were: a) The dose response of C57BL/6 and DBA/2 mice to different amounts of instilled 3-MC. HO and FURST (1974) found that this chemical was more toxic and carcinogenic to NIH-Swiss mice than BaP. b) The age of the animals at the time of treatment, relative to their susceptibility to lung tumor induction.

B. Materials and Methods

I. Carcinogenesis Experiments

Female C57BL/6J, DBA/2J, and NIH-Swiss/Mai mice were quarantined for 2 weeks upon arrival and representative animals were examined for infections. Mice that deviated ±2 g from the average age related body weight for the strain were removed. The remaining animals were divided into groups as in Table 1.

The cage control animals were held for the entire experiment without treatment, while the vehicle controls were given weekly instillations of 0.025 ml 0.2% gelatin-saline solution. Carcinogen-treated mice were given the designated number of weekly instillations of either BaP (Baker Chemical Company) or 3-MC (Eastman Chemical Company), dispersed in gelatin-saline solution by homogenization in a Duall tissue grinder. The purity of the carcinogens was verified by thin layer chromatography. Each carcinogen produced only a single fluorescent spot when developed in the methanol : ethyl ether : water, 4:4:1, solvent system. The carcinogen content of the suspension was monitored periodically with an Aminco-Bowman spectrofluorometer to ensure the uniformity of the dosages. The mice were anesthetized for the instillation procedure by an intraperitoneal injection of pentobarbital equivalent to 60 mg/kg body weight. All animals were observed carefully during the treatments and throughout the 4 week post-treatment period. Except when the condition of dead mice precluded proper diagnosis, all moribund animals were killed and examined. The survivors were randomly distributed into 3 groups for postmortem examination at the third, fifth, and seventh months to analyze the response of the lungs to the carcinogens and the sequence of neoplastic development. The mice were killed with an overdose of pentobarbital (180 mg/kg body weight). Samples of all vital organs were obtained at necropsy and preserved in 10% formalin. The lungs were perfused and inflated for histologic preparation according to the method described by HO and FURST (1973, 1974).

Table 1. Experimental parameters and numbers of mice in each group

	Dosage	Mouse Strain		
Treatment	No. x Amt (mg)	C57BL/6J	DBA/2J	NIH-Swiss/Mai
3-month-old mice				
Cage control	0 x 0	60	60	50
Vehicle control	6 x 0	60	60	50
BaP[a]	6 x 0.5	75	120	125
3-MC[a]	6 x 0.5[b]	75	120	125
3-MC	4 x 0.2	45	20	-
3-MC	4 x 0.3	70	20	-
3-MC	4 x 0.4	85	20	-
3-MC	4 x 0.5	20	-	-
3-MC	4 x 1.0	40	-	-
8-month-old mice[c]				
Vehicle control	4 x 0	22	-	-
3-MC	4 x 0.5	24	-	-
Total number of mice tested		576	360	350

[a]The combined number of mice in 2 experiments.

[b]The same 3-MC dosage as used by NETTESHEIM and HAMMONS, 1971.

[c]The 3 and 8-month-old mice were selected to represent young adults and mature animals.

II. Lung Clearance Study

2 groups of 50 mice of the C57BL/6J, DBA/2J, and NIH-Swiss/Mai strains were utilized. The first group was instilled with 0.3 mg BaP and the second with 0.3 mg 3-MC. Immediately after treatment, 3 mice from each strain in both treatment groups were killed and their lungs were removed for analysis of the carcinogen content. Each set of lungs, excluding the trachea, was homogenized individually in 4.0 ml spectrophotometric grade acetone with a Duall tissue grinder. After 60 min of intermittent shaking, the mixture was centrifuged for 10 min at 500 g to separate the tissue. The supernatant was measured fluorometrically with an Aminco-Bowman spectrofluorometer set at 390 nm activating and 412 nm fluorescent wavelengths for BaP content and 350 nm activating and 400 nm fluorescent wavelengths for 3-MC. Standards were prepared by adding known quantities of the carcinogens to acetone extracts of untreated lungs. On each subsequent day, an equal number of mice were killed and their lungs were similarly assayed. A second instillation of each chemical was given to the remaining mice on the seventh day, repeating the previous procedure.

C. Results

I. Toxicity of BaP and 3-MC

The 3-MC at a dosage of 6 x 0.5 mg was found to be more toxic than BaP in all 3 mouse strains (Table 2), but each strain displayed a characteristic response. The C57BL/6J strain had more survivors than the NIH-Swiss/Mai mice when treated with either chemical. In contrast, the DBA/2J was less affected by 3-MC than the other 2 strains. The maximum tolerable dose of 3-MC for all 3 strains appeared to be 2.0 mg. Increased mortality at greater cumulative doses was observed in 6 x 0.5 mg 3-MC groups, in which most of the deaths occurred after the fifth treatment (2.5 mg). At the 1.0 mg treatment level, 50% of the C57BL/6J mice died soon after the third dose. The average percentage of survivors in the dose-response study was 77% for the C57BL/ 6J mice and 68% for the DBA/2J given the submaximum doses of 3-MC.

Table 2. Percentage of survivors in each experimental group after 10 weeks

Treatment	Dosage No. x Amt (mg)	Mouse Strain		
		C57BL/6J	DBA/2J	NIH-Swiss/Mai
3-month-old mice				
Cage control	0 x 0	100.0	100.0	100.0
Vehicle control	6 x 0	96.9	87.5	100.0
BaP	6 x 0.5	88.0	80.0	82.4
3-MC	6 x 0.5[a]	37.3	68.0	22.4
	4 x 0.2	80.0	80.0	-
	4 x 0.3	68.6	50.0	-
	4 x 0.4	80.0	75.0	-
	4 x 0.5	90.0	-	-
	4 x 1.0	45.0	-	-
8-month-old mice				
Vehicle control	4 x 0	100.0	-	-
3-MC	4 x 0.5	95.8[b]	-	-

[a]Same 3-MC dosage as used by NETTESHEIM and HAMMONS, 1971
[b]Percentage survivors at 60 days.

II. Carcinogenicity of BaP and 3-MC on Mouse Lungs

1 papillary adenoma (alveologenic carcinoma) was found among the C57BL/ 6J mice and 1 adenoma and 1 lymphoma in the DBA/2J mice given 6 x 0.5 mg BaP (Table 3, A-1, B-1). However, 67% of the NIH-Swiss/Mai mouse lungs examined at the seventh month had papillary adenomas (Table 3, C-1). Among all the BaP-treated animals, only 2 of DBA/2J mice developed pulmonary squamous cell metaplasia. There were several mild cases of interstitial pneumonitis and lymphoid hyperplasia in the cage control and vehicle control animals. The NIH-Swiss/Mai control animals had a 2% incidence of solitary papillary adenoma, which was within the normal range for old NIH-Swiss/Mai mice. Epicarditis, a condition common to DBA/2J mice, was found in both treated and untreated animals and may have been a factor in the response of the strain to the carcinogen. 6 weekly instillations of 0.5 mg 3-MC resulted in 37.5% incidence of pulmonary tumors in the C57BL/6J mice, 92% in the DBA/2J mice, and 100% in the NIH-Swiss/Mai mice at the seventh month (Table 3, A-2, B-2, C-2). The predominant tumor observed in the lungs of all 3 mouse strains was papillary adenomas. Histologic evidence indicated that the papillary adenoma may first appear as adenomatous hyperplasia. The latency period before tumor formation was about 60 days in the BaP-treated mice. Tumors in 3-MC-treated mice appeared much sooner and occurred

Table 3. Pulmonary pathology in 3 strains of female mice intra-tracheally instilled with BaP or 3-MC at 3 months of age. (Results are from 3 experiments)

Treatment	Time Exam. (Mo)	Lungs Exam.	Squa. Cell Met.	Tumor Detected						% of Total Lung Tumor
				Adenoma		Adenocarci.		Lymphoma	Squa. Cell Carci.	
				S	M	S	M			
A. C57BL/6J										
1. BaP	3	22	o	o	o	o	o	o	o	0.0
6 x 0.5 mg	5	20	o	1	o	o	o	o	o	5.0
	7	21	o	o	o	o	o	o	o	0.0
2. 3-MC	3	11	5	o	2	o	o	o	o	18.2
6 x 0.5 mg	5	9	o	o	1	o	o	o	1	22.0
	7	8	o	1	2	o	o	o	o	37.5
B. DBA/2J[a]										
1. BaP	1	10[b]	2	o	1	o	o	o	o	10.0
6 x 0.5 mg	3	18	o	o	o	o	o	o	o	0.0
	5	9	o	o	o	o	o	1	o	11.1
2. 3-MC	3	21	1	3	1	o	o	1	o	19.0
6 x 0.5 mg	5	22	2	6	8	o	o	4	2	73.7[c]
C. NIH-Swiss/Mai										
1. BaP	3	34	o	2	2	o	o	o	o	11.8
6 x 0.5 mg	5	32	o	12	3	o	o	o	o	46.9
	7	34	o	11	12	o	o	o	o	67.6
2. 3-MC	1	13[b]	13	o	o	o	o	o	1	7.7
6 x 0.5 mg	3	13	o	o	12	o	o	o	1	92.3
	5	8	o	o	8	1	2	o	o	100.0
	7	7	o	o	7	1	o	o	o	100.0

[a]Experiment in progress.

[b]Moribund mice.

[c]The percentage of total tumor incidence may not reflect the number of tumors in each group, since some lungs may bear more than 1 type of tumors.

Abbreviations: Squa. Cell Met. = squamous cell metaplasia; S = solitary; M = multiple; Adenocarci. = adenocarcinoma; Squa. Cell Carci. = squamous cell carcinoma.

more often as multiple tumors. The adenocarcinomas observed in the NIH-Swiss/Mai mouse lungs may have originated as adenomas.

2 additional types of tumor were noted in the 3-MC experimental groups that were not found in the BaP-treated lungs. Alveologenic squamous cell carcinomas were found in 2 NIH-Swiss/Mai and 2 DBA/2J mice and in 1 C57BL/6J mouse. The criteria for differentiating these tumors from severe metaplasia were pleural and vascular invasion, abundance of mitotic figures, and bizarre cell morphology (Fig. 1). This malignancy appeared as early as 1 month after the initial treatment. Many of the moribund mice examined early in the experiment had small, multi-focal pulmonary squamous cell metaplasias. Macrophages in these lungs were filled with keratinous debris. However, the lungs of survivors

examined at the third, fifth, and seventh months were devoid of such lesions. There were 4 adenocarcinomas among the NIH-Swiss/Mai mice and 4 lymphomas in the DBA/2J mice.

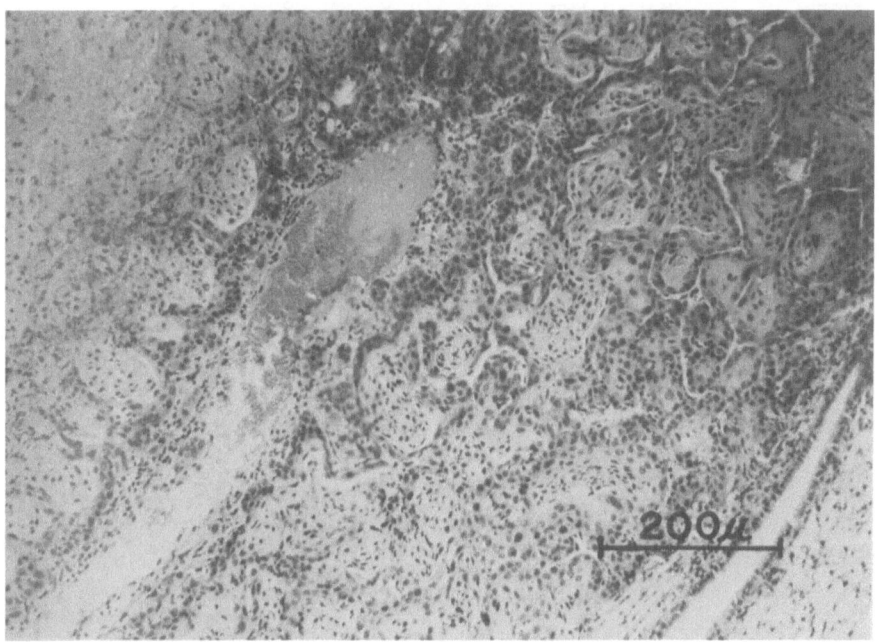

Fig. 1. Photomicrograph showing 3-MC-induced squamous cell carcinoma in C57BL/6J mouse lung. Hematoxylin and eosin stain

III. Dose Response of C57BL/6J and DBA/2J Mice to 3-MC

The majority of the tumors in the C57BL/6J mice inoculated at 3 months did not appear until the fifth month of the experiment regardless of the dosage of 3-MC (Table 4,A). Pulmonary squamous cell metaplasia occurred within a month after the initial treatment, some lesions persisting to the fifth month. Unlike the early metaplastic manifestations observed in lungs treated with 6 x 0.5 mg 3-MC, the later lesions involved large areas of the lobes and may have been precursors of carcinomas. At the 0.2, 0.4, and 1.0 mg per instillation levels, pulmonary squamous cell carcinomas constituted a small percentage of the tumors detected. The total lung tumor incidence declined when animals were given 3-MC at cumulative dose greater than 4 x 0.4 mg. Mice maintained beyond the fifth month exhibited more lung tumors, but the increase was due mainly to papillary adenoma.

The DBA/2J mice had more pulmonary tumors than the C57BL/6J mice comparably treated. Only the 4 x 0.5 mg dose level induced squamous cell carcinomas and lymphomas, in addition to papillary adenomas, by the fifth month (Table 4,C).

Table 4. Dose response of C57BL/6J and DBA/2J mice to 3-MC

Treatment	Time Exam. (Mo)	Lungs Exam.	Squa. Cell Met.	Aden-oma S	M	Adeno-carci. S	M	Lymph-oma	Squa. Cell Carci.	% of Total Lung Tumor
A. 3-month-old C57BL/6J mice										
3-MC	1	7[a]	o	o	o	o	o	o	o	0.0
4 x 0.2 mg	3	11	o	1	o	o	o	o	o	9.1
	5	12	1	o	o	o	o	o	o	0.0
	8	5	o	3	1	o	o	o	1	100.0
4 x 0.3 mg	2/3	2[a]	2	o	o	o	o	o	o	0.0
	1	6[a]	3	o	o	o	o	o	o	0.0
	3	5	o	o	o	o	o	o	o	0.0
	8	15	o	6	3	o	o	o	o	60.0
4 x 0.4 mg	1	8[a]	5	1	o	o	o	o	o	12.5
	3	23	5	o	o	o	o	o	o	0.0
	5	30	1	4	4	o	o	o	2	30.0
	8	5	o	1	3	o	o	o	o	80.0
4 x 0.5 mg	3	6	1	o	o	o	o	o	o	0.0
	5	12	1	3	o	o	o	o	o	25.0
4 x 1.0 mg	3	10	o	o	o	o	o	o	o	0.0
	5	8	o	o	o	o	o	o	1	12.5
B. 8-month-old C57BL/6J mice										
4 x 0.5 mg	2	8	4	2	1	o	o	o	o	37.5
	6	15	o	5	3	o	o	o	4	66.7
C. 3-month-old DBA/2J mice[b]										
4 x 0.2 mg	5	8	o	o	o	o	o	o	o	0.0
4 x 0.3 mg	5	4	o	2	o	o	o	o	o	50.0
4 x 0.4 mg	5	8	1	3	1	o	o	2	1	75.0

[a]Moribund mice.

[b]Experiment in progress.

IV. The Carcinogenic Effect of 3-MC on Mature C57BL/6J Mice

The mature C57BL/6J mice were instilled with the maximum tolerated limit of 3-MC (4 x 0.5 mg) established in the dose-response experiment. Because of the limited number of animals and their age at exposure, examinations were performed at the second and sixth months. The survival rate of the mature mice was 5.8% higher than that of their young counterparts given the same amount of 3-MC. The lungs of the vehicle controls had moderate interstitial pneumonitis and lymphoid hyperplasia. Of the treated mice, 37.5% had papillary adenoma by the second month. The significant finding was the increase in the incidence of pulmonary squamous cell carcinomas at the sixth month (Table 4,B), twice the level of incidence among young mice at any dose level of 3-MC.

V. Clearance Rates of BaP and 3-MC from the Lungs of C57BL/6J, DBA/2J, and NIH-Swiss/Mai Mice

Fluorometric analysis of the mouse lungs immediately after the intratracheal instillation of 0.3 mg of the carcinogens revealed that only 60% of the material reached the lobes. The rest of the inoculum may have remained in the trachea or been immediately expelled. The fraction of the dose deposited in the tracheal lumen could be evacuated intact by the ciliary movement of the respiratory tract epithelium. For this reason, the analytic technique was designed to measure only that portion of the carcinogen that was deposited into the lobes of the lungs. In all 3 mouse strains, BaP was eliminated rapidly from the lungs, less than 1% of it remaining after 96 hours; no detectable amounts were present by the sixth day. There were no measurable rate differences among the 3 strains or between the first and second BaP applications.

The 3-MC was removed from mouse lungs much more gradually than BaP. While 3% of the chemical remained in the NIH-Swiss/Mai and DBA/2J mouse lungs on the sixth day, 15% was detected in the C57BL/6J mice. The clearance rate after the second instillation remained the same for NIH-Swiss/Mai and DBA/2J strains but was accelerated for the C57BL/6J mice. No 3-MC was detectable in lungs of C57BL/6J mice on the fifth day after the second instillation.

D. Discussion

The C57BL/6J and DBA/2J mice were found to be resistant to lung tumor induction by intratracheally instilled BaP. No respiratory tract squamous cell carcinomas were noted upon histopathologic examination in any of the mouse strains after BaP treatment. These results differed from those obtained by other investigators using Syrian golden hamsters and rats, possibly because of the relatively faster rate at which mouse lungs eliminate the chemical. While the hamsters retain over 0.5% BaP in the lungs 21 days after a single treatment (SAFFIOTTI, 1970), mice of all 3 strains reduce instilled BaP to this level by the fifth day. It is uncertain from the results of this study whether the normal clearance mechanism of the mouse respiratory tract or the metabolic action of the induced AHH was more instrumental in the rapid removal process.

Many of the lungs in all 3 mouse strains treated with 3-MC (6 x 0.5 mg) developed squamous cell metaplasia early in the experiment, but only a few squamous cell carcinomas eventually developed in these experimental groups. This difference may be interpreted in 3 ways: a) The 3-MC dosage was insufficient to induce the malignancy. The dose-response experiment with C57BL/6J and DBA/2J mice indicated that a lower rather than a higher 3-MC level was the effective carcinogenic dose. b) Squamous cell metaplasia is a temporary lung tissue response to the toxic effect of 3-MC and is unrelated to malignancy development. Histologic evidence such as the removal of the keratinous debris by the macrophages and the absence of these lesions in the survivors examined at later periods supported this view. c) The animals susceptible to tumor induction by 3-MC may also be less tolerant of the carcinogen; therefore, they became moribund or died before the malignancy had an opportunity to develop. It is possible that the 3-MC induced both the squamous cell metaplasia as a transitional pulmonary tissue response and the lethal effect on the tumor-inducible mice.

The dose-response experiment with C57BL/6J mice indicated that mice given 4 x 0.4 mg to 4 x 0.5 mg of 3-MC had more papillary adenomas and squamous cell carcinomas than mice at any other dose levels. Since there was a proportional increase in the number of survivors, the relative percentage of mice with pulmonary squamous cell carcinomas remained constant. Higher levels of 3-MC resulted in the reduction of both tumor incidence and survivors. Based on the variety and the number of tumors observed plus the smaller amount of the chemical needed to induce these neoplasms, 3-MC must be considered more carcinogenic than BaP in mouse lungs. Nevertheless, all 3 mouse strains showed considerable resistance to squamous cell carcinoma induction by 3-MC.

Supporting the difference in carcinogenicity of BaP and 3-MC, 3-MC had a longer residence time than BaP in the lungs of all 3 strains of mice. The faster pulmonary clearance rate in C57BL/6J mice for the second administration of 3-MC may reflect the increased activity of AHH induced by the first instillation and may explain in part why C57BL/6J mice have the lowest lung tumor incidence found among the 3 test strains. There may be a temporal as well as a dose threshold for chemical and cellular interaction resulting in permanent morphologic changes.

The test population for each of the parameters in this study was too small to lend credence to statistical conclusions, but the data imply that hepatic AHH may not be a suitable indicator of the susceptibility of other organs to polycyclic hydrocarbon carcinogenesis. WIEBEL et al. (1973), using DBA/2 mice with noninducible hepatic AHH, found that the inducible pulmonary AHH level was two-thirds that of the highly inducible C57BL/6 strain. Additionally, the results of this study indicate that the overall pulmonary tumor incidence or the incidence of each category of neoplasms of the 3 mouse strains did not coincide with the respective hepatic AHH inducibility of each strain. Squamous cell carcinoma formation occurred infrequently, but were equally distributed among all 3 strains treated with 6 x 0.5 mg 3-MC. The susceptibility of an individual to tumor development appears to be subjected to several factors, one of which is apparently the age of the animal at the time of initial exposure to a carcinogen. Our preliminary results show that the mature C57BL/6J mice given 4 x 0.5 mg 3-MC had twice as many squamous cell carcinomas as the young adults of the same strain challenged with various amounts of the carcinogen. DIXON et al. (1970) reported that rat pulmonary AHH reaches its highest level at maturity. Similar physiologic changes in the lungs of aging mice may be responsible for the increased number of malignancies observed. The high incidence of papillary adenoma, the formation of adenocarcinomas exclusively in the NIH-Swiss/Mai, and of lymphomas in the DBA/2J strain suggest the additional possibility that chemical carcinogens may be effective only when an individual possesses an inherent tendency to a given disease state. There is a low but predictably consistent incidence of spontaneous adenomas found in the NIH-Swiss/Mai as well as lymphomas found in the DBA/2J mouse lungs in the respective "normal" populations of these strains. Thus, the inducibility of AHH in any tissue may indicate the extent to which a potentially carcinogenic polycyclic hydrocarbon can be converted to the biologically active form, but the final determinant regarding degree and type of tumor susceptibility is more likely a multidimensional matrix of physiologic, genetic, or endogenous viral factors unique to individuals.

Acknowledgements

All pathologic examinations were performed by consultant pathologist
ROBERT KOVATCH, D.V.M. The study was supported by the Council for
Tobacco Research, U.S.A., Inc.

References

DIXON, J.R., LOWE, D.B., RICHARDS, D.E., CRALLEY, L.J., STOKINGER,
H.E.: The role of trace metals in chemical carcinogenesis: Asbestos
cancers. Cancer Res. 30, 1068-1974 (1970).
FIESER, L.F.: Chemistry of natural products related to phenanthrene.
New York: Reinhold 1936.
GREENSTEIN, J.P.: Biochemistry of cancer. New York: Academic Press
1954.
HO, W., FURST, A.: Intratracheal instillation method for mouse lungs.
Oncology 27, 385-393 (1973).
HO, W., FURST, A.: Lung carcinogenesis by benzpyrene instillation.
Proc. West Pharmacol. Soc. 16, 146-149 (1973).
HO, W., FURST, A.: The effect of benzo(a)pyrene and 3-methylcholan-
threne on mouse lungs. Soc. Toxicol Ann. 13, 39 (1974).
KOURI, R.E., SALERNO, R.A., WHITMIRE, C.E.: Relationships between
aryl hydrocarbon hydroxylase inducibility and sensitivity to chemical-
ly induced subcutaneous sarcomas in various strains of mice. J. nat.
Cancer Inst. 50, 363-368 (1973).
NETTESHEIM, P., HAMMONS, A.S.: Induction of squamous cell carcinoma
in the respiratory tract of mice. J. nat. Cancer Inst. 47, 697-701
(1971).
PYLEV, L.N.: Induction of lung cancer in rats by intratracheal insufflation of cancerogenic hydrocarbons. Acta Un. int. Cancer 19,
688-691 (1963),
SAFFIOTTI, U.: Experimental respiratory tract carcinogenesis and its
relation to inhalation exposures. In: Inhalation Carcinogenesis
(M.G. Hanna, ed.), Series 18, pp. 27-51. Springfield, Va.: USAEC
1970.
SAFFIOTTI, U., CEFIS, F., KOLB, L.H.: A method for experimental induction of bronchogenic carcinoma. Cancer Res. 28, 104-124 (1968).
SCHREIBER, H., NETTESHEIM, P., MARTIN, D.H.: Rapid development of
bronchiolo-alveolar squamous cell tumors in rats after intratracheal
injection of 3-methylcholanthrene. J. nat. Cancer Inst. 49, 541-553
(1972).
WIEBEL, F.J., LEUTZ, J.C., GELBOIN, H.V.: Aryl hydrocarbon (benzo(a)
pyrene) hydroxylase: Inducible in extrahepatic tissues of mouse
strains not inducible in liver. Arch. Biochem. Biophys. 154, 292-294
(1973).

Cell-Mediated Immunity after Intratracheal Exposure to 3-Methylcholanthrene, and its Relationship to Tumor Transplant Growth in C3H/f Mai Mice

Charles F. Demoise, Richard E. Kouri, and Carrie E. Whitmire

Department of Experimental Oncology, Viral-Chemical Carcinogenesis Section, Bethesda, MD 20014, USA

ABSTRACT

Immunological deficiencies have often been observed to occur in association with cancer although the exact nature of this relationship
has not been fully characterized. The relative immunocompetence of
an individual definitely plays a major role in the ultimate susceptibility or resistance to cancer. Numerous studies support the concept
that cell-mediated immunity (CMI) is largely responsible for the body's
defense against cancer. Our laboratory is currently interested in the
levels of chemicals at which tumorigenesis occurs in various strains
of mice and whether immunocompetence of the animals is affected.

In this investigation C3H/f Mai mice were intratracheally instilled 4
times at weekly intervals with 500 µg of 3-methylcholanthrene dissolved in a corn oil vehicle. These treatments caused 8% lethality in 30
days; whereas vehicle alone is nontoxic. Effects on CMI were determined 3 days after each treatment by measuring rates of DNA synthesis
with ^{3}H-thymidine in allogeneic and spleen lymphocyte cultures. Spleen,
thymus, and lung weight as well as blood leukocyte counts were measured. Syngeneic and allogeneic tumor transplants were performed on control and test mice to determine whether CMI data is biologically relevant to the process of tumor growth. The CMI and tissue responses
were again evaluated 7, 14, and 28 days after tumor transplantation.

Preliminary data indicates that CMI, as reflected in spleen lymphocyte
responses to phytohemagglutinin, pokeweed mitogen and allogeneic antigen, was suppressed during intratracheal instillations of 3-methyl-
cholanthrene. This effect was most pronounced in response to pokeweed
mitogen and persisted at least 2 weeks after exposures were discontinued. Lymphocyte cultures from mice that received tumor transplants
indicate that the earlier CMI inhibition produced by carcinogenic exposure is not only cancelled but actually enhanced although only
syngeneic transplants were successful. Again, it will be of interest
to follow the kinetics of this effect in the host and compare it to
the rate of tumor transplant growth.

A. Introduction

The intratracheal instillation of polycyclic hydrocarbons in hamsters,
mice, and rats has served as a useful model for studies of respiratory
carcinogenesis (SAFFIOTTI et al., 1968; NETTESHEIM and HAMMONS, 1971;
SCHREIBER et al., 1972; SAFFIOTTI, 1969). Our laboratory is currently
interested in the physiological effects of some of these chemical

carcinogens, intratracheally instilled at concentrations known to induce respiratory malignancies. Evidence has accumulated during the past 15 years that clearly indicates the important role of host immunity in controlling the onset and progression of malignant diseases (MORTON, 1974). In this study as in others, we are characterizing some of the effects of chemical carcinogens on levels of host immunocompetence and their relationships to tumorigenesis.

B. Materials and Methods

I. Animals

Male C3H/f Mai mice 8 weeks old (Microbiological Associates, Walkersville, Maryland) and C57BL/6 Cum mice (Cumberland View Farms, Clinton, Tennessee) of similar age and sex were kept in disposable plastic cages containing corn cob bedding. They were given drinking water containing tetracycline (1 g/liter) and Purine Laboratory Chow ad libitum. A 12-hour lighting cycle was used.

II. Intratracheal Instillation of 3-Methylcholanthrene

C3H/f Mai mice were intratracheally instilled with 3-methylcholanthrene (MCA) according to the technique of HO and FURST (1973). Metofane (Pittman-Moore, New Jersey), an inhalation anesthetic, was used to anesthetize the mice. MCA (500 µg) was dissolved in 0.02 ml of corn oil (CO) and instilled in each of 100 test animals with a 19-gauge blunt needle attached to a Hamilton microliter syringe. A total of 4 such dosages were administered at 1 week intervals. Control mice (100) received only 0.02 ml CO.

III. Transplantation of Tumor Cells

Single-cell suspensions of syngeneic and allogeneic tumor cells from tissue cultures of a MCA induced C3H/f Mai tumor (passage 2) and a spontaneous BALB/c tumor (passage 2)(obtained from Dr. R. MADISON, Microbiological Associates) were diluted in Hanks' Balanced Salt Solution (1×10^7 cells/ml) for transplantation. Syngeneic and allogeneic tumor cells ($1 \times 10^6/0.1$ ml) were inoculated into both MCA and CO exposed mice 2 days after the fourth, and final, intratracheal instillation. These were inoculated subcutaneously over the forehead for ease of palpation and measurement of growth.

IV. Culture Media, Mitogens, and Allogeneic Antigen

The culture media used was RPMI No. 1640 from Microbiological Associates supplemented with 10% heat-inactivated fetal bovine serum, 100 U/ml of penicillin, 100 µg/ml of streptomycin and 200 mM of L-glutamine. Phytohemagglutinin-M (PHA) and pokeweed (PW) mitogens purchased from Difco (Detroit, Michigan), and Gibco (Grand Island, New York), respectively, were reconstituted in sterile-distilled water and used at a final concentration of 1% v/v in culture media. Freshly prepared single-cell suspensions of spleen cells from C57BL/6 Cum mice were exposed to 4,000 R of X-irradiation and served as a source of allogeneic antigen.

V. Spleen Lymphocyte Culture

The relative reactivities of thymus-derived (T) and bone marrow-derived (B) spleen lymphocytes were distinguished *in vitro* by their responses to mitogenic challenge with PHA and PW respectively (ANDERSSON
et al., 1972). T-cell activity was further assessed in the mixed lymphocyte culture (MLC) reaction in response to stimulation by allogeneic
antigen (C57BL/6 Cum spleen cells)(PLATE and MCKENZIE, 1973).

Single-cell suspensions of spleen lymphocytes obtained from 5 individual mice sacrificed at regular intervals after each intratracheal instillation of MCA (3 days post-exposure) and at 7, 14, and 21 days
after transplantation of tumor cells were prepared in the same manner
for all *in vitro* assays of cell-mediated immune (CMI) activity. Spleens
from MCA and CO mice were removed, their capsules opened with scissors,
and the cells teased out into chilled media. The suspension was allowed
to settle briefly to permit removal of connective tissue fragments and
large cell clumps. After 3 centrifugations (1,000 rpm for 10 min) and
rinses, the single-cell suspension of spleen lymphocytes was adjusted
to a density of 6×10^6 cells per ml of media. For mitogen stimulated
cultures, spleen lymphocytes ($6 \times 10^5/1.2$ ml) were pipetted in quadru-
plicate aliquots into wells of Falcon No. 3040 plastic microtiter
plates. PHA and PW were then added to give a final concentration of
1% v/v in each well. Media alone was used for unstimulated controls.

The assay for MLV activity was also set-up with 6×10^5 spleen lymphocytes per 0.2 ml of media per well from MCA or CO mice. Syngeneic
(C3H/f Mai) and allogeneic (C57BL/6 Cum) X-irradiated spleen lymphocytes (6×10^5 cells in 0.2 ml media) were used for antigenic stimulation.

Both mitogenic stimulated and mixed lymphocyte cultures of spleen cells
were incubated at 37°C for 48 hours in a 5% CO_2 atmosphere. One micro
Curie of ^{3}H-thymidine was then added to each culture and incubated an
additional 18 hours. After a total of 66 hours incubation, the cultures
were harvested and the contents of each well were transferred to DEAE
Whatman No. 81 filter pads and allowed to dry. These filters were
washed 4 times with 5% dibasic sodium phosphate, followed by 5 washes
with distilled water, and again dried. Filters were transferred to
vials containing 10 ml of Liquifluor (Beckman Instruments, Fullerton,
California) and counted in a Beckman model LS 250 scintillation counter.
Responses of T and B populations of spleen lymphocytes were expressed
as the difference in counts per minute (ΔCPM) between the unstimulated
and mitogen stimulated cultures. Similarly, in the MLC reaction, the
response of T cells was expressed as the difference in counts per
minute (ΔCPM) between syngeneic and allogeneic antigen stimulated
cultures.

VI. Host Tissue Measurements

Animal weights were obtained on all mice at weekly intervals and at
times when mice were sacrificed for spleen lymphocyte cultures. Pooled
thymuses and individual lung and spleens were weighed. The total number of peripheral blood leukocytes was obtained using a Fisher Auto-
cytometer II (Fisher Instruments, Pittsburgh, Pennsylvania).

C. Results

I. Effects of MCA Exposure and Tumor Transplantation on Animal Weight

Animal weights of CO control and MCA test mice recorded after each
intratracheal instillation and after transplantation of syngeneic and
allogeneic tumor cells are shown in Fig. 1. After 4 exposures and 24
days on test, MCA-mice showed a 10% loss of weight compared to the CO
controls. This effect persisted even after intratracheal instillations
were discontinued, although by day 40 of the mice previously exposed
to MCA did gain weight. It is interesting to observe that mice receiving
syngeneic transplants (5 days after the last MCA treatment) unterwent
a pronounced loss of weight through day 46, 20 days after tumors were
transplanted. As presented later, syngeneic cells grew but allogeneic
tumor cells did not.

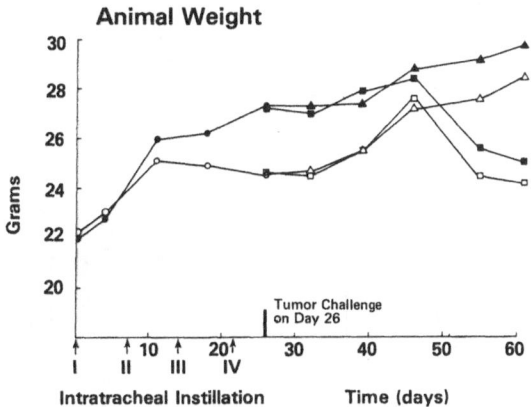

Fig. 1. Weight of mice in
relation to intratracheal
instillation of corn oil
(solid circles) or 3-methyl-
cholanthrene (open circles)
and subsequent transplantation of syngeneic (squares)
or allogeneic (triangles)
tumor cells on day 26. Arrows
indicate times of intra-
tracheal instillation at 0,
7, 14, and 21 days

II. Effects of MCA on Host Tissue Response

Table 1 shows the effects of MCA exposure on thymus, lung, and spleen
weights and on peripheral blood leukocyte counts. All of these tissues
were noticeably altered. Loss of thymus weight ranged from -38% after
1 exposure to -60% after 4, whereas lung weight increased as a function of MCA exposure. Spleen weights were depressed during MCA instillation and rebounded after they were discontinued. Leukocyte
counts appeared to have increased as a function of MCA instillation.

III. Growth of Tumor Transplants

Syngeneic and allogeneic tumor cells were transplanted in CO control
and MCA test mice, but only the syngeneic transplants grew into tumors,
as indicated in Table 2. Tumors were first detected by palpation in
both CO and MCA mice at 10 days after transplantation. It is interesting that tumors in MCA-exposed mice were significantly ($p < 0.01$) smaller
than those in CO mice at 13 days and were also somewhat smaller at 28
days after transplantation.

Table 1. Response of host tissues to 3-methylcholanthrene exposure[a]

| Days on Test | No. of Rx[b] | ORGAN WEIGHT (grams) | | | | | | | | | TOTAL CELLS (x 10^3) | | |
| | | THYMUS | | | LUNG | | | SPLEEN | | | LEUKOCYTES | | |
		C O	MCA	% Change	C O	MCA	% Change	C O	MCA	% Change	C O	MCA	% Change
3	I	.047	.029	−38	.052	.069	+11	.065	.057	−12	3.2	2.9	− 9
10	II	.047	.028	−40	.228	.243	+ 7	.104	.088	−15	6.0	5.7	− 5
17	III	.055	.039	−29	.224	.250	+12	.068	.059	−13	5.0	6.0	+20
24	IV	.055	.022	−60	.214	.236	+10	.064	.061	− 5	4.0	7.0	+75
28	IV	.044	.027	−39	.186	.215	+16	.054	.070	+30	6.7	7.6	+13
35	IV	.033	.034	+ 3	.162	.191	+18	.064	.084	+31	6.6	8.0	+21

[a]Weights and cell totals represented as arithmetic mean of 10 mice

[b]Cumulative number of intratracheal instillations of 500 ug 3-Methylcholanthrene (MCA) in 0.02 ml corn oil (CO)

Table 2. Syngeneic and allogeneic tumor growth in 3-methyl-cholanthrene exposed mice

| Tumor Type[a] | Treatment[b] | Tumor Size (cm) at Days After Transplantation | | | Tumored Mice | |
		10	13	28	No. Tested	(%)
Syngeneic	C O	palpable	0.94	1.91	26/26	(100)
	MCA	palpable	0.75	1.79	26/26	(100)
Allogeneic	C O	no tumor	0.00	0.00	0/26	(0)
	MCA	no tumor	0.00	0.00	0/26	(0)

[a]1 x 10^6 syngeneic (C3H/fMai) or allogeneic (BALB/c) tumor cells were injected subcutaneously in mice five days after the fourth and final intratracheal instillation

[b]Corn oil (C O) alone or 500 ug 3-Methylcholanthrene (MCA) dissolved in C O were administered intratracheally four times at weekly intervals before tumor transplantation

IV. Cell-Mediated Immune Effects of MCA Exposure and Tumor Transplantation

The relative reactivities of T and B spleen lymphocytes were determined *in vitro* with spleens removed from mice both during the intratracheal instillation of MCA and 7, 14, and 21 days after transplantation of tumor cells. Spleen lymphocyte responses to PHA, a T-cell specific mitogen, are shown in Fig. 2. Although some depression of T-cell activity occurred during intratracheal instillation of MCA, it reached significant levels only after the second ($p < 0.02$) and fourth (p 0.01) exposures. This depressed response returned to normal within 3 days after instillations of MCA were discontinued. One may observe that CO instillation in itself lowers T-cell activity after the second and third exposures. Most striking in Fig. 2 was the noticeable enhancement of T-cell reactivity produced by both syngeneic and allogeneic tumor cell transplantation regardless of whether the host was previously exposed to MCA or not. T-cell immune activity also was measured in response to allogeneic antigen in mixed lymphocyte cultures, and these results are shown in Fig. 3. Levels of T-cell reactivity were not effected by MCA exposure, but again were noticeably enhanced by transplantation of syngeneic and allogeneic tumor cells.

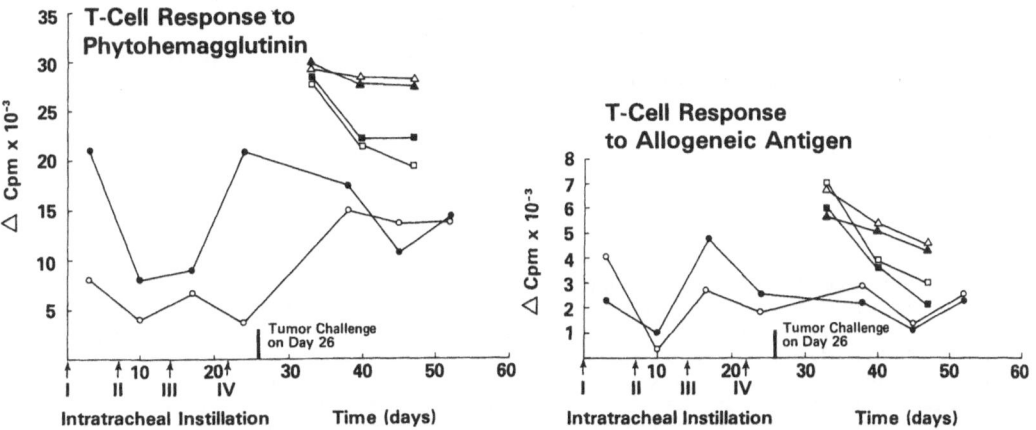

Fig. 2   Fig. 3

Fig. 2. Response of spleen lymphocytes to mitogenic stimulation with phytohemagglutinin after intratracheal instillation of corn oil (solid circles) or 3-methylcholanthrene (open circles) and subsequent transplantation of syngeneic (squares) or allogeneic (triangles) tumor cells on day 26. Arrows indicate times of intratracheal instillation at 0, 7, 14, and 21 days

Fig. 3. Response of spleen lymphocytes in mixed lymphocyte culture to allogeneic antigen after intratracheal instillation of corn oil (solid circles) or 3-methylcholanthrene (open circles) and subsequent transplantation of syngeneic (squares) or allogeneic (triangles) tumor cells on day 26. Arrows indicate times of intratracheal instillation at 0, 7, 14, and 21 days

Whereas T-cell spleen lymphocyte activity was only periodically effected during MCA exposure, bone marrow-derived, B-lymphocyte activity was
significantly depressed as shown in Fig. 4. Pronounced levels of depression occurred after instillations at 0 ($p < 0.0005$), 7 ($p < 0.01$),
14 ($p < 0.025$), and 21 ($p < 0.025$) days and remained depressed for 2
weeks after exposures were discontinued. Both T- and B-cell activity
were stimulated by syngeneic and allogeneic transplanted tumor cells
and again this occurred independent of whether the host had previously
been exposed to MCA or not.

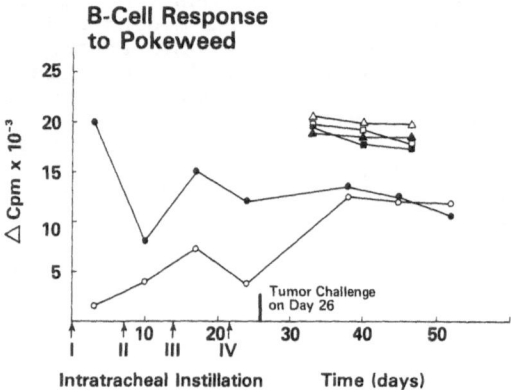

Fig. 4. Response of spleen
lymphocytes to stimulation
with pokeweed mitogen after
intratracheal instillation
of corn oil (solid circles)
or 3-methylcholanthrene
(open circles) and subse-
quent transplantation of
syngeneic (squares) or allogeneic (triangles) tumor
cells on day 26. Arrows indicate times of intratracheal
instillation at 0, 7, 14,
and 21 days

D. Discussion

Contrary to the expectation that MCA exposure might lower host immunocompetence to the point of allowing better growth of transplanted
tumor cells, it instead exhibited a tumor-inhibitory effect, at least
during the early stages of tumor growth. That transplanted syngeneic
tumor cells did not grow as well in mice treated with MCA as in controls treated with CO might be related to the significantly depressed
levels of B-cell activity incurred during the intratracheal instillation of MCA. This immunosuppressive effect might have been sufficient
to influence at least the early stages of tumor growth. MCA is known
to have an immunosuppressive property which impairs the function of
B lymphocyte populations and thereby depresses the level of humoral
antibody (BALL, 1970; STJERNSWÄRD, 1966; STUTMAN, 1969). Others have
shown that antigens elicited on the surface of tumor cells can combine with circulating humoral antibodies to form antigen-antibody
complexes effective in the prevention of tumor cell destruction by
T-cell effector lymphocytes (BALDWIN et al., 1972, 1973; HELLSTRÖM
et al., 1969). This being the case, lower humoral antibody levels
in this study as indirectly suggested by the depressed B-cell activity in MCA exposed mice before tumor cell challenge would have permitted a more effective control of tumor growth. However, it is
also possible that residual MCA in systemic circulation was simply
cytotoxic to transplanted tumor cells and slightly inhibited their
growth. Tumor inhibitory effects have been reported by others and
have been compared to the deleterious action of x-ray, nitrogen
mustard, methotrexate, and other agents on cell proliferation
(HUGGINS and MCCARTHY, 1957; THOMPSON et al., 1960). It is difficult to separate the immunosuppressive and cytotoxic capacities

of various agents (STUTMAN, 1973). Of course, with regard to carcinogenicity, it has already been demonstrated that repeated intratracheal
instillation of MCA in mice eventually produces respiratory malignancies (HO and FURST, 1973b; NETTESHEIM and HAMMONS, 1971). To whatever
degree mouse immunocompetence was altered in this study, it was not
sufficient to overcome a strong histocompatibility barrier and permit
growth of transplanted allogeneic tumor cells.

Cell-mediated immune activity as demonstrated by B- and T-cell responses to mitogenic and allogeneic antigen stimulation was clearly
enhanced by tumor transplantation regardless of any effect of MCA
exposure or tumor growth. The 10% loss of weight by mice exposed to
MCA might have been expected to produce a weakened physiological state
and a specific loss of immunocompetence. Increased weight of lungs in
exposed animals probably was caused by a collection of fluids and infiltration of lymphocytes as an inflamatory response to irritation.
The pronounced loss of weight by thymus tissues in response to MCA
might well have affected alterations in levels of CMI. Peripheral
leukocyte counts were elevated in response to MCA and further reflected chronic irritation of the respiratory tract. However, cell-
mediated immune activity was clearly stimulated in response to tumor
transplantation and appeared to be independent of any previous MCA
induced changes in thymus, lung, spleen, or leukocyte host tissues.

This study suggests that pulmonary exposure to polycyclic hydrocarbons
in mice provides a useful model for characterization of the underlying mechanisms of respiratory carcinogenesis and host immunocompetence.

E. Acknowledgements

We gratefully acknowledge the expert technical assistance of SUSAN
GOSNELL, CINDY MCKINNEY, CHARLES MURRAY, and KENNETH THOURSON. We
thank Dr. ROBERT DONAHUE for a critical reading of the manuscript,
and Mrs. VENTURA for its typing. This work was supported by The
Council for Tobacco Research.

References

ANDERSSON, J., MOLLER, G., SJOBERG, O.: Selective induction of DNA
  synthesis in T and B lymphocytes. Cell. Immunol. 4, 381-393 (1972).
BALDWIN, R.W., EMBLETON, M.J., PRICE, M.R.: Inhibition of lymphocyte
  cytotoxicity for human colon carcinoma by treatment with solubilized
  tumor membrane fractions. Int. J. Cancer 12, 84-92 (1973).
BALDWIN, R.W., PRICE, M.R., ROBINS, R.A.: Blocking of lymphocyte-
  mediated cytotoxicity for rat hepatoma cells by tumor-specific
  antigen-antibody complexes. Nature New Biol. 238, 185-187 (1972).
BALL, J.K.: Immunosuppression and carcinogenesis: Contrasting effects
  with 7,12-dimethylbenzanthracene, benzo(a)pyrene, and 3-methylcholanthrene. J. nat. Cancer Inst. 44, 1-10 (1970).
HELLSTRÖM, I., HELLSTRÖM, K.E., EVANS, C.W., HEPPNER, G.H., PIERCE,
  G.E., YANG, J.P.: Serum mediated protection of neoplastic cells
  from inhibition by lymphocytes immune to their tumor specific antigens. Proc. nat. Acad. Sci. (Wash.) 62, 362-369 (1969).
HO, W., FURST, A.: Intratracheal instillation method for mouse lungs.
  Oncology 27, 385-393 (1973a).
HO, W., FURST, A.: Lung carcinogenesis by benzo(a)pyrene instillation.
  Proc. West. Pharmacol. Soc. 16, 146-149 (1973b).

HUGGINS, C., MCCARTHY, J.J.: Regression of human metastatic mammary cancer induced by 3-methylcholanthrene. Cancer Res. 17, 1028-1032 (1957).

MORTON, D.L.: Horizons in tumor immunology. Surgery 74, 69-79 (1974).

NETTESHEIM, P., HAMMONS, A.S.: Induction of squamous cell carcinoma in the respiratory tract of mice. J. nat. Cancer Inst. 47, 697-701 (1971).

PLATE, J.M.D., MCKENZIE, I.F.C.: "B"-cell stimulation of allogeneic T-cell proliferation in mixed lymphocyte cultures. Nature New Biol. 245, 247-249 (1973).

SAFFIOTTI, U.: Experimental respiratory tract carcinogenesis. Prog. exp. Tumor Res. 11, 302-333 (1969).

SAFFIOTTI, U., CEFIS, F., KOLB, L.H.: A method for the experimental induction of bronchogenic carcinoma. Cancer Res. 28, 104-124 (1968).

SCHREIBER, H., NETTESHEIM, P., MARTIN, D.H.: Rapid development of bronchioloalveolar squamous cell tumors in rats after intratracheal injection of 3-methylcholanthrene. J. nat. Cancer Inst. 49, 541-555 (1972).

STJERNSWÄRD, J.: Age-dependent tumor-host barrier and effect of carcinogen-induced immunodepression on rejection of isografted methylcholanthrene-induced sarcoma cells. J. nat. Cancer Inst. 37, 505-512 (1966).

STUTMAN, O.: Carcinogen-induced immune depression: Absence in mice resistant to chemical oncogenesis. Science 166, 620-621 (1969).

STUTMAN, O.: Immunological aspects of resistance to the oncogenic effect of 3-methylcholanthrene in mice. Israel J. Med. Sci. 9, 217-228 (1973).

THOMPSON, J.S., GURNEY, C.W., KIRSTEN, W.H.: The tumor-inhibitory effects of 3-methylcholanthrene-induced tumors in C3H mice. Cancer Res. 20, 1214-1219 (1960).

The Influence of Carcinogenic Substances Introduced Intratracheally to Several Generations of Experimental Rats

Laima L. Griciute*

Oncological Institute of Lithuanian SSR, Vilnius

ABSTRACT

Among the questions concerning the pathogenesis of bronchogenic cancer the problem of the influence of the carcinogenic substances on the following generations of experimental animals deserves special attention.

Benzo(a)pyrene (5 mg) mixed with Indian ink (1 mg) was introduced intratracheally to 20 young non-inbred laboratory rats (10 males and 10 females). The application was made 3 times at 10-day intervals. One week after the last application the rats were coupled as we tried to avoid the transplacental influence of carcinogenic substances. Their offspring (F_1) at the age of 4-5 weeks was separated from their parents, males and females being kept apart. At the age of 7-8 weeks the offspring received the same amount of carcinogenic substances using the above method. One week after the last application the rats were again coupled. This same method was used for F_2 and F_3. 244 rats were used in this experiment.

We have the impression that bronchogenic cancers occur more frequently in F_2 than in F_3. There also seems to be a slight frequency increase from the original generation up to F_2.

The tumors mainly represented anaplastic carcinomas, arising in all probability, from bronchial glands. In addition to these tumors we also found adenocarcinomas and spinocellular cancer.

Introduction

Experimental evidence exists that indicates that the intratracheal introduction of carcinogenic substances causes the development of bronchogenic cancer in laboratory animals. When considering problems related to bronchogenic cancer, the influence of carcinogenic substances on consecutive generations of experimental animals deserves special attention.

A number of studies have been carried out on the effects of carcinogenic substances on the lungs and other organs of consecutive genera-

---

*Currently Chief of the Environmental Carcinogens Unit, International Agency for Research on Cancer, 150 Cours Albert-Thomas, Lyon 69008, France.

tions of animals. SHABAD (1928) demonstrated that, when subsequent paintings with tar are carried out on F_1- and F_2-generation mice, the frequency of lung adenomas is greater than that in the original generation. SHABAD et al. (1967) also reported an increase in preadenomatous changes in organ cultures of F_2- and F_3-generation fetal mouse lungs obtained from DDT-treated pregnant mice but a decrease in the F_5 generation.

NAPALKOV and ALEXANDROV (1968) noted a higher frequency of thyroid tumors in F_3- and F_4-generation rats treated with 6-methylthiouracyl, though a subsequent decrease was observed in F_5- through F_7-generation controls, after which a new increase occurred. In an experiment with DDT, TURUSOV et al. (1973) observed an increased incidence of lung tumors in F_2- through F_4-generation mice, but not in F_1 or F_5 generations, as compared to the incidence observed in the original generation.

The aim of our experiment was to observe whether carcinogenic substances, when introduced intratracheally, increase the incidence of bronchogenic cancer in consecutive generations of rats.

Materials and Methods

5 mg of benzopyrene, mixed with 1 mg of ink powder and suspended in 0.2 ml of polyglycine, were introduced intratracheally into 20 non-inbred laboratory rats (10 males and 10 females). A total of 3 applications per rat were made at 10-day intervals, each rat receiving a total of 15 mg benzopyrene intratracheally.

One week after the last application, the rats were coupled, since we wanted to avoid the transplacental influence of carcinogenic substances. SHABAD et al.'s data (1964) show that unfixed carcinogenic substances are eliminated from the lungs of animals within the week following administration of the substance.

At 4 to 5 weeks, the offspring (F_1 generation rats) was separated from the parents, males and females being kept apart. At the age of 7 to 8 weeks, the offspring received the same amount of carcinogenic substances as their parents, using the above-mentioned method. One week after the last application the F_1-generation rats were coupled. This same method was employed for F_2- and F_3-generation rats. A total of 244 rats were used in this experiment.

F_1- and F_2-generation rats bred well, but F_3-generation rats did not produce offspring. Many of the F_3 animals died during prenancy without clear pathological changes in the organs. All carcinogen-treated rats were kept until they died spontaneously.

Results and Discussion

Bronchogenic cancer was seen in a number of the rats. The earliest lung tumor was observed 12 months from the beginning of the experiment, and the incidence of lung tumors was based on the number of animals reaching this age. These animals and those with bronchogenic cancer are listed in Table 1. Table 2 shows that the development of tumors in subsequent generations was not accelerated. No sex differentiation was observed.

Table 1.   Rats surviving 12 months from the beginning of experiment

Generation	Number of rats (rats with bronchogenic cancer)
Original	5 rats, of which 1 had bronchogenic cancer
F_1	40 rats, of which 7 (18%) had bronchogenic cancer
F_2	46 rats, of which 12 (26%) had bronchogenic cancer
F_3	14 rats, of which 2 (14%) had bronchogenic cancer

Table 2.   Time of tumor appearance

Generation	Time of appearance (from beginning of experiment)
Original	12 1/2 months
F_1	14 1/2 to 23 months
F_2	14 1/2 to 24 months
F_3	14 1/2 to 15 1/2 months

Histologically, the lung tumors mainly represented anaplastic carcinomas that in all probability originated from bronchial glands (Figs. 1 and 2). JANYSHEVA (1970) and this author found similar tumors in rats following intratracheal administration of small doses of hydrocarbons. The tumors spread peribronchially and perivascularly in the lungs, but metastases in other organs were extremely rare. In addition to these tumors, adenocarcinomas and spinocellular cancer were also observed. Other tumors occurred in the experimental animals, such as reticular sarcoma and mammary carcinoma. No fluctuation in this tumor occurrence was observed in the different generations.

In conclusion, these findings indicate an absence of progressively increased incidence of cancer following administration of benzopyrene. It would appear, however, that bronchogenic cancers occur more frequently in F_2-generation than in F_1- and F_3-generation rats.

Tumor occurrence observed in this experiment fluctuated from a slight increase in the F_2-generation rats to a decrease in F_3-generation rats. These findings concurred with those of SHABAD et al. (1967), NAPALKOV and ALEXANDROV (1968), and TURUSOV et al. (1973).

Further studies should be carried out to ascertain whether our observations on tumor incidence in consecutive generations of rats exposed to carcinogens can be confirmed.

Acknowledgement

The author is grateful to Dr. V. SNIRAS, Mrs. J. PRZANCUZEVICIENE, B. PAKARKLYTE, and O. KAUSILIENE for their competent technical assistance.

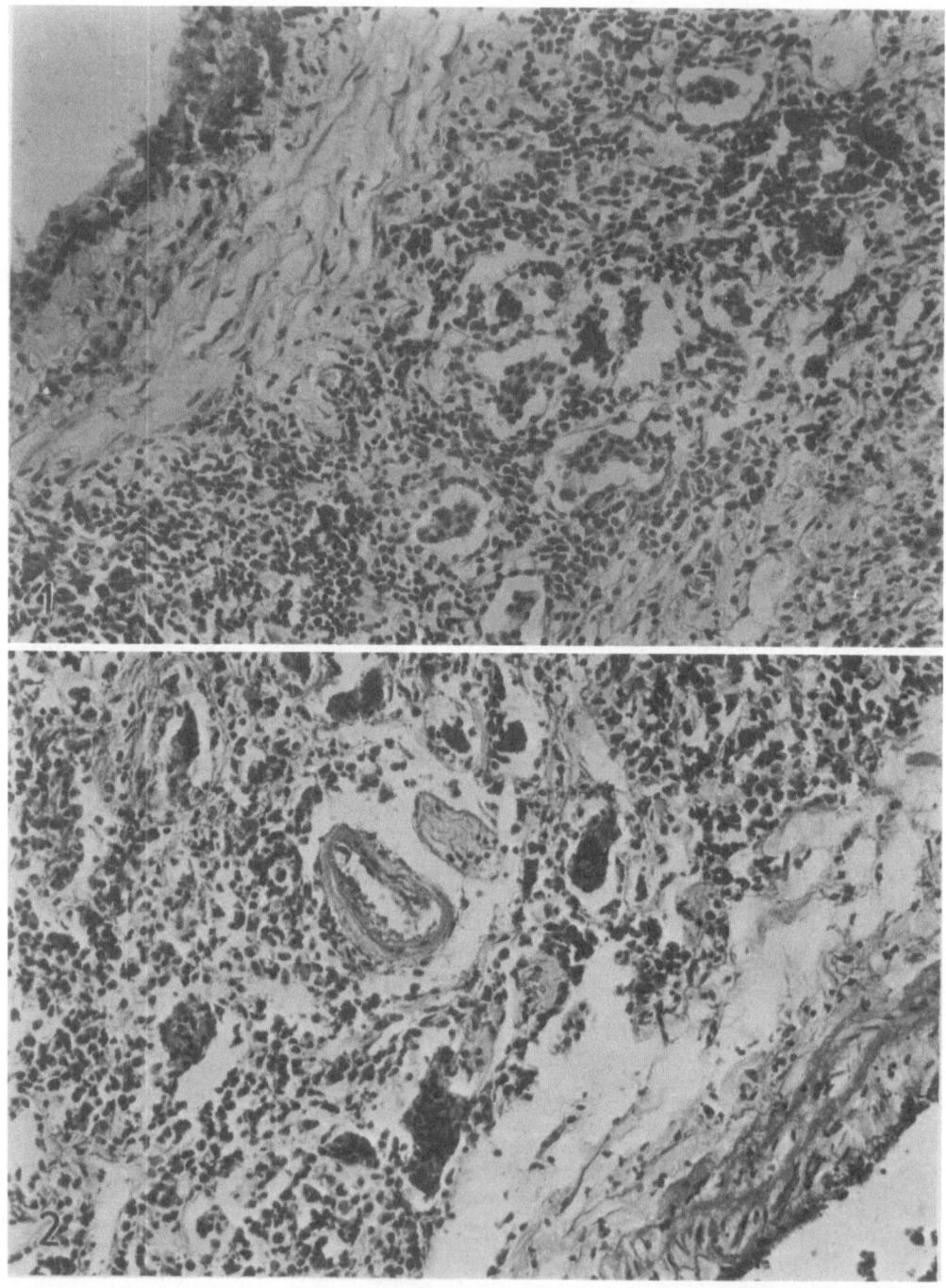

Fig. 1. Anaplastic cell clusters in vicinity of bronchus; ink powder (right upper corner). HE (x 140)

Fig. 2. Anaplastic cell clusters in the lung tissue around a blood vessel. HE (x 140)

References

GRICIUTE, L.: Experimental tumours of the lungs. Monograph Medicina, Moscow, in press.

JANYSHEVA, N.J.: Environmental monitoring of carcinogenic substances. Thesis of Doctorat. Moscow 1970.

NAPALKOV, N.P., ALEXANDROV, V.A.: On the effects of blastomogenic substances on the organism during embryogenesis. Z. Krebsforsch. 71, 32-50 (1968).

SHABAD, L.M.: Experimental tumours of the lungs in mice. Thesis of Doctorat. Leningrad 1928.

SHABAD, L.M., PYLEV, L.N., KOLESNICHENKO, T.S.: The role of soot on the fixation in the lung tissue of carcinogenic substances introduced intratracheally. Vop. Onkol. 6, 65 (1964).

SHABAD, L.M., KOLESNICHENKO, T.S., NIKONOVA, T.V.: The effect of transplacental administration of DDT in·organ cultures of fetal mouse lung tissue. Int. J. Cancer 33, 901-907 (1967).

TURUSOV, V.S., DAY, N.E., TOMATIS, L., GATI, E., CHARLES, R.T.: Tumours in CF-1 mice exposed for 6 consecutive generations to DDT. J. nat. Cancer Inst. 51, 983-997 (1973).

Large-Volume Intratracheal Instillation of Particulate Suspensions to Hamsters*

David W. Baxter and Curtis D. Port

ITT Research Institute, Chicago, IL 60616, USA

ABSTRACT

A technique has been developed that permits the intratracheal instillation of volumes as large as 1.5 ml into the respiratory tract of young adult Syrian golden hamsters. 2 factors are of unique importance for the success of this technique: 1. the use of halothane anesthesia that permits total recovery in as little as 2 minutes, and 2. the use of an intratracheal speculum that seals at the larynx and prevents loss of suspension from the lungs. Suspensions consisting of 2% (w/v) ferric oxide, or benzo(a)pyrene-ferric oxide, in 0.5% gelatin-saline have been instilled with a technique mortality rate of less than 5%. Histopathological examination of the lungs at 4 weeks revealed no significant changes related to the technique. Distribution of a suspension containing black ink was uniform when volumes larger than 1 ml were instilled; smaller volumes were less well distributed. Examination of the gastrointestinal tract within 5 hours after instillation showed that no significant loss of ink suspension from the lungs had occurred. Additional studies are in progress to determine the tumorigenic potential of benzo(a)pyrene-ferric oxide when administered in 2 doses, 7 days apart, of 1.5 ml each (total dose = 30 mg BaP) to the same amount of carcinogen administered in 10 or more doses of 0.25 ml at weekly intervals.

A. Introduction

Experimental respiratory carcinogenesis has been studied in recent years by administering chemical carcinogens directly into the trachea (SAFFIOTTI et al., 1963, 1968; PYLEV, 1961; SHABAD, 1962). The technique described in detail by SAFFIOTTI (1968) was developed to provide "adequate penetration of the carcinogen into the lung tissues to attain a sufficient effective dose at the target site". In order to achieve this goal, BaP was mixed with ferric oxide particles (1:1) and instilled as a saline suspension directly into the trachea, using a 0.25-ml syringe fitted with a blunted 19-gauge needle. When this procedure was repeated 15 times at weekly intervals, a high incidence of bronchogenic carcinoma was produced. The results obtained, however, were dependent upon the total dose administered (SAFFIOTTI et al., 1972a) and the number of administrations carried out (SAFFIOTTI et al., 1972b). In addition, the distribution of the suspension within the respiratory tract was seldom uniform, and regurgitation occurred following in-

---

*This work was supported by IIT Research Institute and by the National Cancer Institute, Contract No. NIH-NCI-72-3292.

stillation of 0.5 ml, the largest volume given. The purpose of this
study was to determine the feasibility of instilling relatively large
volumes (1 to 2 ml) by a modified instillation technique, in order to
increase the dose of the carcinogen administered, increase the distribution of the suspension within the lungs and prevent regurgitation from the lungs into the gastrointestinal tract.

B. Materials and Methods

Male and female Syrian golden hamsters, weighing between 80 and 120 g
were used. The intratracheal instillation technique, described by
MORROW (1972) for use in the rat, was carried out as follows: the hamster was first anesthetized with halothane vapor (approximately 5% in
oxygen) until respiration decreased to less than 5 breaths per minute
and was then suspended by the upper incisor teeth at a 30° angle on an
intratracheal injection support. While the animal was still deeply
anesthetized, an intratracheal speculum was placed through the larynx
into the upper portion of the trachea. The speculum, 65 mm long, was
cut from the tapered end of an Argyle Fr. no. 5 umbilical catheter.
A 20-gauge needle, cut to an appropriate length and blunted, was used
to support the soft plastic speculum during the placement procedure.
Correct placement was verified by the presense of water vapor in the
speculum after the needle had been withdrawn. Instillation of the test
suspension was made with a 1.0 or 2.5 ml disposable syringe fitted
with a 22-gauge catheter (Bardic cutdown catheter, Bard, Inc., Murry
Hill, New Jersey).

With the speculum in place, the hamster was allowed to recover from
the anesthesia to the extent that it responded to touch. At this point,
the catheter was inserted through the speculum and sealed by inserting
the hub of the catheter into the opening of the speculum. When volumes
larger than 1 ml were instilled, the catheter was inserted at end-
respiration to avoid possible "blowback" of the test suspension. Instillation was made by injecting the desired volume from the syringe
and catheter. Any regurgitation from the trachea was contained in the
speculum and later inhaled into the lungs. The speculum was removed
when all of the instillation volume was contained in the lungs and
respiration had returned. The entire procedure was carried out in 5
minutes or less.

I. Mortality and Histopathology Study

A group of 64 hamsters was instilled with 0.5, 1.0, 1.5, or 2.0 ml of
gelatin-saline (0.5% gelatin in 0.9% sterile saline), 0.5% ferric
oxide (ferric oxide no. 8098, Charles Pfizer and Company, Reading,
Pennsylvania) in gelatin-saline or 1.0% ferric oxide in gelatin-saline.
Each animal was weighed weekly and killed at either 2 weeks or 4 weeks
post-instillation for histologic examination of the trachea and lungs.

II. Pulmonary Distribution Study

13 hamsters were instilled with 0.2 to 2.0 ml gelatin-saline + 5%
Pellikan black ink (Günther Wagner, Germany). Each animal was killed
0.5 hours to 5 hours post-instillation and examined for the presence
of ink in both the respiratory and gastrointestinal tracts.

III. Laryngeal and Tracheal Damage Study

12 hamsters were instilled with 1.5 ml gelatin-saline and killed at
intervals between 5 hours and 5 days. The larynx and trachea of each
animal were removed and stained for 1 to 3 minutes with 0.1% methylene
blue and then inspected for gross cellular damage.

C. Results

I. Mortality and Histopathology Study

Of the 64 hamsters instilled in this study, only 3 deaths occurred
prior to sacrifice, and each of these was related to the instillation
procedure itself and not to the volume or type of suspension administered. 2 hamsters died with a perforated trachea (1 on day 0 and 1 on
day 4), and 1 hamster died on day 0 with no gross damage apparent at
autopsy. It is believed that this animal had not sufficiently recovered
from the anesthetic before the instillation (1.5 ml gelatin-saline)
was made. No significant body weight changes or mortality could be
associated with either the volume (0.5 to 2.0 ml) or type of suspension
(0 to 1% ferric oxide in gelatin-saline) administered. Histologic examination of the lungs from these hamsters instilled with 2 ml and killed at 4 weeks showed only minimal pathology. Slight emphysema was seen
in 7 of the 15 animals examined. Slight subacute interstitial infiltrate was seen in 8 of the hamsters. 1 or 2 instances of slight congestion and slight interstitial edema were also seen. Ferric oxide
distribution within individual lobes and between different lobes of
the lungs was judged, on a histologic basis, to be uniform in 8 out
of 10 hamsters given either of the 2 ferric oxide suspensions.

II. Pulmonary Distribution Study

Pellikan ink was toxic when 2 ml of a 5% dilution in gelatin-saline
was administered into the lungs; 1.5 ml or less, however, was well
tolerated.

All animals killed at 0.5 or 5.0 hours after successful instillation
of between 0.2 and 1.5 ml of the ink suspension showed no black color
at the nose, mouth, throat, esophagus, stomach, or small intestine.
1 hamster instilled with 1.5 ml had recovered from the anesthetic at
the time of instillation and immediately regurgitated a portion of the
injected volume over the top of the speculum and into the mouth and
throat. When it was killed 30 minutes later, this animal had ink stains
in the gastrointestinal system extending from the nose and face to the
upper small intestine.

The distribution of ink within the lungs was proportional to the volume
administered (Fig. 1) and 0.2 ml stained a portion of each lobe leaving the periphery of the lungs free of ink (Fig. 1C). The same volume
instilled by the needle technique (SAFFIOTTI et al., 1968) was more
erratically distributed between lobes; the lungs shown in Fig. 1 (A
and B) showed that most of the instillation volume entered the left
lobe. In contrast, instillation volumes in excess of 1 ml and administered through a speculum (Fig. 1, D and F) completely filled
the respiratory tract and resulted in a uniform distribution in each
lobe.

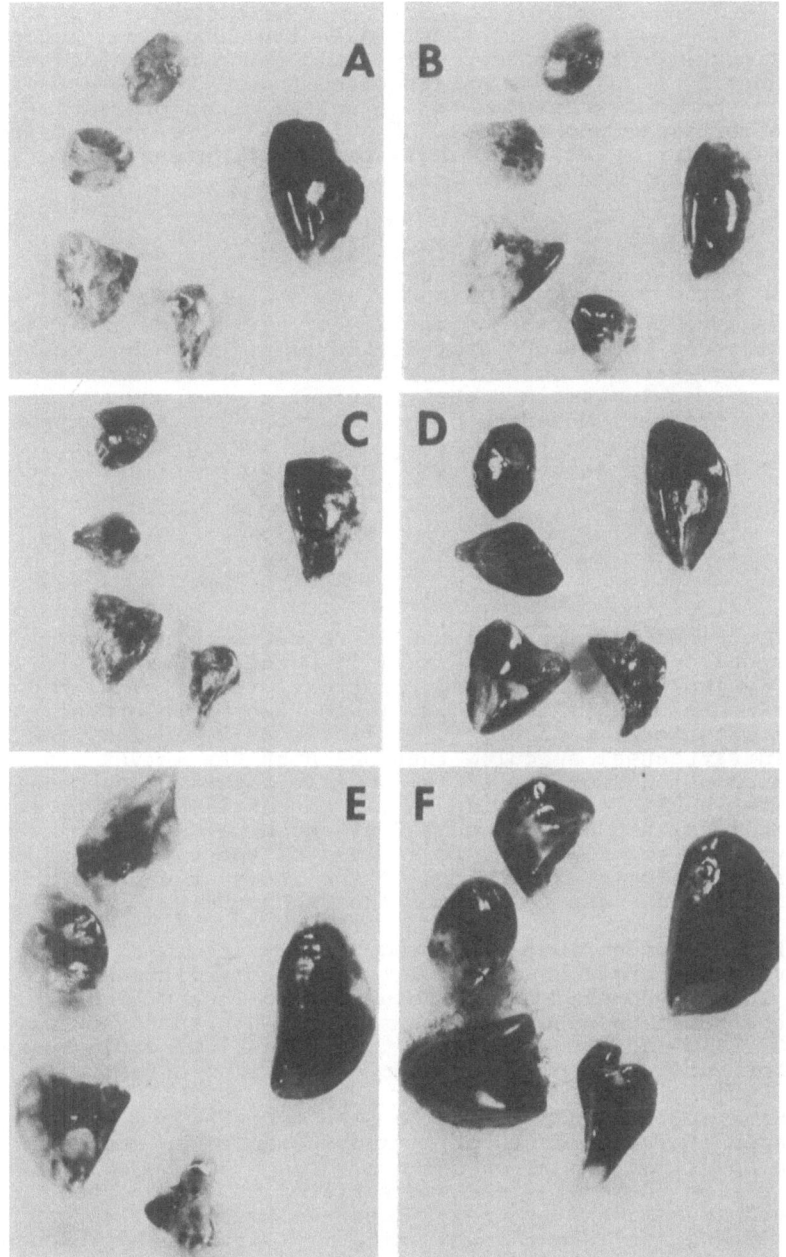

Fig. 1 A-F. Distribution of an ink suspension within the lungs of
adult Syrian golden hamsters. (A) and (B) 0.2 ml administered with a
blunted 19-g needle. (C) through (F) injected volumes administered
through a speculum placed in the trachea. (C) 0.2 ml (compare with
A and B). (D) 1.5 ml. (E) 0.5 ml. (F) 1.0 ml

Several hamsters had relatively clear fluid in the lungs when autopsied, whether at 30 minutes or at 5 hours. This fluid could be drained through the mouth and nose by holding the anesthetized animal upside down and may represent an edematous reaction to the instillation procedure. The hamsters in the mortality and histopathology study (vide supra) also had pulmonary fluid accumulation as indicated by the presence of rales; however, this condition disappeared from between 1 to 3 days after instillation.

III.   Laryngeal and Tracheal Damage Study

Very little damage to the surface epithelium of the larynx and trachea could be demonstrated. The nature of this instillation technique is such that, if damage were to occur, it would most likely occur in the larynx where the speculum seals tightly against the walls, and in the upper half of the trachea. Moderate damage in these areas was apparent at 5 hours and, to a lesser extent, at 24 hours. No significant staining of damaged tissue was detectable at 3 or 5 days post-instillation.

D.   Discussion

The technique described here permits the intratracheal instillation of particulate suspensions as large as 1.5 ml into the respiratory tract of young adult Syrian golden hamsters. 2 factors are of unique importance for the success of this technique: 1. the use of halothane anesthesia which permits total recovery in as little as 2 minutes, and 2. the use of an intratracheal speculum that seals at the larynx and prevents loss of suspension from the lungs. Administration of suspensions containing as much as 1% ferric oxide in 1.5 ml resulted in a technique mortality of less than 5%. Although fluid accumulation was present for several days post-instillation, regardless of the type of suspension given, histopathologic examination of the lungs at 4 weeks revealed no significant changes related to the technique.

Distribution of test suspensions was found to vary according to the volume given. Volumes larger than 1 ml were uniformly distributed throughout the lungs, whereas smaller volumes were less well distributed. Because the hamsters used in these studies were approximately 9 weeks old (80 to 100 g in body weight), less than 1 ml would be required for uniform distribution in younger and smaller animals.

Additional studies are now in progress to determine the tumorigenic potential of benzo(a)pyrene-ferric oxide suspension administered in 2 doses, 7 days apart, of 1.5 ml each (total dose = 30 mg BaP). Preliminary results from these studies have verified those reported above; i.e., technique mortality from 2 large-volume instillations was less than 3%, and ferric oxide was uniformly distributed throughout the lungs of those animals sacrificed for histological examination. In addition, administration of as much as 30 mg of the carcinogen was itself not toxic when administered by the large-volume technique.

References

MORROW, W.G.: A method for intratracheal instillation in the rat. Battelle, Pacific Northwest Laboratories, Annual Report for 1971, BNWL-1650 PT 1, 168, 1972.

PYLEV, L.N.: Experimental induction of lung cancer in rats by intratracheal introduction of 9, 10-dimethyl-1, 2-benzanthracene. Bull. exp. Biol. Med. 52, 99 (1961).

SAFFIOTTI, U., CEFIS, F., KOLB, L.H.: A method for the experimental induction of bronchogenic carcinoma. Cancer Res. 28, 104 (1968).

SAFFIOTTI, U., CEFIS, F., KOLB, L.H., GROTE, M.I.: Intratracheal injections of particulate carcinogens into hamster lungs. Proc. Amer. Ass. Cancer Res. 4, 59 (1963).

SAFFIOTTI, U., MONTESANO, R., SELLAKUMAR, A.R., KAUFMAN, D.G.: Respiratory tract carcinogenesis induced in hamsters by different dose levels of benzo(a)pyrene and ferric oxide. J. Nat. Cancer Inst. 49, 1199 (1972a).

SAFFIOTTI, U., MONTESANO, R., SELLAKUMAR, A.R., CEFIS, F., KAUFMAN, D.G.: Respiratory tract carcinogenesis in hamsters induced by different numbers of administrations of benzo(a)pyrene and ferric oxide. Cancer Res. 32, 1073 (1972b).

SHABAD, L.M.: Experimental cancer of the lung. J. Nat. Cancer Inst. 28, 1305 (1962).

The Intrapleural Route as a Means for Estimating Carcinogenicity*

William E. Smith and Doras D. Hubert

Health Research Institute, Fairleigh Dickinson University, Madison, NJ 07940, USA

ABSTRACT

Intrathoracic tumors have been reported from several laboratories after intrapleural injection of various preparations of mineral substances into experimental animals. Application of information from such studies to problems of pulmonary carcinogenesis involves consideration of whether tumors so induced arise from mesothelial cells of the pleura or from other cells of the lungs or thoracic cage. Another question stems from the fact that direct introduction of test substances into the pleural space does not reproduce natural routes of exposure to inhaled carcinogens, however, the intrapleural route may serve a useful role as a convenient screening procedure in comparison to laborious, repeated intratracheal injections or the large space requirements of inhalation exposures.

In experiments with hamsters exposed to a variety of preparations of asbestiform and other minerals, we have given each animal only a single intrapleural injection. Multiple injections present undesirable variables, since early granulomatous responses to a single injection entail variations in deposition of subsequent injections.

After single intrapleural injection of hamsters, we have seen upward of 80 animals with intrathoracic tumors spreading along pleural surfaces in a manner characteristic of mesotheliomas. For purposes of this paper, these tumors will be designated as mesotheliomas, although we were able to trace their derivation from the mesothelium only in rare cases, most of the tumors being too large to identify their precise origin.

Data from these experiments show that tumor response to chrysotile, amosite, and crocidolite is related to dose. Tumors regarded as mesotheliomas arose in response to preparations of chrysotile containing numerous fibers visible by optical microscopy but not in response to preparations in which the great majority of fibers were visible only by electron microscopy.

*This research was supported by Research Grant EC 00226 from the U.S. Public Health Service and by grants from Johns-Manville Fund and Fannie E. Rippel Foundation.

Introduction

Beginning in 1952, HUEPER and associates reported a series of experiments in which they attempted to utilize the pleural cavity for
study of biologic responses to various minerals that had been associated with pulmonary carcinogenesis in epidemiologic studies of some
occupational groups. Test materials were suspended in lanolin or
gelatin and injected into animals through the supraclavicular fossa
or implanted through thoracotomy. Epidermoid carcinomas, round cell
carcinomas, adenocarcinomas, and sarcomas were reported in lungs of
rats and mice after what was said to be intrapleural deposition of
powdered chromite roast and a number of chromates, whereas no lung
tumors were found in rats exposed by inhalation to chromite ore with
particle size averaging less than 4 μm (HUEPER and PAYNE, 1959, 1960;
HUEPER and CONWAY, 1964). Intrapleural deposition of powdered metallic
nickel and uranium was said to induce sarcomatous responses from the
lung and pleural tissues of rats (HUEPER and CONWAY, 1964). These
sarcomas, however, appear to have been in the thoracic wall or subcutaneous tissues at sites of injection (HUEPER, 1952, 1955; HUEPER
et al., 1952). For intrapleural experiments, multiple injections were
often given over a period of months. Pleural adhesions resulting from
early injections may have caused later injections to be deposited into the lungs, which might account for some tumors described as being
found in the lungs.

HUEPER (1954) found no tumors related to treatment in 25 Osborne-
Mendel rats, each of which received 6 monthly injections of about
15 mg of a preparation of asbestos described as a commercial-grade
medium fiber. This material was suspended in lanolin.

HUEPER and PAYNE (1962) mention a pleural mesothelioma in 1 of 218
"Bethesda black rats" (from the National Institutes of Health) and
state that it is a tumor that appears without any intervention in
rats of that strain. In the same paper, they report an experiment in
which chromic acetate in a gelatin capsule was implanted into the
right pleural cavity of 42 rats and into thigh muscles of 35 rats
of that strain. Aside from 1 tumor at the intramuscular site, they
did not consider tumors occurring elsewhere in these animals to have
any connection with the treatment. These other tumors included 3 mesotheliomas of the pleura.

WAGNER (1962, 1966) has developed a method for intrapleural injections
of materials suspended in saline solution using a needle attached to
a two-way tap introduced under ether anesthesia into the right axilla
of rats at the level of the second teat. One end of the tap is attached
to a capillary manometer, which gives a negative reading when the needle
reaches the pleural cavity. A syringe containing the inoculum is then
attached to the other arm of the tap and a volume of 0.4 ml is injected.

With this technique, WAGNER and BERRY (1969) injected 20 mg of preparations of amosite, crocidolite, chrysotile, and silica into specific
pathogen-free (SPF) Wistar rats. The suspensions in saline were sterilized in an autoclave. There were 96 rats per sample, equally divided
as to sex. With the 3 types of asbestos, they reported tumors that they
diagnosed as mesotheliomas in 38, 61, and 55 rats, respectively. These
tumors ranged in size from large masses enveloping the right lung to
small nodules on the parietal pleura. They were equally distributed
among males and females. Histologically, these tumors were said to
be composed most frequently of spindle cells with occasional clefts
lined by epithelial cells and were therefore considered as mixed-

pattern mesotheliomas. Purely spindle-cell tumors or tumors described as tubulopapillary were less common. In 9 of the rats injected with asbestos, subcutaneous sarcomas were found at injection sites. They were attributed to deposition of the inoculum in the chest wall rather than in the pleural cavity.

In the 96 rats injected with silica, with a particle size of less than 5 μm, about half developed intrathoracic tumors diagnosed as histocytic reticulum cell sarcomas. These tumors are discussed and contrasted with tumors diagnosed as mesotheliomas (WAGNER, 1966). No mesotheliomas were found in 96 control rats injected only with saline solution. These experiments with SPF rats were repeated with standard rats and generally comparable results were obtained.

From subsequent experiments with the same technique, WAGNER et al. (1973) reported that development of mesotheliomas in SPF Wistar rats was approximately proportional to dose of asbestos. In groups of 30 to 35 rats, they found no mesotheliomas in response to a sample of glass fibers, but single mesotheliomas in response to glass powder, nonfibrous aluminum oxide, and barium sulphate, 3 mesotheliomas in response to aluminium silicate fibers, and 18 in response to brucite. They state that their sample of brucite also contained chrysotile.

After intrapleural injection of 1 ml of 1:15 suspensions of asbestos fibers into 102 Sprague-Dawley rats, DONNA (1970) saw tumors in 12 animals after 13 to 20 months. These tumors were described as mesothelial in 3 rats treated with chrysotile, whereas in 4 rats treated with crocidolite and 5 rats treated with amosite, there were said to be undifferentiated pulmonary carcinomas. The possibility that some of the inoculum may have been deposited into the lungs must be considered.

A technique designed to achieve widespread deposition and retention of particulates in the pleural cavity has been developed by STANTON and WRENCH (1972). They suspended preparations of asbestos in liquid gelatin, which was then allowed to harden on a pledget of coarse glass fibers measuring about 30 x 20 x 2 mm. The pledgets were introduced into the left pleural cavity of female Osborne-Mendel (om) rats through a thoracotomy under ether anesthesia. In rats thus treated, they found numerous tumors that they described as pleural mesotheliomas of spindle cell or pleomorphic types, sometimes with tubulopapillary features. In groups of 30 rats treated with pledgets containing 40 mg of UICC (Union Internationale Contre le Cancer) standard reference samples (TIMBRELL, 1969) of chrysotile A, amosite, and crocidolite, tumors designated as mesotheliomas were seen in 15, 15, and 14 animals respectively. Milling of this sample of crocidolite to reduce particle size gave a product that induced mesotheliomas in only 8 animals.

With pledgets containing 10 mg or 1 mg UICC crocidolite, the number of mesothelioma-bearing rats was reported as 11 and 2, respectively. When 10 mg of the same crocidolite was suspended in saline and injected without pledgets of glass fibers, mesotheliomas were found in 9 rats. The closely similar yield of these tumors with and without pledgets indicates no advantage of this special method to influence distribution of particulates within the pleural cavity.

No tumors resulted from control implants of the coarse glass fiber pledgets. Single mesotheliomas were found in groups with pledgets impregnated with 40 mg of glass fibers 1 μm to 25 μm in diameter. In 2 groups treated with 40 mg of glass fibers, 0.06 μm to 3 μm in diameter, 3 and 5 tumors diagnosed as mesotheliomas were found.

Materials and Methods

Our group has carried out experiments in which various preparations of minerals have been injected into the pleural cavity of Syrian golden hamsters. Throughout, we have used male hamsters of the LVG:LAK strain obtained from Lakeview Hamster Colony, Newfield, New Jersey. Test materials have been suspended in 0.9% NaCl solution, sterilized in an autoclave, and injected in a volume of 0.5 ml with a syringe fitted with a 20-gauge needle, except for thick slurries for which an 18-gauge needle was used. Each animal received only 1 injection, which was made into the right chest in the mid-axillary line about 1/4 inch above the lower end of the sternum. Depending on the nature and dose of test materials, granulomatous responses can largely obliterate the pleural cavity within a few weeks. Accordingly, we have not used and do not recommend repeated injections.

In our early work (SMITH et al., 1965b), we "stabbed" the right chest 2 days before injection in an attempt to induce pneumothorax and thus favor intrapleural deposition and spread of inoculum. With experience, we found that comparable deposition and spread can be achieved by direct injection. Hence, preliminary "stabbing" has been omitted in all of our intrapleural work since 1965.

Following attempts at intrapleural injections, part of the inoculum was sometimes found subcutaneously in the chest wall. Sarcomas occasionally arose at such sites. We have not included such subcutaneous tumors in comparing yields of intrathoracic tumors in response to different test materials. To avoid this problem, the occasional animal that shows a subcutaneous swelling at the time of injection is discarded and replaced. With this precaution, examination of trial animals immediately after injection has shown the inoculum in the pleural space. The technique of intrapleural injection is thus not more difficult than the commonly used technique of intraperitoneal injection. No anesthesia is required. The operator holds the animal in 1 hand and makes the injection with the other, holding a finger on the xiphoid to assure proper positioning of the needle.

Results

After intrapleural injection of a carcinogenic dose, we have occasionally seen small tumors whose origin from mesothelium could be traced. The majority of intrathoracic tumors found in our experiments, however, have been large masses whose origin could not be precisely ascertained. Such masses compress the lung, sometimes largely fill the right chest, spread along pleural surfaces, but invade the lungs only superficially. Some penetrate the diaphragm. Occasionally, metastases are found. Gross and microscopic appearance of such tumors in hamsters have been described and illustrated (SMITH et al., 1965a; SMITH et al., 1965b).

In man, mesotheliomas have been described as tumors that spread along mesothelial surfaces and they have been subdivided into epithelial-like, sarcomatous, or mixed types (CHURG and SELIKOFF, 1968). The majority of intrathoracic tumors in our experiments with hamsters appear sarcomatous while others resemble the so-called epithelial or mixed types. Use of the term "mesothelioma" for many experimentally induced tumors reported in animals has been questioned by GROSS (1973) in an exchange of views including STANTON's contribution. For the present, we use the term "mesothelioma" for purposes of comparing experimental yields of malignant tumors that appear to be primary in the chest, spread along mesothelial surfaces, and histologically bear some resemblance to one or another type of tumor presently diagnosed as mesothelioma in man.

Thus defined, we found that the yield of mesotheliomas after intrapleural injection of hamsters was related to the dose of chrysotile or amosite. In groups of 50 hamsters, the number of tumors considered to be mesotheliomas were 9, 4, and 0 in response to 25 mg, 10 mg, and 1 mg chrysotile; 4 and 0 in response to 10 mg and 1 mg amosite (SMITH et al., 1968). No mesotheliomas were found in response to 25 mg of a preparation of talc that contained 50% fibrous tremolite (SMITH, 1973). We saw no mesotheliomas in 100 untreated hamsters maintained as control groups in these experiments.

3 preparations of chrysotile with mean fiber length of 5.3 µm to 6.9 µm, as measured by electron microscopy, were milled to reduce fiber size to mean lengths of 0.37 µm to 0.86 µm. These 6 preparations were tested at a dose level of 25 mg in groups of 50 hamsters each. The 3 original preparations induced extensive pleural adhesions and yielded 8, 9, and 10 mesotheliomas, whereas the 3 samples that had been subjected to further milling induced relatively thin pleural adhesions and no mesotheliomas (SMITH et al., 1972). Fiber diameter in the original preparations averaged 0.18 µm to 0.2 µm and in the milled preparations 0.03 µm to 0.07 µm.

This evidence that carcinogenicity of asbestos is related to physical properties is supported by an as-yet unpublished experiment of ours in which 50 hamsters were given an intrapleural injection of 25 mg serpentine rock dust (antigorite). This material has the chemical composition of chrysotile but is not crystallized in fibrous form. Only 1 mesothelioma resulted.

The following information is available from additional as-yet unpublished experiments with groups of 50 hamsters:

Since the external surface of chrysotile fibers is thought to consist of magnesium hydroxide (SPEIL and LEINEWEBER, 1969), an experiment was designed to ask whether such a surface might play a role in asbestos carcinogenesis. For this purpose, a fibrous magnesium hydroxide (nemalite) was tested. At the 25-mg dose level, no mesotheliomas resulted.

Another experiment was designed to test whether carcinogenic activity might be shown by fibers comparable to asbestos fibers in size but different in chemical composition. For this purpose, we used silicon dioxide fibers with an average diameter of 0.75 µm. At a dose of 10 mg, mesotheliomas developed in 4 hamsters. No mesotheliomas occurred in 50 hamsters injected with borosilicate glass fibers with an average diameter of 5 µm, or in 50 hamsters injected with such glass fibers coated with phenolformaldehyde (a binder used in some preparations of fiberglass).

A standard reference (UICC) sample of crocidolite (TIMBRELL, 1969) was tested in 2 groups of 50 hamsters each. At a dose of 10 mg, it induced mesotheliomas in 10 hamsters. At a dose of 1 mg, it induced mesotheliomas in 2 hamsters. 3 of 50 hamsters developed mesotheliomas after 10 mg of a standard reference (UICC) sample of anthophyllite.

These findings show that intrapleural injection of hamsters with various mineral substances suspended in saline provides a convenient means for

comparison of relative carcinogenicity. In response to the principal
types of asbestos, hamsters have shown a lesser incidence of mesotheliomas than rats, but, as might be expected from the shorter life
span of hamsters, mesotheliomas tend to appear earlier in them than
in rats.

The earliest tumor that we considered a mesothelioma was found in a
hamster examined 151 days after injection of 25 mg chrysotile. In
contrast, the earliest mesothelioma reported in rats by WAGNER and
BERRY (1969) was at 353 days after injection of 20 mg chrysotile,
and the earliest mesothelioma seen in rats by STANTON and WRENCH
(1972) appears to have been at about 350 days after implantation of
a glass pledget containing 40 mg amosite. In tests of UICC crocidolite
at 10 mg, STANTON and WRENCH's data from rats show the earliest mesothelioma at about 560 days when the material was injected in saline
and about 525 days after implantation in a glass pledget, whereas
our test of 10 mg UICC crocidolite in hamsters gave the first mesothelioma at 418 days. By the intrapleural route, the hamster thus
appears to afford a more rapid test model than the rat.

Since tests for carcinogenicity are customarily run over the life span
of test species, the rate at which results can be obtained is of practical importance. To learn whether mice might give useful information
more rapidly than hamsters, we made intrapleural injections of 5 mg
UICC crocidolite suspended in saline into 40 male BALB/c mice. Intrathoracic tumors were found in 3 of these mice at 301, 301, and 340
days. These 3 tumors resemble plasma cell tumors that have been reported in BALB/c mice after intraperitoneal injection of Plexiglass
borings, Plexiglass discs, Millipore filters, or mineral oil (POTTER,
1968). Plasma cell tumors have been reported in White Leghorn fowls
after introduction of tremolite into axillary air sacs (PEACOCK and
PEACOCK, 1966).

Both pleural and peritoneal mesotheliomas have been reported in female
CBA mice after subcutaneous injection of massive (60-mg) amounts of
asbestos in divided doses (ROE et al., 1967). Among 5 groups of 20
mice treated with crocidolite, amosite, or chrysotile there were 6
mice with sarcomas at injection sites and 10 mice with mesotheliomas.
These were distributed among the treatment groups. The lesions diagnosed as mesotheliomas appear to have been small papillomatous proliferations of mesothelial cells. Heavy deposits of fibers were seen
in submesothelial tissues of mice with mesotheliomas. It was thought
that fibers had been actively transported from the subcutaneous site
to the submesothelial site, but subsequent studies by the same group
did not provide evidence for this. Passive movement of fibers along
tissue planes or as a consequence of inflammation and necrosis is now
thought the more probable explanation (ROE, personal communication,
1974).

Discussion

The literature on tumors induced by intraperitoneal injection of
various plastic, metallic and other materials has been reviewed by
HUEPER (1964a) and HUEPER and CONWAY (1964). Discussions of mechanisms
of carcinogenesis by this route and comparison of results of tests by
other routes has been presented by BISCHOFF and BRYSON (1964) and
BRYSON and BISCHOFF (1967, 1969). Most of the tumors reported as experimentally induced at intraperitoneal sites have been sarcomas in

rats. After intraperitoneal implantation of polyurethan foam into Bethesda black rats, HUEPER (1964b) reported tumors including an unspecified number of mesotheliomas, but he also states that peritoneal mesotheliomas occur spontaneously in rats of this strain.

Induction of sarcomas in rats after intraperitoneal injection of asbestos was reported by SCHMÄHL (1958).

KLOSTERKÖTTER and ROBOCK (1970) reported experiments in which they made intraperitoneal injections of 50 mg asbestos into groups of 30 rats. With preparations containing fibers up to 50 μm in length, they found fibrosis in response to chrysotile, amosite, and crocidolite. Mesotheliomas were said to have been found in 2 rats of the group on amosite and in 4 rats of the group on crocidolite. No tumors were found in the chrysotile group. In other groups treated with these 3 samples of asbestos after further milling, there was little fibrogenicity and no tumors. Most particles in these milled products were said to be less than 1 μm in size. The animals were observed for periods of 6 to 12 months.

POTT et al. (1972) reported results from groups of 30 female Wistar rats given 4 intraperitoneal injections of 25 mg UICC chrysotile A or the same material after further milling. Samples were suspended in saline and injected at weekly intervals. The animals were followed for periods up to 2 years. Extensive adhesions were found in the peritoneal cavity of animals given UICC chrysotile but only slight fibrosis in those that had received the milled product. The incidence of tumors was about 40% in both groups, but the first tumor was found at 7 months in the group on UICC chrysotile in contrast to 13 months for the milled product. Most of the tumors were diagnosed as sarcomas but 7 were listed as mesotheliomas.

After intraperitoneal injections of groups of 40 female rats with 6.25 mg, 25 mg, and 100 mg chrysotile, POTT and FRIEDRICHS (1972) found 17, 19, and 16 animals, respectively, with abdominal tumors within 530 days. This apparent plateau of response suggests to us that dose-response studies using intraperitoneal injection may require lesser doses than the intrapleural route. Since the surface area of the peritoneum is much more extensive than the surface area of the pleural cavity, larger numbers of mesothelial cells are at risk.

In testing materials for carcinogenicity in animals, evaluations depend upon observation of tumors of types or at sites not found in controls, or at a frequency or speed of appearance greater than seen "spontaneously" in untreated control animals. For studies on mesotheliomas, there is only limited information on their spontaneous incidence or pathology in animals. A transplantable mesothelioma has been reported in a mouse (SHAPIRO and WARREN, 1949). A mesothelioma was listed among tumors seen in untreated control hamsters (FORTNER, 1961). As mentioned above, both pleural and peritoneal mesotheliomas have been said to occur spontaneously in Bethesda black rats (HUEPER and PAYNE, 1962; HUEPER, 1964b). MORRIS et al. (1961) state that papillary mesotheliomas of the testes or epididymis occurred in 3 Buffalo rats fed N-2-fluorenylacetamide and in 2 untreated control Buffalo rats. Pathologic material from these and other Buffalo rats was studied by H.L. STEWART (personal communication, 1974) who advises that he had not seen spontaneous pleural mesotheliomas but that he had seen mesotheliomas arise spontaneously in that strain from an extension of the peritoneal mesothelium (tunica vaginalis of the testis). He states that these tumors are papillary, sometimes tubular, and they occasionally spread to the peritoneal cavity. In a discussion of spontaneous lesions of rats, RIBELIN and MCCOY (1965)

state that they have seen small papillary tumors along the genital
omentum and serosal surface of the testis or epididymis. The legend
for their photograph of one such tumor describes it as a mesothelioma.
They state that histologically these tumors appear benign and that
they may be found in rats of a number of strains, but most often in
ACI, Buffalo, and om strains.

The cited reports of spontaneous mesotheliomas emphasize need for untreated controls and open avenues for exploration of etiologic mechanisms in testing chemicals for carcinogenicity in cavities lined by
mesothelial tissues. Multiple mesotheliomas have been described in
chickens after injection of MC29 avian leukosis virus (CHABOT et al.,
1970). Resemblance of these virus-induced mesotheliomas in chickens
to cases of multiple mesotheliomas seen in hamsters after injection
of asbestos suggests the possibility that carcinogenic effects of
chemicals associated with mesotheliomas may depend upon stimulation
of a virus (SMITH, in press).

References

BISCHOFF, F., BRYSON, G.: Carcinogenesis through solid state surfaces.
   Prog. exp. Tumor Res. 5, 85-133 (1964).
BRYSON, G., BISCHOFF, F.: Silicate-induced neoplasms. Prog. exp.
   Tumor Res. 9, 77-164 (1967).
BRYSON, G., BISCHOFF, F.: The limitations of safety testing. Prog.
   exp. Tumor Res. 11, 100-133 (1969).
CHABOT, J.F., BEARD, D., LANGLOIS, A.J., BEARD, J.W.: Mesotheliomas
   of peritoneum, epicardium, and pericardium induced by strain MC29
   avian leukosis virus. Cancer Res. 30, 1287-1308 (1970).
CHURG, J., SELIKOFF, I.J.: Geographic pathology of pleural mesothelioma. In: The Lung (A.A. Liebow, D.E. Smith, eds), pp. 284-297.
   Baltimore: Williams and Wilkins 1968.
DONNA, A.: Experimental asbestos tumors induced by chrysotile, crocidolite and amosite in Sprague-Dawley rats. Med. d. Lavoro 61 (1),
   1-32 (1970).
FORTNER, J.C.: The influence of castration on spontaneous tumorigenesis in the Syrian (golden) hamster. Cancer Res. 21, 1491-1498
   (1961).
GROSS, P.: Tumors of the pleura induced with asbestos and fibrous
   glass. J. nat. Cancer Inst. 51, 315-320 (1973).
HUEPER, W.C.: Experimental studies in metal cancerigenesis. I. Nickel
   cancers in rats. Tex. Rep. Biol. Med. 10, 167-186 (1952).
HUEPER, W.C.: Experimental studies in metal cancerigenesis. Tissue
   reactions in rats and rabbits after parenteral introduction of sus-
   pensions of arsenic, beryllium, or asbestos in lanolin. J. nat.
   Cancer Inst. 15, 113-129 (1954).
HUEPER, W.C.: Experimental studies in metal cancerigenesis. IV.
   Cancer produced by parenterally introduced metallic nickel. J. nat.
   Cancer Inst. 16, 55-73 (1955).
HUEPER, W.C.: Macromolecular agents as benign and malignant cell pro-
   liferants. Nat. Cancer Inst. Monograph No. 14, 357-377 (1964a).
HUEPER, W.C.: Cancer induction by polyurethan and polysilicone
   plastics. J. nat. Cancer Inst. 33, 1005-1028 (1964b).
HUEPER, W.C., CONWAY, W.D.: Chemical Carcinogenesis and Cancers.
   Springfield, Ill.: Charles C. Thomas 1964.
HUEPER, W.C., PAYNE, W.W.: Experimental cancers in rats produced by
   chromium compounds and their significance to industry and public
   health. Amer. ind. Hyg. Ass. J. 20, 274-280 (1959).

HUEPER, W.C., PAYNE, W.W.: Experimental studies on chromium compounds. Proceedings of the 13th International Congress on Occupational Health, N.Y., Book Craftsmen Ass., pp. 473-486, 1960.

HUEPER, W.C., PAYNE, W.W.: Experimental studies in metal carcino-genesis: chromium, nickel, iron, arsenic. Arch. Environ. Health $\underline{5}$, 445-462 (1962).

HUEPER, W.C., ZUEFLE, J.H., LINK, A.M., JOHNSON, M.G.: Experimental studies in metal cancerigenesis. II. Experimental uranium cancers in rats. J. nat. Cancer Inst. $\underline{13}$, 291-306 (1952).

KLOSTERKÖTTER, W., ROBOCK, K.: Experimentelle Untersuchungen zum Wirkungsmechanismus von Asbest unter besonderer Berücksichtigung der Faserlänge. Schriftenreihe Arbeitsmedizin, Sozialmedizin, Arbeits-hygiene $\underline{36}$, 111-130 (1970).

MORRIS, H.P., WAGNER, B.P., RAY, F.E., SNELL, K.C., STEWART, H.L.: Comparative study of cancer and other lesions of rats fed N,N'-2,7-fluorenylenebisacetamide or N-2-fluorenylacetamide. National Cancer Inst. Monograph $\underline{5}$, 1-54 (1961).

PEACOCK, P.R., PEACOCK, A.: Asbestos induced tumours in fowls. In: Lung Tumours in Animals (L. Severi, ed.), pp. 571-588. Perugia 1966.

POTT, F., FRIEDRICHS, K.H.: Tumoren der Ratte nach i.p.-Injektion faserförmiger Stäube. Naturwissenschaften $\underline{59}$, 318 (1972).

POTT, E.F., HUTH, F., FRIEDRICHS, K.H.: Tumoren der Ratte nach i.p.-Injektion von gemahlenem Chrysotil und Benzo(a)pyrene. Zbl. Bak-teriologie, Parasitenkunde, Infektionskrankheiten und Hygiene, I Abt. Orig., Reihe B $\underline{155}$, No. 5-6, pp. 463-469 (1972).

POTTER, M.: A resume of the current status of the development of plasma-cell tumors in mice. Cancer Res. $\underline{28}$, 1891-1896 (1968).

RIBELIN, W.E., MCCOY, J.R.: The Pathology of Laboratory Animals, p. 268. Springfield, Ill.: Charles C. Thomas 1965.

ROE, F.J.C., CARTER, R.L., WALTERS, M.A., HARINGTON, J.S.: The pathological effects of subcutaneous injections of asbestos fibres in mice: Migration of fibres to submesothelial tissues and induc-tion of mesotheliomata. Int. J. Cancer $\underline{2}$, 628-638 (1967).

ROE, F.J.C.: personal communication, 1974.

SCHMÄHL, D.: Cancerogene Wirkung von Asbest bei Implantation an Ratten. Z. Krebsforsch. $\underline{62}$, 561-567 (1958).

SHAPIRO, D.M., WARREN, S.: Cancer Innervation. Cancer Res. $\underline{9}$, 707-711 (1949).

SMITH, W.E.: Asbestos, talc and nitrites in relation to gastric cancer. Amer. ind. Hyg. Ass. J. $\underline{34}$, 227-228 (1973).

SMITH, W.E.: Multiple pulmonary carcinomas and mesotheliomas in hamsters. In: Multiple Primary Malignant Tumours (L. Severi, ed.), Perugia, in press.

SMITH, W.E., HUBERT, D.D., BADOLLET, M.S.: Biologic differences in response to long and short asbestos fibers. Amer. ind. Hyg. Ass. J. $\underline{33}$, A162 (1972).

SMITH, W.E., HUBERT, D.D., MILLER, L., BADOLLET, M.S., CHURG, J.: Tests for threshold levels of carcinogenicity of asbestos. In: Internationale Konferenz über die biologischen Wirkungen des As-bestes (Anspach, ed.), pp. 240-242. Dresden 1968.

SMITH, W.E., MILLER, L., CHURG, J., SELIKOFF, I.J.: Mesotheliomas in hamsters following intrapleural injection of asbestos. J. Mt. Sinai Hosp. $\underline{32}$, 1-8 (1965a).

SMITH, W.E., MILLER, L., ELSASSER, R.E., HUBERT, D.D.: Tests for carcinogenicity of asbestos. Ann. N.Y. Acad. Sci. $\underline{132}$, 456-488 (1965b).

SPEIL, S., LEINEWEBER, J.P.: Asbestos minerals in modern technology. Environ. Res. $\underline{2}$, 166-208 (1969).

STANTON, M.F., WRENCH, C.: Mechanisms of mesothelioma induction with asbestos and fibrous glass. J. nat. Cancer Inst. $\underline{48}$, 797-821 (1972).

STEWART, H.L.: personal communication, 1974.

TIMBRELL, V.: Characteristics of the International Union Against
   Cancer Standard Reference Samples of Asbestos. In: Proceedings
   International Conference on Pneumoconiosis, pp. 28-36. Johannes-
   burg 1969.
WAGNER, J.C.: Experimental production of mesothelial tumours of the
   pleura by implantation of dusts in laboratory animals. Nature 196,
   180-181 (1962).
WAGNER, J.C.: The induction of tumours by intrapleural inoculations
   of various types of asbestos dust. In: Lung Tumours in Animals
   (L. Severi, ed.), pp. 589-606. Perugia 1966.
WAGNER, J.C., BERRY, G.: Mesotheliomas in rats following inoculation with asbestos. British J. Cancer 23, 567-581 (1969).
WAGNER, J.C., BERRY, G., TIMBRELL, V.: Mesotheliomata in rats after
   inoculation with asbestos and other materials. Brit. J. Cancer 28,
   173-185 (1973.

Localized Submucosal Bronchial Injections of Carcinogens in Dogs*

Masahiko Okita, Arthur H. Cohen, and John R. Benfield

Departments of Surgery and Pathology, Harbor General Hospital, Torrance, CA 90509, USA

ABSTRACT

The carcinogens, 3,4-benzo(a)pyrene (BaP) in ferric oxide or N-nitroso-N-methylurea (NMU), were injected into the submucosa of the same endobronchial site at weekly intervals in 2 sets of mongrel dogs. Weekly bronchoscopic photography was used to record gross changes, and monthly punch biopsies were taken from the injection sites.

12 dogs were followed. Half had 9 to 15 injections each of 90 mg BaP-ferric oxide, and half had 6 to 9 injections each of 30 mg to 45 mg NMU. 3 dogs died 7 to 12 weeks after the first injection of carcinogen, and 9 continue to be followed, including 5 in the BaP-ferric oxide group and 4 in the NMU group. This report includes results up to 24 weeks after the first injections of BaP-ferric oxide, and up to 16 weeks following the first injections of NMU.

Edema, bronchostenosis, and mucosal irregularities, grossly consistent with neoplasia as it appears bronchoscopically in humans, regularly developed following BaP-ferric oxide injections. Squamous metaplasia accompanied by submucosal inflammation, fibrosis, and pigment deposition was invariably found 8 to 12 weeks after the initial injection of carcinogen. After NMU injections, similar changes were observed but they were slower to occur than after BaP-ferric oxide. Mucosal ulceration, as well as delayed healing of biopsy sites, were among the gross features produced by NMU. All 9 currently surviving dogs have significant mucosal metaplasia.

We conclude that direct recurrent transbronchoscopic submucosal injections of carcinogens is feasible and practical in dogs. The rapidity and reliability with which localized bronchial squamous metaplasia developed suggest that we may be producing a canine lung cancer model.

Introduction

Although the need for innovative research with lung cancer is generally recognized, and the potential value of a large animal bronchogenic carcinoma model is obvious, such a model does not now exist. STAUB and BEATTIE (1965) attempted to produce a canine lung cancer model by

*This project was supported by Grant No. CA 16201, awarded by the National Cancer Institute, and by Grant No. RR 05551, awarded by the Division of Research Resources DHEW.

direct application of carcinogens into the tracheobronchial tree of dogs, but their success was limited. PARK et al. (1972) observed pulmonary neoplasia in beagle dogs after chronic radiation exposure from a plutonium source. The neoplasms produced were not infrequently malignant, but they were certainly not analogous to lung cancers found in humans. Most previous work with experimental pulmonary carcinogenesis has been in small animals such as rats, mice, and hamsters. For example, SAFFIOTTI et al. (1968, 1972) instilled 3,4-benzo(a)pyrene attached to ferric oxide particles into the tracheobronchial tree of Syrian golden hamsters and by this method induced multicentric squamous cell carcinoma in the lungs. N-nitroso-N-methylurea also caused squamous cell carcinomas of the upper respiratory tract in hamsters when instilled intratracheally (HERROLD, 1970), but these tumors were also multicentric and peripheral. The experiments reported here seek to induce specifically localized central pulmonary cancers in dogs analogous to bronchogenic carcinoma in humans.

Materials and Methods

The carcinogens were 3,4-benzo(a)pyrene (BaP) and N-nitroso-N-methylurea (NMU). The BaP was added to equal weights of ferric oxide. The BaP-ferric oxide (Lung Cancer Segment, Carcinogenesis Program, National Cancer Institute) was suspended in normal saline at a concentration of 30 mg/ml. The NMU (Ash-Stevens Company, Detroit, Michigan) was dissolved in saline immediately prior to use either at a concentration of 15 mg/ml or 10 mg/ml, depending upon the stage of the experiment as will be described later.

The experimental groups consisted of randomly selected mongrel dogs weighing 13.6 kg to 26.4 kg. Carcinogens were injected into the submucosa of the proximal end of the right intermediate (accessory) lobe bronchus. Control injections were made into the submucosa at the origin of the diaphragmatic (lower) lobe bronchus of the left lung. The location of the injections is shown in Fig. 1. Group I dogs had weekly submucosal endobronchial injections of 3 ml (90 mg) of BaP-ferric oxide until a total of 1.35 g had been delivered in 15 injections. Because no carcinogen was injected at the time of monthly bronchial biopsies, a total of 20 weeks elapsed between the first and last injections of carcinogen. Control injections into the left tracheobronchial tree of Group I dogs were 3 ml (45 mg) of ferric oxide. Group II dogs had submucosal endobronchial injections of 3 ml of NMU at weekly intervals until a total of 0.510 g of carcinogen had been injected into the right side. For the first 10 weekly injections, a concentration of 15 mg/ml was used, and thereafter the concentration was decreased to 10 mg/ml. No carcinogen was injected at the time of monthly biopsies and to date, 16 weeks have elapsed between the first and last injections of NMU. The weekly injections in this group are currently continuing. The control injections in Group II dogs consisted of 3 ml of normal saline.

The technique for injection of carcinogens required bronchoscopy under general anesthesia with sodium thiopentol, 10 mg/kg, after premedication with ketamine hydrochloride, 10.0 mg/kg. Visualization of the precise location for the site of injections (or biopsies) was accomplished with a rigid fiberoptic telescope (Machida Endoscope Company, Tokyo, Japan). A long, 23 gauge esophageal varices needle (Pilling Company, No. 50-7455) was used to deliver the solutions into the bronchial submucosa.

CANINE PULMONARY CARCINOGENESIS

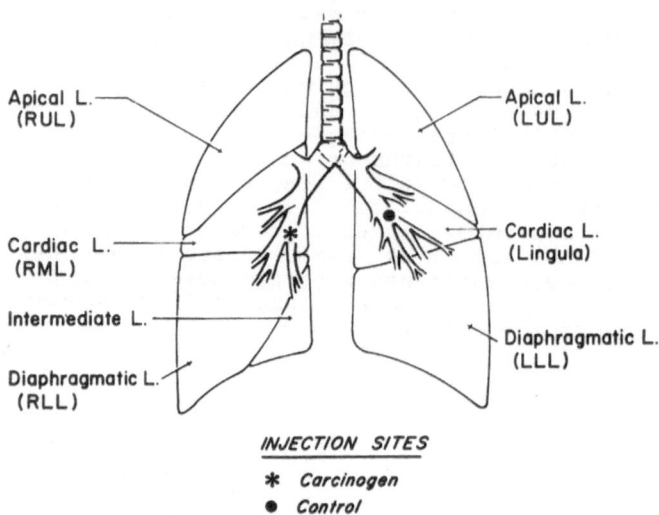

INJECTION SITES

* Carcinogen
● Control

<u>Fig. 1.</u> Sites for submucosal endobronchial injections: Carcinogens were injected at the origin of the right intermediate (accessory) lobes, and control injections were at the origin of the left dia-phragmatic (lower) lobes

The following tests were done before accepting each dog into the study: hemaglobin, hematocrit, total and differential blood leukocyte count, blood chemistries by the use of the simultaneous multiple analyzer (SMA-12), chest x-ray, bronchoscopy, bronchophotography, and biopsy of the proposed injection site. Bronchoscopic biopsies were made with 2 mm forceps of the type usually used with flexible bronchoscopes. Brushings for cytologic examinations were also obtained. All tests were repeated at monthly intervals following the first injection of carcinogens.

Specimens for light microscopy were fixed in 10% neutral buffered for-malin, processed in the usual manner for the preparation of microscopic slides and stained with hematoxylin and eosin.

Results

Our experience with localized submucosal endobronchial injection of single carcinogens in mongrel dogs is summarized in Table 1. We began with 12 dogs, 6 in Group I (BaP ferric oxide) and the remaining 6 in Group II (NMU carcinogen). For causes to be detailed later, 1 dog in Group I died after 9 injections of carcinogen, and 2 dogs in Group II were lost after 7 and 8 injections of NMU, respectively. Although other dogs were added to Groups I and II in order to substitute for the 3 dogs lost in the course of the experiments, these substitutions were too recent to add meaningful data to this report. Therefore, 9 dogs from the original group constitute the current follow-up group beyond 8 weeks after the first injections of carcinogens. The blood tests and chest x-rays obtained as part of the baseline studies, and serially thereafter, remained within normal limits. The bronchial brushing cytologies added nothing to the biopsy data and the remainder of this report will therefore focus upon the bronchoscopic findings and biopsy results.

The endobronchial changes which occurred at the point of injections of carcinogens included mucosal edema, stenosis of the lobar bronchus, and mucosal irregularities consistent with neoplasia. Although each of these changes occurred to some degree in many of the dogs within 4 weeks after the first injection of carcinogens, relatively few significant gross abnormalities were observed before the fourth week after the initial injections. We shall use the word significant to refer to mucosal edema and irregularities that were quite obvious and not subtle. Severe is used to denote changes characterized as extreme. With reference to narrowing of the bronchial lumens, significantly stenotic bronchi were 25% to 75% narrowed. Severely stenotic bronchi were less than 25% patent, or more than 75% narrowed. Stenoses of lesser degrees were generally due to edema, apparent by gross observation of blunted interbronchial spurs.

Group I includes 6 dogs injected endobronchially with BaP-ferric oxide. Results are given in Table 2 and illustrated in Figs 2 and 3. Within 2 weeks after the initial injection, 2 of these dogs (No. 388 and 354) had significant bronchial stenosis. This was primarily due to edema and inflammation. Within 4 weeks, 4 dogs (No. 388, 354, 375, and 378) had grossly apparent bronchial abnormalities at the injection site and 2 (No. 375 and 378) had squamous metaplasia. Those dogs initially having mucosal changes but no squamous metaplasia exhibited hyperplasia of columnar cells. When present, this change appeared a variable period of time prior to the development of squamous metaplasia. By the eighth week, 4 dogs (No. 375, 378, 388, and 421) had squamous metaplasia at the site of injection of carcinogen. In addition to the alterations of the mucosa, abnormalities were evident in the submucosa. By 4 weeks, all dogs had an acute inflammatory reaction characterized by edema, fibrin, and polymorphonuclear leukocyte infiltration. Large deposits of ferric oxide pigment generally were present in the connective tissue but little of it was in macrophages (Fig. 2b). By the time of the bronchial biopsy, 12 weeks after the first injection, all dogs had squamous metaplasia. At the time of this biopsy, 1 dog (No. 397) suffered an anesthetic death. At autopsy, this animal had squamous metaplasia of the lining epithelium and of some bronchial glands at the site of instillation. Pigment in the submucosa and chronic inflammation were also evident. Although patches of bronchopneumonia were present in the right diaphragmatic (lower) lobe, they were considered sufficient to enhance anesthetic risk but not enough to cause death.

The remaining 5 dogs in Group I all displayed significant gross endobronchial abnormalities and all showed evidence of squamous metaplasia on all subsequent bronchial examinations and biopsies. The metaplasia was characterized by typical squamous cells with intercellular bridges and regular, orderly, stratified maturation. At times, however, abnormal maturation as manifested by large, hyperchromatic nuclei in all layers of cells, mitotic figures, and absence of progressive flattening of superficial cells, was evident (No. 375 at 12 weeks, No. 354 at 20 weeks). Once noted, the atypical features (Fig. 4) did not always persist in subsequent biopsies; squamous metaplasia however, once present, did not regress. Although the inflammation process persisted, the intense infiltrate with polymorphonuclear leukocytes was, for the most part, replaced by lymphocytes and few plasma cells. Additionally, beginning with the sixteenth week, dense fibrosis with

Table 1. Summary of experience with localized submucosal endobronchial injections of carcinogens in mongrel dogs

| | | | | Status Last Biopsy | | | | |
| | | | | Gross | | Microscopic | | |
Carcinogen	Dog Number	Number Injections	Number Biopsies	Stenosis	Irreg.	Inflamm.	Fibrosis	Squamous Metaplasia
BaP-ferric oxide	375	15	6	++[a]	++	yes	yes	yes
	378	15	6	++	++	yes	yes	yes
	388	15	6	+[b]	++	yes	yes	yes
	354	15	6	++	++	no	yes	yes
	421	15	6	+	++	yes	yes	yes
	397	9[c]	2	++	++	yes	no	yes
NMU	456	13	4	+	++	yes	no	yes
	464	12	4	+	++	yes	no	yes
	468	13	4	+	++	yes	yes	yes
	471	11	4	0	+	yes	no	no
	455	7[c]	1	+	0	yes	no	no
	465	8[c]	2	0	0	yes	no	no

[a] Severe.
[b] Significant.
[c] Dog died, autopsy findings in text.

Table 2. Incidence and evolution of significant abnormality[a] after localized submucosal endobronchial injection of carcinogens in dogs

Carcinogen	Finding	Time following first injection (weeks)							
		2	4	6	8	12	16	20	24
BaP-ferric oxide Group I	I. Stenosis	2/6	2/6	5/6	5/6	6/6	5/5	5/5	5/5
	A. Inflammation	N.A.[b]	6/6	N.A.	6/6	6/6	4/5	4/5	4/5
	B. Fibrosis	N.A.	0/6	N.A.	0/6	0/6	3/5	3/5	3/5
	II. Mucosal Irregularity	0/6	1/6	3/6	4/6	4/6	5/5	5/5	5/5
	A. Squamous Metaplasia	N.A.	2/6	N.A.	4/6	6/6	5/5	5/5	5/5
NMU Group II	I. Stenosis	2/6	3/6	3/6	1/6	1/4	2/4		
	A. Inflammation	N.A.	5/6	N.A.	5/5	4/4	4/4		
	B. Fibrosis	N.A.	0/6	N.A.	0/5	0/4	1/4		
	II. Mucosal Irregularity	0/6	0/6	1/6	0/5	1/4	2/4		
	A. Squamous Metaplasia	N.A.	1/6	N.A.	1/5	3/4	3/4		

[a] Significant abnormality as defined in text.
[b] Not applicable. No biopsy done.

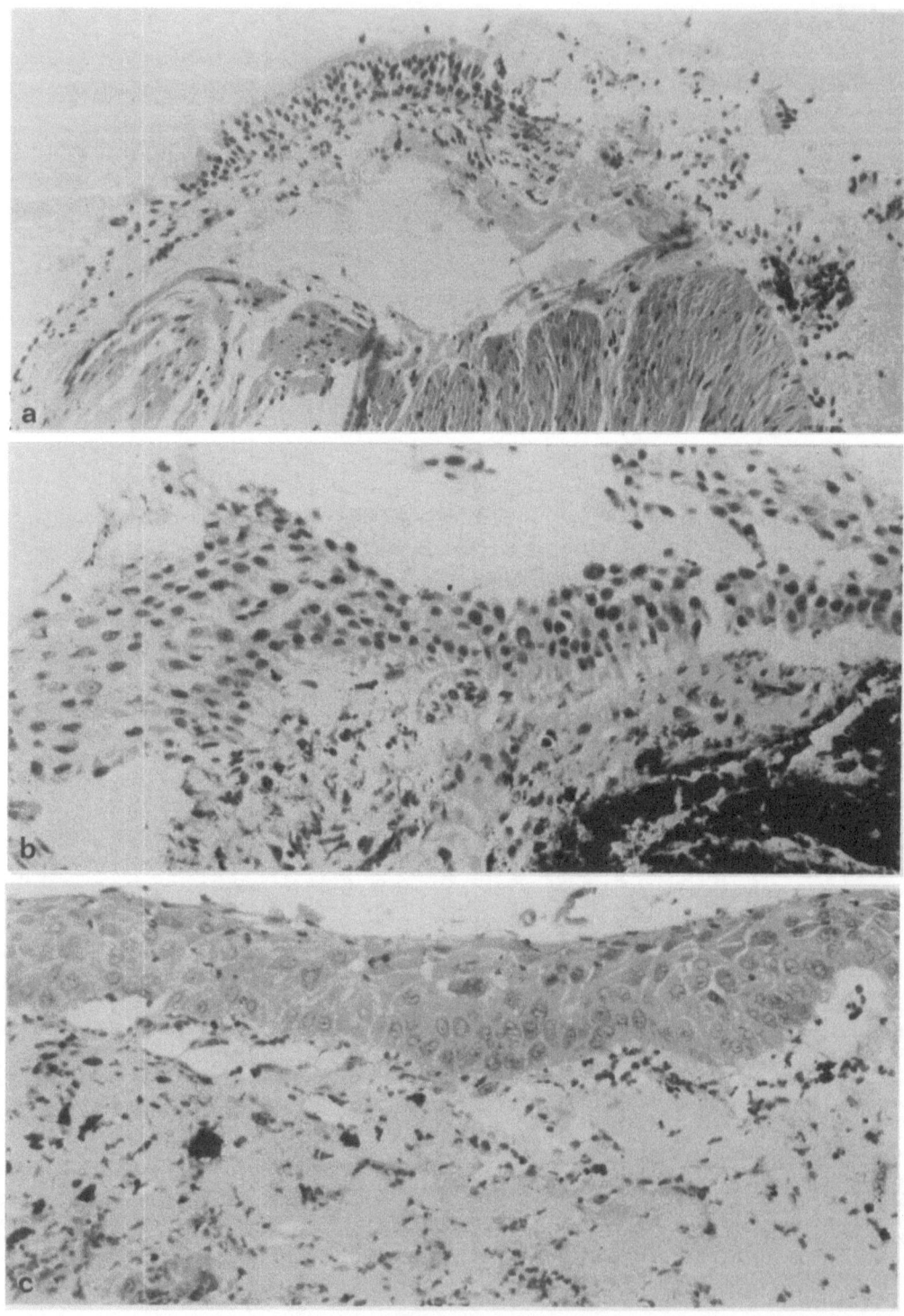

Legend see opposite page

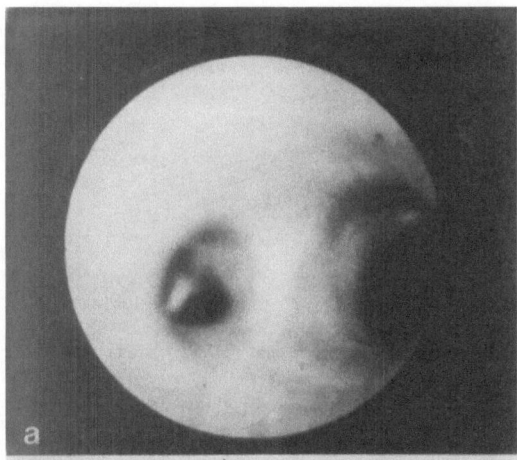

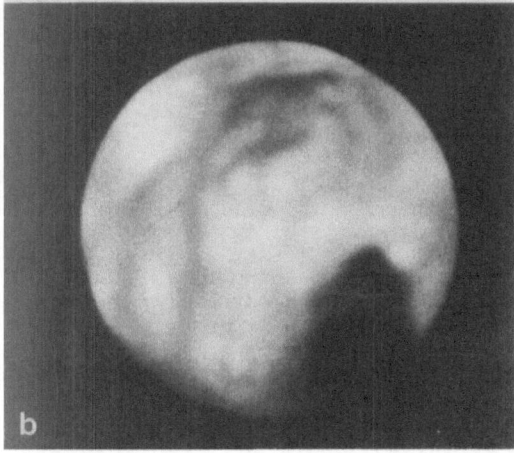

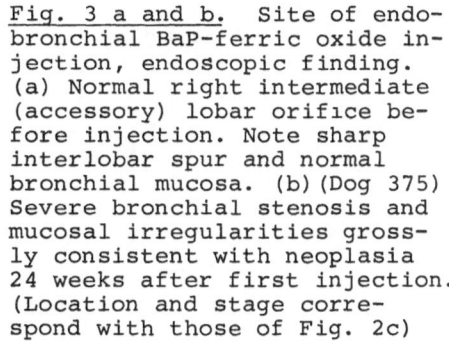

Fig. 3 a and b. Site of endobronchial BaP-ferric oxide injection, endoscopic finding.
(a) Normal right intermediate
(accessory) lobar orifice before injection. Note sharp
interlobar spur and normal
bronchial mucosa. (b)(Dog 375)
Severe bronchial stenosis and
mucosal irregularities grossly consistent with neoplasia
24 weeks after first injection.
(Location and stage correspond with those of Fig. 2c)

expansion and deformity of the submucosa became evident in 3 of the
dogs (No. 375, 378, and 421). It is clear that bronchostenosis at
this point was due primarily to fibrosis and secondarily to edema
and inflammation. By 24 weeks all dogs were similarly affected, and
the most severe exhibited "hyalinization" of the submucosa. While
many large "lakes" of ferric oxide pigment remained, beginning at
the twelfth week much of the pigment was noted in macrophages.

At the present time, as summarized in Table 1, bronchi injected with
BaP-ferric oxide grossly show irregular mucosa covering a narrow
distorted lumen. The mucosa is exuberant and gross findings are consistent with but not diagnostic of neoplasia. Corresponding to this,

Fig. 2. Site of endobronchial BaP-ferric oxide injections. (a) Bronchial biopsy shows normal epithelium, submucosa and muscularis. HE
(x 100). (b)(Dog 378) Bronchial biopsy shows early squamous metaplasia
and large amount of submucosal ferric oxide not ingested by macrophages. HE (x 160). (c)(Dog 375) Bronchial biopsy shows well defined
squamous metaplasia, ferric oxide in macrophages, dense submucosal
fibrosis, and residual inflammation. HE (x 100)

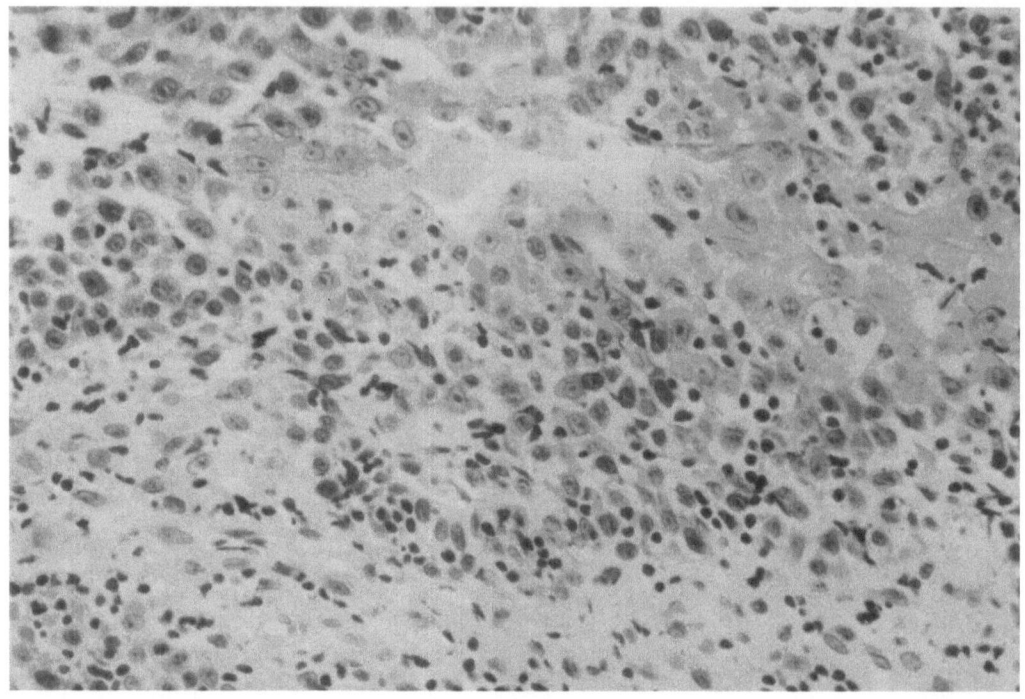

Fig. 4. (Dog 375) Bronchial biopsy shows squamous metaplasia with mild cellular atypia 8 weeks after first BaP-ferric oxide injection. HE (x 200)

the microscopic appearance is that of nonkeratinized, stratified squamous epithelium covering an expanded scarred submucosa containing scattered acute and chronic inflammatory cells and ferric oxide pigment mainly within macrophages (Fig. 2c).

The sites of control injections of ferric oxide in saline in the contralateral lungs of all animals have remained grossly normal, and biopsies from these sites uniformly have revealed normal mucosa and submucosa except for deposits of ferric oxide pigment.

Group II includes 6 dogs injected endobronchially with NMU. These data are given in Tables 1 and 2 and illustrated in Fig. 5. Edema and

Fig. 5. The site of endobronchial NMU injections (Dog. 468) biopsy results. (a) Bronchial biopsy 8 weeks after first injection shows submucosal edema and mild inflammation. There are no significant mucosal abnormalities. HE (x 100). (b) Bronchial biopsy 12 weeks after first injection shows well developed squamous metaplasia and inflammation primarily in the submucosa. HE (x 100). (c) Bronchial biopsy 15 weeks after first injection shows metaplastic epithelium with mild acute and chronic inflammation of the submucosa. HE (x 100).

Note that despite the rather prompt appearance of quite impressive gross abnormalities after NMU injections, squamous metaplasia did not occur as promptly as after BaP-ferric oxide injections as shown in Fig. 2

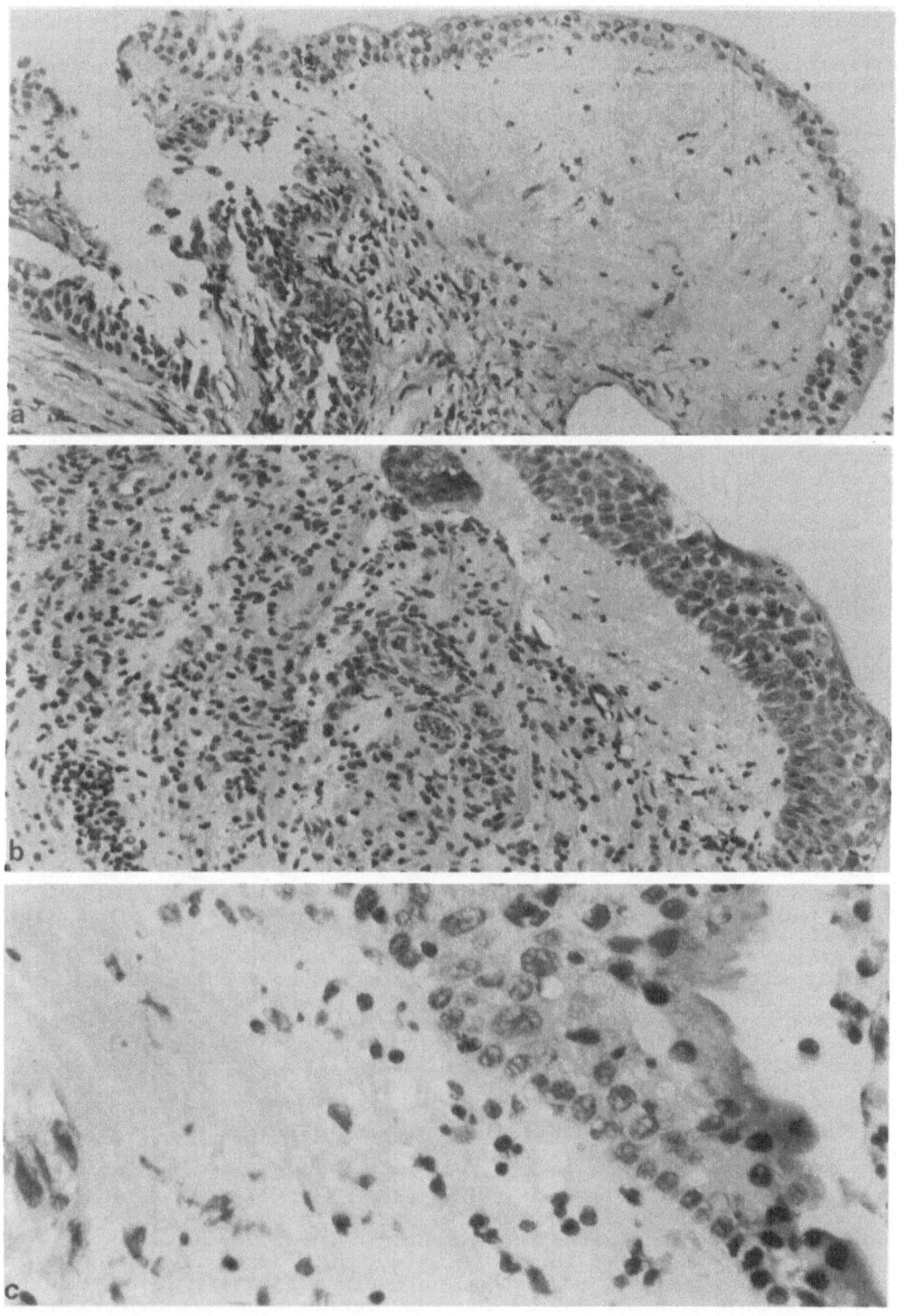

Legend see opposite page

stenosis developed promptly in some dogs, but mucosal irregularities were usually not grossly observed until 12 weeks after the first injections of carcinogen. There was delayed healing of defects caused by biopsies. Squamous metaplasia was noted in 1 dog (No. 465) after 4 weeks and columnar hyperplasia in 2 dogs by 8 weeks. 2 dogs (No. 455 and 465) died 7 and 8 weeks after the first injections of NMU. These dogs expired with similar anatomic findings: there were no abnormalities of mucosal cells, but considerable chronic inflammation was present at the injection sites. Extensive intraalveolar, septal, and perivascular edema with small areas of superimposed fresh hemorrhage and early bronchopneumonia were present in all portions of both lungs. Vascular abnormalities or other anatomic etiologies of this process were undetected either in the lungs or in other organs. Following these deaths, we decreased the concentration of NMU from 15 mg/ml to 10 mg/ml. 2 more dogs (No. 464 and 471) developed squamous metaplasia within 12 weeks at which point 3 of the 4 remaining dogs in this group had significant metaplasia. At the time of this report all of the surviving 4 animals have developed metaplasia. At the last biopsy, 1 dog (No. 471), who had previously shown squamous metaplasia, displayed columnar hyperplasia. Whether this denotes regression of the lesion or merely sampling error has not been determined, although the latter possibility seems likely. In all dogs, an acute and chronic inflammatory infiltrate has been noted in the submucosa, appearing at 4 weeks and remaining through the duration of the experiment to date. In 1 dog (No. 468), submucosal fibrosis was noted at the 16 week biopsy. Thus, the abnormalities observed in NMU treated dogs was less promptly seen than in BaP-ferric oxide treated animals, but both carcinogens caused similar changes.

The sites of control injections of saline into the contralateral bronchial mucosa and submucosa remain normal grossly, and biopsies of these sites showed no abnormalities.

Discussion

Experiments with pulmonary carcinogenesis in animals can be approached either from the viewpoint of evaluating exposures thought to be oncogenic or with the aim of producing models for studies relevant to bronchogenic carcinoma in humans. Although lung cancer is unfortunately common enough in man so that one could fruitfully limit one's attention to patients, we believe that studies in humans and in animals should proceed simultaneously. There can be no argument against the fact that animals can be subjected to trials that would be inappropriate for patients, and it is clear that new information relevant to pulmonary oncogenesis and the management of lung cancer in humans could be derived from a good large animal model.

We have chosen dogs for our experiments because they can undergo essentially all the diagnostic and therapeutic procedures used for patients. Furthermore, previous experiments in our laboratory fortuitously identified 1 canine lobar bronchus apparently free of significant ventilatory collaterals with other lobes (DREWS et al., 1974). We believe this bronchus is therefore particularly well suited for efforts to induce lung cancer in a specific location and that the success of our efforts could provide a unique opportunity to follow pulmonary carcinogenesis serially. The central origin of this bronchus has therefore been selected for the recurrent submucosal injection of proven carcinogens under direct vision; to our knowledge this approach has not been used before. Although BEATTIE and STAUB (1961) instilled carcinogen into canine lower lobe bronchi under direct vision, they used a different carcinogen and did not use submucosal injection.

Lacking precedent, the selection of techniques and dosages was empiric and inferred from the experience of SAFFIOTTI et al. (1968, 1972) and HERROLD et al. (1970). The mechanics of submucosal transbronchoscopic injection have presented little difficulty, but it is noteworthy that the depth of the submucosal injections is clearly a variable and that a small amount (about 0.1 ml) of spill into the distal tracheobronchial tree is almost unavoidable. The concentration of BaP-ferric oxide we selected has been maintained constant throughout the experiments, and the contralateral control injections of ferric oxide produced no significant changes other than the deposition of submucosal pigment. At the time of writing, injections of BaP-ferric oxide have been suspended in order to observe the further evolution of the squamous metaplasia induced. The NMU, known to be a locally direct acting substance that causes ulceration (HERROLD, 1966), led to the apparent death of 2 dogs when employed in concentration of 15 mg/ml, but when the concentration was decreased to 10 mg/ml, it was well tolerated. To investigate the apparent reason for this difference between the tolerance to the 2 concentrations of NMU is outside the scope of our current aims, and we have therefore not pursued this question of dosage further. In summary, concerning the techniques we have selected, it is apparent that they are simple for anyone skilled at endoscopy, that they permit localized submucosal delivery of carcinogens, and that the changes induced were not the result of the repeated trauma of injections and biopsies. Furthermore, we can say with assurance that the 2 mm biopsies made at monthly intervals were neither large enough nor sufficiently numerous inadvertently to excise the total area in which carcinogens had been injected.

The changes observed grossly at the sites of endobronchial injections are worthy of comment beyond the illustrations and the factual information presented earlier in this publication. As might be expected, although gross abnormalities appeared at varying rates in different dogs, there was consistency of pattern both within each group of dogs and between the 2 groups of animals injected with different carcinogens. The BaP-ferric oxide initially caused edema manifested primarily by blunted interbronchial spurs. Within the third month after the initial injection, incomplete bronchial stenosis, appearing grossly more substantive than simple edema, and inflammation began to appear. Thereafter, the sites of injections began to have mucosal irregularities and heaped-up exuberant tissue grossly consistent with neoplasia. By way of contrast, in addition to edema and blunted spurs, the NMU very soon produced grossly, rather impressive, ulcerating endobronchial lesions at the sites of injection. However, to date the microscopic signs of neoplasia from NMU injections have been less impressive than after the injections of BaP-ferric oxide, and NMU injection sites have also differed grossly from those of BaP-ferric oxide in that biopsy defects in the NMU dogs had delayed healing. The progression of changes induced by NMU is in general agreement with the work of HARRIS et al. (1971, 1973), who studied Syrian golden hamsters and also compared the effects of NMU and BaP-ferric oxide. They did not, however, describe the submucosal abnormalities we have seen. There are perhaps the result of submucosal injections of carcinogens and may therefore be a feature of our preparation, more so than in other models which have been studied. Microscopic findings after the 2 carcinogens showed that submucosal edema, inflammation, and fibrosis have been less pronounced after NMU than following BaP-ferric oxide.

In general, we can say that gross findings correlated remarkably accurately with microscopic findings. The mucosal abnormalities we observed by bronchoscopy were reflected by biopsy findings such as hyperplasia, metaplasia, and atypia that were quite similar to changes described by HARRIS et al. (1971, 1973) in their work with hamsters. They first noted epithelial hyperplasia, either preceding or coexisting with squamous metaplasia, followed by metaplastic alterations culminating in neoplasia after a period of atypia. In part, we have been able to reproduce their microscopic results in dogs, and we have added the dimension of serial gross observations by bronchoscopy.

While we have not produced cancers as yet, squamous metaplasia has uniformly been induced. We assume that dogs with squamous metaplasia on their first biopsy after injections of carcinogens had already passed through the hyperplastic phase. Although 3 of our dogs displayed atypical squamous metaplasia, the atypia apparently was transient, for subsequent biopsies have failed to disclose it again. Additionally, in dogs, we have not yet observed true neoplastic cellular proliferation of the type seen in hamsters, but the elapsed time since the onset of our experiments is a smaller portion of the life span of dogs than of hamsters. Besides the mucosal changes, we have documented and serially recorded abnormalities of the submucosa. We have confirmed the observations of HARRIS et al. (1973) that ferric oxide alone does not induce mucosal changes, and we have also noted that the submucosal response is to the carcinogens rather than to ferric oxide alone or the result of the trauma of recurrent injections.

It is neither possible nor fruitful to speculate regarding the future for the preparation we have described. Clearly, we have not yet produced lung cancer in dogs but it is encouraging that we have been able to cause squamous metaplasia so reliably and in such a localized fashion. This makes tenable the unproven hypothesis that squamous cell cancers will eventually evolve. When we are successful, we hope to have reproducible localized squamous cell carcinomas in dogs analogous to those in humans. The new research vistas that such a preparation would make available are indeed exciting.

Acknowledgement

We wish gratefully to acknowledge the help and encouragement we have received from Dr. MICHAEL B. SPORN and Dr. HAROLD L. STEWART of the National Cancer Institute, and from Dr. S.W. NIELSEN of the University of Connecticut. The dedicated technical assistance of EDWIN SHORS, M.A. and THOMAS JENSEN, B.S. is greatly appreciated.

References

BEATTIE, E.J., Jr., STAUB, E.W., CORRELL, N., HASS, G.: Bronchogenic carcinoma produced experimentally in the dog. J. thorac. cardio. Surg. 42, 615-622 (1961).
DREWS, J.A., SHIMADA, K., WHITE, P.H., BENFIELD, J.R.: The pulmonary alveolar macrophage in lung transplantation. Transplantation 17, 319-322 (1974).
HARRIS, C.C., KAUFMAN, D.G., SPORN, M.B., SAFFIOTTI, U.: Histogenesis of squamous metaplasia and squamous cell carcinoma of the respiratory epithelium in an animal model. Cancer Chemother. Rep., Part 3, 4, 43-54 (1973).

HARRIS, C.C., KAUFMAN, D.G., SPORN, M.B., SMITH, J.M., JACKSON, F., SAFFIOTTI, U.: Ultrastructural effects of N-methyl-N-nitrosourea on the tracheobronchial epithelium of the Syrian golden hamster. Int. J. Cancer $\underline{12}$, 259-269 (1973).

HARRIS, C., SPORN, M., KAUFMAN, D., SMITH, J., BAKER, M., SAFFIOTTI, U.: Acute ultrastructural effects of benzo(a)pyrene and ferric oxide on the hamster tracheobronchial epithelium. Cancer Res. $\underline{31}$, 1977-1989 (1971).

HERROLD, K.M.: Carcinogenic effect of N-methyl-N-nitrosourea administered subcutaneously to Syrian hamsters. J. Path. Bact. $\underline{92}$, 35-41.

HERROLD, K.M.: Upper respiratory tract tumors induced in Syrian hamsters by N-methyl-N-nitrosourea. Int. J. Cancer $\underline{6}$, 217-222 (1970).

PARK, J.F., BAIR, W.J., BUSCH, R.H.: Progress in beagle dog studies with transuranium elements at Battelle-Northwest, Vol. 22, pp. 803-810. Northern Ireland: Health Physics Pergamon Press 1972.

SAFFIOTTI, U., CEFIS, F., KOLB, L.H.: A method for the experimental induction of bronchogenic carcinoma. Cancer Res. $\underline{28}$, 104-124 (1968).

SAFFIOTTI, U., MONTESANO, R., SELLAKUMAR, A.R., CEFIS, F., KAUFMAN, D.G.: Respiratory tract carcinogenesis in hamsters induced by different numbers of administrations of benzo(a)pyrene and ferric oxide. Cancer Res. $\underline{32}$, 1073-1081 (1972).

STAUB, E.W., EISENSTEIN, R., HASS, G., BEATTIE, E.J., Jr.: Bronchogenic carcinoma produced experimentally in the normal dog. J. thorac. cardio. Surg. $\underline{49}$, 364-372 (1965).

Studies of Intrabronchial Particle Deposition Using Hollow Bronchial Casts*

Richard B. Schlesinger, Vicki R. Cohen, and Morton Lippmann

Institue of Environmental Medicine, New York University Medical Center, New York, NY 10016, USA

ABSTRACT

The dose to the bronchial epithelium from inhaled carcinogens is unknown. One major reason is that the distribution of the deposited
particles along the bronchial tree has never been adequately determined. We are studying the γ-tagged particle deposition at various
levels in a hollow tracheobronchial tree cast, prepared from a freshly excised human lung, which extends to airways of 2 mm diameter. Three
multiple convergent channel ("focusing") collimators permit measurements in individual airway segments along the bronchial tree. Monodisperse ferric oxide microspheres tagged with ^{99m}Tc are "inhaled" by
the cast which is used repeatedly in tests with various flowrates and
particle sizes. Estimates of the average surface doses to the bronchial
epithelium along the tube lengths and at the bifurcations have been
obtained.

Hollow casts have also been used to determine the deposition patterns
of tantalum powder aerosols used for inhalation bronchography. In this
study, the objective was to determine the optimum flowrate and powder
size for uniform airway coatings deposited during voluntary mouthpiece
breathing.

A. Introduction

Respiratory carcinogens are found in cigarette smoke and in industrial
and community atmospheres, sometimes as droplets of pure materials but
usually as components of otherwise inert particulates. Laboratory
studies have determined many of the biological and chemical properties of some of these carcinogens and general host responses to their
inhalation. Yet the exact dose to the bronchial epithelium is unknown .
because the distribution of deposited particles along the tracheobronchial tree has never been adequately determined. Any realistic dosimetric model must reflect the selective deposition characteristics at
various levels of the tracheobronchial tree, since dose to target
tissues depends upon the amount and distribution of inhaled material
which deposits and is retained at various sites.

*Work described in this paper was supported by NIEHS Grant No. ES-00881
and NCI Contract No. G-73-3855. It is part of a center program supported by NIEHS Center Grant No. ES-00260.

Normally, the tracheobronchial cells are protected by a mucous layer which is propelled in a cephalad direction by beating cilia. Many inhaled irritants, which may coexist with airborne carcinogens, can interfere with the normal functioning of this mucous escalator, resulting in a slowing or actual stasis of mucous flow. The result is a prolonged retention of deposited particulates, causing an increase in both contact time with the epithelium and surface density as more particles accumulate. Increased retention of inhaled carcinogens enhances cell-carcinogen contact, and increases the probability of their interaction. Thus, the incidence of respiratory tract cancer depends on both the concentration of airborne carcinogens and on their pattern of regional deposition. A detailed knowledge of this deposition pattern will permit a better understanding of the relation of carcinogenicity to those characteristics of the inhaled aerosol and respiratory tract which play a role in controlling effective dose to the tissues.

Since the pattern of deposition of inhaled aerosols depends upon particle aerodynamics and anatomical and functional characteristics of the respiratory tract, an experimental system which allows detailed analyses of these parameters is needed. The complex geometry of the tracheobronchial tree cannot be adequately described by any available mathematical model; experimental test systems which accurately reproduce the bronchial structure, while allowing precise control and/or monitoring of the other factors which control deposition, are required for experimental determinations of the deposition pattern.

We have developed a method for the systematic study of particle deposition in human airways, using hollow casts prepared from lungs removed postmortem. Each cast has a unique and constant anatomy. Thus, a test series may be performed to determine the effects of particle aerodynamics and flow rate without the variability due to anatomical differences between lungs inherent in *in vivo* and excised lung studies. Different casts may be used under identical exposure conditions to examine the effects of anatomical variation upon the deposition pattern. In this laboratory, we have used such casts for two different studies: 1. for the determination of the intrabronchial distribution pattern of deposited aerosols and the fractional deposition efficiencies at various branching levels within the tracheobronchial tree, and 2. for the study of the deposition of radioopaque tantalum powder aerosols used in experimental inhalation bronchography.

B. Radioscan Studies of Particle Deposition Patterns

I. Background

There have been very few reports of deposition studies using hollow casts of the human airways. Casts of various areas of the respiratory tract were used by PROETZ (1951) and ERMALA and HOLSTI (1955) to provide a qualitative description of the deposition of cigarette smoke fractions. NELSON and STUART (1970) passed uranium mine aerosols through hollow rubber replicas of a teaching model of the first few generations of the tracheobronchial tree; the model was then cut into sections and deposited activity measured in each. A similar measurement technique was used by MARTIN and JACOBI (1972) to study the deposition of submicron radioactive aerosols in hollow idealized plastic models of the tracheobronchial tree extending through the segmental bronchi.

The method developed in this laboratory consists of the use of collimated NaI scintillation detectors to view small sections of the tracheobronchial tree systematically, following exposure of the cast to radio-
actively-tagged aerosols under various constant "inspiratory" flow
schemes. The aerosols consist of ferric oxide microspheres tagged with
the short-lived (T 1/2 = 6 hr), γ-emitting radioisotope ^{99m}Tc. Use of
a scanning measurement technique with a short-lived isotope allows
each unique cast to be used repeatedly for tests under various exposure conditions. The aerosols are produced by one of two methods:
1. by a spinning disk generator for particles with aerodynamic diameters $\geq$ 1 μm ($\sigma g \leq$ 1.1) (LIPPMANN and ALBERT, 1967), or 2. by an Environmental Research Corporation atomizer-impactor generator for those in
the 0.3 μm range ($\sigma g \sim$ 1.6) (WHITBY et al., 1965). The cast is suspended
within a Plexiglas "artificial thorax" during exposure to test aerosol, while a constant flow is drawn through it. Prior to each test,
the cast is coated with a thin layer of silicone oil to simulate the
mucus.

In a previous publication (SCHLESINGER and LIPPMANN, 1972), we described the deposition at each branching level for 1.7 μm to 12.2 μm
(aerodynamic diameter) particles at 30 liters/min in 3 Silastic casts
extending from the trachea through the segmental bronchi. The deposition pattern was determined by scanning the casts using a 1 inch diameter NaI scintillation detector with a 1 cm x 3 cm slit collimator.

In a more detailed study, currently in progress, we are using an improved collimated detection system and hollow laryngeal casts in
series with hollow silicone rubber tracheobronchial tree casts extending to airways of 2 mm diameter.

II. Preparation of The Hollow Casts

Tracheobronchial tree casts are prepared by pouring melted wax (a
mixture of Freeman Manufacturing Company waxes 120A and 120B) into
lungs which have been fixed in formalin fumes at approximately 3/4
total lung capacity and then air-dried (BLUMENTHAL and BOREN, 1959).
After the wax hardens, the tissue is dissolved in NaOH and the wax
cast pruned up to branches no smaller in diameter than 2 mm. The
length, midpoint diameter, and branching angle were measured for each
branching segment of this wax cast. A unique identification number
was assigned to each branch, using the binary numbering system of
PHALEN et al. (1974).

The hollow cast was made by coating the wax with a clear silicone
rubber (Dow-Corning Dispersion Coating 92-009). The cast was placed
in an oven and the wax core allowed to run out. All bronchial endings
were then opened. The hollow cast is very flexible and allows bend-
ing without breakage. A photograph of this cast is shown in Fig. 1.

A realistic system for depositon studies should include the larynx
but, since the shape of the glottis and its associated structures
changes with respect to the velocity of inspiration, laryngeal geometry should not be constant if a range of flow rates is to be used.
Based upon single cineradiograph frames of laryngeal and vocal cord
movement during various types of inspiratory breathing patterns and
radiograms and tomograms of the larynx (NEGUS, 1947; GRANT, 1951;
ARDRAN et al., 1953; FINK et al., 1956; MEYERSON, 1964), 3 hollow
larynxs were modeled from a cadaveric larynx, with the true and false
vocal cords representative of their geometry at the ranges of inspiratory flow rates used in this study.

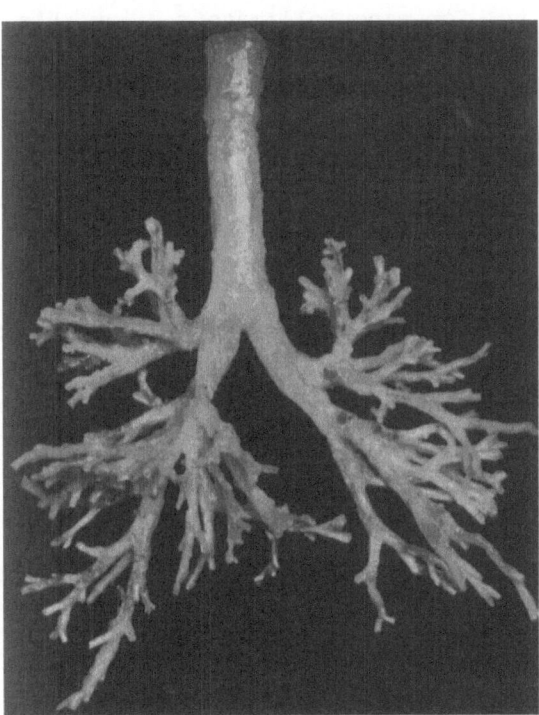

Fig. 1. Photograph of the hollow cast used in current radioscan studies

III. Measurement of The Distribution of Deposited Particles

The accurate, extensive mapping of the distribution of deposited activity within a cast using short-lived isotopes necessitates relatively short counting times, high statistical reliability, and good spatial resolution. These factors are limited by the sensitivity and field of view characteristics of the collimated detector. A new collimator design was developed, since the slit collimator used previously was inadequate for viewing very small areas with great sensitivity.

Although all collimators make some compromise between resolution (breadth of response) and sensitivity (counts per minute per unit activity), properly designed multiple convergent channel ("focusing") collimators offer the best compromise for volume scanning (NEWELL et al., 1952; FRANCES et al., 1955). This type of collimator consists of a block of shielding material, e.g., lead, containing many channels separated by septa and angled so that projections of the fields of view of all of the channels become superimposed at a certain distance, the focal length, from the front face of the collimator. Sensitivity and resolution are maximal around the focus; the former depends primarily upon the number of channels, and the latter on channel diameter.

A characteristic of focusing collimators is that they exhibit a certain "depth of field", i.e., their response is fairly constant and the resolution high over a certain volume within the focal region. This "volume focus" characteristic is essential for the current work, since the bronchi being analyzed are not flat sources in 1 plane but, as with any volume source, may be considered to be surfaces of activity in different planes. It is necessary to be able to detect activity from deposits which are both on the near and far side of the crystal face, preferably with equal sensitivity. Focusing collimators allow this to be done while viewing the sample from only 1 direction.

Three collimators for a 3 inch diameter NaI scintillation detector, having channels of 1.0 cm, 0.5 cm, and 0.2 cm diameter respectively, were designed and constructed for the current test series. The channels are arranged in a hexagonal array around a center hole.

The total volumetric response of each of the collimators was determined by analyzing the response to a point source of ^{99m}Tc moved systematically within the field of view in both the lateral and longitudinal directions with respect to the collimator axis. Point source response data are fundamental measures of a collimator's performance and completely determine the spatial resolution for collimators such as these, where response is symmetrical around the collimator axis. The count rate at each point was recorded and then expressed as a percent of the maximum rate. Points exhibiting equal count rates were joined to give isoresponse contours of the collimator's field of view (Fig. 2); these contours are actually cross sections of isoresponse surfaces which are cylindrically symmetrical about a vertical axis through the center of the collimator. Each branch segment which is to be analyzed is placed at a specific working distance in front of the collimator face such that the entire segment volume falls within the volume defined by the 90% contours. Thus, all of the aerosol which deposited on the entire section will be counted with ≥ 90% efficiency.

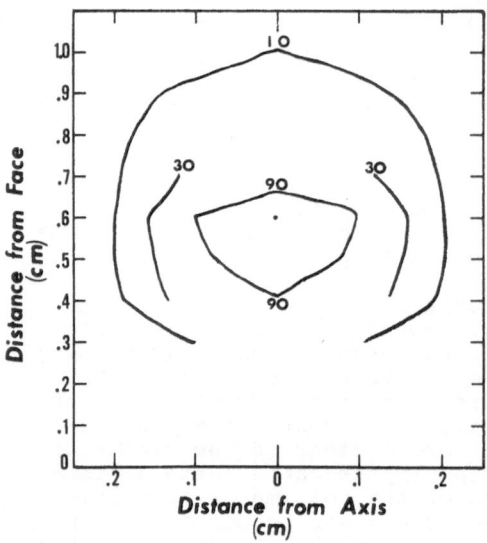

Fig. 2. Isoresponse contours of the 127-channel (0.2 cm channel diameter) collimator for a point source of ^{99m}Tc in air

The photomultiplier signals are processed by a 100-channel pulse height analyzer, and read out through a serial converter which sums only those pulses corresponding to the major peak of γ-emission from ^{99m}Tc and rejects pulses from background and scattered photons. The detector itself and the hollow casts are housed within a specially designed low background chamber.

Each branching segment in which deposition is measured is divided into two kinds of regions, i.e., "length" and "bifurcation", for which separate measurements are made. The "length" region of relatively long branches is further divided into two or more counting regions. The diameter of the branch section determines the collimator which is used to measure deposited activity.

All bronchi with diameters ≥ 0.5 cm are analyzed. For branches with smaller diameters a statistical sampling technique was used to select those to be counted, so as to give an accurate and realistic portrayal of the deposition profile along the cast. The total cast contains 432 bronchial segments and, of these, deposited activity was routinely measured in 83. Separate analysis of bifurcations and lengths and separation of longer segments into more than I counting region resulted in a total of 160 separate counting sections.

IV. Selective Deposition, Dose, and Cancer Pathogenesis

One of the applications of deposition data obtained from casts is the comparison of deposition sites to sites of cancer origin.

In a previous study (SCHLESINGER and LIPPMANN, 1972), the mean deposition efficiencies for 1.7 μm to 12.2 μm particles in the 5 lobar bronchi were compared with data from several studies (SIMONS, 1937; FRIED, 1948; GARLAND, 1961; GARLAND et al., 1962) which reported the frequency of involvement of each of these lobar bronchi as sites of origin of primary bronchial carcinoma. A correlation was found between deposition efficiency and frequency of involvement as a site of cancer origin. Particles in the same size range make up a large part of the mass in atmospheric aerosols in the many cities where pollution is dominated by combustion of coal and fuel oil (PASCERI and FRIEDLANDER, 1965).

The region within the tracheobronchial tree with the highest frequency of primary cancer extends from the main bronchi through the segmental bronchi. Within this area, cancers tend to originate at bifurcations (KOTIN and FALK, 1959; AUERBACH et al., 1961). SCHLESINGER and LIPPMANN (1972) and BELL (1974) showed that these branch points are sites of selective deposition, where surface concentrations of deposited particles may be quite high. In addition to being subjected to a heavy dose of carcinogen by direct deposition, HILDING (1957) suggests that branch points are regions of slower movement of the moving mucous blanket, which adds further to the residence time of carcinogens which deposit within these regions or are being carried through them on the moving mucus.

Data from the current test series strengthens the association between localized regions of selective deposition and primary cancer sites. New experimental data on the percentage of the deposition in a given airway segment of generations 1 through 4 which occurs in the region including the bifurcation under various exposure conditions are presented in Table 1.

In order to relate experimental deposition efficiency data for our hollow bronchial cast to actual dose to bronchial epithelium, the surface area over which the deposit is spread must be taken into account. Preliminary estimates of relative doses to tissues within the bifurcation regions of the high cancer risk bronchial generations have been calculated. The total deposition occurring within the bifurcation and length regions of generations 1 through 4 were divided by the respective total surface areas to give the average dose for

Table 1. Average percentage of deposition in an airway segment which occurs at the bifurcation under various exposure criteria

Generation[a]	15 liters/min[b]				30 liters/min	60 liters/min		
	7.0 μm[c]	4.4 μm[c]	3.1 μm[c]	0.28 μm[c]	0.26 μm[c]	8.0 μm[c]	4.8 μm[c]	2.6 μm[c]
1	42.9	41.3	40.1	32.8	38.2	60.4	52.1	58.1
2	61.3	53.2	64.0	63.1	51.6	68.3	48.1	65.3
3	63.7	59.1	55.9	56.3	55.1	72.9	55.5	53.1
4	55.9	56.0	46.3	38.9	38.7	62.8	60.2	58.7

[a] A generation represents the number of branchings below the trachea that itself is generation 0.
[b] Constant inspiratory flow.
[c] Aerodynamic diameter.

each region. The ratios of average dose to the bifurcation regions to
that along the tube lengths are presented in Fig. 3.

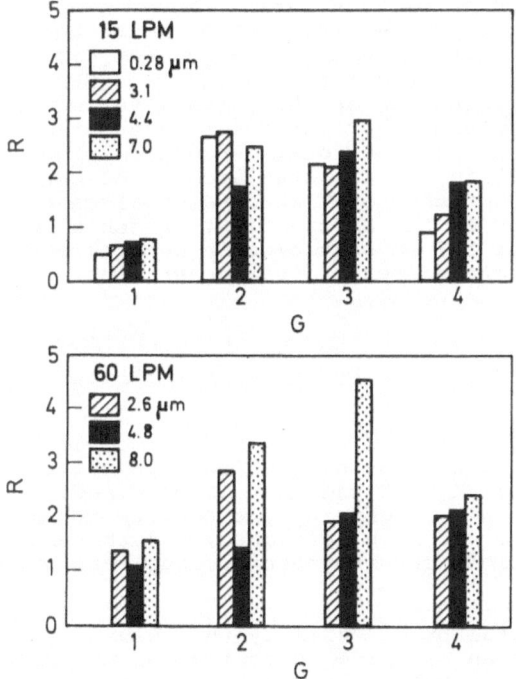

Fig. 3. Ratio (R) of average surface dose to bifurcation regions to the average surface dose to length regions for branching generations (G) 1 through 4

Generally, the average surface dose is lowest in generation 1, peaks
in generation 2 or 3, and then falls off in generation 4. This pattern
of relative dose is similar to the pattern concerning the sites of
cancer origin within this region. On the average, for every 10 primary
lung cancers, only 1 arises in the main bronchi (corresponds to generation 1), 6 arise in the lobar and segmental bronchi (corresponds to
generations 2, 3 and a small fraction of 4), and only 3 arise distal
to the segmental bronchi (most of generation 4, and beyond)(VEEZE,
1968). Thus, the primary sites of bronchogenic cancer are distributed
in a similar fashion to particle deposition sites within the tracheobronchial tree.

The 0.28 and 0.26 μm median diameter aerosols used in the current
study have distributions similar to that reported for cigarette smoke
(KEITH and DERRICK, 1960; PORSTENDÖRFER, 1971). As shown in Table 1,
these small particles also deposit preferentially at airway bifurcations. Thus, the local dose from cigarette smoke aerosol at the bifurcations within the high cancer risk bronchial generations may be
due primarily to direct particle deposition at these sites.

Since the actual deposition sites are not evenly distributed over the
entire surface area, the bifurcation regions include areas with surface densities both higher and lower than the average. Using an idealized model of the first bifurcation, BELL (1974) measured the concentration of latex particles deposited on the surfaces within this region. He found that the deposition was highest around the carina.

BELL's technique involves microscopic scanning of the surfaces and provides data on the distribution of particles as a function of distance from the carina, with a resolution of a fraction of a millimeter. Combining his fine structure deposition data with our quantitative assay of total deposition within the bifurcation region permits an integrated overview which neither technique alone can provide. We have applied the deposition pattern around the carina from BELL's profile contours to the actual surface area of the carinal region of the first bifurcation of our hollow cast. For particles in the range of 0.37 µm to 5.7 µm, from 67% to 94% of the total deposition within the bifurcation region occurred within a local area around the carina which accounted for only about 25% of the total internal surface area of the entire bifurcation. In terms of the entire first bronchial generation, 26% of the total deposit of 5.7 µm particles in generation 1 occurs in only 8% of the entire surface area of this generation.

C. Deposition of Radioopaque Aerosols for Inhalation Bronchography

Tantalum powder has recently been introduced as a contrast medium for bronchography which does not produce the side effects associated with currently used iodinated materials and one that is more radioopaque (NADEL et al., 1968). It is not in general use because routine delivery and exposure criteria have not been developed, and the exact amount of powder necessary for optimal bronchographic visualization is unknown.

The production of a clinically useful bronchogram by the voluntary inhalation of powdered tantalum is an exercise in controlled particle deposition. The ideal inhalation protocol would result in a fairly uniform coating of the bronchial tree down to about the eighth branching level with a minimum of penetration beyond the terminal bronchioles. This creates limitations with respect to the particle deposition mechanisms which may be utilized, inasmuch as a uniform surface distribution using currently available size fractions of tantalum powder may be obtained only by use of gravitational sedimentation. A study was performed to determine the patient position and breathing pattern which would favor production of the most uniform upper airway deposition pattern of tantalum and the minimum surface density of powder on the airways necessary for optimal bronchography.

An initial determination of the optimal inhalation protocol giving the desired deposition pattern was made by performing deposition calculations using various inspiratory flow rates and available tantalum powder size fractions. The protocol was then verified experimentally by exposing a cast of the larynx and tracheobronchial tree to tantalum under these calculated "optimal" conditions.

The initial experimental exposure conditions were a constant 8 liters/min inspiratory flow rate and a tantalum aerosol having a mass median aerodynamic diameter of 9.2 µm (σ_g = 1.41). The cast was exposed to the powder while in a horizontal position in order to maximize gravitational settling. The degree of uniformity obtained for a tantalum coated airway cast within a sugar-filled chest phantom is shown in Fig. 4. Tantalum clearly outlined unobstructed airways. Optimal visualization was found to require ~8 mg/cm^2 of powder, corresponding to a uniform layer 4.9 µm thick. Surface density was determined by washing out the tantalum powder from those branches having optimal radiographic visibility.

In our initial radiographs, a rice-filled Plexiglas thorax was used to simulate the chest cavity, and grains of rice became lodged in certain airways. After tantalum inhalation, these simulated "lesions" were clearly delineated. In some instances, rice caused complete occlusion of the airway. These occluded airways are seen as sites of unusually heavy deposits, and airways distal to them are relatively devoid of tantalum.

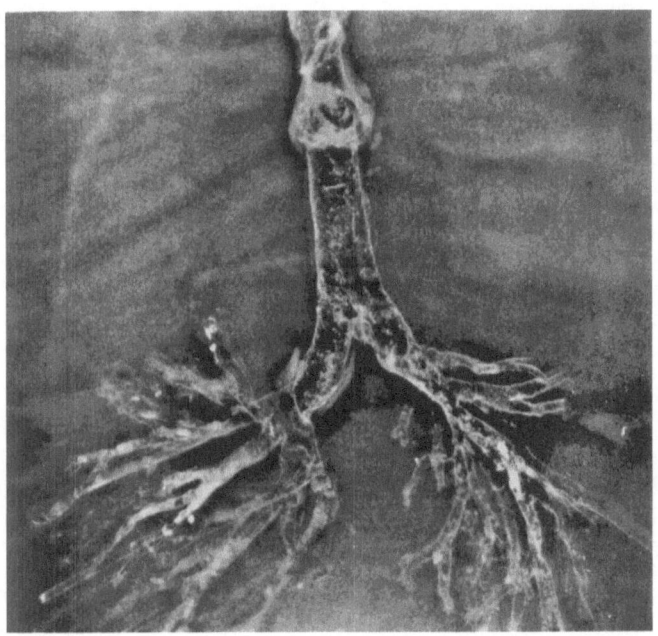

Fig. 4. Bronchogram of a hollow cast within a sugar-filled chest phantom. Note that rice grains partially occlude some airways and completely occlude others

Use of a hollow cast has allowed determination of the exact amount of deposition within specific bronchi and demonstrated that a suitably uniform surface density may be achieved by inhalation of preclassified powder under strictly controlled exposure conditions.

D. Conclusion: Hollow Casts as Systems for Studying Particle Deposition

Hollow casts of the human airways are excellent systems for the study of respiratory tract particle deposition mechanisms. Their use enables fine spatial resolution, allowing the detailed determination of intra-bronchial deposition patterns for any exposure condition, and they avoid a number of complications inherent in *in vivo* testing: variation in respiratory flow rate during exposure, counting errors of deposited particles due to large masses of adjacent tissue which absorb and scatter radiation, and the presence of extraneous counts from activity in the head and stomach.

Although casts are a very realistic system, they are not completely true to life. They have constant-caliber airways, while the bronchi actually change in diameter during a respiratory cycle. Intrathoracic pressure differentials *in vivo* influence the distribution of ventilation in the lungs and resultant distribution of particles being carried by the airstream. The presence of lower airways *in vivo*, which are not present in the cast, also influences the flow pattern in proximal airways. Yet, within these limitations systematic studies using casts provide a valuable complement to *in vivo* deposition studies. Coordination of the results will assist in the realistic interpretation of cast deposition patterns.

There are many additional studies which could be advantageously performed using hollow casts of the human airways. The effect of sinusoidally varying inspiratory flows during exposure to aerosols is of interest. Deposition could be studied in casts produced from diseased lungs, since pathology may change the normal geometry and air flow pattern, resulting in a shift in the deposition pattern. For therapeutic aerosols, the pattern of deposition may be critical in achieving the desired effects; deposition in normal lungs and its alteration in diseased ones must therefore be accounted for. The pattern of deposition of hygroscopic particles, such as those in cigarette smoke, could also be studied efficiently in casts.

The comprehensive study of respiratory tract carcinogenesis requires a multifaceted approach involving identification and analysis of specific carcinogens, study of target tissue metabolism and its relation to local tissue dose, study of the interaction of particulates with the lung, and, of course, determination of the sites of ultimate deposition since the primary requirement for exertion of any effect is deposition and retention within the lungs. The deposition pattern depends on many variables, and studies using hollow bronchial casts can help to clarify many of them.

References

ARDRAN, G.M., KEMP, F.H., MANEN, L.: Closure of the larynx. Brit. J. Radiol. 26, 497-509 (1953).
AUERBACH, O., STOUT, A.P., HAMMOND, E.C., GARFINKEL, L.: Changes in bronchial epithelium in relation to cigarette smoking and in relation to lung cancer. New Engl. J. Med. 265, 253-267 (1961).
BELL, K.A.: Aerosol deposition in models of a human lung bifurcation. Ph.D. Thesis. California Institute of Technology 1974.
BLUMENTHAL, B.J., BOREN, H.G.: Lung structure in 3 dimensions after inflation and fume fixation. Amer. Rev. Tuberc. 79, 764-772 (1959).
ERMALA, P., HOLSTI, L.R.: Distribution and absorption of tobacco tar in the organs of the respiratory tract. Cancer 8, 673-678 (1955).
FINK, B.R., BASEK, M., EPANCHIN, V.: The mechanism of opening of the human larynx. Laryngoscope 66, 410-425 (1956).
FRANCIS, J.E., Jr., BELL, P.R., HARRIS, C.C.: Medical scintillation spectrometry. Nucleonics 13, 82-88 (1955).
FRIED, B.M.: Bronchiogenic carcinoma and adenoma. Baltimore: Williams and Wilkins 1948.
GARLAND, L.H.: Bronchial carcinoma. Lobar distribution of lesions in 250 cases. Calif. Med. 94, 7-8 (1961).

GARLAND, L.H., BEIER, R.L., COULSON, W., HEALD, J.H., STEIN, R.L.:
The apparent sites of origin of carcinomas of the lung. Radiology
78, 1-11 (1962).

GRANT, J.C.B.: Respiratory system. In: Cunningham's Textbook of
Anatomy (J.C. Brash, ed.), pp. 685-726. London: Oxford 1951.

HILDING, A.C.: Ciliary streaming in the bronchial tree and the time
element in carcinogenesis. New Engl. J. Med. 256, 634-640 (1957).

KEITH, C.H., DERRICK, J.C.: Measurement of the particle size distribution and concentration of cigarette smoke by the conifuge. J.
Colloid Sci. 15, 340-356 (1960).

KOTIN, P., FALK, H.L.: The role and action of environmental agents in
the pathogenesis of lung cancer. I. Air pollutants. Cancer 12,
147-163 (1959).

LIPPMANN, M., ALBERT, R.E.: A compact electric-motor driven spinning
disc aerosol generator. Amer. ind. Hyg. Ass. J. 28, 501-506 (1967).

MARTIN, D., JACOBI, W.: Diffusion deposition of small-sized particles
in the bronchial tree. Hlth Phys. 23, 23-29 (1972).

MEYERSON, M.C.: The human larynx. Springfield, Ill.: C.C. Thomas 1964.

NADEL, J.A., WOLFE, W.G., GRAF, P.D.: Powdered tantalum as a medium
for bronchography in canine and human lungs. Invest. Radiol. 3,
229-238 (1968).

NEGUS, V.E.: Certain anatomical and physiological considerations in
paralysis of the larynx. Proc. Roy. Soc. Med. 40, 849-853 (1947).

NELSON, I.C., STUART, B.O.: Radon daughter deposition in the respiratory tract. In: Battelle Pacific Northwest Laboratory Annual Report,
Vol. II, pt. 2, p. 67. 1970.

NEWELL, R.R., SAUNDERS, W., MILLER, E.: Multichannel collimators for
gamma-ray scanning with scintillation counters. Nucleonics 10,
36-40 (1952).

PASCERI, R.E., FRIEDLANDER, S.K.: Measurement of the particle size
distribution of the atmospheric aerosol: II. Experimental results
and discussion. J. Atmos. Sci. 22, 577-584 (1965).

PHALEN, R.F., YEH, H.C., RAABE, O.G.: Animal models for inhalation
studies. Presented at American Industrial Hygiene Conference, Miami
Beach, Florida, 12-17 May, 1974.

PORSTENDÖRFER, J.: Untersuchungen zur Frage des Wachstums von inhalierten Aerosolteilchen im Atemtrakt. Aerosol Sci. 2, 73-79 (1971).

PROETZ, A.W.: Air currents in the upper respiratory tract and their
clinical importance. Ann. Otol. (St. Louis) 60, 439-467 (1951).

SCHLESINGER, R.B., LIPPMANN, M.: Particle deposition in casts of
the human upper tracheobronchial tree. Amer. Ind. Hyg. Ass. J. 33,
237-251 (1972).

SIMONS, E.J.: Primary carcinoma of the lung. Chicago: Year Book
Publishers 1937.

VEEZE, P.: Rationale and methods of early detection in lung cancer.
Assen: Van Gorcum and Co. 1968.

WHITBY, K.T., LUNDGREN, D.A., PETERSON, C.M.: Homogeneous aerosol
generators. Int. J. Air Water Pollution 9, 263-277 (1965).

The Distribution and Retention of Selected Metals in Rat Tissue after Inhalation of Cadmium Oxide Aerosols*

Phyllis D. Kaplan, M. Blackstone, and N. Richdale

The University of Cincinnati, College of Medicine, Department of Environmental Health, Kettering Laboratory, Cincinnati, OH 45219, USA

ABSTRACT

As part of a study to determine the binding of cadmium ions to cellular components of the lung and kidney after inhalation of its oxide aerosol, the retention and distribution of cadmium, zinc, and copper were measured as a function of exposure level and time. The animals were sacrificed on a periodic basis and their tissues analyzed for the metals with the aid of atomic absorption spectrophotometry. The retention of cadmium, based on calculations of the amount inhaled, was measured and found to be relative to the ambient concentration within the inhalation chamber. The concentrations of the metals in each organ were primarily related to the length of the exposure. Homogenization of each organ, followed by subcellular fractionation through differential centrifugation, was used to demonstrate the steady increase in concentration of all 3 metals within the cytoplasm of the cells.

A. Introduction

The relationship between elevated levels of cadmium in the lung and pulmonary emphysema or bronchitis has been noted for years (BAADER, 1951; FRIBERG, 1950; FRIBERG et al., 1971; HIRST et al., 1973a; SNIDER et al., 1973; KAZANTZIS et al., 1963). Most recently, SNIDER et al. (1973) experimentally induced centrilobular emphysema in rats with cadmium chloride aerosols. These studies, relating exposure to cadmium with lung disease, have not been followed by more detailed work directed towards elucidating the mechanisms of toxicity of cadmium in the lung.

Although several workers have followed the subcellular distribution of cadmium in a variety of organs and others have monitored its absorption into the blood stream and subsequent redistribution into other body compartments following other routes of administration, little information has been available on the absorption, internal distribution, and elimination of cadmium from the lung after inhalation exposures (SHAIKH and LUCIS, 1972a, 1972b; WEBB, 1972a, 1972b; NORDBERG et al., 1972; LUCIS et al., 1972; NORDBERG and PISCATOR, 1972; GRIFFIN, 1970).

*This work was sponsored by the National Institute of Occupational Safety and Health, Grant No. 2R01 OH 00347-04, Public Health Service, Department of Health, Education, and Welfare.

The present work was undertaken in order to evaluate the response of
the lung to cadmium oxide aerosols. Cadmium was measured after varying exposure periods and located with respect to its subcellular distribution and associations. Its subcellular distribution in the lung
was then compared with that occurring simultaneously in the kidney
so that respiratory absorption, distribution, and clearance could be
related to several parameters, amongst which, molecular binding and
organ pathology were considered the most important.

B. Materials and Methods

I. Experimental Animals

All animals used were white male Sprague-Dawley rats 3 months old
at the commencement of the inhalation experiments. Initial body
weights were ~200 g to 250 g and were about 450 g at time of death.

Animals were maintained in stainless steel cages in air conditioned
quarters on standard laboratory chow (Purina) with tap water ad libitum.

II. Reagents and Glassware

All chemicals used for analyses were ultra pure or reagent grade. All
water used was glass distilled 3 times. All glassware was boiled in
aqua regia, followed by rinsing in distilled water, soaking in 1%
(w/v) edetic acid, and rinsing again 5 to 10 times.

Buffers composed of (0.25 m) sucrose and (0.001 m) Tris, pH 7.4, were
prepared daily. Concentrated stock solutions of the metals and all
other solutions were prepared as previously described (KAPLAN et al.,
1973).

III. Inhalation Chambers and Aerosol Generation

The animal exposure chambers used (Young and Bertke, Cincinnati, Ohio)
possessed an internal volume of 12 ft^3 with a conical top feed and
bottom exit. The aerosols were generated by passing nebulized cadmium
acetate through a 600°C oxidation furnace. The effluent air stream was
cooled by a series of condensers, so that the final temperature entering the chamber ranged from 38°C to 45°C (HORSTMAN et al., 1973). The
effluent from the chamber was passed through an absolute filter prior
to venting. During the exposure periods, aerosol particles in a known
volume of air from the exposure chamber were collected on Millipore
filters for metal analyses by atomic absorption spectrophotometry. The
size distribution of the aerosol in the chamber was measured using a
7 stage Anderson impactor with the 47 mm Millipore backup filter
(FLESCH et al., 1967). All stages were analyzed for metals using
atomic absorption spectrophotometry. The chemical composition of the
particles was verified by x-ray analysis and electron spectroscopy
for chemical analysis (ESCA)(Dr. BILL MODDEMAN, University of Dayton).
Both methods demonstrated the absence of cadmium acetate. The analyses
performed with the aid of electron spectroscopy indicated that approximately 30% by weight of the oxide was present in a 2:1 ratio of cadmium to oxygen, rather than the 1:1 ratio expected.

IV. Preparation and Fractionation of Tissue

Using a previously published technique (KAPLAN et al., 1973), anaesthetized rats were opened and their lungs perfused through the heart with the homogenizing medium to remove the blood. The lungs were then washed via tracheal cannulation to remove alveolar macrophages, lung surfactant, and any remaining cadmium oxide particles. These were then stripped of the bronchi, rinsed, weighed, pressed, and homogenized. Kidneys were rinsed, weighed, and transferred directly to the cold homogenization medium. The respective organs for each experiment were pooled prior to homogenization and fractionation.

The homogenization and fractionation procedure was an adaptation of standard techniques (REISS, 1966; VATTER et al., 1968; O'HARE et al., 1971, UMBREIT et al., 1964; HOGEBOOM et al., 1948). The whole homogenate was subjected to differential centrifugation to separate the subcellular components. In the initial experiments, the excised lung or kidney tissue was homogenized in 9 volumes buffer. The homogenates were centrifuged at 1,000 g for 10 minutes, 1,700 g for 5 minutes, 12,000 g for 10 minutes, and 100,000 g for 60 minutes. The respective fractions were examined by light and electron microscopy for verification of morphological purity. In later work, the tissue was homogenized in 5 volumes of buffer followed by centrifugation at 10,000 g for 10 minutes and 100,000 g for 60 minutes. All fractions were lyophilized and weighed prior to further analyses. The final supernatant fractions were usually analyzed immediately but could be stored at -4°C without alteration in their metal concentrations.

V. Tissue Analyses

Metal analyses were performed on a Perkin-Elmer 403 Atomic Absorption Spectrophotometer equipped with a Boling triple slot burner and an air/acetylene flame. Sensitivity of the instrument for cadmium, zinc, and copper was 0.01 ppm at 1% absorption.

All tissue samples were solubilized with dimethyldidodecylammonium hydroxide (Soluene[100]) in toluene or tetramethylammonium hydroxide in methanol prior to analyses. Solubilization required 24 hours at 60°C in a shaking incubator (KAPLAN et al., 1973). After digestion the samples were diluted 2 1/2 times their volume with solvent and analyzed directly. The quantity of sugar present in the supernatants made solubilization in toluene impracticable. Instead, these fractions were hydrolysed in a 1:50 (w/v) ratio of 24% tetramethylammonium hydroxide and brought to volume with methanol. Reagent blanks and standard curves were analyzed concurrently. Both internal and external standards were used.

VI. Inhalation Experiments

The inhalation procedures used were those established by BINGHAM et al. (1968). Animals were housed within the chambers in compartmentalized stainless steel racks (1 compartment per rat) for the duration of the exposure period, after which they were returned to their regular quarters. Exposure periods lasted 7 to 8 hours per day, 5 days per week for a total duration of 1 1/2 to 9 months. Control rats for each experiment were simply maintained in their regular quarters for the duration of the experiment. Initial experiments were conducted on 10 control and 10 exposed animals. The numbers have been increased for the work in progress.

C. Results and Discussion

I. Precision of Analyses

The analytical procedure used permits a maximum precision of $\pm$ 3% for the metal analyses. The minimum varied from $\pm$ 10% to 15% on specific occasions. Table 1 illustrates this point. The fraction that has been chosen for illustration was the precipitate from centrifugation at 1,700 g, which contains some whole cells, larger cell fragments, and nuclei (see below). Since this was a relatively heterogeneous mixture and since all organs were pooled for sample analyses, the figures shown represent the average precision obtainable with this method. Zinc concentrations did not vary in this fraction of either organ after these short term exposures. The arithmetic mean for the summation of the control and exposed groups was 39.17 $\pm$ 1.83 µg/g and 57.53 $\pm$ 2.14 µg/g in the lung and kidney respectively.

II. Subcellular Distribution of Cadmium in Control and Exposed Groups

5 morphological entities were separated and defined by the homogenization and differential centrifugation process. They correspond to the same subcellular components widely cited in the literature (THIERS and VALLEE, 1957) and are as follows: fibrous connective tissue, whole cells and heavy fragments, nuclei and smaller cell fragments, mitochondria and lysosomes, microsomes, soluble supernatant (or, cytosol).

Although cadmium values in control animals were very low and subject to a great deal of statistical variation until the animals were 8 months old, it was clear that of the cadmium present in the lung and kidney before exposure, the vast majority resided in the fibrous tissue and cell membranes. Since the kidney contains relatively little fibrous material, the percentage of the total kidney cadmium in this fraction is concomitantly lower.

Once animals were exposed to the aerosol, cadmium was rapidly redistributed largely into the soluble supernatant where it reached a plateau in the lung after 6 months; however, it was still rising in the kidney at 9 months. Although the concentrations of cadmium in the lung and kidney fibrous tissue were increasing steadily with exposure, these fractions represented less than 15% of the lung total and less than 10% of the kidney total at any time. The other fraction that contained a substantial amount of cadmium by virtue of its weight was the heterogeneous mixture of cells, large fragment and nuclei; in the lung, the value rose from 10% to 30%; for the kidney, it decreased simultaneously with the increase noted above in the supernatant (45% to 16%).

III. Cadmium, Zinc, and Copper Distribution as a Function of Exposure to Cadmium Oxide Aerosols

Figs 1, 2, and 3 illustrate the changes in total and supernatant metal content for both organs with respect to time. Lacking paired control data for the last 2 exposure periods, it is difficult to assign a change in copper values related to cadmium oxide exposure (Fig. 3). In so far as data has been gathered for Fig. 2, there is a clear rise in the zinc content of the lung supernatant with that of cadmium. Zinc and cadmium values plateau at the same point in time. Since the cadmium content plateaus in the lung, Fig. 1 has been used to calculate its

Table 1. Analytical variation in metal concentrations[a] within a lung and kidney fraction[b] (arithmetic mean $\pm$ standard error)

Exposure Period, Weeks	Cadmium μg/g $\pm$ S.E.		Zinc μg/g $\pm$ S.E.		Copper μg/g $\pm$ S.E.	
	Lung	Kidney	Lung	Kidney	Lung	Kidney
Controls[c]						
–	0.78 $\pm$ 0.14	0.89 $\pm$ 0.18	40.25 $\pm$ 2.20	55.925 $\pm$ 3.06	1.41 $\pm$ 0.29	8.42 $\pm$ 0.82
–	< limit	0.34 $\pm$ 0.09	46.38 $\pm$ 2.05	58.067 $\pm$ 4.07	1.60 $\pm$ 0.16	6.69 $\pm$ 1.22
–	0.35 $\pm$ 0.05	1.00 $\pm$ 0.17	21.18 $\pm$ 2.19	64.625 $\pm$ 4.57	1.82 $\pm$ 0.05	21.70 $\pm$ 1.24
–	0.57 $\pm$ 0.07	1.04 $\pm$ 0.12	44.90 $\pm$ 2.46	56.675 $\pm$ 2.28	2.42 $\pm$ 0.13	23.25 $\pm$ 2.22
–	2.99 $\pm$ 0.12	3.72 $\pm$ 0.23	45.17 $\pm$ 7.47	49.00 $\pm$ 4.54	3.97 $\pm$ 0.26	19.40 $\pm$ 2.88
Exposed						
5.8	13.80 $\pm$ 2.98	2.32 $\pm$ 0.21	43.07 $\pm$ 1.41	52.70 $\pm$ 7.08	1.45 $\pm$ 0.17	3.18 $\pm$ 0.37
6.2	17.05 $\pm$ 0.18	3.64 $\pm$ 0.17	32.47 $\pm$ 7.06	63.40 $\pm$ 2.68	3.11 $\pm$ 0.05	12.53 $\pm$ 1.25
6.8	12.30 $\pm$ 0.18	3.80 $\pm$ 0.25	45.93 $\pm$ 2.20	62.55 $\pm$ 2.06	2.90 $\pm$ 0.09	27.38 $\pm$ 2.10

[a] Concentrations are based on micrograms per gram dry weight for 4 to 16 separate analyses.

[b] The fraction used for this table was composed of whole cells, cell fragments and nuclei. (See text)

[c] The first 3 sets of control animals are age paired with the exposure group given. The second 2 sets are part of a longer exposure experiment.

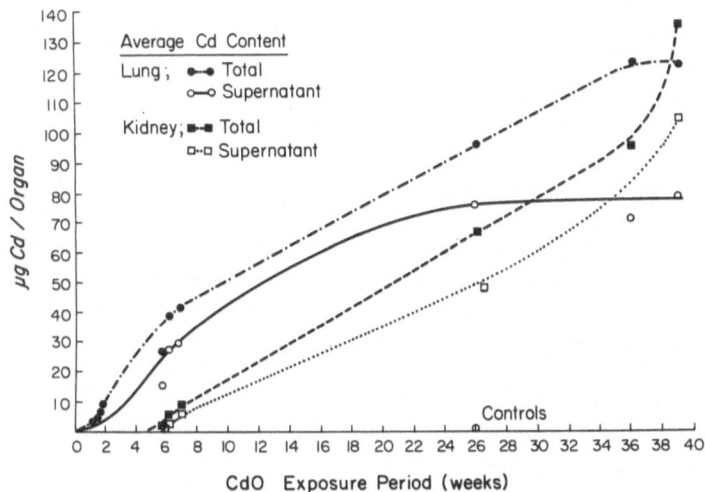

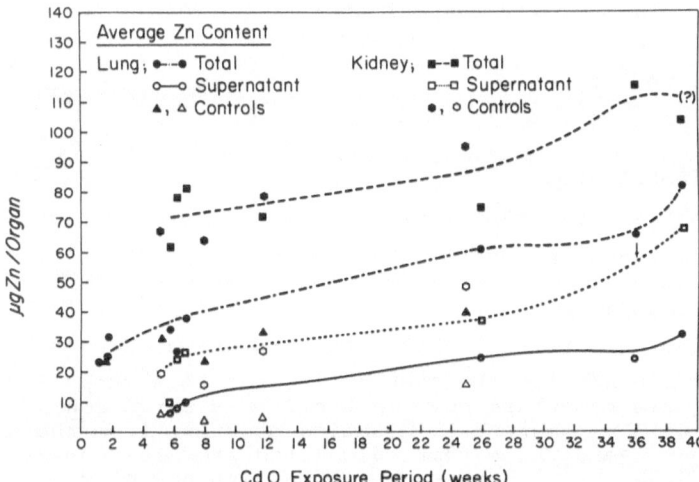

rate of absorption and its overall elimination constant from the lung.
In addition, the halftime for cadmium saturation and an apparent volume of distribution have been estimated. Using the standard kinetic
treatment for "drug" absorption and elimination in a body component
(GOLDSTEIN et al., 1968) where initially:

$$d(Cd)/dt = A - k_e (Cd)$$

A   = rate of absorption
k_e = overall elimination constant
(Cd) = amount of Cd present
t   = time

and the rate of absorption is assumed to be first order and proportional to the exposure level as long as the mechanism is not saturated, one can calculate an absorption rate of 8.33 μg/week from the
initial slope where (Cd) is very small and d(Cd)dt = A. At this point,
the percent cadmium absorbed of that inhaled is 13.2% for the whole

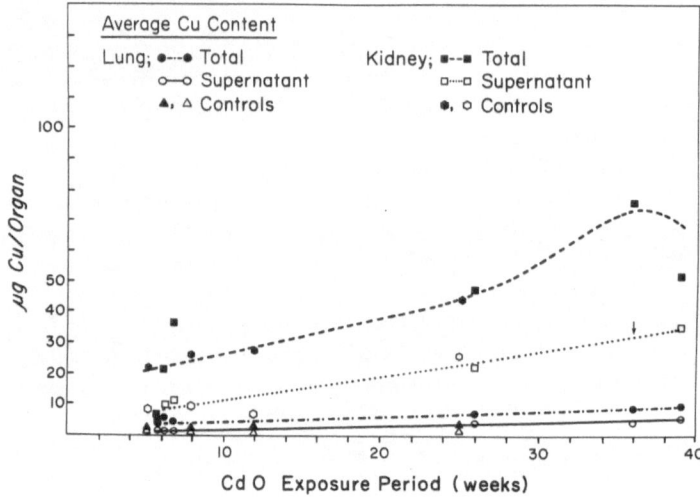

Fig. 3

lung; for the supernatant, A = 6.25 µg/week and the percent absorbed is 9.9%.

When cadmium has plateaued (t→oc):

$$(Cd) = \frac{A}{k_e \; V_d}$$

V_d = volume of distribution

and when (Cd) is at half its plateau level,

$$\ln \frac{(Cd) t \; 1/2}{(Cd) \; plateau} = \ln 1/2 = -k_e t \; 1/2$$

∴ t 1/2 = 0.693/k_e

t 1/2 = the time to reach half the saturation value

t 1/2 is measured as 9.2 weeks for the supernatant and 14.4 weeks for the whole lung. It may lie somewhere between the 2 on a curve constructed from more data. The apparent elimination constant from the supernatant is 0.075 per week, while that calculated from the curve for the whole lung is 0.05 per week. The approximate volume of distribution at plateau level is 0.91 to 0.94 of the total lung.

Since the rate of accumulation of cadmium in the kidney appears to be first order and equal to 3.05 µg per week, the amount present in the kidney can be calculated and compared with the amount eliminated by the lung during the linear absorption period. This has been done. During this period, the kidney contains about 94% of that eliminated by the lung after an accumulation lag of about 4 weeks. After lengthier exposures, as the concentration in the lung increased,

$$(Cd)_t = \frac{A}{k_e \; V_d} \; (1 - e^{-k_e t}).$$

Using the overall elimination constant calculated from the lung supernatant curve as being more accurate, a volume of distribution of 0.94, an exposure period of 26 weeks, and an absorption rate of 8.65 µg per week (to compensate for a larger lung surface area in older animals), the calculated amount of cadmium present is 104 µg, versus the 96.8 µg found. The absorption rate then, for 200 g to 400 g rats, must be between 8.3 to 8.6 μg per week as long as the exposure level is 150 μg/m^3 or above. The calculated percent retained of that inhaled is about 2.5% for both supernatant and whole lung in this time period.

IV. Cadmium Retention by the Lung and Kidney

The above calculations compare favorably with those obtained by direct measurement in Table 2. From the initial slope, one calculates an absorption of 13% of that inhaled and measures a retention of 8% to 10% for the entire lung; for the supernatant, the respective values are 10% versus 7%. After 36 weeks, the lungs should have absorbed approximately 307 μg Cd^{++}, of which 122.36 μg (40.6%) is found. The kidneys should have accumulated 96.4 μg versus the 95.05 measured (31.6%), allowing one to estimate that the remainder of the body contains the 84 μg (28%) absorbed through the lungs. The calculated percent absorption of that inhaled would be 9.8% without excretion. Including the lung elimination constant brings the retention value to 2.5% for the lung, versus the 4.3% given in Table 2.

All retention values in Table 2 have been derived by using a respiratory volume of 0.08208 m^3/day for a 400 g rat with tidal volume of 2 cc and a respiratory rate of 85.5/minute. Deposition estimations have been omitted. It is clear from Table 2 as well as Fig. 1 that the lung, as a compartment, becomes saturated whereas the kidney does not. The relative dependence of the retention figures on the exposure levels is also evident. Since the absorption rate is fairly constant, the higher level exposures greatly exceed the lung absorption capacity.

V. Pathology

The lungs of a total of 13 rats were examined. Seven of these animals were sacrificed at different times because of clinical pulmonary disease. Of the 3 animals examined after short exposure periods, 2 exhibited peribronchial and alveolar hyperplasia, with 1 focus of interstitial fibromuscular change about the alveoli. Of the 7 rats suffering murine pneumonia, 3 exhibited emphysema and focal pulmonary edema along with fulminating bronchitis and bronchiolitis. Bacterial cultures were taken from the bronchiolar mucus of 1 animal, and 4 organisms were isolated: a gram positive, β-hemolytic diplococcus; a gram positive α-hemolytic cocci; a gram negative short rods; and a staphylococcus. The last 3 animals submitted for pathological examination all possessed severe, chronic bronchitis. Subpleural emphysema was present; however, it was not possible to decide if this occurred because of the intercurrent disease or because of the exposure to cadmium.

More detailed examination of additional pulmonary tissue from this exposure period are being conducted to resolve this question.

D. Summary

As part of a study to determine the binding of cadmium ions to subcellular components of the lung and kidney after inhalation of its oxide aerosols, the retention and distribution of cadmium, zinc, and copper were measured as a function of exposure level and time. The concentration of cadmium in the lung and kidney was found to be a

Table 2. Cadmium retention by the lung and kidney as a function of exposure level and time to cadmium oxide aerosols[a]

Exposure Period Weeks	Mean Exposure Level[b] μg Cd++/m³	Calculated Inhaled Cadmium[c] μg	Total Cadmium Recovered, μg — Lung	Total Cadmium Recovered, μg — Kidney	Calculated Retention of Inhaled Cadmium, % — Lung Tot.Org.[d]	Lung Supernat.	Kidney Tot.Org.[d]	Kidney Supernat.
Control	0	0	0.43					
1.3	102.8	56.98	3.68		6.4			
1.4	51.0	33.02	4.29		14.1			
1.7	52.4	39.21	7.68		21.6			
1.8	52.1	44.87	9.67		25.1			
Control	0	0	0.33	0.59				
5.8	153.0	340.36	26.55	2.94	7.8	4.59	0.85	0.37
6.2	153.0	381.67	38.66	5.55	10.1	7.16	1.45	0.67
6.6	153.0	417.70	41.42	9.67	9.9	7.04	2.30	1.47
Control	0	0	1.33	2.86	–	–	–	–
26	319.8	3131.62	95.79	66.41	3.1	2.41	2.10	1.48
36	226	3076.29	122.36	95.05	4.3	2.30	3.00	–
39	348	4454.57	121.00	135.29	2.72	1.77	3.04	2.43

[a] The particle mass median diameter is 0.15 μ with 97% being less than 0.94 μ.

[b] The arithmetic mean is calculated from the summation of all samples periods divided by their number. Samples were collected on a 47 mmHA Millipore filter and analyzed for Cd++ with the aid of atomic absorption spectrophotometry.

[c] The figures presented are based on a respiratory volume of 0.01026 m³/hr times the number of exposure hours, times the mean concentration of Cd++/m³.

[d] Total, or whole, organ figures are the summation of the metal ion content in each subcellular fraction of that organ.

[e] The control animals are age paired for each exposure period with the exception of the last 2.

function of several variables amongst which absorption rate, exposure
level, and time exerted the greatest influence. Thus, animals exposed
to similar amounts of cadmiumd distributed over different periods of
time were found to contain more cadmium when the exposure period was
extended. This has been attributed to a fairly constant absorption
rate at these exposure levels, all of which were above saturation. A
concomitant increase in zinc was observed in both organs; however,
copper levels do not appear to differ significantly from the controls.
The preliminary pathology reports indicate that after 9 months exposure, pulmonary emphysema is present.

E. Acknowledgements

We should like to express our gratitude to Dr. ELLEN O'FLAHERTY for
a discussion of the kinetic treatment and Drs. K. STEMMER and R. RITTER-
HOF for the pathology report.

References

BAADER, E.W.: Die chronische Kadmiumvergiftung. Dtsch med. Wschr. 76,
484 (1951).

BINGHAM, E., PFITZER, E., BARKLEY, W., RADFORD, E.P.: Alveolar macrophages. Reduced number in rats after prolonged inhalation of lead
sesquioxide. Science 62, 1297-1299 (1968).

FLESCH, J.P., NORRIS, C.H., NUGENT, A.E.: Calibrating particulate
air samplers with monodisperse aerosols: Application to the Anderson
Cascade Impactor. Amer. ind. Hyg. Ass. J. 28, 507-   (1967).

FRIBERG, L.: Health hazards in the manufacture of alkaline accumula-
tors with special reference to chronic cadmium poisoning. Acta med.
scand. 238, Suppl. 240, 7-124 (1950).

FRIBERG, L., PISCATOR, M., NORDBERG, G.: Cadmium in the environment.
Chemical Rubber Co., Cleveland 1971.

FRIBERG, L., PISCATOR, M., NORDBERG, G., KELLSTROM, T.: Cadmium in
the environment, II. Prepared for: Office of Research and Monitoring, U.S. Environmental Protection Agency, Washington, D.C. 20460,
1973.

GOLDSTEIN, A., ARONOW, L., KALMAN, S.M.: Principles of drug action;
The basis of pharmacology. ch 4. New York: Harper and Row 1968.

GRIFFIN, R.B.: Cadmium, lead, and copper distribution in cadmium
dosed rats. The University of Michigan, Ph.D. Thesis, Ann Arbor,
Univ. Microfilms, Inc. 1970.

HIRST, R.N., PERRY, H.M., GRUZ, M.G., PIERCE, J.A.: Elevated cadmium
concentration in emphysematous lungs. Amer. Rev. Resp. Dis. 108,
30-39 (1973).

HOGEBOOM, G.H., SCHNEIDER, W.C., PALADE, G.E.: Cytochemical studies
of mammalian tissues. J. biol. Chem. 172, 619-639 (1948).

HORSTMAN, S., BARKLEY, W., LARSON, E., BINGHAM, E.: Aerosols of lead,
nickel, and cadmium. A method of generating soluble and insoluble
compounds. Arch. Environ. Hlth 26, 75-77 (1973).

KAPLAN, P.D., BLACKSTONE, M., RICHDALE, N.: Direct determination of
cadmium, nickel, and zinc in rat lungs. Arch Environ. Hlth 27,
387-389 (1973).

KAZANTZIS, G., FLYNN, F.V., SPOWAGE, J.S., TROTT, D.G.: Renal tubular malfunction and pulmonary emphysema in cadmium pigment workers.
Quart. J. Med. 32, 165 (1963).

LUCIS, O.J., LUCIS, R., SHAIKH, Z.A.: Cadmium and zinc in pregnancy and lactation. Arch. Environ. Hlth $\underline{25}$, 14-22 (1972).

NORDBERG, G.F., PISCATOR, M.: Influence of long-term cadmium exposure on urinary excretion of protein and cadmium in mice. Environ. Physiol. Biochem. $\underline{2}$, 37 (1972).

NORDBERG, G.F., PISCATOR, M.: Influence of long-term cadmium exposure on urinary excretion of protein and cadmium in mice. Environ. Physiol. Biochem. $\underline{2}$, 37 (1972).

O'HARE, K.H., REISS, O.K., VATTER, A.E.: Esterases in developing and adult rat lung. J. Histochem. Cytochem. $\underline{19}$, 97-115 (1971).

REISS, O.K.: Studies of lung metabolism. J. Cell Biol. $\underline{30}$, 45-57 (1966).

SHAIKH, Z.A., LUCIS, O.J.: Biological differences in cadmium and zinc turnover. Arch. Environ. Hlth $\underline{24}$, 410-418 (1972a).

SHAIKH, Z.A., LUCIS, O.J.: Cadmium and zinc binding in mammalian liver and kidneys. Arch. Environ. Hlth $\underline{24}$, 419-425 (1972b).

SNIDER, G.L., HAYES, J.A., KORTHY, A.L., LEWIS, G.P.: Centrilobular emphysema experimentally induced by cadmium chloride aerosol. Amer. Rev. Resp. Dis. $\underline{108}$, 40-47 (1973).

THIERS, R.E., VALLEE, B.L.: Distribution of metals in subcellular fractions of rat liver. J. biol. Chem. $\underline{226}$, 911-920 (1957).

UMBREIT, W.W., BURRIS, R.H., STAUFFER, J.F. (Eds): Manometric Techniques, pp. 183-184. Minneapolis: Burgess Publishing Co. 1964.

VATTER, A.E., REISS, O.K., NEWMAN, J.K., LINDQUIST, K., GROENEBOER, E.: Enzymes of the lung. J. Cell Biol. $\underline{38}$, 80-98 (1968).

WEBB, M.: Binding of cadmium ions by rat liver and kidney. Biochem. Pharmacol. $\underline{21}$, 2751-2765 (1972a).

WEBB, M.: Protection by zinc against cadmium toxicity. Biochem. Pharmacol. $\underline{21}$, 2767-2771 (1972b).

Conception and Methods of Experimental Studies in Germany to Estimate the Carcinogenic Burden by Air Pollution in Man

D. Schmähl and K. G. Schmidt

Deutsches Krebsforschungszentrum, Institut fur Toxikologie und Chemotherapie
Heidelberg, W.-Germany

ABSTRACT

The lecture describes tasks and organization of a working group of
the Federal Ministry of the Interior of Germany on "Investigations
on the Carcinogenic Burden by Air Pollution in Man". In our institute
it could be shown in dropping experiments in 3400 female NMRI-mice
that noncarcinogenic hydrocarbons are not able to compensate the
effect of carcinogenic hydrocarbons, and that a mixture of carcinogenic PAH is more active than only 1 substance of the mixture. Probably an overall synergism is present.

Introduction

In 1969/70, a commission was formed by the Ministry of the Interior,
Federal Republic of Germany, in order to carry out scientific investigations which could provide a background of information, eventually
leading to the establishment of legislation to reduce carcinogenic
components in air pollution.

The intention of the commission was to assess the risk by carcinogenic constituents of air pollution to man and to determine tolerated
concentration levels of such substances in the air by means of chemical identification and biological testing (SCHMÄHL, 1973). Because
the necessary individual projects of our group were so many, the investigations were first restricted to 1 source of emission; this
approach seemed advantageous from another standpoint: we hoped to
overcome expected methodological difficulties in the first model. We
chose automobile exhaust gases, since they contribute a large proportion of the emissions, particularly in urban areas, contain carcinogenic components and can be standardized relatively easily. Other
important emission sources, such as heating, energy provision, and
other firing plants, are to be included in future studies.

In choosing suitable methods of investigation, certain restrictions
had to be adopted. For example inhalation of polluted air in a corresponding environment or in specially conditioned rooms is a good choice
for animal experiments because of the physiological mode of application and the good comparability with human conditions. However, the
long time of preparation, high costs of investment, and limited number of possible tests did not permit use of this method for routine
investigations of individual questions. Therefore, more simple test
models, such as epicutaneous skin dropping and subcutaneous injection
were used, with simultaneous, parallel studies with selected material

(i.e., PAH) carried out by the more complicated methods in order to compare the different test models. For this purpose, experiments with epicutaneous dropping, subcutaneous injection, intratracheal instillation, and inhalation were started. By means of "conversion factors" that can be derived from the different results of the above experiments it should be possible to transmit findings of more simple tests to the conditions of the respiratory tract. The order of these tests is described in Fig. 1.

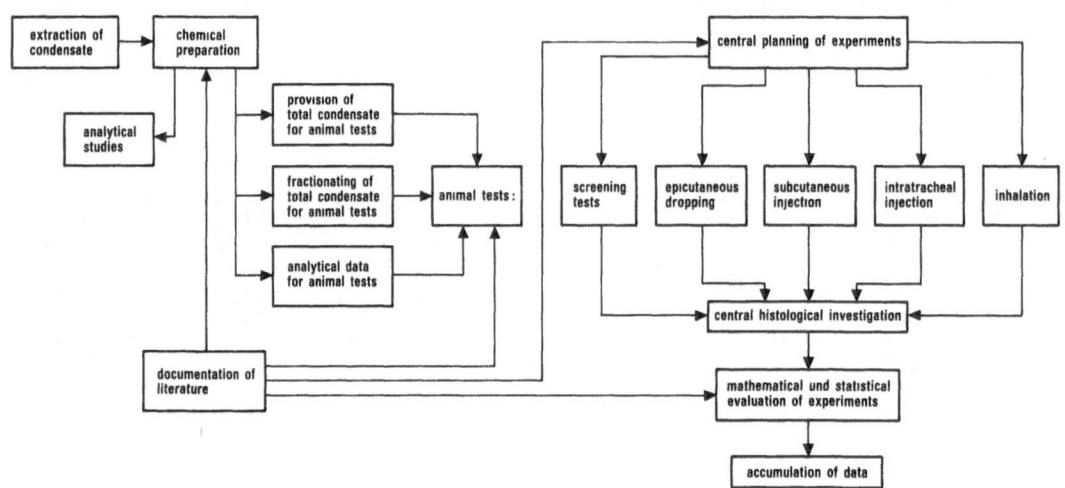

Fig. 1. Test program

The condensates of automobile exhaust gas were gained by a repeatedly modified method at the Federal Institute for Materials Testing in Berlin[a] and the Biochemical Institute for Environmental Carcinogens of the University of Hamburg[b]. In this method, vehicles are driven on a role-test-stand in a certain driving cycle, the so-called Europe Test, in order to imitate engine behavior in town traffic. By a combined cooling and filter system the gas and particle phase of the exhaust gas stream are separated. The actual condensate is produced from filter and cleansing liquids in Hamburg. In addition to providing the material for the animal tests, the Hamburg group[c] investigated the influence upon the composition of condensate when combustion conditions in motor and fuel (e.g., regulation of carburetor, oil, petrol) were altered. The most essential preliminary result of these studies is the fact that the content of PAH in exhaust gas depends substantially upon the working temperature of the motor, i.e., with cold start about 20 times as much of these compounds are emitted into the atmosphere compared to driving with warm motor and high speed.

---

[a]Bundesanstalt für Materialprüfung (BAM), 1 Berlin 45, Unter den Eichen 87.

[b]Biochemisches Institut für Umweltcarcinogene, 207 Ahrensburg, Sieker Landstr. 19.

[c]Deutsche Gesellschaft für Mineralölwissenschaft und Kohlechemie e.V., 2 Hamburg 1, Steindamm 71 and Biochemisches Institut für Umweltcarcinogene, 207 Ahrensburg, Sieker Landstr. 19.

The biological effects of exhaust gas condensate were investigated at
the Vaselin-Werk, Hamburg[d], the Medical College, Hannover[e], the Institute of Air Hygiene and Silicosis Research, Düsseldorf[f], the Institute of Hygiene of the University of Mainz[g], and the Institute of
Forest Botany of the University of Freiburg[h]. Both the condensate and
its fractions as well as a mixture of selected pure PAH, which have
been identified in the exhaust gas, were examined by epicutaneous
dropping and subcutaneous injection. Furthermore, experiments with
intratracheal injection and inhalation of only 1 carcinogen, benzo(a)-
pyrene (BaP), were initiated to provide for calculation of the previously mentioned "conversion factor". Finally the suitability of
various types of "pilot" tests for carcinogenicity (e.g., sebaceous
glands suppression test, genetic investigations) was experimentally
investigated.

The planning and evaluation of all experiments was carried out at the
Institute of Mathematics of the College of Technology, Hannover[i],
where the experimental data are also stored. Optimal information of
all examiners was achieved by continuous documentation of literature
at the Institute of Hygiene, Mainz. Before describing the results of
our institute, it should be noted that a part of the hitherto performed work was published in the English language in Zentralblatt für
Bakteriologie und Hygiene, I. Abt. Orig. B. 158, 1-95 (1973).

At the Institute of Toxicology and Chemotherapy, German Cancer Research Center, Heidelberg[j], we are investigating whether PAH, contained in various aerosols of air mixtures and known from the literature as carcinogenic or noncarcinogenic, inhibit, promote, or do not
influence each other in their biological effects. Previous investigations have suggested such effects (FALK et al., 1964; WATTENBERG, 1966;
VAN DUUREN and MELCHIONNE, 1969). In an extensive model experiment,
the PAH listed in Table 1 were examined in 3400 female NMRI-mice.
These PAH are contained in automobile exhaust gas (AEG) as well as in
cigarette smoke (CS) and preservation curing smoke (PCS); in the
latter, the proportions of the PAH in the individual media is different. We assumed the analytically measured quantity of benzo(a)pyrene
to equal 1 and listed the remaining hydrocarbons according to their
proportion to BaP (Table 1).

We attempted to examine (a) whether the 4 carcinogenic hydrocarbons
were more potent carcinogens than BaP alone, (b) whether the hydrocarbons assumed to be noncarcinogenic were in fact noncarcinogenic

---

[d] Vaselin-Werk, Biochemisches Laboratorium, 2 Hamburg 11, Worthdamm
13-29.

[e] Medizinische Hochschule Hannover, Abteilung für exp. Pathologie,
3 Hannover-Kleefeld, Karl-Wiechert-Allee 9.

[f] Institut für Lufthygiene und Silikoseforschung der Universität,
4 Düsseldorf, Gurlittstr. 53.

[g] Hygiene-Institut der Universität, 65 Mainz, Hochhaus am Augustusplatz.

[h] Institut für Forstbotanik der Universität, 78 Freiburg/Br., Bertoldstr.
17.

[i] Institut für Mathematik der Technischen Universität, 3 Hannover,
Welfengarten 1.

[j] Institut für Toxikologie und Chemotherapie am Deutschen Krebsforschungszentrum, 68 Heidelberg, Im Neuenheimer Feld 280.

142

Table 1. Quantities of PAH in condensates of cigarette smoke (CS),
automobile exhaust gases (AEG), and preservation curing smoke (PCS)
(in relationship to benzo(a)pyrene (BaP))

	CS	AEG	PCS
Phenanthrene	16.5	27.0	7.4
Anthracene	5.3	8.5	2.3
Fluoranthene	7.7	10.8	4.2
Pyrene	19.0	13.8	4.4
Benzoanthracene*	2.8	1.4	2.6
Chrysene	4.3	1.2	1.1
Benzofluoranthene*	1.8	0.9	2.5
Benzopyrene	0.8	0.6	0.8
Benzo(a)pyrene*	1.0	1.0	1.0
Dibenzanthracene*	0.7	0.7	0.8
Benzoperylene	0.6	3.1	0.6

*Carcinogenic PAH.

Table 2. Tumors produced by hydrocarbons in condensate of automobile
exhaust gas

	NCPH[a]				CPH[b]			CPH+NCPH			BaP			Solvent[d]
	1[c]	3	9	27	1	1.7	3	1	1.7	3	1	1.7	3	
animals still alive	59	57	63	52	37	33	20	49	34	7	52	54	39	52
carcinomas	–	–	–	–	1	4	1	3	3	5	–	–	–	–
papillomas	–	–	1	6	13	17	10	19	18	2	3	4	13	–
animals died	41	43	37	48	63	67	80	51	66	93	48	46	61	48
carcinomas	–	–	–	3	8	25	50	14	33	56	–	5	23	–
papillomas	–	–	–	–	4	5	9	2	7	7	1	–	5	–
total number of carcinomas	–	–	–	3	9	29	51	17	36	61	–	5	23	–
total number of papillomas	–	–	1	6	17	22	19	21	25	9	4	4	18	–
total number of skin tumors	–	–	1	9	26	51	70	38	61	70	4	9	41	–

Interim report on experiments in female NMRI-mice for carcinogenic
activity of PAH of automobile exhaust condensates in comparison with
benzo(a)pyrene (BaP)
Method: Skin dropping twice weekly in µg quantities
Time period: October 1972 - March 1974

[a]NCPH = noncarcinogenic polycyclic hydrocarbons (Table 1)
[b]CPH = carcinogenic polycyclic hydrocarbons (Table 1)
[c]Dosage is related to benzo(a)pyrene in the different mixtures of the
hydrocarbons as indicated in Table 1
[d]Solvent = acetone

Table 3. Tumors produced by hydrocarbons in condensate of cigarette smoke

	NCPH[a]				CPH[b]			CPH+NCPH			BaP			Solvent[d]
	1[c]	3	9	27	1	1.7	3	1	1.7	3	1	1.7	3	
animals still alive	56	53	54	47	54	40	16	46	32	6	52	54	39	52
carcinomas	–	–	1	1	1	1	3	1	1	–	–	–	–	–
papillomas	–	1	2	10	7	14	9	12	20	4	3	4	13	–
animals died	44	47	46	53	46	60	84	54	68	94	48	46	61	48
carcinomas	–	1	–	8	8	24	57	13	31	72	–	5	23	–
papillomas	–	–	–	4	1	5	3	4	3	–	1	5	–	–
total number of carcinomas	–	1	1	9	9	23	60	14	32	72	–	5	23	–
total number of papillomas	–	1	2	14	8	10	12	16	23	4	4	4	4	–
total number of skin tumors	–	2	3	23	17	44	72	30	55	76	4	9	41	–

Interim report on experiments in female NMRI-mice for carcinogenic activity of PAH of cigarette smoke condensates in comparison with benzo(a)pyrene (BaP)
Method: Skin dropping twice weekly in µg quantities
Time period: October 1972 - March 1974

[a]NCPH = noncarcinogenic polycyclic hydrocarbons (Table 1)
[b]CPH = carcinogenic polycyclic hydrocarbons (Table 1)
[c]Dosage is related to benzo(a)pyrene in the different mixtures of the hydrocarbons as indicated in Table 1
[d]Solvent = acetone

when applied in a mixture, and (c) whether the total mixture of all 11 hydrocarbons inhibits, promotes, or leaves uninfluenced the carcinogenic effect of the carcinogenic hydrocarbons. Groups of 100 animals each were treated twice weekly by dropping the PAH in acetone to the shorn skin of the back. In previous tests we had detected that in this mouse strain the BaP-dosage of 1.7 µg twice weekly leads to up to 20% squamous cell carcinomas (SCHMIDT et al., 1973). The induction period of the tumors amounted to ~420 days when a total dosage of ~200 µg BaP was given. In the present experiment the dosage of 1.7 µg BaP was assumed to be a "medium" dosage in order to note effects promoting the formation of tumors.

The preliminary results of this study are demonstrated in Tables 2, 3, and 4. The most essential finding was the fact that the mixture of carcinogenic and noncarcinogenic hydrocarbons was active in the same way as the mixture of carcinogenic hydrocarbons alone. In no case was an inhibition of the carcinogenesis by the noncarcinogenic hydrocarbons present. Furthermore, it is obvious that compared to the application of BaP alone the mixture of the carcinogenic hydrocarbons is nearly twice as active. This was equally true for automobile exhaust gas, cigarette smoke and preservation curing smoke condensate. Application of solvent alone did not produce tumors.

144

Table 4. Tumors produced by hydrocarbons in condensate of preservation curing smoke

	NCPH[a]				CPH[b]			CPH+NCPH			BaP			Solvent[d]
	1[c]	3	9	27	1	1.7	3	1	1.7	3	1	1.7	3	
animals still alive	55	49	48	50	44	36	6	48	27	21	52	54	39	52
carcinomas	-	-	-	-	-	2	-	1	-	2	-	-	-	-
papillomas	-	-	2	4	14	19	5	13	15	13	3	4	13	-
animals died	45	51	52	50	56	64	94	52	73	79	48	46	61	48
carcinomas	-	-	-	2	15	22	60	13	31	62	-	5	23	-
papillomas	-	-	-	1	4	5	4	8	9	4	-	-	5	-
total number of carcinomas	-	-	-	2	15	24	60	14	31	64	-	5	23	-
total number of papillomas	-	-	2	5	18	24	9	21	24	17	4	4	18	-
total number of skin tumors	-	-	2	7	33	48	69	35	55	81	4	9	41	-

Interim report on experiments in female NMRI-mice for carcinogenic activity of PAH of preservation curing smoke condensates in comparison with benzo(a)pyrene (BaP)
Method: Skin dropping twice weekly in µg quantities
Time period: October 1972 - March 1974

[a]NCPH = noncarcinogenic polycyclic hydrocarbons (Table 1)
[b]CPH = carcinogenic polycyclic hydrocarbons (Table 1)
[c]Dosage is related to benzo(a)pyrene in the different mixtures of the hydrocarbons as indicated in Table 1
[d]Solvent = acetone

The fact that application of the 2 highest doses of noncarcinogenic PAH produced few local papillomas and carcinomas may be of particular interest. This effect may be related to the use of chrysene and benzo-(a)pyrene, which in some reports were described to have weak carcinogenic properties.

In conclusion, the most remarkable result of our study was the observation that a clear syncarcinogenesis is present when the effect of a mixture of carcinogenic PAH is compared with only 1 carcinogenic PAH, in this instance benzo(a)pyrene. Noncarcinogenic hydrocarbons do not reduce the syncarcinogenic effect observed when added to the mixture.

References

DUUREN, B.L. VAN, MELCHIONNE, S.: Inhibition of tumorigenesis. Prog. exp. Tumor Res. 12, 55-94 (1969).
FALK, H.L., KOTIN, P., THOMPSON, S.: Inhibition of carcinogenesis. Arch. Environ. Hlth 9, 169-179 (1964).
SCHMÄHL, D.: Investigations on the carcinogenic burden by air pollution in man. Preface. Zbl. Bakt., I. Abt. Orig. B. 158, 1-3 (1973).

SCHMIDT, K.G., SCHMÄHL, D., MISFELD, J.: Experimental investigations to determine a dose-response relationship and to estimate a threshold dose of benzo(a)pyrene in the skin of 2 different mouse strains. Zbl. Bakt., I. Abt. Orig. B. 158, 62-68 (1973).

VAN DUUREN, B.L., MELCHIONNE, S.: Inhibition of tumorigenesis. Prog. exp. Tumor Res. 12, 55-94 (1969).

WATTENBERG, L.W.: Chemoprophylaxis of Carcinogenesis. A Review. Cancer Res. 26, 1520-1526 (1966).

Experimental Carcinogenicity and Bioassays of Automobile Exhaust Condensate and Its Polycyclic Aromatic Hydrocarbons

Horst Brune

Beratungsforum fur Praventivmedizin und Umweltschutz GmbH, Hamburg, W.-Germany

ABSTRACT

Experiments and activities of members of the German governmental research group are presented in addition to those reported by SCHMÄHL
(1974) in these proceedings.

The description of the biomathematic model for planning and evaluation
of experiments is followed by data on the interaction of polycyclic
aromatic hydrocarbons (PAH) from the automobile exhaust condensate
(AEC). With subcutaneous application similar findings were observed
as previously demonstrated by SCHMÄHL (1974), who administered the
test substances epicutaneously. There was no inhibition effect of
tumor development by combining noncarcinogenic PAHs with carcinogenic
ones.

Intratracheal instillations of BaP have been done to clarify dose-
response-relationships. The clearance rate of PAHs from the respiratory tract was investigated as well as the influence exerted by different solvents. A new constructed apparatus for chronic inhalation
studies with a convenient particle size is described.

According to a fractionating scheme for AEC the relation of the solvent to AEC and its fractions as well as acute and subchronic toxicity of those substances were tested.

As a screening method for biological activities of the AEC and its
PAHs the sebaceous gland suppression test was used. It demonstrated
an approximately 20-times greater acticity on the basis of BaP applied
for AEC than for BaP alone.

Other experiments administering AEC and its fractions epicutaneously,
subcutaneously and as intratracheal instillation are not yet completed. Analytical studies of the total ratio of PAHs to AEC have
been performed. 15 up to now unknown PAHs with 4 to 7 rings were
found, which we assumed possible carcinogens. Their carcinogenicity
will be studied in screening tests and chronic experiments.

Introduction

The organization of our research group, the extent of the technical
and chemical work accomplished by GRIMMER et al. (1973), as well as
results obtained in animal experiments on the synergism of carcinogenic polycyclic aromatic hydrocarbons (PAH) present in the automobile

exhaust condensate (AEC) have been presented by SCHMÄHL (1974) in these proceedings.

In this paper, additional experiments are presented which were performed by several members of our research group which include:

BORNEFF and PFEIFFER, Hygiene-Institut, Universität Mainz.
GRIMMER, Institut für Umweltcarcinogene, Hamburg.
KIMMERLE, Bayer A.G., Toxikologische Abteilung, Wuppertal.
MISFELD, Institut für Mathematik der Technischen Universität Hannover and TIMM, Institut für Mathematik der Universität Bremen.
MOHR, Institut für experimentelle Pathologie, Medizinische Hochschule Hannover.
POTT and TOMINGAS, Medizinisches Institut für Lufthygiene und Silikose-forschung, Düsseldorf.
STÖBER, Aerobiologisches Institut, Fraunhofergesellschaft, Grafschaft.

The experiments are mainly designed to establish which components of AEC produce carcinogenic effects either alone or in combination and which constituents must be eliminated in order to reduce tumor development caused by AEC in experimental animals. These questions can only be answered if it can be clarified whether the different substances cause additive, overadditive, or inhibiting effects.

Report and Evaluation of Animal Experiments

As a model for the planning and evaluation of these animal experiments, the 3 concepts of MISFELD and TIMM (1973) were employed that had been designed to investigate other compounds. These concepts are:

- determination of the relative effectiveness,
- evaluation of constituent effects,
- analysis of the total effect in relation to separate effects.

The potency of the PAH is assumed as the principal cause for carcinogenic effects demonstrated in animal experiments. As representative of this class of chemicals, which are present in AEC at about 315 µg/g, benzo(a)pyrene (BaP) has been used in the animal experiments. The tumorigenic effects of BaP, cigarette smoke, and AEC were demonstrated by LEE and O'NEILL (1971), WYNDER and HOFFMANN (1962), DAY (1967), and GRIMMER et al. (1973)(see Table 1) according to the method of MISFELD and TIMM (1973), who compared them as follows:

1. AEC is 10 times more active than cigarette smoke condensate.
2. BaP is 12,000 times more active than cigarette smoke condensate.
3. BaP is 1,200 times more active than AEC.

It can be estimated that the amount of BaP present in AEC would by itself produce only 3.8% of the AEC effect. In this respect, the additive effect of the BaP-free AEC amounts to 96.2% of the total effect of the unaltered AEC.

The known carcinogens and those substances recognized as noncarcinogenic PAH present in the AEC were studied at the German Cancer Research Center and also by PFEIFFER (1973).

In Table 2 the results of PAH interaction after subcutaneous application are demonstrated; the relative concentrations of the 10 PAHs used in the mixtures was adjusted to those in AEC. BaP and DBA were used

148

Table 1. Induction of tumors in mice with benzo(a)pyrene, (BaP),
automobile exhaust condensate, and cigarette smoke condensate

Substance	Dose per application (in mg)	Animals with tumors (in %)	Weight portion of BaP	Reference
Benzo(a)-pyrene	$2 \cdot 10^{-3}$ $4 \cdot 10^{-3}$ $8 \cdot 10^{-3}$ $16 \cdot 10^{-3}$	4.0 15.3 37.7 73.7	1	LEE and O'NEILL (1971)
Automobile exhaust condensate	7.1 14.2 35.4 46.7	4.0 50.0 50.0 60.0	$3.15 \cdot 10^{-5}$	WYNDER and HOFFMANN (1962)
Cigarette smoke condensate	7.5 15.0 37.5 49.5	0 6.0 18.0 34.0	$0.7 \cdot 10^{-6}$	WYNDER and HOFFMANN (1962)
Cigarette smoke condensate	25.0 50.0 100.0	12.0 25.0 31.9	$1.08 \cdot 10^{-6}$	DAY (1967)
Automobile exhaust condensate	to calculate	≈50	$4.2 \cdot 10^{-5}$	GRIMMER (personal communic. 1974)

Table 2. Number of tumors at the end of experiment (114th week after
treatment). 2 carcinogenic compounds used: benzo(a)pyrene (BaP)
(3-100 µg), 1,2,5,6-dibenzanthracene (DBA)(2-75 µg) and a mixture
of both compounds. 10 noncarcinogenic compounds used: 1,2-benzo(a)-
pyrene, 1,2-benzanthracene, phenanthrene, anthracene, pyrene, fluoranthene, chrysene, perylene, 1,12-benzperylene, and coronene; dose
adjusted relative concentration in AEC (PFEIFFER, personal communication 1974)

group BaP dose	number of tumors	group DBA dose	number of tumors	group BaP+DBA	number of tumors	group 10 PAH	number of tumors	group 12 PAH	number of tumors
3,12 µg	20	2,35 µg	57	BaP+DBA	56	10 PAH	30	12 PAH	62
6,25 µg	53	4,7 µg	67	BaP+DBA	68	10 PAH	28	12 PAH	69
12,5 µg	66	9,3 µg	59	BaP+DBA	71	10 PAH	33	12 PAH	73
25,0 µg	72	18,7 µg	74	BaP+DBA	80	10 PAH	37	12 PAH	83
50,0 µg	84	37,5 µg	83	BaP+DBA	83	10 PAH	37	12 PAH	76
100,0 µg	95	75,0 µg	85	BaP+DBA	91	10 PAH	22	12 PAH	95

as test substances either alone, combined, or in combination with 10
different noncarcinogenic PAH. It appeared that no inhibition of tumor
development was observed when 10 noncarcinogenic substances were administered simultaneously with the 2 carcinogens, as previously demon-

strated by SCHMÄHL (1974). The absence of a dose-response relationship and the incidence of tumors caused by PAHs deemed noncarcinogenic
is unexplainable. It is possible that the group receiving high doses
died too early to develop tumors. This experiment, however, is not
yet completed, and the results will be evaluated later statistically.

HILFRICH et al. (1973) have investigated the effects of BaP alone
when intratracheally instilled to Syrian golden hamsters. Table 3 demonstrates that the average survival rate decreased as the administered dose was increased. The animals of the highest dose groups (3.91 mg
and 9.77 mg) lived only about 3 or 4 weeks. The animals of the lowest
dose groups (0.1 mg to 0.25 mg) lived longer than 30 weeks and the
control groups lived still longer.

Table 3. Summary of findings after intratracheal treatment of Syrian
golden hamsters with different weekly dosages of benzo(a)pyrene.
(MOHR, personal communication 1974)

treatment (application weekly)	number of animals	animals with tumors of the respiration tract (%)			medium survival time (weeks) (from/to)	medium survival time of tumor bearing animals (weeks) (from, to)
		benign	malignant	total		
controls	29	0 (0)	0 (0)	0 (0)	36,6 (8-72)	-
0,1 mg BaP	28	0 (0)	2 (7)	2 (7)	33,9 (2-61)	54,5 (54-55)
0,25 mg BaP	24	0 (0)	14 (58)	14 (58)	33,8 (8-56)	42,2 (28-56)
0,63 mg BaP	30	2 (7)	14 (47)	16 (53)	17,6 (4-34)	21,3 (17-34)
1,56 mg BaP	30	3 (10)	3 (10)	6 (20)	8,3 (2-12)	9,7 (6-12)
3,91 mg BaP	30	1 (3)	1 (3)	2 (7)	3,9 (2-7)	6,0 (5-7)
9,77 mg BaP	30	0 (0)	0 (0)	0 (0)	3,3 (2-5)	

Regarding the induction of tumors, the first bronchiogenic tumor was
induced in an animal of the 3.91-dosage group after 4 weeks and in
one of the 1.56-mg dosage group after 5 weeks. The first neoplasm of
the trachea was a papilloma diagnosed 9 weeks after beginning treatment with 1.56 mg BaP. The groups receiving the lowest dosages developed the most tumors because of the higher survival time. The groups receiving either 0.25 mg or 0.63 mg BaP and living 18 to 30 weeks demonstrated the highest tumor rate, with 30% tumors in the trachea and
50% in the lungs.

In an inhalation model experiment, KIMMERLE, EBEN, and GRIMMER (personal communication 1974) tested how much retained fluoranthene was
present in the trachea and in the lungs of Syrian golden hamsters.
The trachea retained 2/3 the total amount of applied chemical while
1/3 remained in the bronchioles and alveoli. In additional studies,
the same authors clarified the speed of clearing the respiratory tract
of fluoranthene and the influence exerted by different solvents (water,
acetone, polyethylene-glycol, and n-tricapryline). Thereby it became
clear that already 24 hours after exposure, no detectable amount of
fluoranthene remained in the respiratory tract and that one attains
better deposition results with DMSO as a solvent as compared to results with the others employed.

Table 4. Elimination of fluoranthene from trachea and lung of hamsters after inhalation period of 1 hour. Solvent: dimethylsulfoxide (DMSO). Killing directly after exposure period. (KIMMERLE, EBEN, and GRIMMER, personal communication 1974)

mg fluoranthene/m^3 air	average values of 5 hamsters μg fluoranthene/animal	
	trachea	lung
22,3	1,3	0,6
77,2	2,9	1,4
278,6	17,4	9,5

The elimination of DBA and BaP after intratracheal instillation in hamsters was demonstrated by POTT and TOMINGAS (personal communication 1974). They found that BaP was more quickly cleared from the respiratory tract than was DBA.

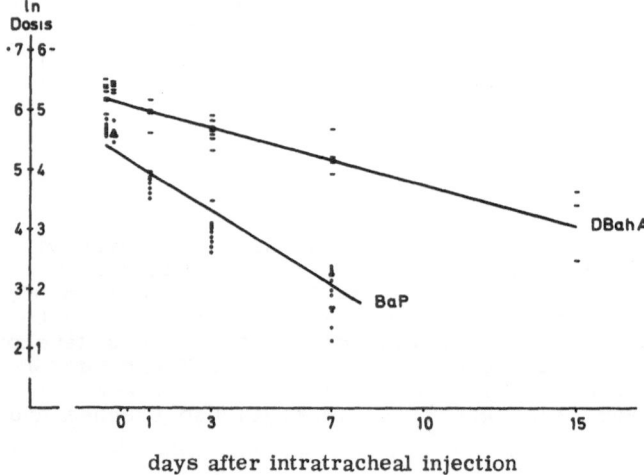

days after intratracheal injection

Fig. 1. Elimination of dibenz(a,h)anthracene (DBahA) and benzo(a)-pyrene (BaP) from the lung and trachea of Syrian golden hamsters after intratracheal injection of 400 μg of a polyaromate in 0.2 ml NaCl solution. (POTT and TOMINGAS, personal communication 1974)

Chronic inhalation studies can only be performed now that former great technical difficulties have begun to be solved. The apparatus employed is composed of an aerosol generator, an isolated animal maintenance chamber, and an inhalation exposure chamber. In the generator constructed by STÖBER (personal communication 1974), PAH is generated as an aerosol by evaporation of the particular constituent material and its condensation on airborne nuclei of NaCl. This generator is applicable to all substances that vaporize below 300°C and do not decompose at this temperature.

Fig. 2 shows a sample of pyreneaerosol that has a high mass concentration with an average particle diameter of 1.4 μm. The aerosol concentration was determined gravimetrically at 1 g/m³. When a medium
mass concentration is present (Fig. 3), the average particle diameter
falls to 0.48 μm. Here we have an aerosol concentration of 60 mg/m³.
This particle size is convenient for inhalation experiments, and the
aerosol concentration can be regulated by adjusting the vaporizing

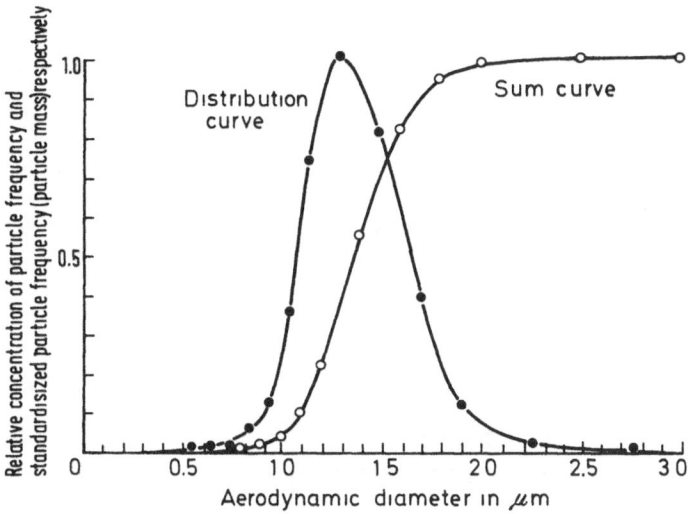

Fig. 2. Distribution of particle size of a pyreneaerosol of high
mass concentration. (Taken from HOCHRAINER, 1974)

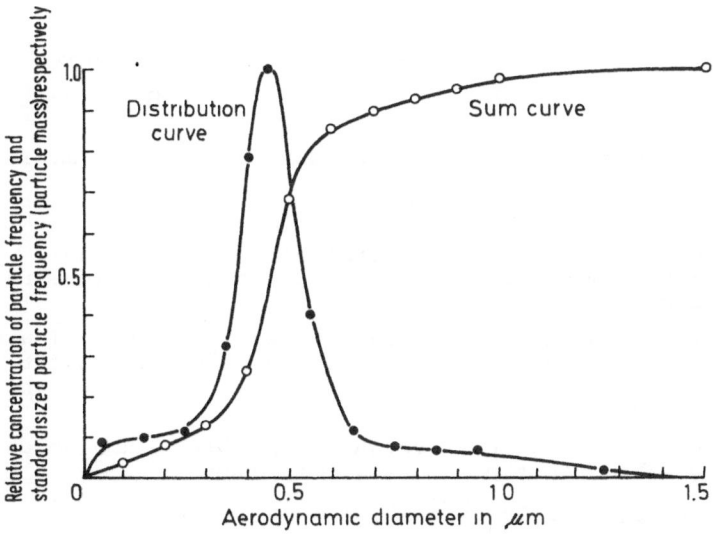

Fig. 3. Distribution of particle size of a pyreneaerosol of medium
mass concentration. (Taken from HOCHRAINER and STÖBER, 1974)

temperature and the volume of the stream. At KIMMERLE's institute
different PAHs present in AEC and their combinations will be used in
inhalation experiments. The animals live in the above-mentioned isola-
tor and are exposed to the aerosol 5 times weekly in such a way that
only the frontal part of the head is exposed while the rest of the
body is protected from contamination.

Instructions on the construction and utilization of the generator
(HOCHRAINER and STÖBER, 1974) and the total apparatus (KIMMERLE) will
soon be published.

The AEC and its fractions, as well as the pure PAH, will be tested in
various institutes. For the testing of a constituent effect, the
scheme of GRIMMER (personal communication 1974) will be employed
(Fig. 4).

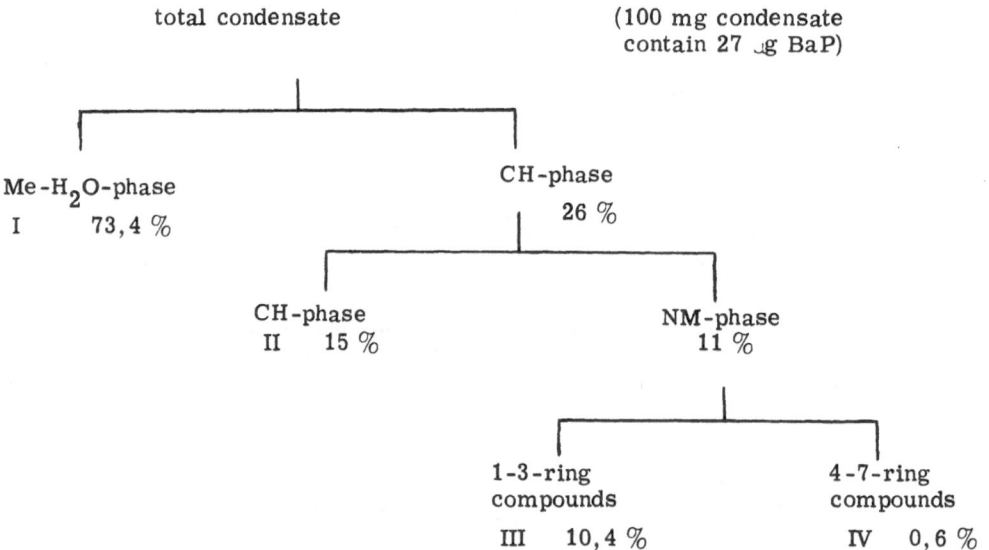

__Fig. 4.__ Fractionating scheme. (Taken from GRIMMER, personal communication 1974)

1. Total condensate is extracted with 90% methanol and cyclohexane
in equal amounts for 2 to 3 minutes, the phases separated, cyclohexane
above and methanol below.

2. The cyclohexane Phase I is then extracted 3 times with equal amounts
of nitromethane and cyclohexane; in this way, the PAHs remain almost
selectively in the lower nitromethane Phase (e.g., BaP 97%), with the
cyclohexane Phase II above.

3. The nitromethane Phase is then run through a sephadex column which
separates the 1-3 ring PAHs from the 4-7 ring compounds.

In our laboratories, we next tested the relation of the solvent to
the AEC and some of its fractions by epicutaneous and subcutaneous
application. Those substances tested were water, physiological saline,
gelatin, tylose, 10% watery calf serum albumin, ethynol, vegetable oil,

methanol, acetone, tetrahydrofurane, n-tricapryline alone and in combination with gelatine, tylose, and ethynol as well as dimethylsulfoxide (DMSO). A moleculare solution of AEC was not possible with any
of the 15 tested solvents. Treating the mixtures with ultramax- and
supersonic apparatus resulted in an irreversible rubber-like clotted
mass.

The subcutaneous application of AEC was best accomplished by suspend-
ing it in 10% watery calf serum albumin (Behring) which is an ambiv-
alent medium for the hydrophilic and lipophilic constituents of AEC,
this suspension was carefully homogenized in a Potter vessel. We
attained the best suspension with DMSO, which will be used for the
epicutaneous applications.

The nitromethane Phase, as an example, is injectable only with n-
tricapryline, but for painting, DMSO is utilized. The subcutaneous
maximal tolerable dose of AEC is 5-mg substance suspended in 0.5-ml
serum albumin. The single injection of more than 2% condensate suspension in serum albumin results in the demarcation and rejection of the
substance by ulceration in but a few days. The fractions suspended
in n-tricaprylin were tolerable up to a 20% suspension of the AEC
constituent. After daily paintings of 0.3 ml of a 25% AEC suspension
in DMSO, we observed no irritations.

To date, no specific short-term test exists for carcinogenicity; however, several authors have established a good correlation between the
results of the sebaceous gland suppression test (SGST) and chronic
studies on carcinogenesis with the use of PAH and cigarette smoke condensate. We have also employed this test in our laboratories with
equal success over the last 7 years as an aid in estimating the biological activation of cigarette smoke condensate and fractions. Therefore, we have also chosen this test to screening the activity of AEC
and BaP (Table 5).

At this point I would like to emphasize that the correlations between
the SGST and chronic studies can be applied only to PAH and cigarette
smoke condensate and perhaps AEC; no other carcinogen can be evaluated.

3 groups of 20, about 40-day-old CFLP mice (during the nongrowing phase
for hair) were treated 3 times at 2-day intervals with 0.05 ml of the
suspended test substance. The application was applied to the dorsal
skin in the flank area 1 to 1.5 cm wide. 3 days after the last painting, the animals were sacrificed and the treated skin section excised
and prepared for histology. Depending on the biological activity of
the tested substance, the sebaceous glands were microscopically identified and we counted up to 100 hair follicles per slide. Experience has
demonstrated a dose-response relationship that can be statistically
analyzed and evaluated. However, in the very low dosage groups, the
evaluation is somewhat difficult. The mean and the upper and lower
limits of the confidence range of the average values were determined
by the logit-transformation method. The application and evaluation
are encoded.

These values have been reproduced, and they demonstrate an approximately 20-times greater biological activity on the basis of BaP applied
for AEC in group 3 than for BaP only in group 6. Additional tests with
AEC, the aforementioned fractions thereof, and BaP at different concentrations are still being evaluated. Corresponding chronic experiments will likewise be performed by us. One completed experiment demonstrates that the BaP in AEC is 4 or 5 times as effective as BaP
alone (Table 6). This experiment is being repeated. In addition, the

Table 5. Sebaceous glands suppression test with automotive exhaust gas. 20 CFLP-mice per group; treatment: 3 x 0.05 ml of test substance in 1 week. The mean value and the upper - and lower - tolerance line of the trust range of the mean values were determined by logit-transformation of the individual values

Substance	Sebaceous glands suppression (%)		
	upper tolerance line	mean value	lower tolerance line
Exhaust gas cond.containing 0.0961 mcg BaP in 0.05 ml DMSO (related to 10 mcg BaP/anno)	34.7	27.1	20.7
Exhaust gas cond.containing 0.288 mcg BaP in 0.05 ml DMSO (related to 30 mcg BaP/anno)	41.6	33.1	25.6
Exhaust gas cond.containing 0.865 mcg BaP in 0.05 ml DMSO (related to 90 mcg BaP/anno)	69.3	56.8	43.3
Benzo(a)pyrene 3.84 mcg BaP in 0.05 ml DMSO (related to 400 mcg BaP/anno)	28.6	22.9	18.1
Benzo(a)pyrene 7.68 mcg BaP in 0.05 ml DMSO (related to 800 mcg BaP/anno)	39.1	31.5	24.7
Benzo(a)pyrene 16.5 mcg BaP in 0.05 ml DMSO (related to 1716 mcg BaP/anno)(BaP 1:3000 in DMSO)	63.5	50.0	36.5

95% statistical certainty.

condensate fractions according to the scheme by GRIMMER as mentioned above are being administered alone and in recombination at 2 or 3 dosage levels.

Parallel studies with subcutaneous application are being performed by POTT (personal communication 1974), and MOHR is instilling AEC at several dose levels to hamsters intratracheally.

Regarding these 3 studies, no results have yet been compiled, because too few animals have died to establish reliable correlations.

An important finding remains to be mentioned: it is definitive that GRIMMER (personal communication 1973) has established the total ratio of PAH to AEC by use of a capillary gas chromatography on a high-capacity column in combination with a mass spectrometer. By this method he found about 135 PAHs present in an amount greater than 2.5 µg/g condensate.

30 substances were found with 4 to 7 rings, 15 of which are known while for the other 15, only the molecular weights have been reported where-

Table 6. Results of experiments with epicutaneous and subcutaneous application of automotive exhaust condensates and benzo(a)pyrene in CFLP-mice. Duration of treatment: up to 99 weeks

Application	Single dose d		Effective number of animals	Local tumors	Medium induction time of tumors (weeks)
2x weekly ep.appl. exhaust gas condensate annual dosage related					
to 10 mcg BaP	0.0961	μg	64	2	68.5 (50-87)
30 mcg BaP	0.288	μg	67	0	-
90 mcg BaP	0.865	μg	77	17	44.4 (29-71)
2x weekly ep.appl. BaP solution in DMSO annual dosage related					
to 200 mcg BaP	1.92	μg	72	9	60.6 (40-88)
400 mcg BaP	3.84	μg	74	18	48.2 (15-75)
800 mcg BaP	7.68	μg	87	66	46.2 (32-67)
1x sc.injection of BaP in n-tricapr. annual dosage related					
to 12.5 mcg BaP			73	14	39.8 (20-71)
25 mcg BaP			83	40	33.9 (16-82)
50 mcg BaP			85	63	28.4 (16-84)
Control of solvent 2x weekly ep.appl. of 0.05 ml DMSO			90	0	-
1x sc.injection of 0.5 ml n-tricapr.			77	3	38.3 (24-47)

as their structures remain to be determined. Since we must assume that these substances are possible carcinogens, we intend to screen them as soon as possible and test their carcinogenicity in chronic experiments. This is especially important, because among these substances there are some that are present in amounts 10 times larger than the amount of BaP.

GRIMMER is developing and establishing special collecting experiences and analytical methods, so that the influence of the metallic compounds in AEC on the carcinogenicity of PAH can be tested.

References

DAY, T.D.: Carcinogenic action of cigarette smoke condensate on mouse skin. Brit. J. Cancer 21, 56-81 (1967).
GRIMMER, G., HILDEBRANDT, A., BOEHNKE, H.: Sampling and analytics of polycyclic hydrocarbons in automobile exhaust gas. Zbl. Bakt., I. Abt. Orig. B. 158, Heft 1, 22-49 (1973).
HILFRICH, J., BRESCH, H., MISFELD, J., MOHR, U.: Investigation on the carcinogenic burden by air pollution man V. Tumors of the respiratory tract in Syrian golden hamsters after intratracheal instillation of benzo(a)pyrene. Zbl. Bakt., I. Abt. Orig. B. 158, Heft 1, 59-61 (1973).

HOCHRAINER, D., STÖBER, W.: A generator for the production of organic aerosols of narrow particle size distribution for inhalation tests with experimental animals. Zbl. Bakt., I. Abt. Orig. B. 159, Heft 2, (1974).

LEE, P.N., O'NEILL, J.A.: The effect of time and dose applied on tumor incidence rate in benzopyrene skin painting experiments. Brit. J. Cancer 25, 759-770 (1971).

MISFELD, J., TIMM, J.: Investigation on the carcinogenic burden by air pollution in Man. I. Mathematical planning of experiments. Zbl. Bakt., I. Abt. Orig. B. 158, 4-21 (1973).

PFEIFFER, E.H.: Investigations on the carcinogenic burden by air pollution in Man VII. Studies on the oncogenetic interaction of polycyclic aromatic hydrocarbons. Zbl. Bakt., I. Abt. Orig. B. 158, 69-83 (1973).

SCHMÄHL, D.: Conception and methods of experimental studies in Germany in estimate the carcinogenic burden by air pollution in man. In: These proceedings.

WYNDER, E.L., HOFFMANN, D.: A study of air pollution carcinogenesis (III. Carcinogenic activity of gasoline engine exhaust condensate). Cancer 15, 103-108 (1962).

Session II   Multifactorial Respiratory Carcinogenesis and Related Bioassays

Chairman: Paul Nettesheim

Biology Division, Oak Ridge National Laboratory, Oak Ridge, TN, USA

Review and Introductory Remarks: Multifactorial Respiratory Carcinogenesis*

Paul Nettesheim

Oak Ridge National Laboratory, Biology Division, Oak Ridge, TN 37830, USA

The title of this session suggests that the interaction of the etiological agent - the carcinogen - with the target, leading to the development of neoplasia, is not a simple one and furthermore, that the
modalities involved are crucial in determining the outcome of this
interaction. What evidence do we really have that one individual is
more prone than another to develop lung cancer, either because of
some genetic predisposition, because of his age, dietary habits, or
because of some injury to his respiratory tract. I think we must ad-
mit that the "multifactorial" pathogenesis of cancer is still largely
hypothetical, and that we have mostly circumstantial evidence for its
existence and role in the induction of bronchogenic carcinoma (or almost any other neoplasia) in *man*. However, I think that whatever direct
or indirect evidence there is, is suggestive enough to justify a
systematic search for the role of predisposing, conditioning, or enhancing factors or synergisms in the pathogenesis of lung cancer. We
need to ask ourselves by which mechanism(s) we can reasonably suspect
the carcinogenesis process to be decisively influenced, and what experimental tools and approaches we have available to investigate and
test the various hypotheses. Some possible interactions of host and
environmental factors with tumor induction and progression are summarized in Fig. 1. The underlying premise is that the carcinogen is an
"external" physical, chemical, or viral agent. We are asking: With
carcinogen-exposure taking place, what, if anything, will increase
or decrease the chance that the process of carcinogenesis is effectively triggered and allowed to run its fatal course? Obviously, carcino-
gen-dose is one important factor and a rather complicated one, since
the relationship between exposure and dose at the level of the macromolecular target is likely to be subject to many modifying factors:
factors influencing distribution, penetration, and clearance; metabolic
activation, detoxification, and the final interaction of the ultimate
carcinogen with the molecular target site or sites. However, it is
generally agreed that, with initiation having been allowed to occur,
the final course is not yet set. Repair mechanisms, growth regulators,
and cellular or humoral defenses (against emerging neoplastic cells)
during the post-initiation phase of tumor-induction constitute another
series of intervening factors that have the potential to disrupt the
chain of events. And whether these mechanisms are functioning at optimum efficiency or not may indeed influence the outcome decisively.

While the scheme of modifying factors outlined in Fig. 1 applies
generally to the process of carcinogenesis, it takes on specific fea-

---

*Research supported jointly by the National Cancer Institute and the
U.S. Atomic Energy Commission under contract with the Union Carbide
Corporation.

158

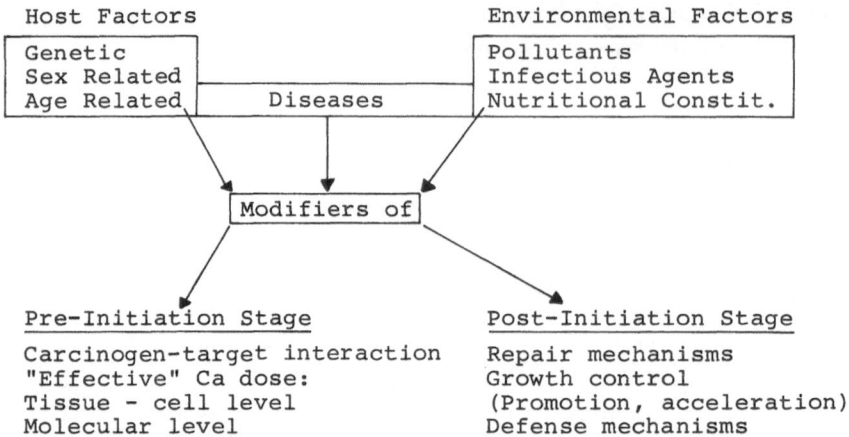

Fig. 1. Potential modifiers of induction and progression of the neoplastic process

tures when applied to different organ systems because of the unique anatomical, physiological, and metabolic characteristics typical of each organ. This constitutes the need for "organ-specific" cancer research that has to investigate a unique set of problems and to develop experimental approaches tailored to its own need.

A glance at the program of this meeting shows which "modifiers" are currently being investigated in respiratory tract carcinogenesis. The effort so far seems to be mostly concentrated on environmental factors. This type of work makes rather severe demands on our capability to control and manipulate experimental conditions. It has been and still is difficult enough to test and measure the carcinogenic potency of tobacco smoke under conditions which have at least some resemblance to human exposure. To study modifying factors of respiratory tract carcinogenesis is infinitely more difficult. This will become clear in what I hope will develop into a spirited discussion of the possible role of noncarcinogenic particles in respiratory carcinogenesis: are such particles cofactors, and if so, what is the mechanism? Is the observed effect more than a laboratory artifact?

An example of the difficulties we encounter, due to the inadequacy of our experimental models, is investigations into the role of infectious agents in the pathogenesis of lung cancer. To my knowledge, KOTIN and his colleagues (KOTIN, 1966) were the first to investigate this problem systematically. They described the development of squamous cell tumors in mice exposed to influenza viruses and synthetic smog. Their data also show a reduction in the incidence of pulmonary adenomas in mice which are infected with influenza viruses. In a similar study, we found no squamous cell tumors but an increase in pulmonary adenomas in smog-exposed mice and this effect of smog was - as in KOTIN's experiments - abolished by virus infection (NETTESHEIM et al., 1970). At the time, we interpreted this effect of viral infection as a permanent reduction in the amount of target tissue, due to the extensive pneumonia with subsequent scarring. We continued to work on the possible relationship of infection and lung cancer, using different experimental approaches and looking at different aspects of the problem. We found an enhancement of the nitrosamine-induced lung tumor response in rats by chronic murine pneumonia (SCHREIBER et al.,

1972); in mechanistic studies, we found long-lasting inhibition of particle clearance in mice succumbing to viral pneumonia (CREASIA et al., 1973); suppression of arylhydrocarbon hydroxylase activity during viral pneumonia (CORBETT et al., 1973); and reduction in the capability to respond to antigen during certain phases of viral infection (NETTESHEIM and WILLIAMS, 1974; NETTESHEIM et al., 1974). All of these observations seem compatible with the notion that some respiratory infections might precondition the host for lung cancer. However, we were still puzzled by KOTIN's and our own findings, which showed a depression of the pulmonary adenoma response by viral infection. We wondered whether the suppression seen in these studies would also occur when a different method of tumor-induction was chosen that could be applied in different temporal relationships to the inoculation of the animals with viruses. Specific-pathogen-free Balb/C mice were inoculated with a nonlethal but infectious dose of either PR_8-influenza virus or Sendai virus at different time intervals before or after intraperitoneal injections of Urethan (3 daily injections of 1 mg/g body weight). The number of pulmonary adenomas was determined 4 months after Urethan administration (Table 1). Only animals showing serological and/or morphological evidence of viral infection were included in the study. With both viruses, a significant reduction in the adenoma response was seen when the viral inoculation was performed 9 days before (and perhaps 3 days before and 1 day after) the start of Urethan injection. At all other time intervals, the viral infection did not alter the Urethan-induced tumor incidence. Thus, the suppressive effect of the viral infection, seen in the previous inhalation studies, could be reproduced in the Urethan system. We had to conclude that our previous interpretation as to a possible mechanism for this suppression (permanent loss of target tissue) was probably wrong, since no suppres-

Table 1. Effect of viral infection on the urethan induced pulmonary adenoma response in BALB/c mice[a]

Time of viral inoculation (in days)	Type of virus	Mean number of tumors per mouse			
		Urethan and virus	Urethan only	Virus only	Vehicle only
-60	Sendai	11.1 ± 0.7	12.2 ± 0.7	0.2	0
	PR8	10.2 ± 0.8	11.7 ± 0.9	0	0
-21	Sendai	10.3 ± 1.0	11.1 ± 0.5	0.1	–
	PR8	11.9 ± 0.9	13.6 ± 1.2	0.1	–
- 9	Sendai	6.9 ± 0.9	12.3 ± 1.3	–	–
	PR8	4.0 ± 0.9	11.2 ± 1.0	–	–
- 3	Sendai	all died	–	–	–
	PR8 (5m)	4.2 ± 1.0	–	–	–
+ 1	Sendai	all died	–	–	–
	PR8 (4m)	3.5 ± 0.9	–	–	–
+30	Sendai	14.6 ± 0.9	13.2 ± 1.2	0	–
	PR8	13.1 ± 1.0	12.0 ± 1.7	0	–
+90	Sendai	11.2 ± 0.9	11.5 ± 0.8	0.1	0.1
	PR8	12.7 ± 1.3	12.4 ± 1.9	0.1	0

[a]Urethan was injected at 0-time; viral inoculation was performed before (-) or after (+) urethan injection. Data are based on 15 mice per group except on days -3 and +1. Mice were killed 4 months after urethan injection.

sion was seen when the viral infection occurred several weeks before or after the Urethan exposure. Instead, we concluded that the observed effect might be an indication of interference of the massive inflammatory process (between 1 to 3 weeks after viral inoculation) with carcinogen metabolism, or of a *temporary* loss of target cells (Type II, alveolar cells).

So we are presently left with the dilemma that 2 studies with 2 different systemic carcinogens and 2 different types of infectious agents give opposite results: 1 shows an enhancement (SCHREIBER et al., 1972), the other a suppression, of the tumor response. Of course, there are considerable differences in the experimental design between the 2 studies which might also be responsible for this discrepancy. The point is that I think we will not be very successful in studying in depth the possible interaction of infectious agents and carcinogens unless we learn to select the exact same target site for both agents, and learn to control the dose at that site for each, both in acute- as well as in chronic-exposure studies. I think that we will come across similar problems in the course of this session, as we hear about studies dealing with interaction of different environmental agents in lung cancer induction.

References

CORBETT, T.H., NETTESHEIM, P.: Effect of PR-8 viral respiratory infection on the benzo(a)pyrene hydroxylse activity in BALB/c mice. J. nat. Cancer Inst. 50, 778-782 (1973).
CREASIA, D.A., NETTESHEIM, P., HAMMONS, A.S.: Impairment of deep lung clearance due to infection with influenza virus. Arch. Environ. Hlth 26, 197-201 (1973).
KOTIN, P.: The influence of pathogenic viruses on cancer induced by inhalation. In: Canadian Cancer Conference, Vol. 6, pp. 475-498. London: Pergamon Press 1966.
NETTESHEIM, P., HANNA, M.G., Jr., DOHERTY, D.G., NEWELL, R.F., HELLMAN, A.: Effects of chronic exposure to artificial smog and chromium oxide dust on the incidence of lung tumors in mice. In: Inhalation Carcinogenesis (M.G. Hanna, Jr., P. Nettesheim, J.R. Gilbert, eds), AEC Symposium Series No. 18, pp. 302-320. Oak Ridge, Tennessee: U.S. Atomic Energy Commission, Division of Technical Inf. 1970.
NETTESHEIM, P., SCHREIBER, H., CREASIA, D.A., RICHTER, C.B.: Respiratory infections and the pathogenesis of lung cancer. In: Recent Results in Cancer Research, Vol. 44, pp. 138-157. Proceedings of a Conference held in Düsseldorf, Germany, March 23-25, 1972. Berlin, Heidelberg, New York: Springer 1974.
NETTESHEIM, P., WILLIAMS, M.L.: Induction of the humoral antibody response via the respiratory tract. Ann. N.Y. Acad. Sci. 221, 220-233 (1974).
SCHREIBER, H., NETTESHEIM, P., LIJINSKY, W., RICHTER, C.B., WALBURG, H.E., Jr.: Induction of lung cancer in germfree, specific-pathogen-free, and infected rats by N-nitrosoheptamethyleneimine: enhancement by respiratory infection. J. nat. Cancer Inst. 49, 1107-1114 (1972).

Morphogenesis of Experimental Lung Tumors in Hamsters: The Effects of Carrier Dust*

Frej Stenbäck

Eppley Institute for Cancer Research, University of Nebraska Medical Center, Omaha, NB 68105, USA

ABSTRACT

In this paper, the biological and morphological characteristics of lung tumors induced in hamsters by subcutaneous injections of diethyl-nitrosamine (DEN) and intratracheal instillations of benzo(a)pyrene (BaP) and the effect of carrier dusts, such as ferric oxide (Fe_2O_3), are discussed. These results are compared with alterations induced with other polycyclic hydrocarbons such as 7H-dibenz(c,g)carbazole, dibenz(a,i)pyrene, and various other carrier dusts in previous studies, as well as environmental agents, cigarette smoke condensate, and gasoline exhaust. In the present study, DEN induced tumors (mostly papillary) of the upper respiratory tract. The distribution and types of tumor induced by intratracheal instillations of polycyclic hydrocarbons and dusts in the larynx, trachea, and lungs (i.e., papillomas, squamous cell carcinomas, adenomas, and adenocarcinomas), depended on both the carrier agent and carcinogen to a varying degree, and bore no relation to particle size or retention time. The intratracheal instillation method offers a reliable means of inducing respiratory tumors similar to those in man, using chemicals found in our environment.

A. Introduction

Efforts to design a model system for experimental lung tumor induction, producing tumors similar to those of man, have been met with limited success for many years. Intrathoracic injection of carcinogens into rats, for example, produced a high mortality and resulted in lesions quite specific to the system used (STANTON and BLACKWELL, 1961). Nor were quantitatively satisfactory neoplastic responses induced in inhalation studies where the experimental situation is more comparable to the human exposure (AUERBACH et al., 1970). 2 classes of compounds have, however, proven effective in systemic lung tumor induction studies, namely, the carbamates, particularly ethylcarbamate (urethan), and the nitrosamines, especially diethylnitrosamine (DEN) (DRUCKREY et al., 1967; MONTESANO and SAFFIOTTI, 1968). A significant step forward was made toward the design of a sensitive, reliable method of lung tumor induction, devoid of harmful side effects, when SAFFIOTTI et al. (1968) induced lung tumors in the Syrian golden hamster by intratracheal instillations of polycyclic hydrocarbons such as benzo(a)pyrene (BaP), in combination with an inert dust, ferric oxide (Fe_2O_3).

*Supported by U.S. Public Health Service contract PH 43-NCI-E-68-959 from the National Cancer Institute.

This paper presents results from studies on the morphogenesis of lung
tumor formation and the relationship to carcinogen and carrier dust
used, as well as the use of this method in studies of environmental
hazards. Systemic applications of DEN and intratracheal instillation
of polycyclic hydrocarbons such as BaP with Fe_2O_3 as the carrier dust
are compared with previously published results obtained using other
carrier dusts as well as polycyclic hydrocarbons such as dibenz(a,i)
pyrene (DB(ai)P), 7H-dibenz(c,g)carbazole (DBC), and 9,10-dimethyl
(1,2)benz(a)anthracene (DMBA) with Fe_2O_3 in Syrian golden hamsters
(SELLAKUMAR and SHUBIK, 1972; STENBÄCK and SELLAKUMAR, in press (a),
in press (b); STENBÄCK et al., in preparation).

B. Material and Methods

Randomly bred Syrian golden hamsters from the Eppley Colony were used,
housed in plastic cages on San-i-cel bedding and given Rockland or
Wayne pelleted diet and water ad libitum.

The compounds BaP and DEN were obtained from Aldrich Chemical Company
(Milwaukee, Wisconsin); Fe_2O_3 from Fischer Scientific Company (Fair-
lawn, New Jersey); saline solution (0.2% sodium chloride, sterile,
nonpyrogenic) from Baxter Laboratories, Inc. (Morton Grove, Illinois)
and Brevital sodium (sodium- di-1-methyl-5-allyl-5 (1-methyl-2-pentynyl)
barbiturate) from Eli Lilly & Company (Indianapolis, Indiana). The
gasoline exhaust condensate was prepared by the Dow Chemical Company,
Indianapolis, Indiana. The particle size determinations were performed by Coulter Company, Hialeah, Florida.

The exhaust condensate was given 3 mg in 0.2 ml saline 4 times for 4
weeks to 40 animals. Another group of 20 animals received 100 μg tobacco tar in 0.2 ml saline once a week for 13 weeks. 1 mg DEN was injected subcutaneously for 12 weeks, in 38 animals. Using the method
of SAFFIOTTI et al. (1968), 3 mg BaP and 3 mg Fe_2O_3 were given weekly for 15 weeks to 48 hamsters.

Animals were weighed weekly, and those in poor condition were isolated
and left to die spontaneously, or were killed when moribund. Autopsies
were performed on all animals, except for a few lost through cannibalism. At autopsy, the trachea was ligated and the lungs were removed
en bloc while still fully expanded; the organs were then fixed in 10%
buffered formalin. Histological sections were prepared from each lung
lobe and the larynx, trachea, stem bronchi, and any other organs showing gross pathology. Sections were stained with hematoxylin-eosin and
special stains as needed. Glutaraldehyde (2.5% in Sorensen's buffer)-
fixed specimens were divided into 1 x 1 x 3 mm sections, washed in
Sorensen's buffer, and post-fixed in 1% buffered osmium tetroxide for
1 hour. They were dehydrated with increasing concentrations of ethanol
and embedded in Epoxy resin 502. The semithin (1'μ) sections were
stained with toluidine blue. Pale, gold-colored sections on formvar
coated grids, contrasted with uranyl acetate and lead citrate, were
studied with a Philips SM2 electron microscope.

C. Results

I. Treatment with DEN

Repeated subcutaneous injections of DEN induced a large number of
upper respiratory tract tumors, as shown in Fig. 1a. The nasal cavity
tumors were of several different types - papillomas, squamous cell
carcinomas, esthesioneuroepitheliomas, adenomas, and adenocarcinomas
of adenomatous, papillary, or tubular types. The laryngeal tumors were
squamous cell papillomas, with a fibrous stalk covered by a flattened
epithelium, as well as squamous cell carcinomas of various differentia-
tions. Villous papillomas of the trachea, with epithelium occasionally
containing columnar cells (Fig. 1b) were also common. The peripheral
lung lesions seen in a number of animals (Fig. 1c) were composed of
cords or islets of tightly arranged small cells with rounded basophilic
nuclei, faintly staining cytoplasm, and distinct cell borders. The
superficial cell layers were occasionally flattened; however, horn
pearls, keratinization, or unequivocal intercellular bridges did not
occur. Some lesions showed papillary or acinar structures, with a
scanty fibrous stroma. The lumen contained weakly staining mucin substances. The epithelium surrounding these structures consisted of
cuboidal basophilic cells, rarely showing secretory activity (Fig. 1c).
The lesions were always clearly delineated, with no signs of infiltration into surrounding lung tissue or formation of metastases.

In Syrian golden hamsters, the respiratory tract is the main target
for the carcinogenic effect of DEN, regardless of the route of administration (HERROLD, 1964a, 1964b). The neoplastic response to
subcutaneous administrations of DEN, however, varies with the different segments of the respiratory tract, but shows a proclivity for
the upper respiratory tract, as opposed to the bronchioalveolar
tract (MONTESANO et al., 1968, 1970).

Tracheal tumors in man are rare, and thus far only about 400 cases
have been reported (STEIN and VOLK, 1959; KAUFMAN and KLOPSTOCK, 1963;
HAJDU et al., 1970). Why this situation exists is unclear, since
laryngeal and bronchial carcinomas are common in man. This is true
despite the fact that the trachea, larynx, and bronchi are sequentially
situated and histologically similar (HOUSTON et al., 1969; RANKE et
al., 1962). In man, exophytic bronchial cancers, including verrucous
and papillary carcinomas, represent a small group with a favorable
prognosis (SHERWIN et al., 1962; RAKOV et al., 1963; SMITH and DEXTER,
1963). A positive correlation between cigarette smoking and the development of epidermoid tracheal carcinoma in the trachea has been suggested
(HAJDU et al., 1970).

The nature of the peripheral lung tumors seen in DEN-treated hamsters
has been a subject of considerable discussion. The morphological picture of peripheral tumors has been considered indicative of alveolar
cell origin (FERON, 1972). FERON has also suggested that autotrans-
plantation of papillary material into the alveoli may be responsible
for the peripheral adenomas. This view has been supported by others,
who base their opinion on the similarity of morphological structure,
as well as the exclusive appearance in animals with tracheal papillomas
(STENBÄCK et al., 1973) seen also in these studies.

II. Treatment with BaP/Fe$_2$O$_3$

Repeated intratracheal instillations of polycyclic hydrocarbons, such
as BaP with Fe$_2$O$_3$ as carrier dust, showed that the neoplastic progres-

164

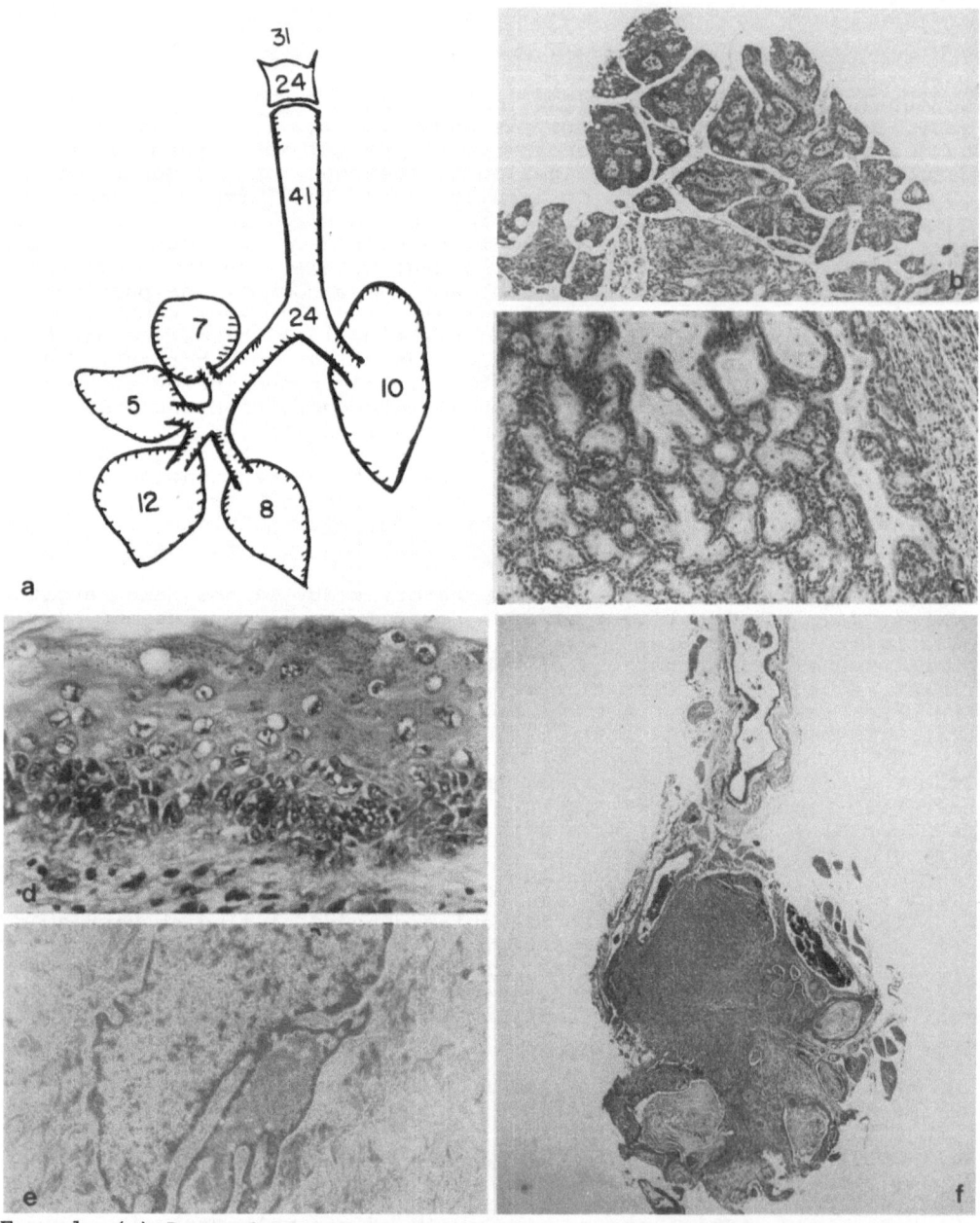

Fig. 1. (a) Distribution of DEN induced tumors. (b) Tracheal papilloma composed of scanty fibrous tissue and proliferating epithelium. HE (x 28). (c) Adenosquamous lesion with epithelial cells in a glandular arrangement. HE (x 96). (d) Bronchial mucosa covered by keratinizing squamous epithelium. HE (x 40). (f) Squamous cell carcinoma obliterating tracheal lumen. HE (x 7.6). (e) High-power view of squamous cell carcinoma cells, with hyperchromatic indented nucleus and numerous tonofilaments in the cytoplasm. Lead citrate-uranyl acetate (x 15.200)

sion at the tracheobronchial epithelium followed 2 main lines. The predominant feature of the epithelium of animals treated 2 to 5 times with BaP/Fe$_2$O$_3$ was squamous metaplasia, whereby the regular columnar cells were replaced by multiple layers of regularly built epithelial cells comparable to those induced by DMBA and Fe$_2$O$_3$ (Fig. 1d). Continued treatment introduced dysplastic features with irregular stratification, variability in cellular shapes, sizes, and nuclei, and disturbed polarization. Ultrastructural studies showed intracellular keratohyalin granules and tonofilaments, deranged mitochondria, and irregular, indented hyperchromatic nuclei (Fig. 1e). Ultimately a number of squamous cell carcinomas with variable degrees of keratin formation and differentiation occurred (Fig. 1f).

Carcinogens such as BaP, as well as DMBA, induced a prominent epithelial proliferation, starting as squamous metaplasia and causing most tumors to be of squamous type (STENBÄCK and SELLAKUMAR, in press). Several studies have stressed the significance of epithelial metaplasia for the development of bronchial cancer (AUERBACH et al., 1957; SANDERUD, 1958). HARRIS et al. (1971), using a BaP/Fe$_2$O$_3$ mixture, reported that squamous metaplasia and hyperplasia occurred only when both agents were used together. Carcinoma *in situ* documentation of the primary origins of epidermoid cancer has been associated with invasive cancer in man (BLACK and ACKERMAN, 1952). However, there is as big an incidence of *in situ* cancer in the trachea as there is of bronchial cancer, despite the difference in tumor incidence (AUERBACH et al., 1957; IDE et al., 1959).

The squamous cell carcinomas seen in these studies could be divided into 4 groups as follows: 1. well-differentiated tumors with excessive keratin formation containing large horn cysts; 2. poorly differentiated tumors with eosinophilic polygonal cells and intercellular bridges, but scanty keratin formation; 3. anaplastic tumors composed of basophilic round cells; and 4. a spindle cell type, with few intercellular bridges, scanty cytoplasm, and a sarcomatoid pattern.

The spindle cell tumors resembled true carcinosarcomas in certain aspects, although similar to spindle cell tumors found in the esophagus (TALBERT and CANTRELL, 1963), pharynx, and larynx of man (SHERWIN et al., 1962). Epidermoid lung tumors in man represent a clearly defined group closely related to cigarette smoking (KREYBERG, 1962). Peritracheal sarcomas have been found in hamsters (FERON, 1972), whereas in man only single reports for findings of fibrosarcomas and leiomyosarcomas have been published (SHAW et al., 1961; DeMATTEIS and ANGELETTI, 1965).

Another pattern of neoplastic progression induced by treatment with BaP and Fe$_2$O$_3$ was pseudoglandular formations of the tracheobronchial epithelium. Ultrastructural studies revealed intraepithelial glandlike structures, including cilia in metaplastic epithelium (Fig. 2a); these lesions were rare. Proliferation of columnar or cuboidal cells of the bronchioles in adenomatoid patterns without mucin production (Fig. 2b) similar to the bronchiol adenomatoid lesions of man, were also seen in the BaP/Fe$_2$O$_3$ treated animals. The size of the lesions varied considerably; some showed only a few acinar formations around a bronchiole, while others spread extensively into adjacent lung tissue. The presence of bronchiol epithelial proliferations around dust deposits was also common (Fig. 2c) although not in direct association with tumor formation. Adenocarcinomas were not very frequent, showing glandular acinar or tubular formation with scanty mucin producing columnar cells (Fig. 2d).

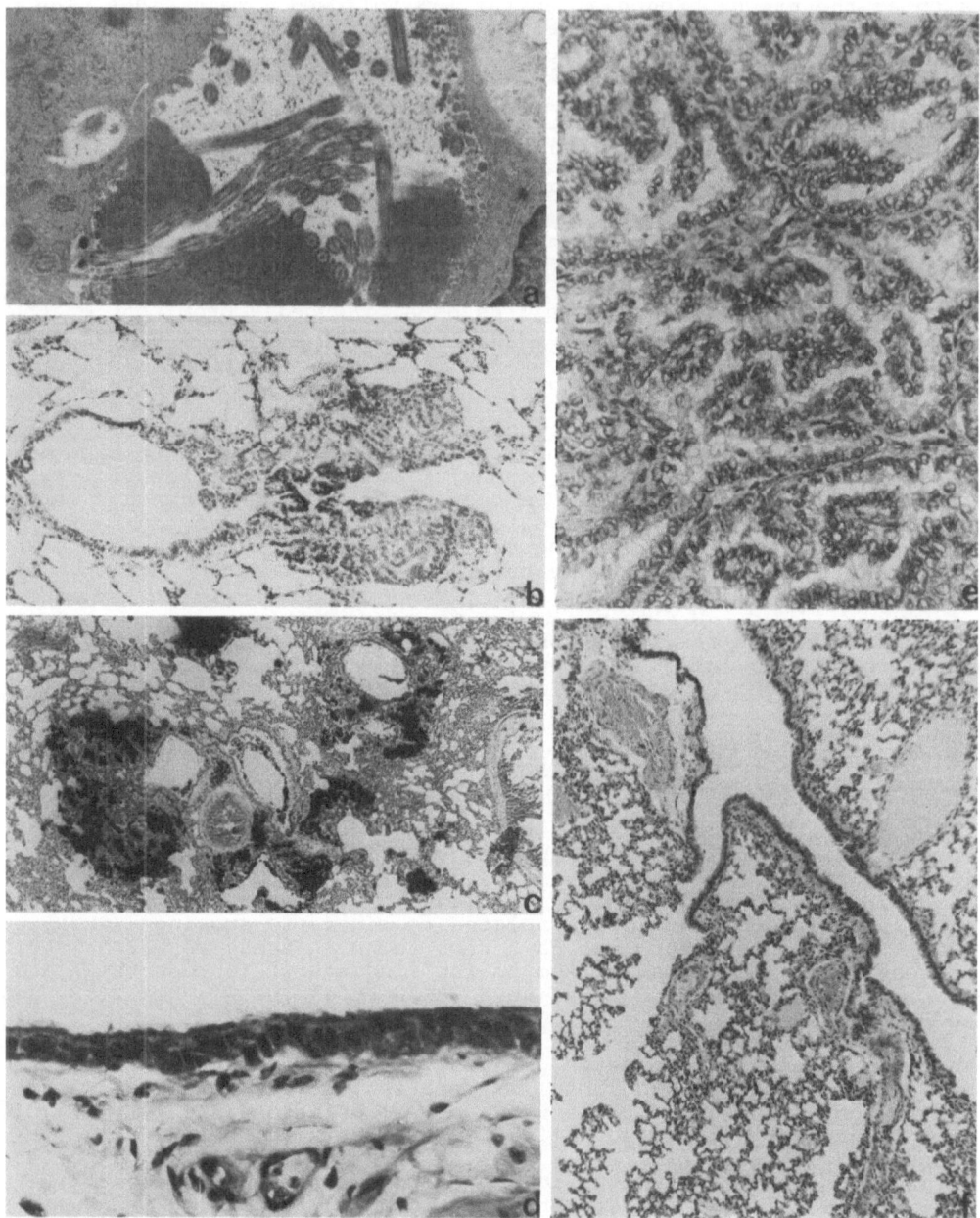

Fig. 2. (a) Intraepithelial cyst formation with ciliated cells in BaP/Fe$_2$O$_3$-treated hamster tracheobronchial epithelium. Uranyl acetate-lead citrate (x 9.600). (b) Bronchial adenomatoid lesion with pro-liferation of regular cells growing along the alveolar surfaces. HE (x 84). (c) Accumulations of Fe$_2$O$_3$ and proliferation of bronchiolar-epithelium in Fe$_2$O$_3$ treated hamster lung. HE (x 20). (d) Adenocarcinoma composed of cuboidal, scanty mucin secreting cells, with acinar and

The neoplastic nature of the peribronchial adenomatoid lesion has been a matter of controversy. These lesions have been reported in hamsters after carcinogen applications (SAFFIOTTI et al., 1968), but also have been noted in healthy animals, in those suffering from inflammatory conditions (KOTIN and WISELY, 1963), and in dogs following cigarette smoking. These bronchiolar lesions are not uncommon in the human; 1 report sets the rate at 11.9% of 1,799 reported cases (BERG et al., 1969).

Human adenocarcinomas are mostly peripherally located and often are associated with pulmonary scars, consisting of polygonal or cylindrical cells with definite papillae, or with glands that are not always mucin-secreting (BENNETT et al., 1969). Bronchioalveolar tumors in man grow along the alveolar lining, without destroying lung parenchyma (BENNETT et al., 1969; DELARUE et al., 1972). The relationship between incidence of adenocarcinomas and cigarette smoking has been shown (HAMMOND et al., 1970), although less clearly than for squamous cell carcinomas, perhaps relating to the lower incidence of adenocarcinomas in man (KREYBERG, 1962).

Efforts to define preneoplastic alterations of prognostic significance in lung tumorigenesis have met with limited success (STENBÄCK et al., 1973). Findings have included metaplasia, squamous cell, transitional and mucous metaplasia, as well as cilia cytophtoria and micropapillomatosis. These are mainly nonspecific and occur also in inflammatory and toxic states (STENBÄCK et al., 1973).

III. Treatment with Environmental Agents

The pathological alterations induced by tobacco tar were mostly attributed to the toxic properties of the treating agent. The tracheobronchial epithelium remained relatively unchanged, with only slight epithelial detachment and decrease in microvilli (Fig. 2e). The alveoli evidenced more distinct abnormalities, exhibiting hemorrhages with occasional accumulations of lymphocytes, monocytes, and leukocytes.

Animals receiving gasoline exhaust treatment with condensates dissolved in saline, 3 mg/application showed well-preserved lungs. A slight hyperplasia of the lower respiratory tract epithelium occurred in combination with interstitial cell proliferation. In tracheal areas where the epithelium was low, cells containing large nuclei and a few cilia occurred, though epithelial necrosis and exfoliation were uncommon.

Hamsters receiving 0.2 ml of the undiluted condensate showed tracheobronchial epithelium with epithelial atrophy, micropapillomatosis, and squamous and transitional cell metaplasia. Local collapse of the alveolar structure, increase in cellularity of the interstitial tissue, and mobilization of alveolar macrophages were also observed (Fig. 2f). The liver exhibited hydropic degeneration, and the kidney tubular epithelium was partially necrotic, with hemorrhages in the interstitial tissue and glomeruli.

---

papillary structure. HE (x 230). (e) Epithelial disorganization, nuclear enlargement, and lack of cilia in tobacco-tar-treated hamster tracheobronchial epithelium. HE (x 360). (f) Gasoline-exhaust-condensate-treated hamster lung, showing minimal pathological changes, slightly increased interstitial cellularity, and enlarged bronchial epithelial cells. HE (x 64)

168

D. Discussion

In studies of environmental hazards, the amount of particulate used
and the nonspecific toxic effects observed are significant. BaP/Fe$_2$O$_3$
is carcinogenic in doses of 15 to 45 mg/animal (SAFFIOTTI et al.,
1972), while decreasing the dose to 1 to 2 mg is only marginally
effective. However, small doses of DMBA (0.9 mg/animal) proved effective (STENBÄCK and SELLAKUMAR, in preparation). The dose-related
injury, carcinogenic effect on injured epithelium, and possible overload of the dust clearance mechanism may account for the results. The
morphological characteristics of tumors are also dose-related. At the
0.5 mg dose level, DB(a,i)P produces mainly squamous cell carcinomas,
the 1 mg dose leads to an increase in anaplastic carcinomas (STENBÄCK
and SELLAKUMAR, in press). The survival rate, the occurrence of other
diseases, as well as the toxicity of the compounds used, affects the
morphology of the tumors, as indicated in Fig. 3 where the incidence
of malignant tumors is directly related to the rate of survival.

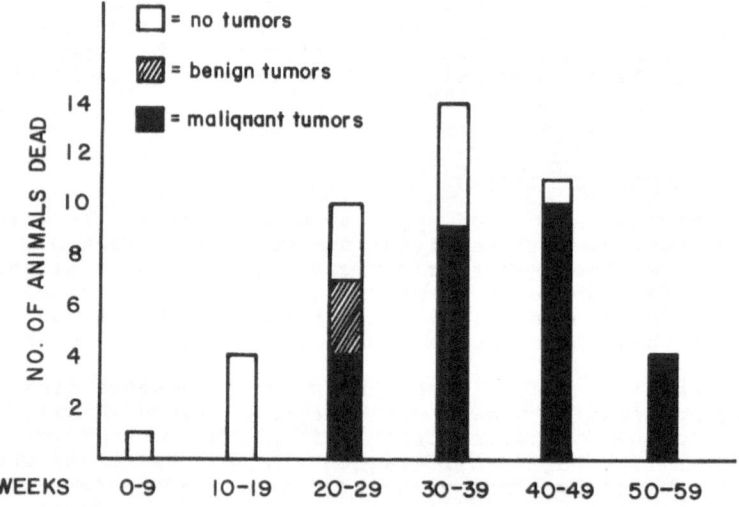

Fig. 3. Incidence of tumors in relation to age of animal at death.
Modified from reference STENBÄCK and SELLAKUMAR, in press (a)

The histological tumor types induced by polycyclic hydrocarbon infiltration differ, depending both on the carcinogen and the carrier
dust (Fig. 4). BaP alone (FERON, 1972) induced a number of different
tumor types, with mixed adenosquamous tumors being common. However,
the type of tumor may depend on the animal strain, as well as the
classification criteria of lesions; the occurrence of mixed tumors
has long been the subject of dispute (KREYBERG, 1967). In previous studies, DBC and DB(a,i)P induced mainly squamous tumors, whereas BaP,
with MgO and silica gel as carrier dusts, induced a higher number of
papillomatous and glandular tumors [HENRY et al., 1973; SELLAKUMAR and
SHUBIK, 1972; STENBÄCK and SELLAKUMAR, in press (a and b)]. The localization also varied with the type of carcinogen and carrier dust (Fig.5).
BaP alone, BaP/Fe$_2$O$_3$, and DBC/Fe$_2$O$_3$ induced tracheal tumors, while,
with MgO and silica gel as carrier agents mainly induced tumors of the
peripheral bronchi and lung. This was also the case with DB(a,i)P.

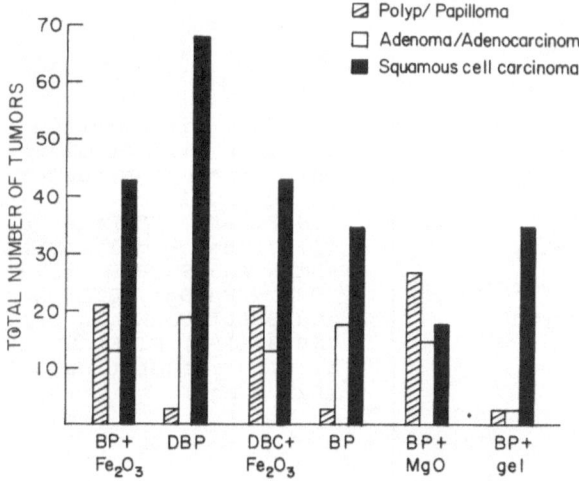

Fig. 4. Type of tumors induced by different carcinogens and carrier dust. Modified from FERON (1972)(BaP), HENRY et al. (1973)(BaP + gel), SELLA-KUMAR and SHUBIK (1972) (DBC + Fe2O3), STENBÄCK and SELLAKUMAR (in press) (DB(a,i)P), STENBÄCK et al. (in preparation)

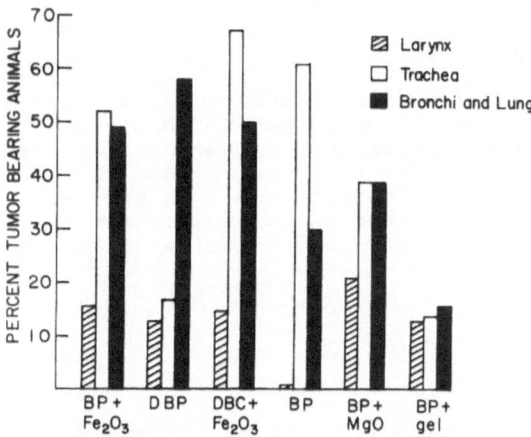

Fig. 5. Localization of respiratory tumors induced by different carcinogens and carrier dusts. Modified from FERON (1972)(BaP), HENRY et al. (1973)(BaP + gel), SELLAKUMAR and SHUBIK (1972)(DBC + Fe2O3), STEN-BÄCK and SELLAKUMAR (in press)(DB(a,i)P), STENBÄCK et al. (in preparation) (BaP + MgO)

The distribution of the particle size, as shown in Fig. 6, also plays a role. The tumorigenic effect of BaP alone in FERON's (1972) studies, for example, has been explained as due to the presence of large particles. However, a definite correlation does not seem obvious, because the large particle sizes in the BaP, DB(a,i)P, and DBC experiments, and the smaller particle sizes used in the BaP/gel and BaP/Fe2O3 studies, failed to correlate in terms of both location and tumor type. Another possible explanation for the variance in tumor distribution is the rate of clearance of BaP from the lung. Large doses of the compound in gelatin produced a sizeable number of peripheral tumors, and in such cases the clearance of BaP was slow (HENRY et al., 1973). The elimination of particles deposited in the respiratory bronchioles and alveoli is dependent upon particle load (SAFFIOTTI et al., 1965). The tumor incidence and localization is also affected by the absorption ability, type of particles, and surface activity of the hydrocarbon/dust complex, the significance of which remains to be determined. The tumors observed in the laryngeal and tracheal segments could be attributed to the combination of tissue damage and deposition of carcinogen in these areas, either by regurgitation or during

170

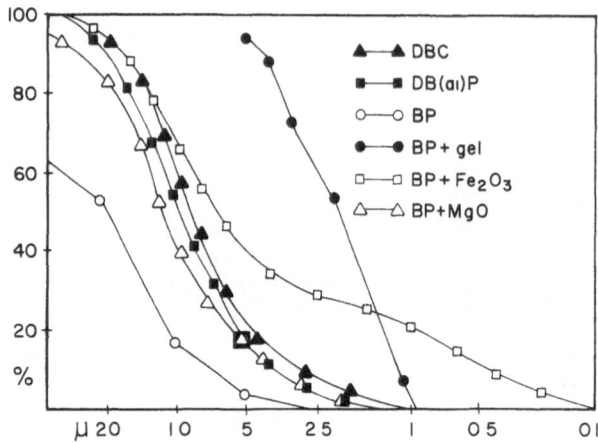

Fig. 6. Distribution of particle size of different carcinogens and carrier dusts. Modified from FERON (1972(BaP), HENRY et al. (1973)(BaP + gel), SELLA-KUMAR and SHUBIK (1972) (DBC + Fe_2O_3), STENBÄCK and SELLAKUMAR (in press) (DB(a,i)P), STENBÄCK et al. (in preparation) (BaP + MgO)

instillation. FERON (1972), using large particles of BaP only induced mainly tracheal tumors at sites of BaP concentration. Thus, the low incidence of peripheral tumors may be ascribed to the small dose and rapid removal of small particles.

The results presented here show that lung tumors in animals are inducible by combination of 2 agents, one of which may not be carcinogenic alone but affects the neoplastic progression. The intratracheal instillation method produces tumors similar to those in man, the location and type depending upon the carcinogen as well as carrier agent. This method is also applicable to studies on environmental agents, the limitations depending on the dose and toxicity of the agent.

E. Acknowledgement

The author wishes to acknowledge the cooperation of Dr. A. SELLAKUMAR in performing these studies, as well as the assistance of Mr. J. ROWLAND, the editorial assistance of Mrs. M. SUSMAN, and the photography of Messrs. A. WASHINGTON and W. WILLIAMS.

References

AUERBACH, O., GERE, J.B., FORMAN, J.B., PETRICK, T.G., SMOLIN, H.J., MUEHSAM, G.E., KASSOUNY, D.V., STOUT, A.P.: Changes in the bronchial epithelium in relation to smoking and cancer of the lung: A report of progress. New Engl. J. Med. 256, 97-104 (1957).
AUERBACH, O., HAMMOND, E.C., KIRMAN, D., GARFINKEL, L.: Effects of cigarette smoking on dogs. II. Pulmonary neoplasms. Arch. Environ. Hlth 21, 754-768 (1970).
BENNETT, D.E., SASSER, W.F., FERGUSON, T.B.: Adenocarcinoma of the lung in men. A clinicopathologic study of 100 cases. Cancer 23, 431-439 (1969).
BERG, J.W., SCHOTTENFIELD, D., HUTTER, R.V.P.: Histology, epidemiology end results. In: The Memorial Hospital Cancer Registry. New York: Memorial Hospital for Cancer and Allied Diseases 1969.

BLACK, H., ACKERMAN, L.V.: The importance of epidermoid carcinoma *in situ* in the histogenesis of carcinoma of the lung. Ann. Surg. 136, 44-55 (1952).

DELARUE, N.C., ANDERSON, W., SANDERS, D., STARR, J.: Bronchioloalveolar carcinoma. A reappraisal after 24 years. Cancer 29, 90-97 (1972).

DEMATTEIS, A., ANGELETTI, C.A.: Primary fibrosarcoma of the lung. Path. Microbiol. 27, 129 (1965).

DRUCKREY, H., PREUSSMANN, R., IVANKOVIC, S., SCHMÄHL, D.: Oranotrope carcinogene Wirkungen bei 65 verschiedenen N-nitroso-Verbindungen und BD-Ratten. Z. Krebsforsch. 69, 103-201 (1967).

FERON, V.J.: Respiratory tract tumors in hamsters after intratracheal instillations of benzo(a)pyrene alone and with furfural. Cancer Res. 32, 28-36 (1972).

HAJDU, S.I., HUVOS, A.G., GOODNER, J.T., FOOTE, F.W., Jr., BEATTIE, E.J.: Carcinoma of the trachea. Clinicopathologic study of 41 cases. Cancer 25, 1448-1456 (1970).

HAMMOND, E.C., AUERBACH, O., KIRMAN, D., GARFINKEL, L.: Effects of cigarette smoking on dogs. I. Design of experiment, mortality, and findings in lung parenchyma. Arch. Environ. Hlth 21, 740-753 (1970).

HARRIS, C.C., SPORN, M.B., KAUFMAN, D.G., SMITH, J.M., BAKER, M., SAFFIOTTI, U.: Acute ultrastructural effects of benzo(a)pyrene and ferric oxide on the hamster tracheobronchiol epithelium. Cancer Res. 31, 1977-1989 (1971).

HENRY, M.C., PORT, C.D., BATES, R.R., KAUFMAN, D.G.: Respiratory tract tumors in hamsters induced by benzo(a)pyrene. Cancer Res. 33, 1585-1592 (1973).

HERROLD, K.M.: Induction of olfactory neuroepithelial tumours in Syrian hamsters by diethylnitrosamine. Cancer 17, 114-121 (1964a).

HERROLD, K.M.: Effect of the route of administration on the carcino-genic action of diethylnitrosamine. Brit. J. Cancer 18, 763-767 (1964b).

HOUSTON, H.E., PAYNE, W.S., HARRISON, E.G., OLSEN, A.M.: Primary cancers of the trachea. Arch. Surg. 99, 132-140 (1969).

IDE, G., SUNTZEFF, V., COWDRY, E.V.: A comparison of the histo-pathology of tracheal and bronchiol epithelium of smokers and non-smokers. Cancer 12, 473-484 (1959).

KAUFMAN, G., KLOPSTOCK, R.: Papillomatosis of respiratory tract. Amer. Rev. Resp. Dis. 88, 839 (1963).

KOTIN, P., WISELY, D.V.: Production of lung cancer in mice by in-halation exposure to influenza virus and aerosols of hydrocarbons. Prog. exp. Tumor Res. 3, 186-215 (1963).

KREYBERG, L.: Histological lung cancer types - A morphological and biological correlation. Acta path. microbiol. scand. Suppl. 157, 1-92 (1962).

KREYBERG, L.: Histologic typing of lung tumors. Geneva: World Health Organization 1967.

MONTESANO, R., SAFFIOTTI, U.: Carcinogenic response of the respiratory tract of Syrian golden hamsters to different doses of diethylnitro-samine. Cancer Res. 28, 2197-2210 (1968).

MONTESANO, R., SAFFIOTTI, U., SHUBIK, P.: The role of topical and systemic factors in experimental respiratory carcinogenesis. In: Inhalation Carcinogenesis (M.G. Hanna, Jr., P. Nettesheim, J.R. Gilbert, eds), AEC Symposium Series no. 18, pp. 353-371. Oak Ridge, Tennessee: U.S. Atomic Energy Commission, Division Technical Inf. 1970.

RAKOV, A.I., TSCHOUKOREVA, N.K., WAGNER, R.I.: Forms of growth of bronchial cancer and their clinical significance. Acta Un. int. Cancer 19, 1322-1325 (1963).

RANKE, E.J., PRESLEY, S.S., HOLINGER, P.H.: Tracheogenic carcinoma. J.A.M.A. 182, 519-522 (1962).

172

SAFFIOTTI, U., BORG, S.A., GROTE, M.I., KARP, D.B.: Retention rates
of particulate carcinogens in the lungs. Chicago Med. Sch. Quart.
24, 10-17 (1964).
SAFFIOTTI, U., CEFIS, F., KOLB, L.H.: A method for the experimental
induction of bronchogenic carcinoma. Cancer Res. 28, 104-124 (1968).
SAFFIOTTI, U., CEFIS, F., KOLB, L.H., SHUBIK, P.: Experimental studies
of the conditions of exposure to carcinogens for lung cancer induction. J. Air Pollut. Control Ass. 15, 23-25 (1965).
SAFFIOTTI, U., MONTESANO, R., SELLAKUMAR, A.R., CEFIS, F., KAUFMAN,
D.G.: Respiratory tract carcinogenesis in hamsters induced by
different numbers of administrations of benzo(a)pyrene and ferric
oxide. Cancer Res. 32, 1073-1081 (1972).
SAFFIOTTI, U., SELLAKUMAR, A.R., MONTESANO, R., KAUFMAN, D.B.:
Respiratory tract carcinogenesis induced in hamsters by different
dose levels of benzo(a)pyrene and ferric oxide. J. nat. Cancer Inst.
49, 1199-1204 (1972).
SANDERUD, K.: Squamous metaplasia of the respiratory tract epithelium.
An autopsy study of 214 cases. 4. Relation to bronchial carcinoma.
Acta path. microbiol. scand. 44, 329-344 (1958).
SELLAKUMAR, A., SHUBIK, P.: Carcinogenicity of 7H-dibenzo(c,g)carbazole
in the respiratory tract of hamsters. J. nat. Cancer Inst. 48,
1641-1646 (1972).
SHAW, R.R., PAULSON, D.L., KEE, J.L., LOVETT, V.F.: Primary pulmonary
leiomyosarcomas. J. thorac. cardio. Surg. 41, 430-436 (1961).
SHERWIN, R.P., LAFORET, E.G., STRIEDER, J.W.: Exophytic endobronchial
carcinoma. J. thorac. cardio. Surg. 43, 716-730 (1962).
SMITH, J.F., DEXTER, D.: Papillary neoplasms of the bronchus of low-
grade malignancy. Thorax 18, 340 (1963).
STANTON, M.F., BLACKWELL, R.: Induction of epidermoid carcinoma in
lungs of rats: A "new" method based upon deposition of methylcholanthrene in areas of pulmonary infarction. J. nat. Cancer Inst.
27, 375-407 (1961).
STEIN, A.A., VOLK, B.M.: Papillomatosis of trachea and lung: Report
of a case. Arch. Path. 68, 468-474 (1959).
STENBÄCK, F., FERRERO, A., SHUBIK, P.: Synergistic effect of
diethylnitrosamine and different dusts on respiratory carcinogenesis in hamsters. Cancer Res. 33, 2209-2214 (1973).
STENBÄCK, F., SELLAKUMAR, A.: Squamous metaplasia and respiratory
tumors induced by intratracheal instillations of 7,12-dimethyl-
benz(a)anthracene in Syrian golden hamsters. Europ. J. Cancer 8
[in press (a)].
STENBÄCK, F., SELLAKUMAR, A.: Respiratory carcinogenesis using
dibenz(a,i)pyrene. Z. Krebsforsch. [in press (b)].
STENBÄCK, F., SELLAKUMAR, A., SHUBIK, P.: Magnesium oxide as carrier
dust in benzo(a)pyrene induced lung carcinogenesis. (In preparation).
STEWART, H.L.: Pulmonary tumors in mice. In: Physiopathology of
Cancer (F. Homburger, ed.). New York: Hoober & Harper 1953.
TALBERT, J.L., CANTRELL, J.R.: Clinical and pathologic characteristics
of a carcinosarcoma of the esophagus. J. thorac. Surg. 45, 1-12
(1963).

Role of Particles in Respiratory Carcinogenesis Bioassay

Mary C. Henry[1], Curtis D. Port[1], and David G. Kaufman[2]

[1]Life Sciences Division, IIT Research Institute, Chicago, IL 60616, USA
[2]Lung Cancer Branch, Division of Cancer Cause and Prevention, National Cancer Institute, Bethesda, MD 20014, USA

ABSTRACT

In animal models of lung cancer induction, metallic dust particles have been used to increase the lung retention of carcinogens and enhance tumor development. The influence of the physical characteristics of the carcinogen-dust combination on lung tumor induction was investigated in a Syrian hamster model where benzopyrene(BP)-ferric oxide suspensions were given by intratracheal instillation.

The size of the dust particle, the size of the carcinogen-dust aggregates and physical association markedly influenced onset and incidence of lung tumors. The probability of tumor-bearing animals at weeks of experiment was greater when BP was attached to small particles (0.5 to 5 µm) than to larger sizes (5 to 30 µm). A mixture of small and large ferric oxide particles with carcinogen produced a higher tumor incidence than the carcinogen-larger particle preparation. Methods of preparation influenced the size of carcinogen-dust aggregates and development of epidermoid carcinomas. Larger aggregates were present after low-temperature precipitation of BP onto the dust than after grinding the 2 substances together in a mortar. The former preparation produced a faster onset and greater probability of tumor-bearing animals. Simple mixing of the carrier dust and carcinogen in a vehicle did not produce a physical association and treated hamsters had a very low lung tumor yield. The presence of ferric oxide particles less than 0.5 µm enhanced the induction of peripheral respiratory tract carcinomas. Without the carrier dust only larger doses of BP can initiate the neoplastic process.

The rate of BP elution from different size particles and aggregates *in vivo* was examined. Physical association of the carcinogen and dust slowed the lung clearance of BP but retention rates did not correlate with particle size.

In this model system, the presence of the dust in lung did not influence tumor induction by nitrosamines, whether given systemically or intratracheally. Lung tumors were induced by the intratracheal instillation of dimethylnitrosamine.

A. Introduction

Laboratory models for the study of respiratory tract carcinogenesis have been reported by a number of investigators (KUSCHNER, 1968; PYLEV et al., 1969; SAFFIOTTI et al., 1968). Their success in demon-

strating lung tumor induction by benzo(a)pyrene (BaP) was ascribed
to techniques that permitted adequate penetration and retention of
the hydrocarbon. A high incidence of bronchogenic carcinomas was obtained in Syrian golden hamsters by SAFFIOTTI (1969), with intratracheal instillation of BaP attached to ferric oxide. The insoluble
dust was considered to act as a carrier and to facilitate the retention of the carcinogen in the lung tissue, although other studies
suggest that the dust particles may have a co-carcinogenic effect
(HARRIS et al., 1971; NETTESHEIM, 1972). In studies with a systemic
respiratory carcinogen, diethylnitrosamine (DEN), hamsters pretreated
with low doses of DEN, followed by intratracheal instillation of
ferric oxide, responded with a much higher incidence of lung tumors
than did hamsters treated with DEN alone (MONTESANO et al., 1970).
Intratracheal instillation of the ferric oxide in combination with
DEN also increased the neoplastic response in the hamster respiratory
tract (FERON et al., 1972).

The carcinogenic response in the BaP-ferric oxide model is dependent
on such physical and physicochemical factors as particle size and
amount of carcinogen retained in the lung. Preliminary experiments
have indicated the marked effect of particle size distribution on
the retention of BaP in the lung (SAFFIOTTI, 1970). The present studies
examined the relationship of the physical properties of BaP-ferric
oxide preparation, dose of carcinogen delivered into the lung, and
histologic changes in the respiratory tract to the lung tumor incidence produced by these preparations in the Syrian golden hamster.
The effects of dust in the lung and particle size on carcinogenic
action of nitrosamines were also investigated.

B. Physicochemical Properties of BaP-Ferric Oxide Mixtures

I. Methods of Preparation

The preparations listed in Table 1 were selected from a series of experiments designed to investigate the effects of method of preparation, particle size distribution, and absence of the inert dust on
BaP-carcinogenic potential. Coated mixtures were prepared by nuclea-
tion of the carcinogen on the particle at low temperature. The BaP
and dust were ground together in a mullite mortar for 30 minutes to
produce Mixture 5. Mixture 6 was prepared by ball-milling BaP in 0.5%
gelatin for 7 days. 50% (by mass) of the uncoated ferric oxide particles used to prepare Mixtures 1, 4, and 5 were within the 0.5 to 1 μm
range. Mixtures 2 and 3 size ranges were adjusted so that, by number,
90% or more fell within the ranges specified.

II. Dose of Carcinogen

The proportion of BaP recovered from the dry BaP-dust mixtures was
approximately 50% of the total sample weight. The concentrations (%)
of BaP in suspension, listed in Table 1, are based on these measurements. The actual dose of BaP delivered into the lung, however, was
less than the expected dose. These values were determined by delivery
of 0.2 ml into a test tube, and the results were verified by analysis
of BaP-content in hamster lungs immediately after intubation. For
most mixtures, the carcinogen dose instilled was 40% to 50% of the
expected dose, but only 1/5 of the BaP in the mixture suspended in
saline (Mixture 4) was delivered through the syringe. The variance

Table 1. Benzo(a)pyrene preparations used in carcinogenesis bioassays

Mixture[a]	Method[b]	Size range Fe$_2$O$_3$ particles (μm)	Vehicle[c]	Concentration of BaP (%)	No. of weekly treatments	mg BaP per treatment[d] theor.	delivered[e] (mean±SE)	Calculated total dose (mg BaP)
1. BaP Fe$_2$O$_3$		0.1-5		1.0	30	2	0.87 ±0.07	26
2. BaP Fe$_2$O$_3$	Coated	0.5-1	Gelatin	2.0	30	4	1.44 ±0.22	43
3. BaP Fe$_2$O$_3$		2-5		2.0	30	4	1.52 ±0.26	46
4. BaP Fe$_2$O$_3$		0.1-5	Saline	2.0	10	4	0.81 ±0.23	8
5. BaP Fe$_2$O$_3$	Ground	0.1-5	Gelatin	1.0	30	2	0.91 ±0.09	27
5. BaP	Ball-milled	-	Gelatin	-	8	-	13.3 to 15.5	111

[a]Ratio of BaP to ferric oxide was 1:1

[b]Described by SAFFIOTTI, 1970; HENRY et al., 1973; HENRY and KAUFMAN, 1973

[c]Gelatin concentrations were 0.5% in saline

[d]Volume instilled was 0.2 ml

[e]Values determined by spectrophotometric analyses of 5 replicate samples taken from 7 to 30 suspensions; amount delivered through a syringe and 19-gauge needle after vortex mixing

among replicate samples suspended in saline was greater than that for
the other mixtures suspended in gelatin. Only the delivered dose is
given for the BaP-gelatin mixture (6), since this material was prepared as a suspension and losses occurred in preparation. Thus, for
these experiments, the total doses instilled into hamster lungs ranged
from 8 to 111 mg (Table 1).

III.   Size Distribution

Size distributions of the BaP-ferric oxide and BaP-gelatin aggregates
were determined by microscopic examination and sedimentation. The
percentages of aggregates in 3 size ranges were determined by number
(frequency) and mass (weight) for the mixtures in suspension, passed
through a 19-gauge needle (Table 2). The suspensions were mixed for
30 seconds to 1 minutes by vortex and the material immediately drawn
up into the syringe and then delivered. Excessive vortex mixing, continuous stirring on a magnetic stirrer, or dispersion by an ultrasonic
probe were found to markedley alter particle size distribution or to
remove the BaP from the ferric oxide (DAVIES, 1974, unpublished observations). Size distributions for a few of the dry powders were also
measured. The coated mixtures, containing small ferric oxide particles
and suspended in gelatin (1, 2, and 5), had a greater number of particles <3 μm. Aggregates in the BaP-gelatin mixture were 5 μm or less,
with 50% in the 0.5 to 1.0 μm size range. The coated mixture in saline
(4) had fewer small particles and the saline did not appear to wet
the aggregates and allow for dispersion as well as did the gelatin
vehicle. The combination of larger ferric oxide particles (2 to 5 μm)
and BaP shifted the aggregate size distribution to the 3 to 15 μm
range. The dry powders had a greater number of large aggregates, suggesting that mixing and shearing broke down these larger sizes. There
were no large particles of BaP in the coated particles. The dry-ground
mixture, however, had 1 quarter of the large particles (> 15 μm) as
crystals of BaP without ferric oxide. After suspension and delivery,
the number of large BaP crystals was half that present in the dry
powder. The differences between frequency and mass size distributions
represent the greater weight of the heavier particles.

IV.   Lung Clearance of Benzopyrene

Because increased retention in the lung and higher tumor incidences
have been reported when BaP is administered with particulate materials
and the amount of carcinogen retained depends on the size of particles
and their absorptive capacity, we examined the persistence of BaP in
the respiratory tract after intratracheal instillation of BaP-dust
mictures with different physical properties. Benzopyrene-coated ferric
oxide particles of different sizes and mixtures prepared by different
methods were examined and lung clearance of the carcinogen coated on
particles was compared to BaP retention after administration in a
gelatin vehicle without particles. Among the coated BaP-ferric oxide
preparations, there was no significant difference in lung clearance
of the carcinogen regardless of particle size (0.1-5, 0.5-1, 2-5,
5-10, 15-30 μm), but BaP retention was significantly greater when
administered with carrier particles than when in a gelatin vehicle.
The carcinogen in a ground mixture was initially cleared at a slower
rate, possibly due to the large crystals of BaP present in this preparation. When BaP is not physically attached to the particle (mixture),
its rate of clearance is similar to BaP administered in a gelatin
vehicle (104 vs 72 min). The ferric oxide particles in the suspension
may have inhibited lung clearance mechanisms to a slight degree. These

results suggest that, depending on the physical state of the preparations, different clearance mechanisms are involved.

Table 2. Size distributions of ferric oxide and for BaP aggregates

Mixture (Ferric oxide particle size, μm)	Percent of aggregates in size range (μm)[a]					
	Number			Mass		
	<3	3-15	>15	<3	3-15	>15
1. Coated (0.1-5)	95 (24)[b]	4 (31)	1 (45)	5.5 (0.3)	25.5 (5.6)	70.0 (94.1)
2. Coated (0.5-1)	80 (29)	20 (71)	0 (0)	3.6 (0.3)	96.4 (99.7)	0 (0)
3. Coated (2-5)	51	44	5	0.7	75.3	24
4. Coated, saline (0.1-5)	60	35	5	0.2	16.4	83.4
5. Ground (0.1-5)	92 (35)	6 (59)	2 (6)	2.4 (0.2)	21.0 (47.2)	76.7 (52.6)
6. BaP-gelatin	83	17[c]	0	5.5	94.5	0

[a]Size distribution determined on samples mixed by vortex and passed
through 19-gauge needle
[b]Numbers in parentheses are size distributions of dry powders
[c]All aggregates 5 μm or less

C. Aggregate Distribution in Tissue Sections

After 16 to 19 treatments with Mixture 1, and also from 6 to 7 weeks
after the end of treatment, large-particle aggregates occluding the
bronchioles were found in sections of hamster lung tissue (Fig. 1).
Small aggregates were present in the respiratory bronchioles, alveolar
ducts, and alveoli. Although most of the particles were located in
macrophages, small aggregates lay free in the lower airway lumens.
Lung sections from hamsters, treated with BaP-coated ferric oxide
particles in the size ranges 0.5 to 1 (Fig. 2) and 2 to 5 μm (Fig. 3),
also showed the presence of large aggregates in the bronchi and
respiratory bronchioles. The epithelium of these ducts, as well as
the trachea, showed hyperplasia and focal squamous metaplasia. Particles in the lung parenchyma were present in alveolar macrophages.

Hamsters necropsied after 10 treatments with Mixture 4 showed particles present in alveolar macrophages and also extra-cellular in
the lower airways. There were numerous large aggregates in bronchioles,
which were made up of ferric oxide-laden macrophages, as well as
ferric oxide alone (Fig. 4). The epithelium in the vicinity of the
aggregates showed hyperplasia and squamous metaplasia. The entire
length of the trachea showed epithelial hyperplasia and focal squamous
metaplasia.

Large-particle aggregates were not present in hamsters instilled with
Mixture 5. The distribution of particles in the lung after instillation of this preparation has been described in detail by SAFFIOTTI
et al. (1968). Similar patterns were seen in these studies, although

178

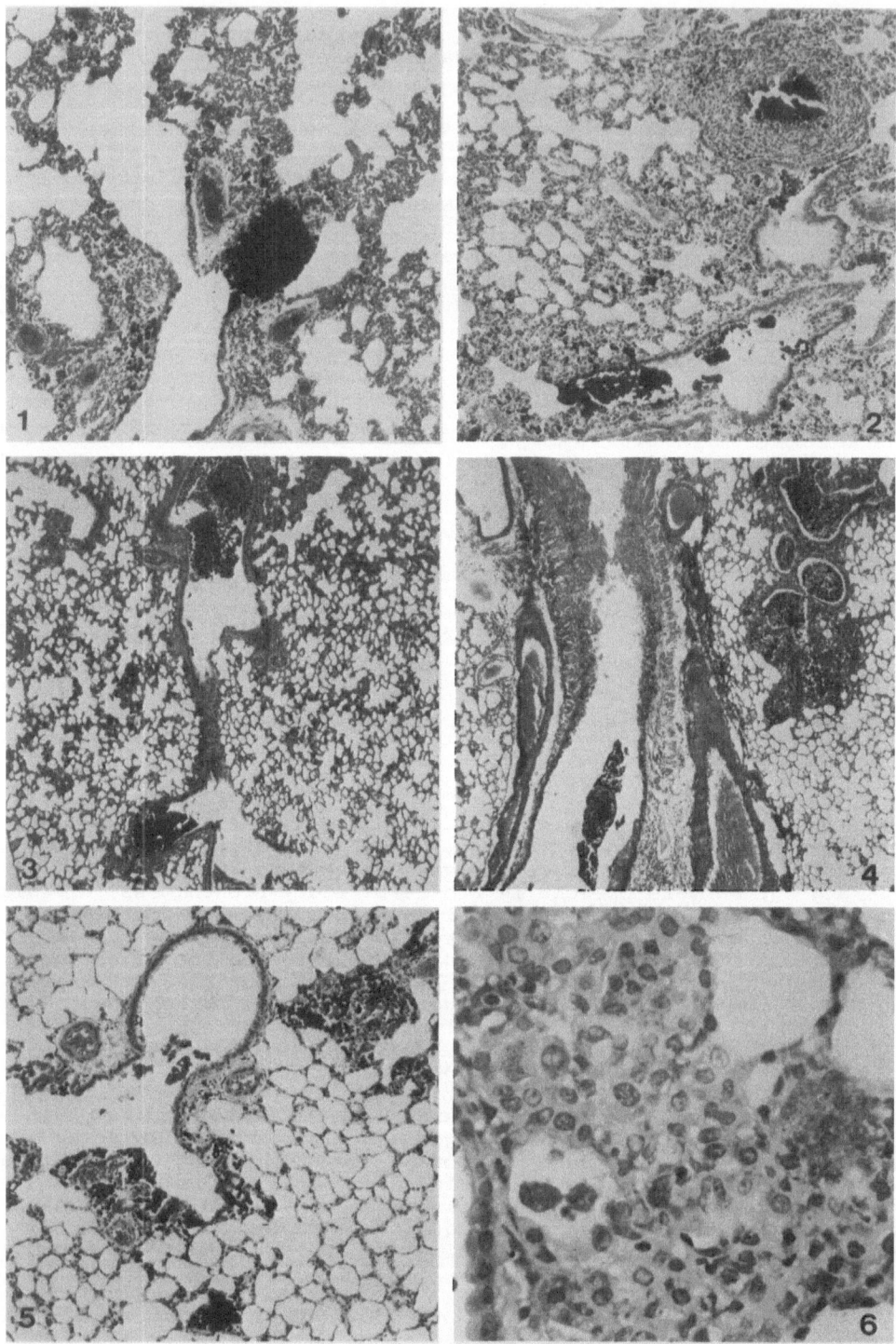

Legend see opposite page

a few animals had small-particle clumps in bronchioles, with an associated squamous metaplasia and keratinization after 14 to 20 instillations (Fig. 5). Animals dying after the end of treatment had normal
epithelial lining in the bronchi and bronchioles. Hyperplasia and
squamous metaplasia of the tracheal epithelium were observed in animals
dying during treatment.

The histologic changes in hamsters intubated with the BaP-gelatin mixture (6) have been described (HENRY et al., 1973). The lungs were
filled with numerous macrophages containing a yellowish-brown pigment
(Fig. 6). Tracheal epithelium was devoid of cilia, congested, and had
undergone squamous metaplasia with exuberant cornification.

D. Tumor Incidence

The effect of these different physicochemical properties on induction
of malignant tumors, and their locations in different segments of
the respiratory tract, are depicted in Figs 7-10. The predominant
tumor-type was the squamous cell carcinoma; a few adenocarcinomas
were observed in the bronchi and lung parenchyma. In most groups,
only a few tracheal polyps and peripheral adenomas were observed,
and their inclusion in the calculations of tumor incidence did not
affect the comparisons. The actuarial computational method used to
correct for animals actually at risk has been reported in detail
(SAFFIOTTI et al., 1972).

I. Larynx

Only a few tumors were induced in the larynx (Fig. 7) in all groups,
and the greatest probability for laryngeal tumors was in hamsters
which were treated with Mixture 1.

II. Trachea

The trachea was the most frequently-affected site and showed the
earliest onset of tumor formation, in all but the BaP-gelatin group
(Fig. 8). This mixture also induced tracheal polyps in 7 animals. BaP-
coated ferric oxide particles in the narrow size range of 0.5 to 1 µm
produced the earliest onset and highest probability of tumor-bearing
animals. Tumor incidence was slightly less in hamsters treated with
larger dust particles (2 to 5 µm) and in those treated with the coated
mixture containing particles < 0.5 µm. These results do not correlate
with BaP-dose since the coated preparations with the narrow size
distributions (Mixtures 2 and 3) contained from 1.6 to 1.7 times the
carcinogen of Mixture 1. The smaller ferric oxide particles (<2 µm)
appeared to enhance the carcinogenic potential of BaP. Tumor induction after instillation of the ground preparation showed a different

Figs 1-6. Hamster lung subjected to intratracheal instillation of
(1) BaP-ferric oxide mixture 1, 0.1 to 5 µm particle size, coated,
HE (x 70); (2) BaP-ferric oxide mixture 2, 0.5 to 1 µm particle size,
coated, HE (x 70); (3) BaP-ferric oxide mixture 3, 2 to 5 µm particle
size, coated, HE (x 30); (4) BaP-ferric oxide mixture 4, 0.1 to 5 µm
particle size, coated, suspended in saline, HE (x 30); (5) BaP-ferric
oxide mixture 5, 0.1 to 5 µm particle size, ground, HE (x 70); (6)
BaP-gelatin mixture 6, HE (x 460)

180

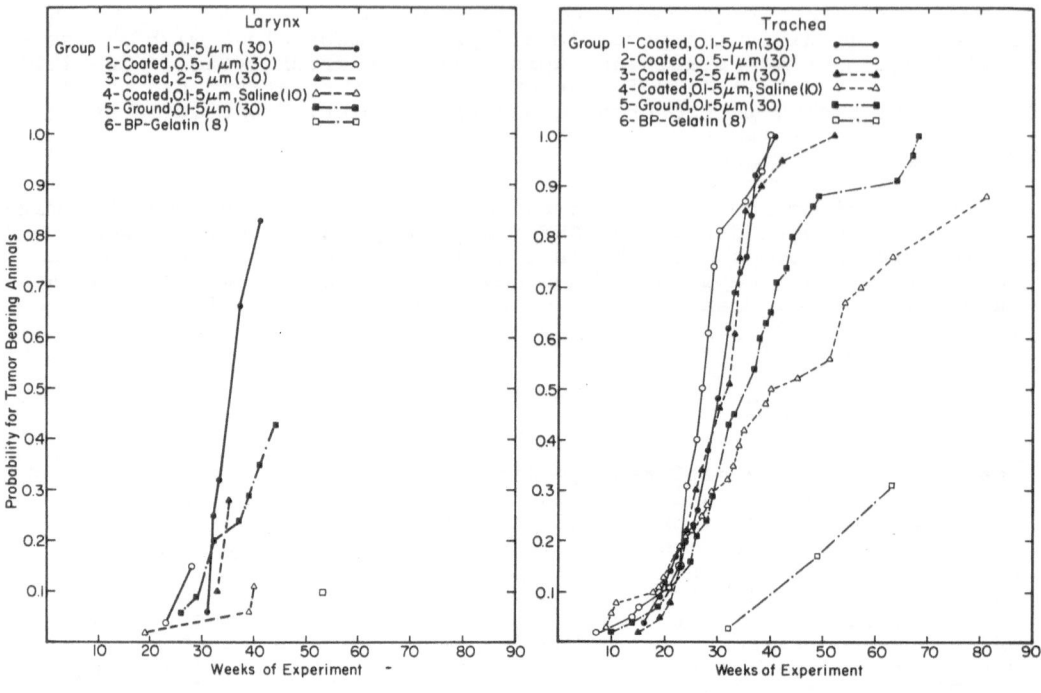

Fig. 7   Fig. 8

Figs 7 and 8. Probability of hamsters bearing (7) laryngeal and
(8) tracheal tumors

pattern. Tracheal tumors were present at 10 weeks, but thereafter
mortality due to the neoplastic process was delayed, relative to
animals which received the coated mixtures, and especially the coated
preparation with the same ferric oxide size-distribution and approximately the same dose of carcinogen (Mixture 1). Hamsters which received the lowest total dose of carcinogen (coated mixture suspended
in saline) showed the greatest overall latency for neoplastic change.
Those animals which died early with tracheal tumors may have received
a larger dose. As indicated, there was a large variance in delivered-
dose of this preparation.

III. Bronchi

Onset of tumor formation and number of tumor-bearing animals decreased
in groups treated with ferric oxide particles < 0.5 μm (Fig. 9). Only
3 animals given Mixture 1 carried neoplasms in this region. 2 bronchogenic carcinomas were observed in animals intubated with large doses
of BaP-gelatin. Tumor induction in animals receiving the ground mixture (5), or the coated mixture suspended in saline (4), was significantly delayed, relative to tumor induction in those intubated with
coated particles in gelatin (Mixtures 2 and 3). These results demonstrate that, in contrast to the lack of a marked dose effect in
induction of tracheal tumors, there were substantial changes in bronchial tumor incidence, relative to dose. A greater amount of carcinogen was received by the animals treated with Mixtures 2 and 3, compared to the other BaP-ferric oxide mixtures, and these hamsters show-

ed a shorter latency and a greater incidence of bronchial tumors. Other factors, however, may influence the neoplastic process in this region. Localization of BaP-ferric oxide aggregates in the respiratory tract, aggregate size, and retention time of the BaP in these areas may also have influenced bronchial tumor induction, regardless of dose. Large aggregates in the bronchi and respiratory bronchioles were commonly present in tissue sections from hamsters treated with the Mixtures 1, 2, and 3, which induced early onset of the neoplastic process. Only small partice clumps were observed in animals intubated with mixtures producing a longer tumor latency.

IV. Peripheral Lung

Only 2 peripheral lung tumors resulted from Mixture 2 and 1 from Mixture 3 (Fig. 10). In the other groups, tumor latency was greater than that for other regions of the respiratory tract. This was the only site where there was a significant tumor incidence in hamsters instilled with the small BaP-gelatin aggregates. Tumor incidence in this region was greatest in the groups that received carcinogen adsorbed to ferric oxide particles < 0.5 μm. The aggregates formed from these particles coated with BaP were small enough to deposit in the peripheral lung but the carcinogen dose was probably less than that present in other regions.

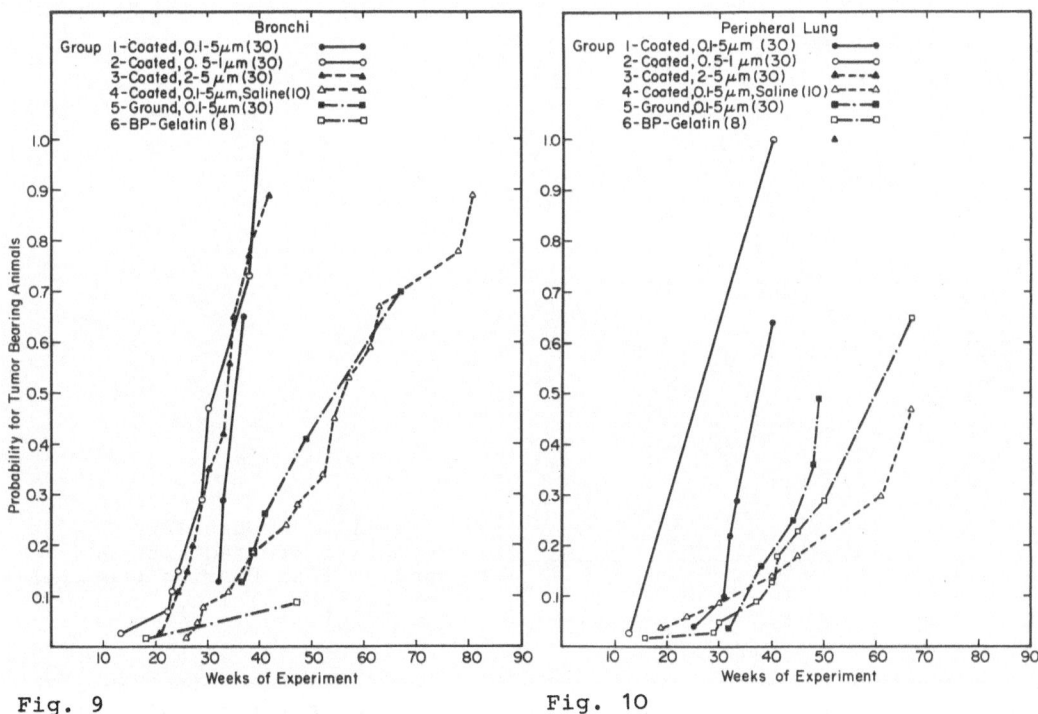

Fig. 9   Fig. 10

Figs 9 and 10. Probability of hamsters bearing (9) bronchial and (10) peripheral lung tumors

E. Effect of Particles on Induction of Lung Tumors by Nitrosamines

To investigate the effects of different metallic dusts and various particle sizes on lung tumor induction diethylnitrosamine (DEN), low doses (0.5 mg) of the nitrosamine were injected subcutaneously, weekly for 12 weeks, followed by 30 weekly intratracheal instillations of the dust in 0.5% gelatin. This dose of DEN induces primarily upper respiratory tract tumors (MONTESANO and SAFFIOTTI, 1968). The 4 particle size ranges were 0.5 to 1, 2 to 5, 5 to 10, and 15 to 30 µm for each of the 5 dusts, carbon, ferric oxide, aluminium oxide, cobalt oxide, and nickel oxide. Control groups for each experiment received the DEN treatment, followed by 30 treatments with the vehicle. The results of these experiments illustrate the variability that may occur in duplicate experiments, even when the same experimental protocol is used for the control groups. As Fig. 11 shows, there was a high incidence of tracheal and peripheral lung tumors in all the control groups. In general, there were no significant differences in onset of tumor formation, tumor incidence at weeks of experiment, and site of tumor formation in the respiratory tract among the gelatin and 4 particle size groups for each dust.

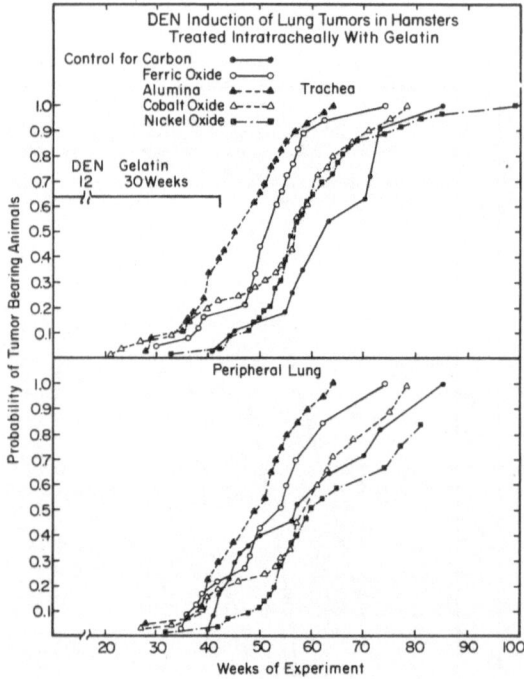

Fig. 11. Probability of hamsters treated with DEN and gelatin bearing tracheal or peripheral lung tumors

The greatest difference in time-to-onset of tumor formation among the control groups was 20 weeks in the control groups for the alumina and the carbon experiments. Tracheal tumors were observed earlier than parenchymal tumors in the ferric oxide and cobalt oxide controls, whereas the reverse was observed in the other control groups. For the control group in the carbon experiment, the probability for peripheral lung tumors was higher than that for tracheal tumors from weeks 40 through 70. The percentage of animals bearing only peripheral lung tumors ranged from 3% in the positive control groups for the alumina, cobalt, and nickel oxide experiments, to 28% in the control group of the carbon study.

The variation in results among the 5 gelatin control groups may be due to differences in the health status or unknown physiologic parameters in the separate colonies of hamsters used in the 5 experiments. Serum antibody titers to 11 murine viruses were negative for all the groups at 0 time, except for the colony used in the alumina experiment. In these animals, significant levels of antibody to GDVII were present (REED et al., 1974), and these animals had the shortest survival time. The results of these experiments suggest that any alteration in, or disturbance of, the normal status of lung tissue in the hamster markedly increases its sensitivity to tumor induction by DEN.

The effects of dust particles on tumor induction by dimethylnitrosamine (DMN) were also investigated. In these experiments, low doses (0.2 mg) of the carcinogen were instilled intratracheally in 0.5% gelatin alone or in combination with ferric oxide particles in the size range 0.1 to 5 μm, for 10 or 25 treatments. There were no differences in tumor induction between groups, or between doses. Thus, for this nitrosamine also, the presence of dust particles in lung had no influence on tumor induction.

F. Discussion

In the experimental model for lung tumor induction by intratracheal instillation of a BaP-ferric oxide mixture, dose-response relationships have been shown to be important in attaining a high tumor incidence (MONTESANO et al., 1970). The number of intubations, dosage-per-administration, and frequency of treatment have all been shown to influence time-to-onset and number of tumors. In the studies considered here, the actual dose of carcinogen administered, method of preparation, aggregate size distribution, and localization in the respiratory tract are considered important. These data will facilitate comparisons of different methods of treatment and results of different laboratories.

The discrepancies between expected- and delivered-doses in these experiments emphasize the necessity of verifying the actual dose present after treatment. Methods of suspension and dispersion can also influence the physical characteristics of the delivered material. Prolonged vortex-mixing can remove the carcinogen from the dust particles and increase the amount of BaP delivered (BAXTER, unpublished observations). Ultrasonic dispersion leads to unpredictable dissociation of the carcinogen and carrier dust and larger BaP-ferric oxide aggregates (DAVIES, 1974, unpublished observations). Examination of different vehicles indicates that the gelatin particles aid in the dispersion of the mixtures, whereas saline suspensions contain larger particle sizes and the delivered carcinogen dose is less predictable.

Respiratory tract tumors can be induced without the carrier dust, but only with very large doses of BaP in particles ranging from 0.3 to 5 μm, and tumor incidence is low. With this regimen, primarily peripheral neoplasms are present after treatment. The low tumor yield may be related to the more rapid lung clearance of these particles than

of BaP adsorbed-to-carrier particles (HENRY et al., 1973). Intratracheal administration of BaP-ferric oxide mixtures, in which the
carcinogen is not attached to the dust, also results in a low tumor
yield and lower BaP-retention in the lung than that after administration of coated or ground preparations (HENRY et al., unpublished observations). Although lung retention of the carcinogen is important
in the carcinogenic dose-response relationship, the total amount
present in the respiratory tract may not give an accurate estimate of
the dose acting at a specific site (HENRY and KAUFMAN, 1973).

As shown in the studies reported here, the differences in total tumor
incidence and localization of the neoplastic response in the respiratory tract can be influenced by the physicochemical properties of
the mixtures. A strict dose-response relationship was not apparent
in these studies, since hamsters which received doses differing by
almost twofold, had similar tumor incidence. High tumor incidence
and reduced survival rates were associated with mixtures containing
the majority of ferric oxide particles <1 μm. In these groups, large-
particle aggregates were found occluding bronchioles. The smaller
particles in association with the carcinogen may have a greater tendency to form these aggregates. With this association, a larger amount
of carcinogen is held in localized areas to initiate the neoplastic
process. Thus, although tumor induction is related to the dose of
carcinogen, the physical characteristics of the BaP-ferric oxide mixture and, consequently, the amount of carcinogen concentrated in a
local site, can markedly affect tumor incidence and distribution in
the respiratory tract.

G. Acknowledgement

This work was performed under Contract No. N01 CP 92148, Carcinogenesis, Division of Cancer Cause and Prevention, National Cancer
Institute, National Institutes of Health. The mixtures used in this
study and analyses of their size distribution, were provided by Mr.
R. DAVIES, Chemistry Division, IIT Research Institute.

References

FERON, V.J., EMMELOT, P., BOSSENAAR, T.: Lower respiratory tract
    tumours in Syrian golden hamsters after intratracheal instillations
    of diethylnitrosamine alone and with ferric oxide. Europ. J. Cancer
    8, 445-449 (1972).
HARRIS, C.C., SMITH, J.M., SPORN, M.B., SAFFIOTTI, U.: Acute ultra-
    structural effects of benzo(a)pyrene on the hamster respiratory
    epithelium. Proc. Amer. Ass. Cancer Res. 12, 13 (1971).
HENRY, M.C., KAUFMAN, D.G.: Clearance of benzo(a)pyrene from hamster
    lungs after administration on coated particles. J. nat. Cancer Inst.
    51, 1961-1964 (1973).
HENRY, M.C., PORT, C.D., BATES, R.R., KAUFMAN, D.G.: Respiratory
    tract tumors in hamsters induced by benzo(a)pyrene. Cancer Res. 33,
    1585-1592 (1973).
KUSCHNER, M.: The causes of lung cancer. Amer. Rev. Resp. Dis. 98,
    573-590 (1968).
MONTESANO, R., SAFFIOTTI, U.: Carcinogenic response of the respiratory
    tract of Syrian golden hamsters to different doses of diethyl-
    nitrosamine. Cancer Res. 28, 2197-2210 (1968).

MONTESANO, R., SAFFIOTTI, U., SHUBIK, P.: The role of topical and
    systemic factors in experimental respiratory carcinogenesis. In:
    Inhalation Carcinogenesis (M.G. Hanna, Jr., P. Nettesheim, J.R.
    Gilbert, eds), AEC Symposium Series no. 18, pp. 353-371. Oak Ridge,
    Tennessee: U.S. Atomic Energy Commission, Division of Technical Inf.
    1970.
NETTESHEIM, P.: Respiratory carcinogenesis studies with the Syrian
    golden hamsters: a review. Prog. exp. Tumor Res. <u>16</u>, 185-200 (1972).
PYLEV, L.N., ROE, F.J.C., WARWICK, G.P.: Elimination of radioactivity
    after intratracheal instillation of tritiated 3,4-benzopyrene in
    hamsters. Brit. J. Cancer <u>23</u>, 103-115 (1969).
REED, J.M., SCHIFF, L.J., SHEFNER, A.M., HENRY, M.C.: Antibody levels
    to murine viruses in Syrian hamsters. Lab. Anim. <u>24</u>, 33-38 (1974).
SAFFIOTTI, U.: Experimental respiratory tract carcinogenesis. Prog.
    exp. Tumor Res. <u>11</u>, 302-333 (1969).
SAFFIOTTI, U.: Experimental respiratory tract carcinogenesis and its
    relation to inhalation exposures. In: Inhalation Carcinogenesis
    (M.G. Hanna, Jr., P. Nettesheim, J.R. Gilbert, eds), AEC Symposium
    Series no. 18, pp. 27-54. Oak Ridge, Tennessee: U.S. Atomic Energy
    Commission, Division of Technical Inf. 1970.
SAFFIOTTI, U., CEFIS, F., KOLB, L.H.: A method for the experimental
    induction of bronchogenic carcinoma. Cancer Res. <u>28</u>, 104-124 (1968).
SAFFIOTTI, U., MONTESANO, R., SELLAKUMAR, A.R., KAUFMAN, D.G.:
    Respiratory tract carcinogenesis in hamsters induced by different
    numbers of administration of benzo(a)pyrene and ferric oxide.
    Cancer Res. <u>32</u>, 1073-1078 (1972).

Effect of Particulate Benzo(a)pyrene Carrier on Carcinogenesis in the Respiratory Tract of Hamsters*

Robert L. Farrell[1] and G. W. Davis[2]

[1]Department of Veterinary Pathology, University of Georgia, Athens, GA 30602, USA
[2]Department of Veterinary Pathobiology, Ohio State University, Columbus, OH 43210, USA

ABSTRACT

A series of experiments was designed with the objectives: (1) to determine if particle size is a factor in the carcinogenic response of the respiratory tract of hamsters exposed to benzo(a)pyrene (BaP) adsorbed to particles of ferric oxide, aluminum oxide, or carbon; and (2) to determine the relationship of particle size to the degree of carcinogenic response at different levels of the respiratory tract.

4 particle size ranges (0.5 to 1.0 μm; 2 to 5 μm; 5 to 10 μm, and 15 to 30 μm) of each particle type (ferric oxide, aluminum oxide, and carbon), with and without adsorbed BaP, were tracheally instilled weekly for 25 weeks in 8-week old Syrian hamsters.

In the 4 BaP-ferric oxide groups (50 per group), squamous metaplasia was first observed in the tracheal epithelium at 19 weeks after the first instillation, in the 0.5 to 1 μm size range group. In these 4 groups there were 64 animals with 79 tumors in the trachea; well differentiated squamous carcinomas occurred in the trachea in 47 tumor-bearing animals as well as 1 undifferentiated carcinoma and 1 adenocarcinoma.

There were 50 bronchogenic squamous carcinomas in all 4 groups and 2 anaplastic carcinomas in the 0.5 to 1.0 μm particle size group. In the periphery of the lung there were 2 squamous carcinomas and 1 anaplastic carcinoma. In the 4 aluminum oxide-BaP groups, tumors occurred later and less often than in the ferric oxide-BaP group. There were 19 carcinomas that developed in all segments of the respiratory tract of 17 animals, compared to 107 carcinomas in 89 animals in the ferric oxide-BaP groups, and 134 carcinomas in 92 animals in the carbon groups. In the 4 control groups of each of the 3 particle types no primary tumors or squamous metaplasia were observed on gross or microscopic examination of the respiratory tract. The difference between the incidence of tumors in the ferric oxide-BaP and carbon-BaP groups compared to the aluminum oxide-BaP groups was interpreted to be a difference in surface activity of the various particle types.

---

*Preparation of particulates and determination of particle size distribution was done by R. DAVIES, Illinois Institute of Technology Research Institute, Chicago.

A. Introduction

Particles that elicit minimal reaction from the lung may serve as
effective carriers of carcinogenic chemicals to pulmonary epithelium.
HENRY et al. (1973) found that each segment of the respiratory tract
of hamsters with the exception of the bronchi had a similar incidence
of tumors following repetitive intratracheal instillation of uniform
colloid suspension of BaP.

In another study in hamsters (SAFFIOTTI et al., 1972), a high tumor
incidence was ascribed to adequate penetration of tracheally instilled
BaP adhered to ferric oxide particles. The ferric oxide served as a
carrier and facilitated the penetration and retention of BaP. In
further studies (SAFFIOTTI et al., 1972), a positive dose-response
relationship was found when repeated instillations of ferric oxide-
BaP were made.

The role of vehicles and carriers of airborne carcinogens needs clari-
fication. The relationship of particle size to the segment of the
respiratory tract affected is not known. Also it is not known whether
the surface activity of an inert particle is a factor in carcinogenesis with particle carried carcinogen.

A series of experiments were designed with these objectives: (1) to
determine if particle size is a factor in the carcinogenic response
of the respiratory tract of hamsters exposed to benzo(a)pyrene adsorbed to particles of ferric oxide, aluminum oxide, or carbon; and
(2) to determine the relationship of particle size to the degree of
carcinogenic response at different levels of the respiratory tract.

B. Materials and Methods

The design of the experiments to study the effects of the particulate
was the same for each type of particulate. 4 size ranges (0.5 to 1.0
μm, 2 to 5 μm, 5 to 10 μm, 15 to 30 μm) of particles (HENRY and KAUF-
MAN, 1973), with and without adsorbed benzo(a)pyrene (BaP). These were
instilled into 8 groups of 50 (25 male, 25 female) Syrian hamsters
each. Intratracheal instillations were made, using the technique of
SAFFIOTTI et al. (1968), once a week for 25 consecutive weeks.

In the 4 control groups, each animal received 0.2 ml of 2% (by weight)
particles in 0.5% gelatin-in-saline suspension (gel-saline). In the
4 BaP groups, each animal received 0.2 ml of 2% particles and 2% BaP
(adsorbed to the particles) in gel-saline.

Necropsies were performed on animals that died or were killed in ex-
tremis. Tissues were fixed in 10% buffered formalin, sectioned at
6 μm, and stained with hemotoxylin and eosin.

The method of KAPLAN and MEIER (1968) was used to compute the cumulative probability of observing a respiratory tract tumor at time of
death. The method is described by SAFFIOTTI et al. (1972).

I. Ferric Oxide and Benzo(a)pyrene

Cumulative deaths are shown in Fig. 1 (they can be compared with those
of other groups using Figs 2 and 3). The causes of death were partial

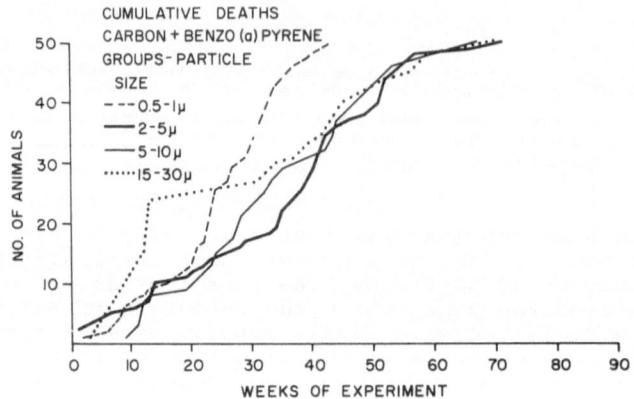

Fig. 1

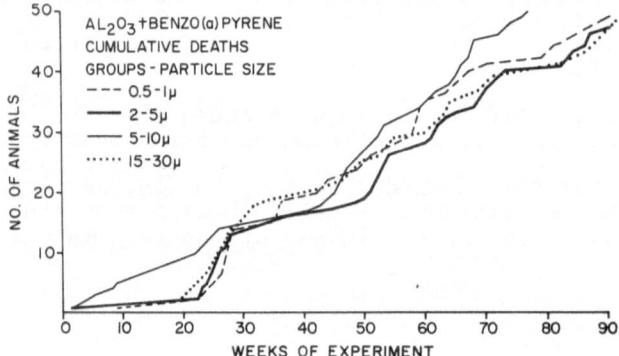

Fig. 2

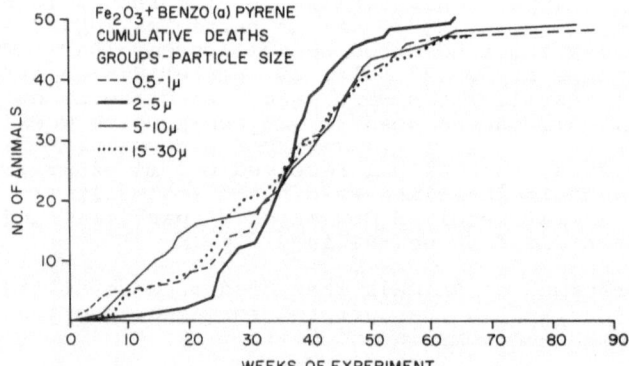

Fig. 3

obstruction of the lumens of the trachea and bronchi by metaplastic and neoplastic cellular proliferations, enteric infections with secondary septicemia, and pneumonia. In the 4 ferric oxide gel-saline groups, no primary tumors or squamous metaplastic changes were observed in the respiratory tracts of 181 animals.

In the 4 BaP-ferric oxide groups, squamous metaplasia was first observed in the tracheal epithelium at 19 weeks following the beginning of treatment in the 0.5 to 1.0 μm size range group. These areas tended to occur in patches (Fig. 4) but sometimes were more extensive when associated with squamous carcinoma (Fig. 5). In these 4 groups, there were 64 animals with 79 tumors in the trachea, more than any other segment of the respiratory tract. Of these, 52 were well-differentiated squamous carcinomas (Figs 5 and 6), 1 was an undifferentiated carcinoma (0.5 to 1.0 μm group), and 1 was an adenocarcinoma (5 to 10 μm group).

Bronchogenic tumors were the next most numerous. There were 50 bronchogenic squamous carcinomas in all groups; there were 2 anaplastic carcinomas in the 0.5 to 1.0 μm particle size group.

In the bronchioles, 4 tumors were bronchiolar adenocarcinomas. The periphery of the lung contained 2 squamous carcinomas, 1 anaplastic carcinoma, and 1 malignant lymphoma (infiltrating).

Some of the neoplasms were mixtures of cell types and patterns. Figs 7 to 9 show an anaplastic carcinoma from an animal in the 0.5 to 1.0 μm ferric oxide + BaP group having areas of squamous change and adenomatous formations. Squamous changes were occasionally seen in adenocarcinomas (Figs 10 and 11).

The probability of tumors occurring 4 in the larynx, trachea, bronchi, bronchioles, and alveoli is indicated in Fig. 12 (for comparison see Figs 13 and 14). Distribution and percent of tumors is shown in Table 1. The percent of tumor-bearing animals (TBA) in the 4 ferric oxide-BaP groups was 51, 51, 46, and 50 in the 0.5 to 1 μm, 2 to 5 μm, 5 to 10 μm, and 15 to 30 μm groups, respectively. The percent of TBA with carcinomas was 45, 38, 27, and 36 in the respective groups.

II. Aluminum Oxide and Benzo(a)pyrene

Cumulative death rates are shown in Fig. 2.

In the 4 aluminum oxide gel-saline groups, no primary tumors or squamous metaplasia were observed in 187 animals.

In the 4 aluminum oxide-BaP groups, tumors occurred later in the experiment and less often than in the ferric oxide-BaP groups (Figs 12 and 13). There were 19 carcinomas that developed in all segments of the respiratory tract of 17 animals compared to 107 carcinomas in 89 animals in the ferric oxide-BaP groups. The distribution of these tumors is shown in Table 2.

The probability of tumors occurring 4 in the larynx, trachea, bronchi, bronchioles, and alveoli is indicated in Fig. 13.

The percent of TBA in the 4 aluminum oxide-BaP groups was 24, 17, 21, and 25 in the 0.5 to 1.0 μm, 2 to 5 μm, 5 to 10 μm, and 15 to 30 μm groups, respectively. The percent of TBA with carcinomas was 13, 4, 15, and 4 in the respective groups (Table 2).

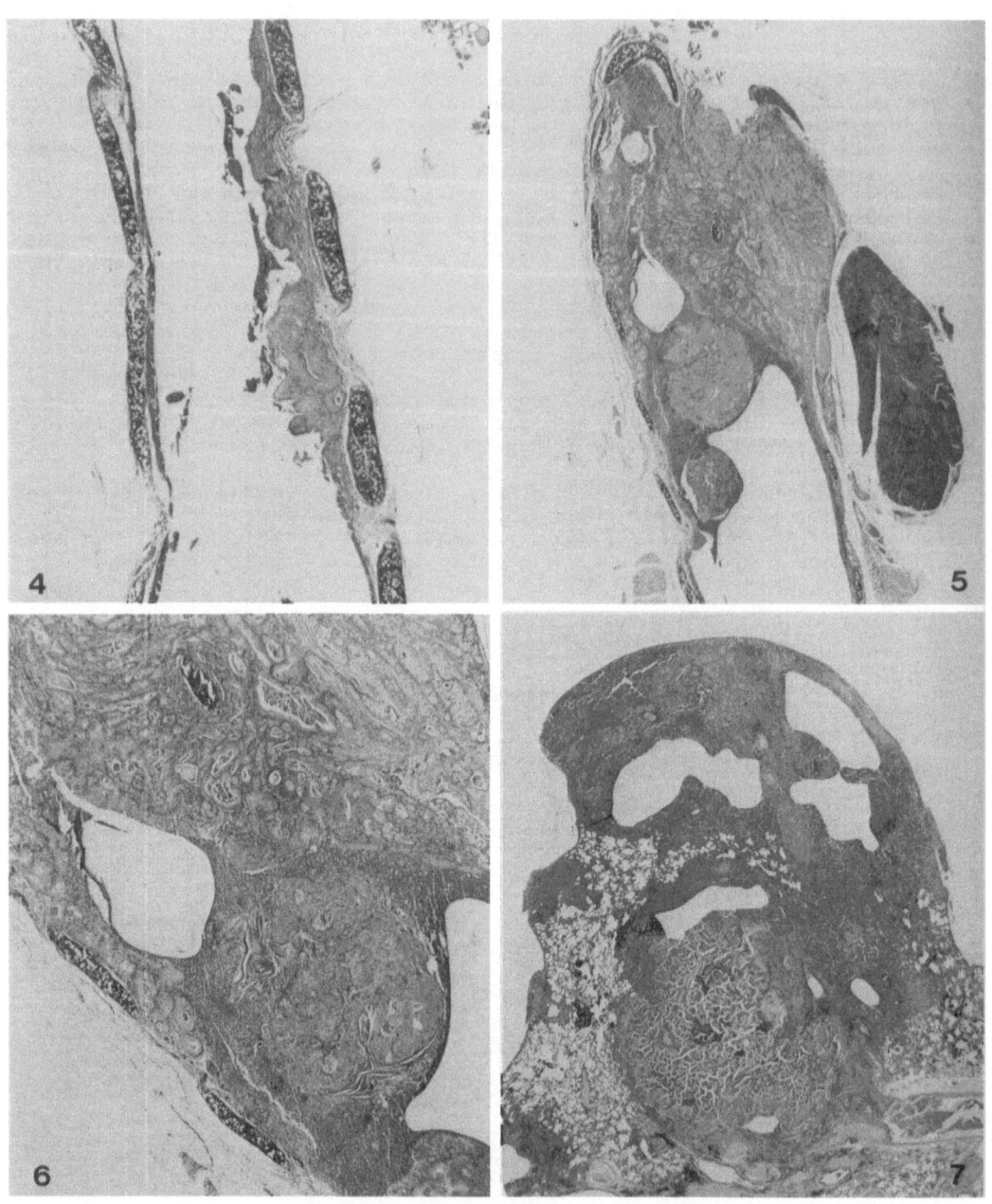

Fig. 4. Squamous metaplasia in the trachea of a hamster that died 21 weeks after the beginning of a projected 25 week intratracheal in-stillation of 5 to 10 μm Fe_2O_3 and benzo(a)pyrene. HE (x 24)

Fig. 5. Squamous carcinoma penetrating and destroying the tracheal wall of a hamster that died 33 weeks after start of treatment with 25 weekly tracheal instillations of 0.5 to 1.0 μm Fe_2O_3 and benzo(a)pyrene. Squamous metaplastic change of the epithelium can be seen adjacent to the carcinoma. HE (x 10.5)

Fig. 6. Detail of Fig. 5, showing keratinized pearls and a remnant of cartilage in the location of the former tracheal wall. HE (x 24)

Fig. 7. Anaplastic carcinoma in the lung of a hamster treated with 0.5 to 1.0 μm Fe_2O_3 and benzo(a)pyrene for 25 weeks. The animal died 44 weeks after start of treatment. HE (x 10.5)

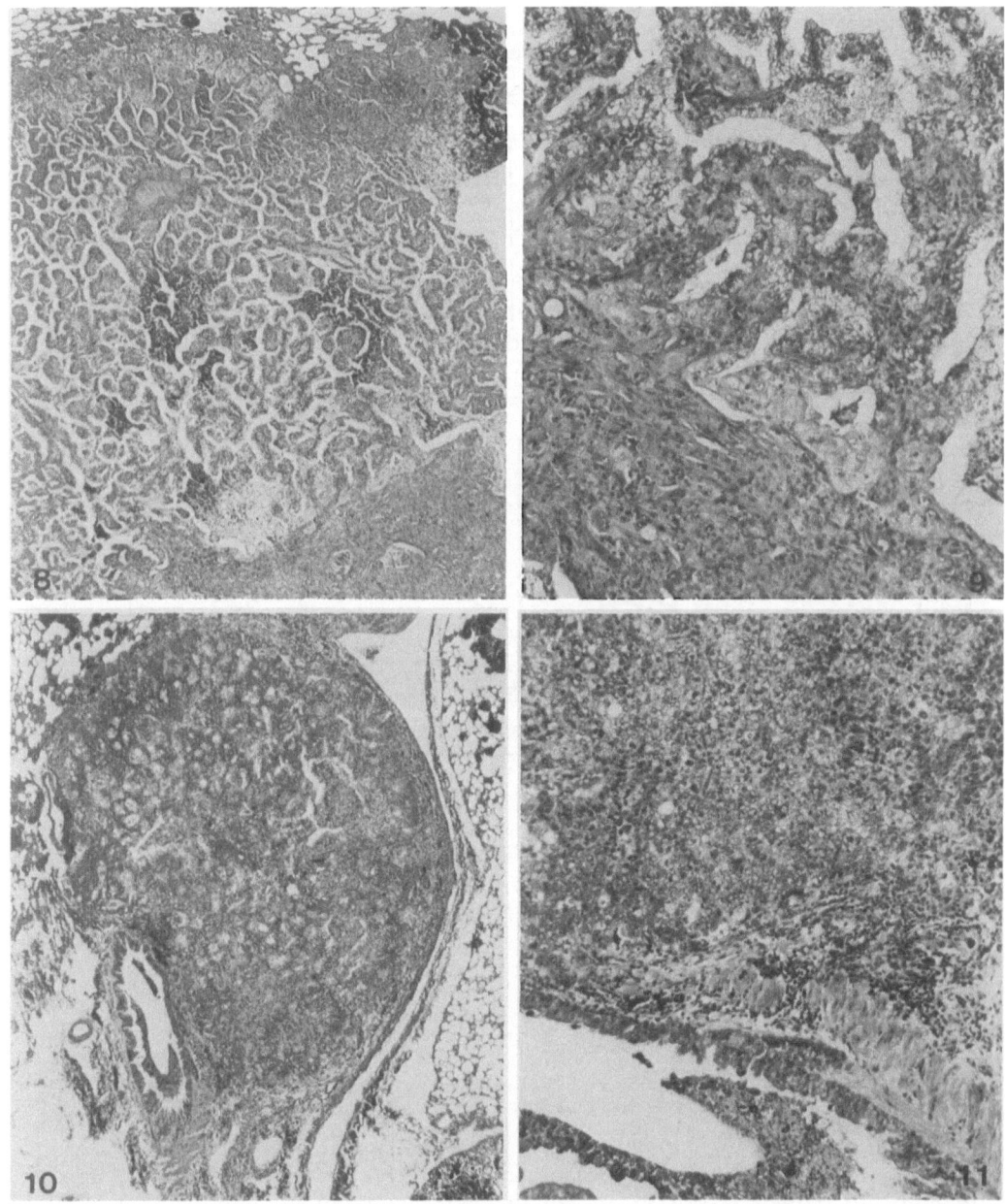

Fig. 8. Anaplastic carcinoma, showing area of adenomatous pattern
adjacent to and blending with an area with squamous differentiation.
Same animal as Fig. 7. HE (x 94)
Fig. 9. Detail from Fig. 8, showing adjacent adenomatous and squamous
patterns of anaplastic carcinoma. HE (x 94)
Figs 10 and 11. Bronchiolar adenocarcinoma in the lung of a hamster
that died 33 weeks after start of treatment with 25 weekly tracheal
instillations of 2 to 5 μm Fe_2O_3 and benzo(a)pyrene. The adenomatous
pattern is shown (Fig. 10) with squamous changes (Fig. 11). HE (x 94)

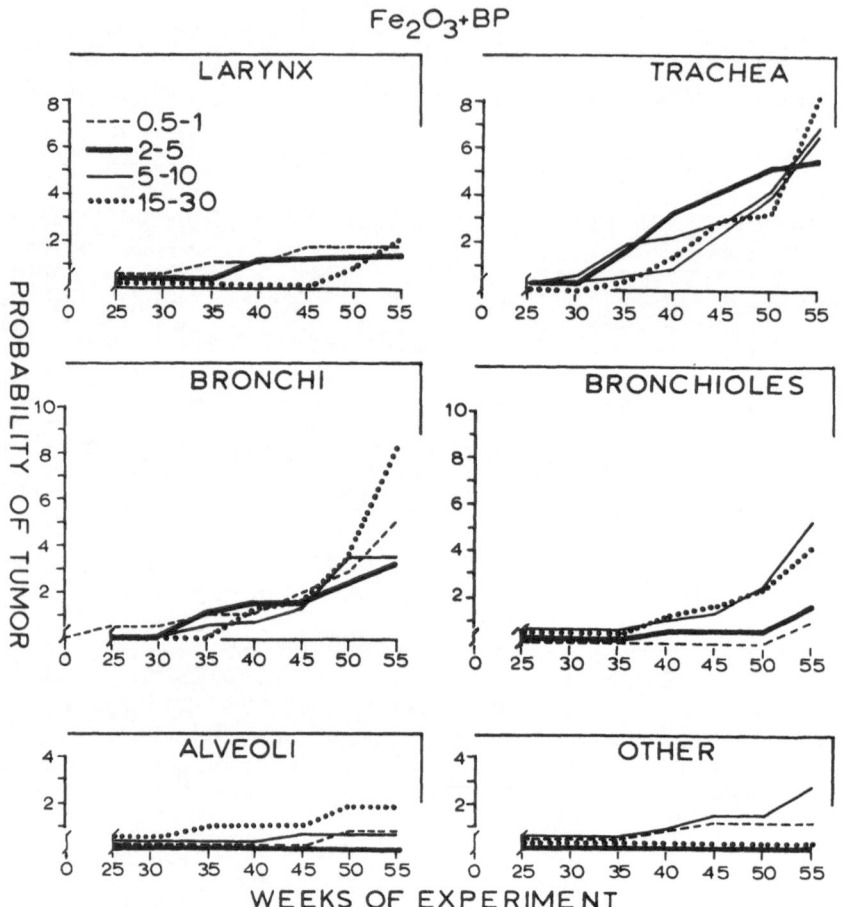

Fig. 12

III. Carbon and Benzo(a)pyrene

The cumulative death rate are shown in Fig. 3.

No primary tumors or squamous metaplasia were observed on gross or microscopic examination in the respiratory tract of animals in the 4 carbon-gel-saline groups.

Papillomas and squamous carcinomas were often seen in the trachea and bronchi of these animals. Occasionally squamous carcinoma was seen to arise in a bronchiole or in areas of marked "bronchiolar adenomatoid lesions". Bronchiectasis, which occurred often, was sometimes so marked that most of the lobe in which the ectatic bronchus occurred was displaced or replaced. The effected bronchus usually was distended with keratinous detritus mixed with purulent exudate (Fig. 15).

In the 4 carbon-BaP groups, squamous metaplasia was observed in the trachea and main bronchi between 10 weeks (0.5 to 1.0 µm groups) and 14 weeks (2 to 5 µm group). In these groups there was a total of 92 animals with one or more primary tumors of the respiratory tract (81 of these had one or more carcinomas). The total number of respiratory

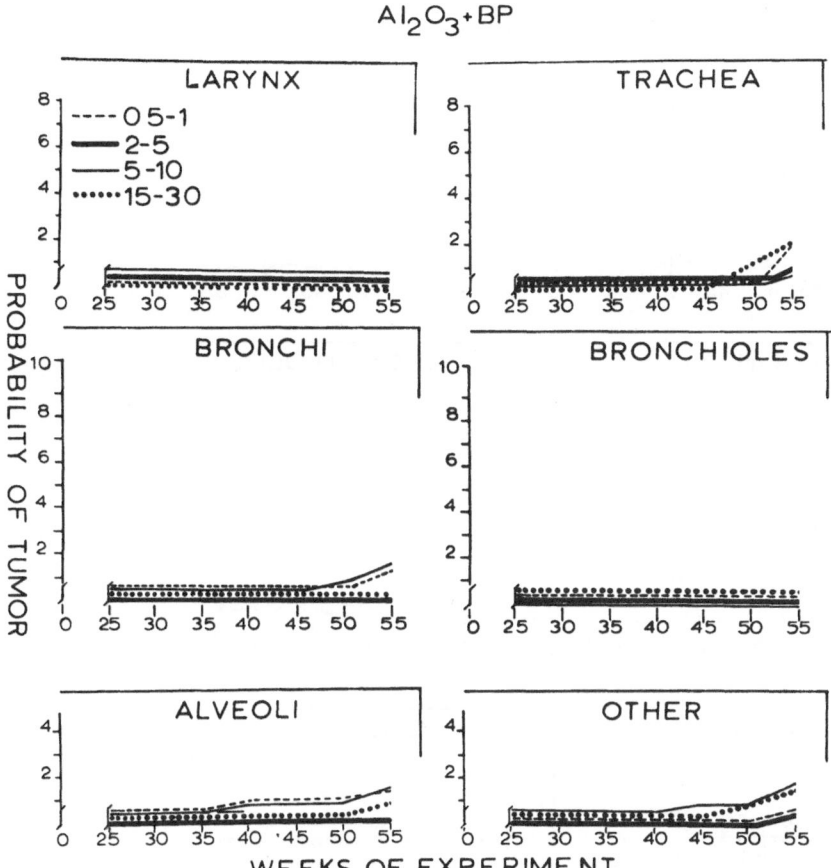

Fig. 13

tract tumors were divided among the 4 particle size groups as follows: 0.5 to 1.0 μm, 60 tumors (47 carcinomas); 2 to 5 μm, 26 tumors (22 carcinomas); 5 to 10 μm, 59 tumors (41 carcinomas); and 15 to 30 μm, 29 tumors (24 carcinomas). The distribution and probability of these tumors within segments of the respiratory tract are shown respectively in Table 3 and Fig. 14.

The percent of TBA in the 4 carbon-BaP groups was 70, 37, 54, and 36 in the 0.5 to 1.0 μm, 2 to 5 μm, 5 to 10 μm, and 15 to 30 μm. The percent of TBA with carcinomas was 52, 31, 52, and 36 in the respective groups.

194

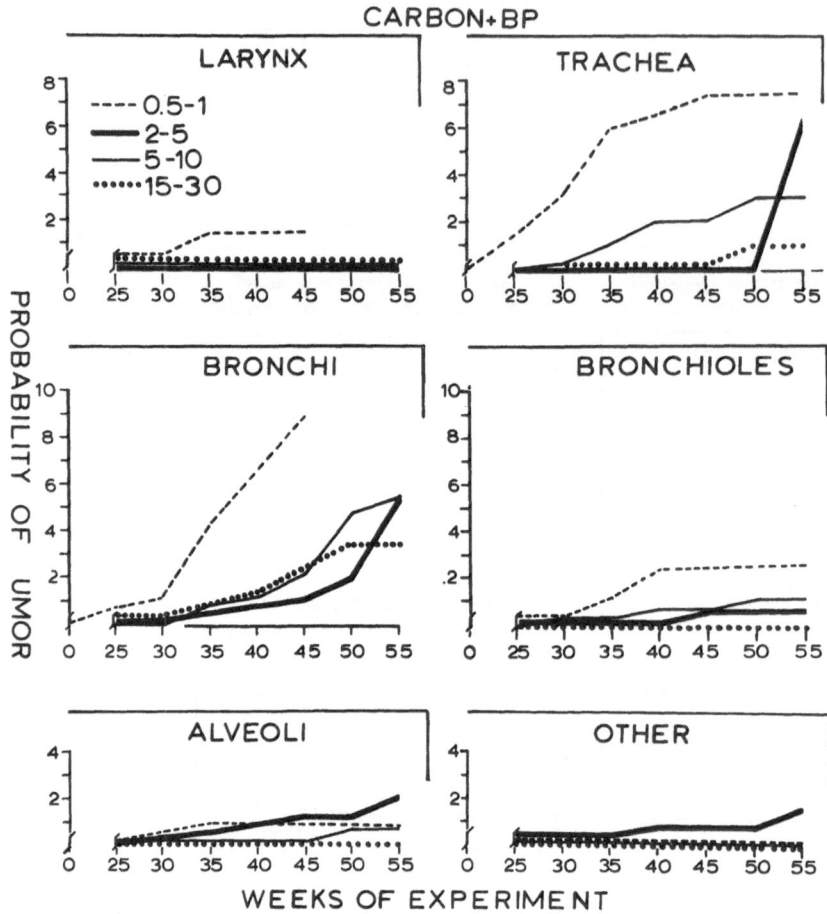

Fig. 14

C. Discussion

There were differences in the carcinogenic effects of the particulates of ferric oxide, carbon (nut shell charcoal), and aluminum oxide when BaP was adsorbed to the different particulates.

In all segments of the respiratory tract there were 134 carcinomas in 81 carbon-BaP (C-BaP) tumor-bearing animals (TBA), 107 carcinomas in 69 ferric oxide-BaP (Fe-BaP) TBA, and 19 carcinomas in 17 aluminum oxide-BaP (Al-BaP) TBA.

During the first 25 week instillation period in the 0.5 to 1.0 μm particle size groups there were 13, 5, and 24 deaths in the Fe-BaP, Al-BaP, and C-BaP groups (Tables 1, 2, 3) respectively. The carbon produced more pneumoconiosis than did the ferric oxide or aluminum oxide and probably made the animals more susceptible to bacterial pneumonia and enteritis.

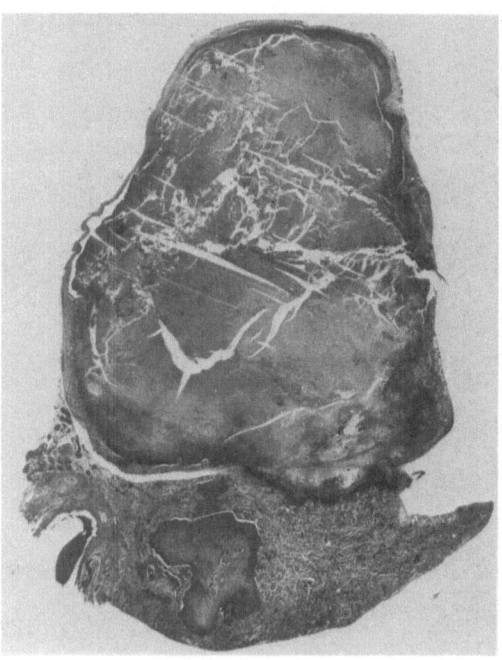

Fig. 15. Bronchiectasis in the diaphragmatic lobe of the lung of a female hamster treated with 2 to 5 μm carbon and benzo(a)-pyrene for 25 weeks. The animal died 46 weeks after the start of treatment. The contents of the ectatic bronchus consists of friable detritus of keratin and purulent exudate. HE (x 3)

HENRY and KAUFMAN (1973) investigated the clearance of particles of ferric oxide, aluminum oxide, and carbon coated with benzo(a)pyrene from hamster lungs and found that BaP was cleared much more slowly from carbon-treated animals and that there was a positive correlation between particle size and retention rate.

In the present study the animals in the C-BaP 0.5 to 1.0 μm group began to develop carcinoma before, in greater numbers, and in a shorter time than did the animals in the Fe-BaP 0.5 to 1.0 μm group. It is possible that the number of carcinomas would have been even larger if the animals in the C-BaP group had survived the 25 week instillation period as well as those in the C-BaP group.

The probability for the presence of tumor-bearing animals varied between the respective particle size groups.

The probability of the occurrence of tumors in various segments of the respiratory tract of animals in the Fe-BaP, Al-BaP and C-BaP groups are shown in Figs 12, 13, and 14, respectively. The probability of tumor-bearing animals was greater in the C-BaP 0.5 to 1.0 μm group than in the Fe-BaP 0.5 to 1.0 μm group. In the 15 to 30 μm particle groups the probability for tumor-bearing animals was greater in the Fe-BaP group than in the C-BaP group. This reversal of relative probability trends in C-BaP (0.5 to 1.0 μm) over Fe-BaP (0.5 to 1.0 μm) compared to Fe-BaP (15 to 30 μm) over C-BaP (15 to 30 μm) may have been due to a greater long-term retention of ferric oxide than of carbon above 2 μm particle size after the 25 week instillation period.

The bronchiectasis observed in many of the animals that developed carcinomas in the C-BaP groups occurred more often and more extensively when compared to this lesion in the Fe-BaP animals (Fig. 15). In the C-BaP animals, the ectatic bronchi were greatly distended with keratin detritus and, often, purulent exudate.

Table 1. Distribution of tumors in respiratory tract of hamsters treated with benzo(a)pyrene and ferric oxide

Group/Particle Size	Larynx	Trachea	Bronchi	Bronchioles	Alveoli	Other	Tumor-Bearing/Total No. Necropsied	Per Cent
0.5 to 1 µm	3[a] (1)[b]	19 (16)	11 (10)	1 (1)	1 (1)	2 (1)	25/49 (22)/49	51.0 44.8
2 to 5 µm	3	18 (14)	8 (8)	2	0	0	24/47 (18)/47	51.0 38.0
5 to 10 µm	0	13 (9)	8 (3)	8 (2)	1 (1)	4 (2)	22/48 (13)/48	45.8 27.0
15 to 30 µm	2	14 (10)	13 (12)	7 (1)	2 (1)	4 (4)	22/44 (16)/44	50.0 36.0

[a] Number of animals with tumors in this location
[b] Number of animals with carcinoma

Table 2. Distribution of tumors in respiratory tract of hamsters treated with benzo(a)pyrene and aluminum oxide

Group/Particle Size	Larynx	Trachea	Bronchi	Bronchioles	Alveoli	Other	Tumor-Bearing/Total No. Necropsied	Per Cent
0.5 to 1 µm	0	5[a] (4)[b]	2 (1)	0	2 (1)	4 (1)	11/45 (6)/45	24.0 13.0
2 to 5 µm	0	5 (1)	0	0	1	2 (1)	8/48 (2)/48	17.0 4.0
5 to 10 µm	1	3 (2)	4 (4)	0	2 (1)	4 (2)	10/47 (7)/47	21.0 15.0
15 to 30 µm	1	5 (1)	3 (1)	1 (1)	4	4 (1)	12/48 (2)/48	25.0 4.0

[a] Number of animals with tumors in this location
[b] Number of animals with carcinoma

Table 3. Distribution of tumors in respiratory tract of hamsters treated with benzo(a)pyrene and carbon

Group/Particle Size	Larynx	Trachea	Bronchi	Bronchioles	Alveoli	Other	Tumor-Bearing/Total No. Necropsied	Per Cent
0.5 to 1 μm	2[a] (1)[b]	27 (18)	16 (16)	2 (2)	3 (3)	0	32/46 (24)/46	70.0 52.0
2 to 5 μm	0	3 (2)	13 (11)	2 (2)	8 (7)	2 (1)	18/49 (15)/49	37.0 31.0
5 to 10 μm	0	11 (4)	22 (22)	3 (3)	5 (5)	0	26/48 (25)/48	54.0 52.0
15 to 30 μm	0	8 (5)	16 (16)	1 (1)	2 (1)	1	17/47 (17)/47	36.0 36.0

[a]Number of animals with tumors in this location
[b]Number of animals with carcinoma

The number of carcinomas (17) in all Al-BaP groups was markedly lower than in the comparable Fe-BaP (113) and C-BaP (113) groups. The amount of pneumoconiosis observed microscopically was also lower. The degree of retention of particles may be related to the relative susceptibility of the lung to bacterial infection.

References

HENRY, M.C., KAUFMAN, D.G.: Clearance of benzo(a)pyrene from hamster lungs after administration on coated particles. J. nat. Cancer Inst. 51, 1961-1964 (1973).

HENRY, M.C., PORT, C.D., BATES, R.R., KAUFMAN, D.G.: Respiratory tract tumors in hamsters induced by benzo(a)pyrene. Cancer Res. 33, 1585-1592 (1973).

KAPLAN, E.L., MEIER, P.: Nonparametric estimation from incomplete observations. J. Amer. Statist. Ass. 53, 457-481 (1958).

SAFFIOTTI, U., CEFIS, F., KOLB, L.H.: A method for the experimental induction of bronchogenic carcinoma. Cancer Res. 28, 104-124 (1968).

SAFFIOTTI, U., MONTESANO, R., SELLAKUMAR, A.R., CEFIS, F., KAUFMAN, D.G.: Respiratory tract carcinogenesis in hamsters induced by different numbers of administrations of benzo(a)pyrene and ferric oxide. Cancer Res. 32, 1073-1081 (1972).

Chemical Induction of Lung Carcinomas in Rats*

William H. Blair

Department of Research, Mercy Hospital and Medical Center, Chicago, IL 60616, USA

ABSTRACT

Lung carcinomas were induced in rats with intratracheal instillations
of benzo(a)pyrene in combination with ferric oxide suspended in sterile
saline. The development of lung tumors was followed by sequential sacrifice and histologic observation of the lung and other involved tissues. Lung lesions were early squamous metaplasia without keratinization, followed by metaplasia with keratinization which developed into
microtumors. The microtumors progressed to visible masses and appeared as highly differentiated squamous cell keratinizing tumors with
limited local invasion and no distant metastases. With time the tumors
appeared less well differentiated with the presence of local invasion
and extension to the pleura. In the late stages of tumorigenesis the
chest wall, diaphragm and liver were invaded by the induced epidermoid
carcinoma. Metastases were seen in the liver, pancreas, kidney, adrenal
and lymph nodes. In addition to the epidermoid carcinoma, adenocarcinoma, and small cell anaplastic (oat cell like) carcinoma were observed. The small cell tumors were found in approximately 20% of the
rats and were associated with a sudden weight loss and death of animals.

Introduction

The development of an animal model for the study of lung cancer is
necessary in order to elucidate the genesis of the disease process.
Instillation of polycyclic hydrocarbons in mice (NETTESHEIM and
HAMMONS, 1971), rats (PYLEV, 1962; SHABAD, 1962), and hamsters (DELLA-
PORTA et al., 1958; HERROLD and DUNHAM, 1962) have resulted in the
production of lung neoplasms. A drawback of the early work was the
low yield of tumor induction.

Recently SAFFIOTTI and his co-workers (SAFFIOTTI, 1969; SAFFIOTTI et
al., 1968) combined benzo(a)pyrene (BaP) with ferric oxide in saline
for instillation into hamster lungs. He achieved a high yield of lung
tumors which are described as primarily bronchogenic in origin.

This author has induced lung carcinoma in laboratory rats with BaP
and 7,12-dimethylbenz(a)anthracene combined with ferric oxide (BLAIR
et al., 1972, 1973). This paper will summarize some of the significant

*This investigation was supported by Research Funds from Mercy Hospital
and Medical Center.

pathology seen in rats after lung exposure to the polycyclic hydrocarbon BaP.

Materials and Methods

Male and female Sprague-Dawley rats were treated 15 times with once-
weekly intratracheal instillations of BaP, with ferric oxide as a
carrier dust. Each instillation consisted of 3 mg of hydrocarbon and
3 mg of carrier dust in 0.1 ml of saline. Prior to instillation of
the hydrocarbons the rats were lightly anesthetized with ether.

To study the effects of carrier dust, ferric oxide in saline was also
instilled in both male and female rats. Chest X-rays were taken after
3 months to monitor the development of lung tumors.

Intentional sacrifice from the fifth week on was performed to monitor
sequential lung alterations. The lung tissue, stomach, large and small
intestines, thoracic lymph nodes, pancreas, adrenal, kidney, spleen,
and thymus were fixed in formalin, embedded in paraffin, and stained
with hematoxylin and eosin for microscopic observation. Microscopic
observations were made on a Nikon Apophot photomicroscope and representative photomicrographs were taken.

Results

Clinically, the rats appeared to be normal during the instillation
phase of the experiment (15 weeks) with normal appearance and weight
gain. By 4 to 5 months, weight loss was observed and the animals were
subject to spells of dyspnea. Chest X-rays confirmed the presence of
lung neoplasms. After 6 months, some rats had rapid weight loss, nasal
hemorrhage, and expired within 2 weeks after the onset of symptoms.

At autopsy after 5 months, massive multiple keratinizing lesions of
the lung were found. They were subpleural, nonencapsulated, and whitish
in color. In several rats, obvious tumor nodules were seen on the liver,
kidney, chest wall, and lymph nodes.

Microscopic observation reveals epidermoid carcinoma in the majority
of rats after 5 months. At earlier times, the neoplasm appears somewhat benign, with proliferating squamous cells producing keratin and
no local extension of the tumor (Fig. 1). With time, the tumor produces
less keratin and becomes pleomorphic in appearance and locally invades
the lung parenchyma. This is followed by invasion of pleura, chest
wall (Fig. 2) and diaphragm. Metastases can be observed in the regional
lymph nodes (Fig. 3), kidneys (Fig. 4), adrenals (Fig. 5), and liver
(Fig. 6). The metastatic lesions appear as either highly differentiated
or poorly differentiated epidermoid carcinoma.

Adenocarcinoma, bronchiolo-alveolar, and bronchial cylindromas were
also observed. In addition, a small-cell anaplastic carcinoma was
seen, which appears similar to oat-cell carcinoma. The cells are small,
dark, pleomorphic with little or no cytoplasm having ovoid and spindle-
shaped nuclei (Figs 7 and 8). The cells appear to grow in sheets and
are locally invasive.

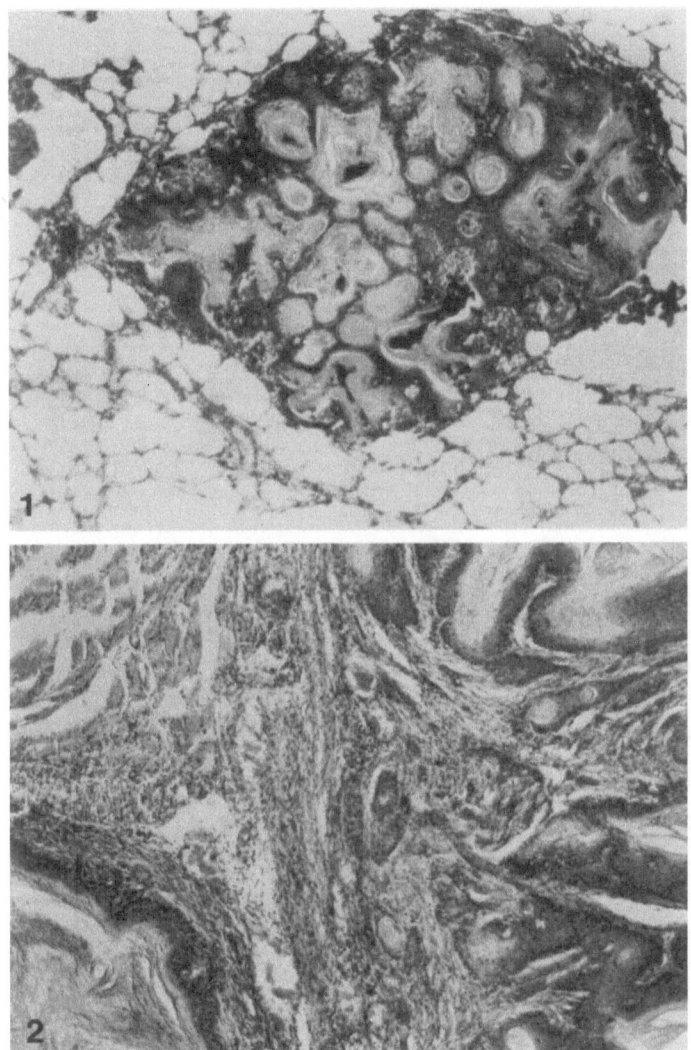

Fig. 1. Early lung tumor with squamous metaplasia and keratin formation. No invasion tendency. Hematoxylin and eosin (HE) stain. (x 16)

Fig. 2. Epidermoid carcinoma (right) invading through pleura into
chest cavity (lower left) and intercostal muscles (upper left).
HE stain (x 16)

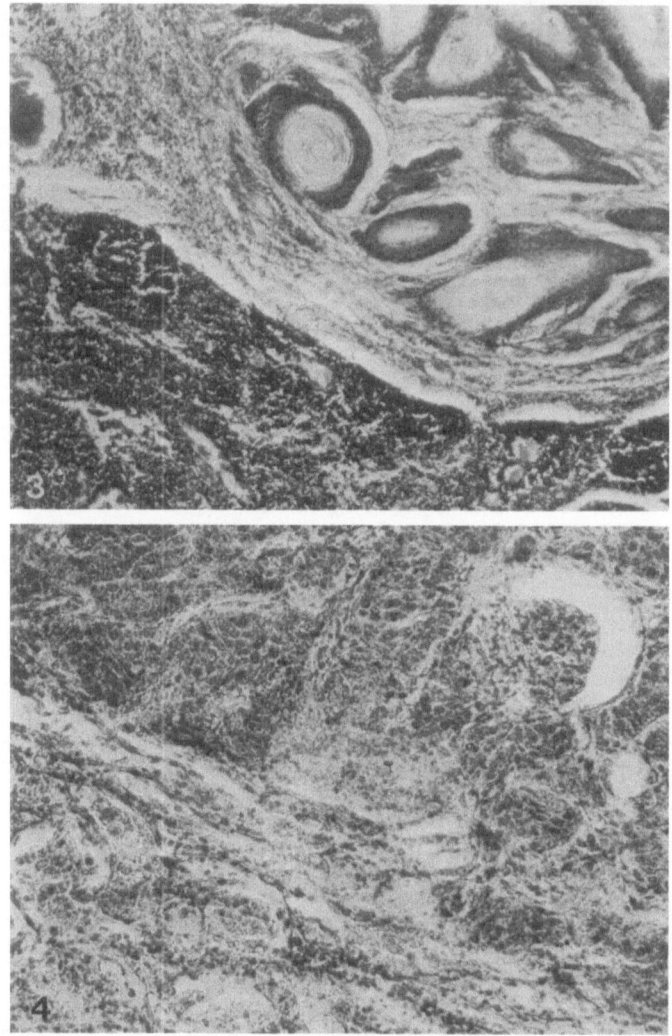

Fig. 3. Epidermoid carcinoma invading upper pole of paraortic lymph node. HE stain (x 16)

Fig. 4. Metastatic poorly differentiated epidermoid carcinoma to the kidney (upper field). HE stain (x 40)

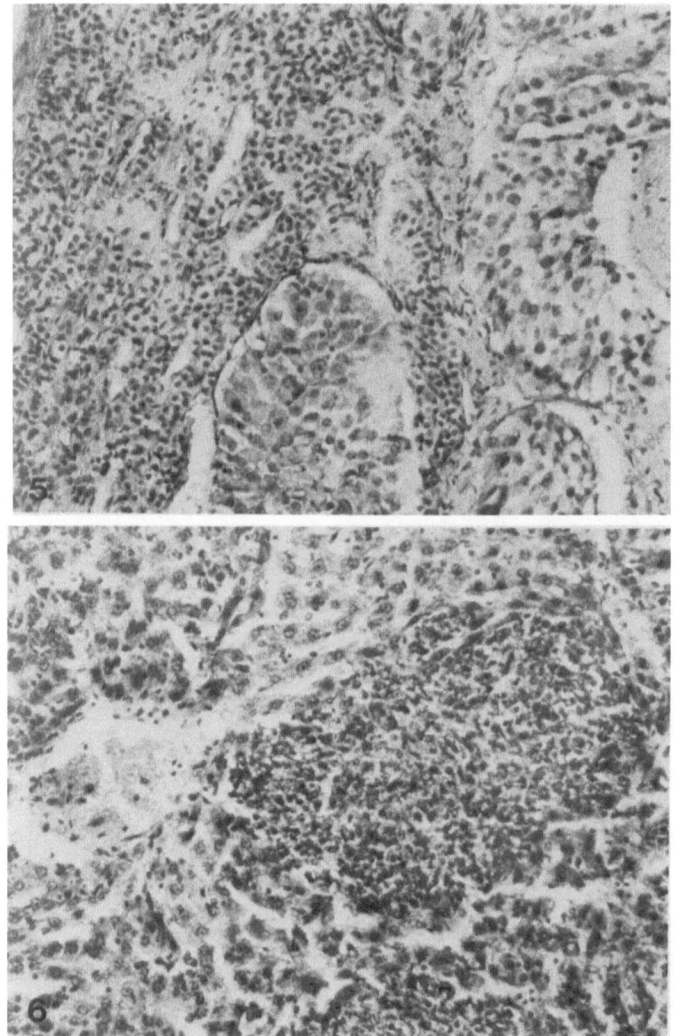

Fig. 5. Adrenal metastasis of epidermoid carcinoma which occupies
the medulla (left) pressing the cortical tissue to the capsule.
HE stain (x 16)

Fig. 6. Liver metastasis of poorly differentiated epidermoid carcinoma. HE stain (x 40)

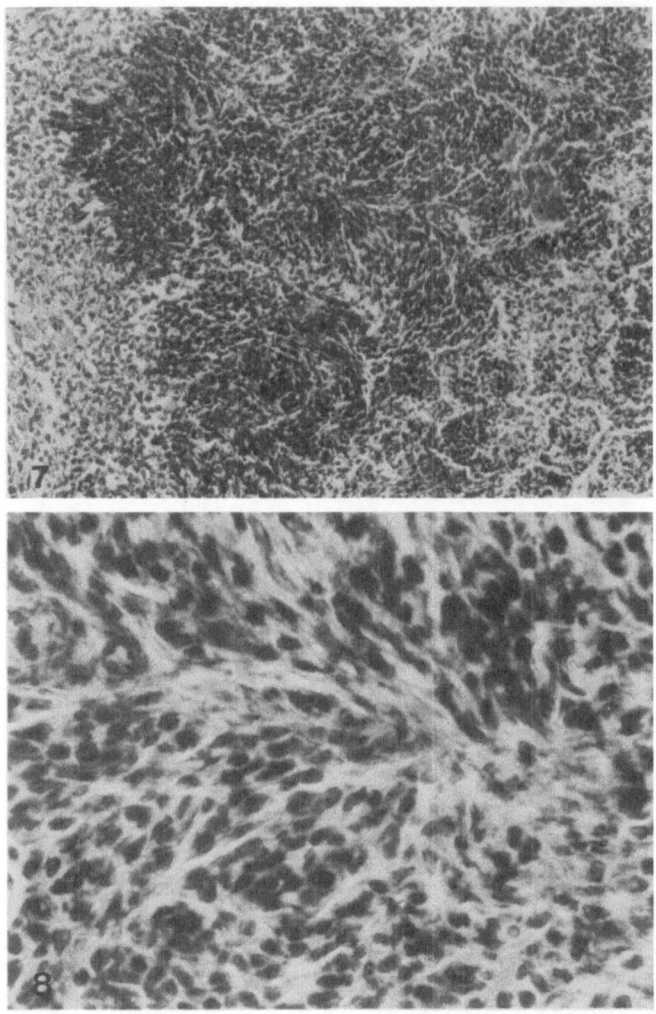

Fig. 7. Small-cell anaplastic ("oat cell like") carcinoma arising in the lung parenchyma. HE stain (x 40)

Fig. 8. Magnification of an area in Fig. 7 with pleomorphic, streaming small cells. HE stain (x 160)

Most of the lesions in the lung appear to develop first in the alveolar and bronchiolo-alveolar epithelium, while the bronchogenic lesions develop at a later time period. Table 1 summarizes the types of lung tumors found after treatment with BaP and ferric oxide.

Rats treated with ferric oxide only developed localized histiocytic foci which remained unchanged during the experiment.

Table 1. Tumor distribution in rats treated with BaP and ferric oxide (100 rats)

Tumor Type	Rats with Lung Tumors	
	Number	Mean Survival (months)
Epidermoid carcinoma		
Well differentiated	47	18
Poorly differentiated	40	14
Adenocarcinoma	11	18
Small cell anaplastic carcinoma	20[a]	12
No lung tumor	5[b]	24[c]

[a]18 of the rats with small cell tumors also exhibited epidermoid or adenocarcinoma in other areas of lung tissue.

[b]Areas of pulmonary squamous metaplastic microtumors were seen in 3 of 5 rats.

[c]Experiment terminated at 24 months with intentional sacrifice.

Discussion

Treatment of rats with BaP and ferric oxide results in rapid development of lung tumors. The initial tumors appear morphologically as benign lesions but take on malignant characteristics with time. In some animals, a small-cell anaplastic tumor is seen which appears similar to oat-cell carcinoma in humans.

The tumors appear to develop in the alveoli or bronchiolo-alveolar region of the lung. This observation is not in agreement with the findings of PYLEV (1962) and SHABAD (1962) or with the earlier work of NISKANEN (1949). Those authors indicated a bronchogenic site of tumor origin in their hydrocarbon treated rats. Recently SCHREIBER et al. (1972) reported a bronchiolo-alveolar origin of tumors in rats treated with 3-methylcholanthrene.

Laboratory rats appear to be very sensitive to the development of lung tumors after exposure to polycyclic hydrocarbons. They develop tumors rapidly and survival time of the rats is sufficient for the tumor to invade and metastasize to distant organs. In addition, a small-cell anaplastic (oat-cell like) tumor is observed in rats after 6 months. This tumor has not previously been described in laboratory animals (SAFFIOTTI, 1969). This author and colleagues have suggested (1972, 1973) that the rat may be an ideal animal for lung carcinogenesis studies.

References

BLAIR, W.H., CHEN, K.C., BASAVARAJ, H.K.: Induction of squamous neoplasia in rats with a benzo(a)pyrene-ferric oxide mixture. Proc. Amer. Ass. Cancer Res. 13, 74 (1972).

BLAIR, W.H., OTERO, N., RAO, H.: Development of lung neoplasms in rats treated with 7,12-dimethylbenz(a)anthracene. Proc. Amer. Ass. Cancer Res. 14, 497 (1973).

DELLAPORTA, G., KOLB, L., SHUBIK, P.: Induction of tracheobronchial carcinomas in the Syrian golden hamster. Cancer Res. 18, 592 (1958).

HERROLD, K.M., DUNHAM, I.J.: Induction of carcinoma and papilloma of the tracheobronchial mucosa of Syrian hamsters by intratracheal instillation of benzo(a)pyrene. J. nat. Cancer Inst. 28, 467 (1962).

NETTESHEIM, P., HAMMONS, A.S.: Induction of squamous cell carcinoma in the respiratory tract of mice. J. nat. Cancer Inst. 47, 697 (1971).

NISKANEN, K.O.: Observations on metaplasia of the bronchial epithelium and its relation to carcinoma of the lung; pathoanatomical and experimental researches. Acta path. microbiol. scand. Suppl. 80, 1-80 (1949).

PYLEV, L.N.: Induction of lung cancer in rats by intratracheal instillation of carcinogenic hydrocarbons. Acta U.N. Int. Cancer 688 (1962).

SAFFIOTTI, U.: Experimental respiratory tract carcinogenesis and its relation to inhalation exposures. In: Inhalation Carcinogenesis (M.G. Hanna, ed.), pp. 27-51. AEC Symposium Series 17. Gatlinburg: Tennessee 1969.

SAFFIOTTI, U.: Experimental respiratory tract carcinogenesis. Int. Symp. on Carcinogenesis Testing, Boston, Mass., 1967. Drugs Exp. Tumor Res. VII, pp. 302-333. Basel, New York: Karger 1969.

SAFFIOTTI, U., CEFIS, F., KOLB, I.H.: A method for the experimental induction of bronchogenic carcinoma. Cancer Res. 28, 104 (1968).

SCHREIBER, H., NETTESHEIM, P., MARTIN, D.: Rapid development of bronchiolo-alveolar squamous cell tumors in rats after intratracheal injection of 3-methylcholanthrene. J. nat. Cancer Inst. 49, 541 (1972).

SHABAD, L.M.: Experimental cancer of the lung. J. nat. Cancer Inst. 28, 1305 (1962).

Synergistic Effects of Benzo (a) pyrene and N-Methyl-N-Nitrosourea on Respiratory Carcinogenesis in Syrian Golden Hamsters*

David G. Kaufman and Russell M. Madison

Lung Cancer Branch, National Cancer Institute, and Microbiological Associates, Inc., Bethesda, MD 20014, USA

ABSTRACT

Sequential intratracheal administrations of benzo(a)pyrene plus ferric oxide and N-methyl-N-nitrosourea to Syrian golden hamsters resulted in a greater tumor response than that expected as the additive effect of tumor responses induced by each carcinogen alone. Mortality was accelerated in groups receiving both carcinogens. The extents of the synergistic tumor responses and the increased mortality rates related to the specific sequence of carcinogen administrations. Squamous cell carcinoma was the predominant type of tumor induced; the average latency of these tumors was reduced by the sequential carcinogen treatments. The high mortality and rapid tumor development resulted in numerous early deaths of hamsters bearing a spectrum of epithelial lesions. A sequence of stages in the histogenesis of squamous cell carcinomas is suggested based on these observations.

Introduction

The induction of bronchogenic carcinomas in Syrian golden hamsters by the intratracheal instillation of benzo(a)pyrene (BaP) absorbed to ferric oxide (Fe_2O_3) particles and suspended in saline solution (SAFFIOTTI et al., 1968), has been a widely used model for the study of lung cancer. Tumors induced by this experimental method resemble the majority of human lung cancers in both location and morphologic characteristics. Previous studies have demonstrated the relationship between the quantity and the fractionation of the administered carcinogen and the resulting tumor incidence (SAFFIOTTI et al., 1972a, 1972b). Furthermore, the studies on the role of the ferric oxide (SELLAKUMAR et al., 1973; HENRY et al., 1974) and the rate of clearance of BaP from the respiratory tract (HENRY and KAUFMAN, 1973) have helped to characterize better the properties of this system. The morphologic features of tumor development in this system have been documented by both transmission (HARRIS et al., 1971) and scanning electron microscopy (PORT et al., 1973).

N-methyl-N-nitrosourea (NMU) has also been demonstrated to be an effective carcinogen for the respiratory tract when administered by intratracheal instillation (HERROLD, 1970). Ultrastructural features

---

*This work was performed in part under Contract No. NO1-CP-02199, from Division of Cancer Cause and Prevention, National Cancer Institute, National Institutes of Health.

of the histogenesis of these tumors has also been the subject of study (HARRIS et al., 1973). The tumors observed in these studies were predominantly epidermoid carcinomas and the larynx and trachea were the most frequently affected sites.

In contrast to these experimental studies in animals, bronchogenic carcinoma in man is generally presumed to be the result of environmental exposures to a number of carcinogens. Thus, further information regarding the effect of concurrent or sequential exposures to more than 1 carcinogen may provide further insight into the causation of lung cancer in man. In the present study we have compared the carcinogenic effects of sequential administration of both BaP plus Fe_2O_3 and NMU in comparison to the administration of either BaP plus Fe_2O_3 or NMU alone. These 2 carcinogens were chosen because of their demonstrated effectiveness as respiratory carcinogens. Differences in number and latency of the tumors induced were sought as indications of interaction of the 2 carcinogens.

Materials and Methods

Male Syrian golden hamsters were obtained from Mammalian Genetics and Animal Production Section, Division of Cancer Therapy, National Cancer Institute. They were housed in polycarbonate cages on Bed-O-Cobs (Anderson Cob Mills, Inc.), generally in groups of 6. They were fed Purina Lab Chow (Ralston Purina Company) and given water ad libitum.

BaP (Aldrich Chemical Company) was hand-ground with an equal quantity of Fe_2O_3 (Type R3098; Charles Pfizer, Inc.) in a mullite mortar. This preparation of BaP adsorbed to Fe_2O_3 was suspended in sterile 0.15 M NaCl solution immediately prior to administration. NMU (Ash-Stevens, Inc.) was dissolved in sterile 0.015 M Na-Citrate, pH 6.5 buffer containing 0.15 M NaCl and used within 30 min of preparation. Hamsters were anesthetized by intraperitoneal injection of sodium methohexital (Eli Lilly and Company) dissolved in 0.15 M NaCl. They received intratracheally instillations of 0.2 ml volume using previously reported methods (SAFFIOTTI et al., 1968). 5 groups of hamsters of 10 to 12 weeks of age were treated with BaP plus Fe_2O_3 and/or NMU according to the experimental protocol specified in Table 1. Individual intratracheal doses contained either 5 mg BaP plus 5 mg Fe_2O_3 or 0.5 mg NMU.

Animals were observed and weighed weekly. They were allowed to die spontaneously or were killed when moribund, with the exception of 3 hamsters in Group 1 surviving at week 80 which were electively sacrificed. All hamsters except a few lost through cannibalism were autopsied and studied histologically. The technique used for autopsy and for fixation of the lungs was that previously reported (SAFFIOTTI et al., 1968).

Results

Survival rates for the 5 experimental groups are reported in Table 2. Despite the fact that Groups 3 to 5 received the same total dose of both carcinogens, differences were observed in their survival rates. Bronchopneumonia, often with progression to lobar confluence in 1 or more lobes, was a common finding in hamsters dying during the treat-

Table 1. Schedule of intratracheal treatment of Syrian golden hamsters with BaP plus Fe_2O_3 and/or NMU

Groups	Initial number of hamsters	Weekly treatments during weeks	
		1 - 10	11 - 20
1	30	5 mg BaP + 5 mg Fe_2O_3[a]	None
2	26	0.5 mg NMU[b]	None
3	30	5 mg BaP + 5 mg Fe_2O_3	0.5 mg NMU
4	30	0.5 mg NMU	5 mg BaP + 5 mg Fe_2O_3
5	30	5 mg BaP + 5 mg Fe_2O_3 and 0.5 mg NMU, altern. weeks[c]	

[a] 5 mg BaP plus 5 mg Fe_2O_3 suspended in 0.2 ml of sterile 0.15 M NaCl solution was administered by intratracheal instillation.

[b] 0.5 mg NMU dissolved in 0.2 ml of sterile 0.015 M Na-Citrate, pH 6.5 buffer containing 0.15 M NaCl was administered by intratracheal instillation.

[c] BaP plus Fe_2O_3 was administered on week 1 and every second week thereafter for a total of 10 times; NMU was administered on week 2 and every second week thereafter for a total of 10 times.

Table 2. Survival rates of Syrian golden hamsters following intratracheal treatment with BaP plus Fe_2O_3 and/or NMU

Group[a]	Initial number of hamsters	Number of survivors at experiment weeks							
		10	20	30	40	50	60	70	80
1	30	29	27	24	19	15	10	7	3[b]
2	26	25	23	20	17	13	7	2	0
3	30	26	25	19	12	1	0	-	-
4	30	28	8	0	-	-	-	-	-
5	30	30	17	2	0	-	-	-	-

[a] The treatment schedules for Groups 1 to 5 are specified in Table 1.
[b] The 3 surviving animals at 80 weeks were sacrificed. All 3 hamsters were found to have malignant tumors of the respiratory tract.

ment period in Groups 4 and 5. Group 3, in which there was a much lower mortality during the treatment period, also appeared to have an accelerated rate of death as compared to Groups 1 and 2 which received only a single carcinogen.

Tumors were found in all 5 Groups, but the incidence and number of tumors varied considerably among the Groups (Table 3). The majority of the tumors were squamous cell carcinomas.

Table 3. Respiratory tract tumor induction in Syrian golden hamsters
following intratracheal treatment with BaP plus Fe_2O_3 and/or NMU

Group[a]	Effective number of hamsters[b]	Number of tumor bearing hamsters	Number of tumors	Average number of tumors in tumor bearing hamsters
1	27	18	39	2.2
2	25	7	7	1.0
3	27	18	30	1.7
4	26	13	14	1.1
5	27	19	42	2.2

[a]The treatment schedules for Groups 1 to 5 are specified in Table 1.
[b]Initial number of hamsters less those lost through cannibalism.

Groups 1 and 5 had comparable incidences and numbers of tumors and
the average number of tumors in each case was 2.2 in animals bearing
tumors. The incidence and multiplicity of tumors in Group 3 was slightly lower, and in Groups 2 and 4, substantially lower. Since survival
rates in the 5 Groups varied considerably, the relative risk for death
with a respiratory tract tumor present was calculated with an actuarial
method as previously described (SAFFIOTTI et al., 1972a). This method
offers a measure of tumor incidence as related to the number of animals
actually at risk at a given time after the start of the experiment. The
results of this analysis are presented in Fig. 1. When the effects of
the numerous early deaths from bronchopneumonia are removed from the
consideration of incidence, Group 4 actually has the highest relative
risk of dying with a tumor as a function of time. The relative rate of
mortality of tumor bearing hamsters in Group 5 is only slightly lower

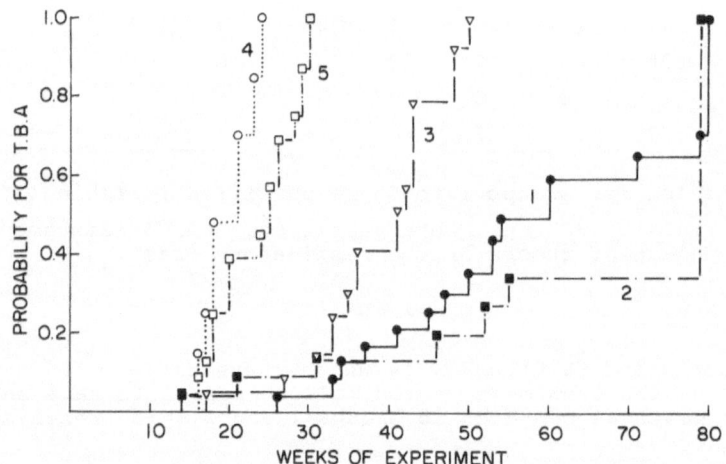

Fig. 1. Probabilities for the observation of a respiratory tract
tumor at death: Group 1, ●——●; Group 2, ■–··–■; Group 3, ▽———▽;
Group 4, o·····o; Group 5, □–···–□

Table 4. Distribution and mean latency of tumors of Syrian golden hamsters following intratracheal treatment with BaP plus Fe_2O_3 and/or NMU

Group[a]	Effective Number of hamsters[b]	Number of tumors at each site				Mean latent period (weeks)[c]			
		Larynx	Trachea	Bronchi	Lung	Larynx	Trachea	Bronchi	Lung
1	27	8	14	12	5	49	59	58	66
2	25	2	4	1	0	54	40	31	–
3[d]	27	11	12	7	0	38	37	41	–
4	26	7	6	1	0	20	18	24	–
5	27	15	25	2	0	24	23	20	–

[a] The treatment schedules for Groups 1 to 5 are specified in Table 1.
[b] Initial number of hamsters less those lost through cannibalism.
[c] Arithmetic average of the weeks of experiment at which each tumor was seen.
[d] There were also 2 tumors of the nasal cavity with a mean latency of 46 weeks found in this Group.

than in Group 4, but that for Group 3, which received the same total carcinogen dose, is considerably lower. In Groups 1 and 2, the majority of deaths of hamsters bearing tumors occurred later.

The distribution of tumors in the respiratory tract and the mean latency for the development of tumors at these various locations is reported in Table 4. As in previous studies using BaP plus Fe_2O_3 (SAFFIOTTI, 1970), the greatest number of tumors in Group 1 were in the bronchi with a slightly lower incidence in the trachea. In this Group, tumors of all sites showed a long average latent period; tumors of the larynx appeared slightly earlier and those of the lung periphery somewhat later than those in the trachea and bronchi. The majority of tumors in Groups 3 to 5 were in the larynx and trachea and the latency of the tumors was considerably shorter than in Group 1. Tumors of the lung periphery were not seen in Groups 2 to 5.

The results in Fig. 1 and Table 4 show that deaths of hamsters bearing tumors occurred with a shorter latency in Groups 3 to 5, which received both carcinogens, than in Groups 1 and 2, which received only 1. If the differences in relative rates of deaths of tumor bearing hamsters relates just to the difference in total carcinogen dose, then combining the tumor responses induced independently by the 2 carcinogens (Groups 1 and 2) should give a curve corresponding to those observed for Groups 3 to 5. Thus, we wished to determine whether 2 carcinogens act independently (additive effect) or whether there was interaction between them (synergistic effect). We employed the data from Groups 1 and 2 to derive expected probabilities for tumor bearing deaths with both BaP plus Fe_2O_3 (starting week 1) and NMU (starting week 11) in a group initially composed of 27 hamsters. The derived probability curve (1+2) is compared in Fig. 2 with that observed (Group 3) for such treatment. The difference between these curves is a measure of the interaction between the 2 carcinogens and, thus, is a further indication of synergism. Comparison of Group 4 with an appropriate derived group (e.g., NMU first, etc.) shows greater divergence than in Fig. 2. This latter result may be some-

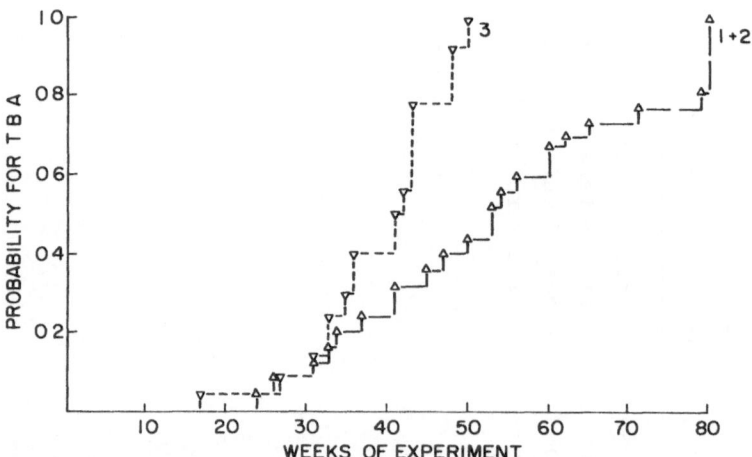

Fig. 2. Probabilities for the observation of a respiratory tract tumor at death. Results observed for Group 3 (∇---∇) are compared for those expected for comparable treatment with BaP plus Fe_2O_3 and NMU as derived from the results in Groups 1 and 2 ($\triangle$—$\triangle$)

what exaggerated since in some cases, small early tumors were detected in animals dying with bronchopneumonia.

The very high carcinogen dose received by Groups 3 to 5 produced a
great multiplicity of lesions particularly in the trachea and larynx.
This, coupled with the rapid mortality in these groups, provided many
examples of early changes and premalignant lesions. From this material,
there appears to be a progressive sequence of changes which may relate to the histogenesis of squamous cell carcinomas of the respiratory tract under these experimental conditions. Figs 3 to 9 illustrate
a few of these lesions. Typical squamous metaplasias with regular
alignment of basal cells (Fig. 3) were frequently found among animals
dying during the treatment period. In many lesions there was irregulari-
ty of the basal cell layer with foci in which basal cells were increased
in number forming small nodular areas (Fig. 4). In these areas the
orientation of basal cells was related to the peripheral expansion of
the nodule rather than the epithelial axis and suggested a slightly
increased proliferation rate of the basal cells in these areas. In
some cases these nodules achieved much greater size (Fig. 5), but
preserved their spherical character with distinct relationships between stroma and epithelium along convex borders. In other cases,
the downgrowth of basal cells was in the form of narrow pegs of cells
penetrating underlying stroma, often in complex networks of pleomorphic poorly-oriented cells, but with distinct demarcation between
epithelium and stroma (Fig. 6). The growth characteristics of these
penetrating cells presumably are different than those just forming
nodules of growth near the original basal cell level. Perhaps this
altered growth is indicative of a stage of progressive loss of growth
control exerted on the basal cells by the stroma. Penetrating cells
of other lesions deeply and extensively infiltrated the supporting
stroma, often with extensive networks and clusters of cells far from
the overlying epithelium. The surface area of the interface of stroma
and epithelium becomes extensive and indistinct and mitoses become
more numerous. Perhaps at this point the normal growth restraint
exerted by the stroma on the epithelium has been largely or completely lost. Frankly invasive squamous carcinomas, generally seen somewhat later, infiltrated muscle (Fig. 7) and grew through the membranous
areas between cartilages (Fig. 8). In 1 tumor in the present study,
there was also a small area of invasion of cartilage (Fig. 9). More
extensive documentation of the benign and malignant lesions of the
respiratory tract and other sites in this study will be presented
in the future.

214

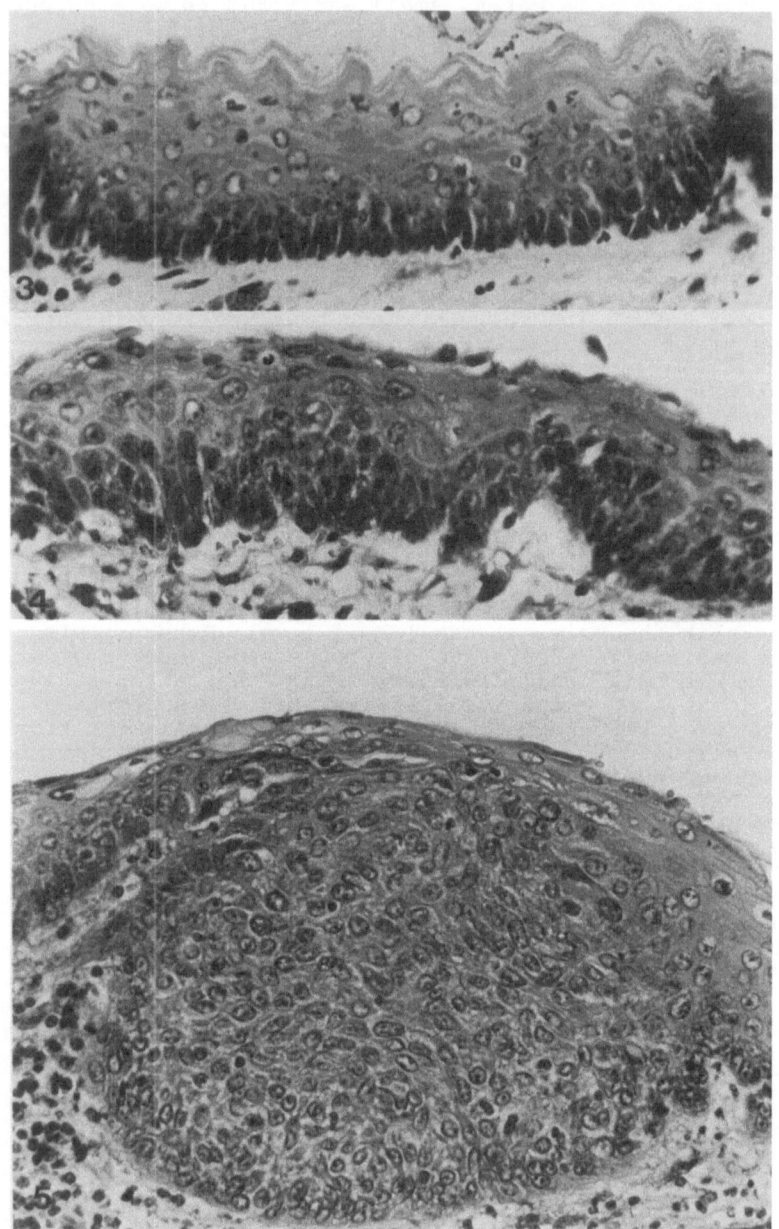

Fig. 3. Squamous metaplasia of the larynx. Note regularity of level and orientation of basal cells. HE (x 200)

Fig. 4. Squamous metaplasia of the larynx. Small variations in orientation and depth of basal cells with formation of nodules. HE (x 200)

Fig. 5. Squamous metaplasia of the larynx with large spherical nodule of basal cell proliferation. HE (x 200) .

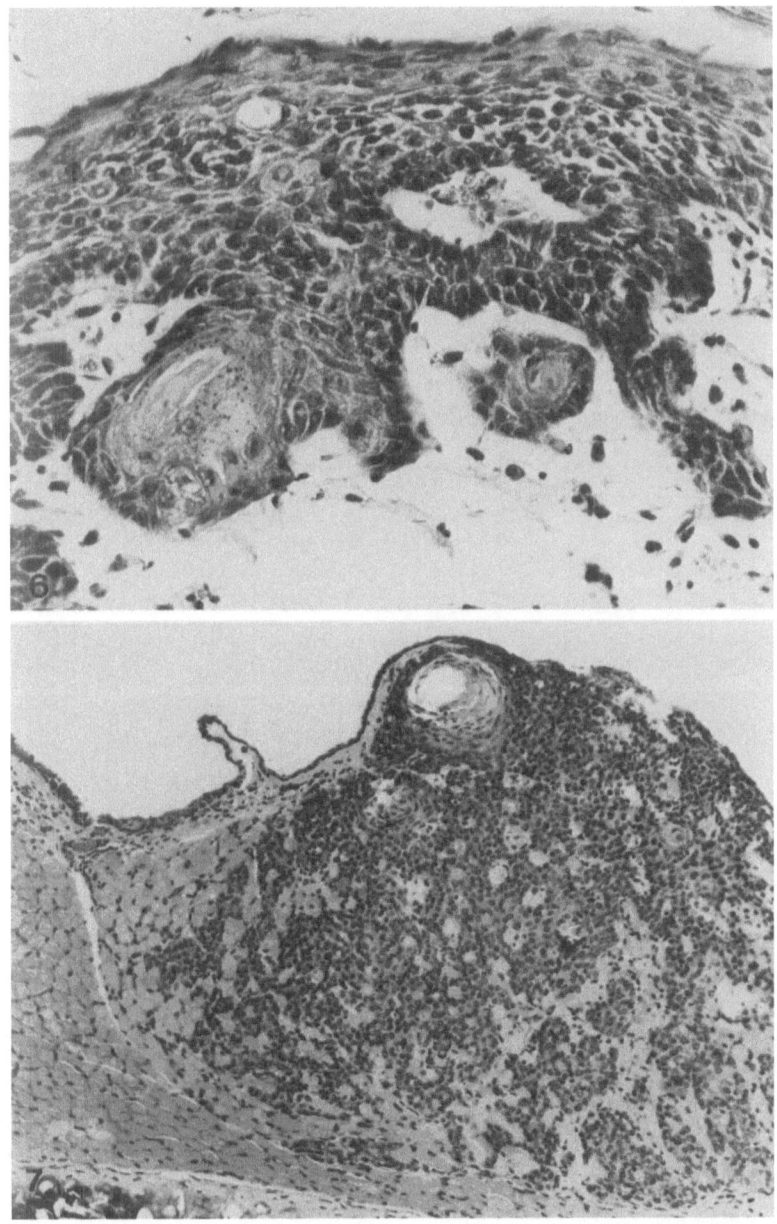

Fig. 6. Pseudoepitheliomatous hyperplasia (leukoplakia) of the larynx. Nodular and peg-like downgrowth of pleomorphic basal cells. HE (x 200)

Fig. 7. Squamous carcinoma of larynx invading intrinsic laryngeal muscle. HE (x 80)

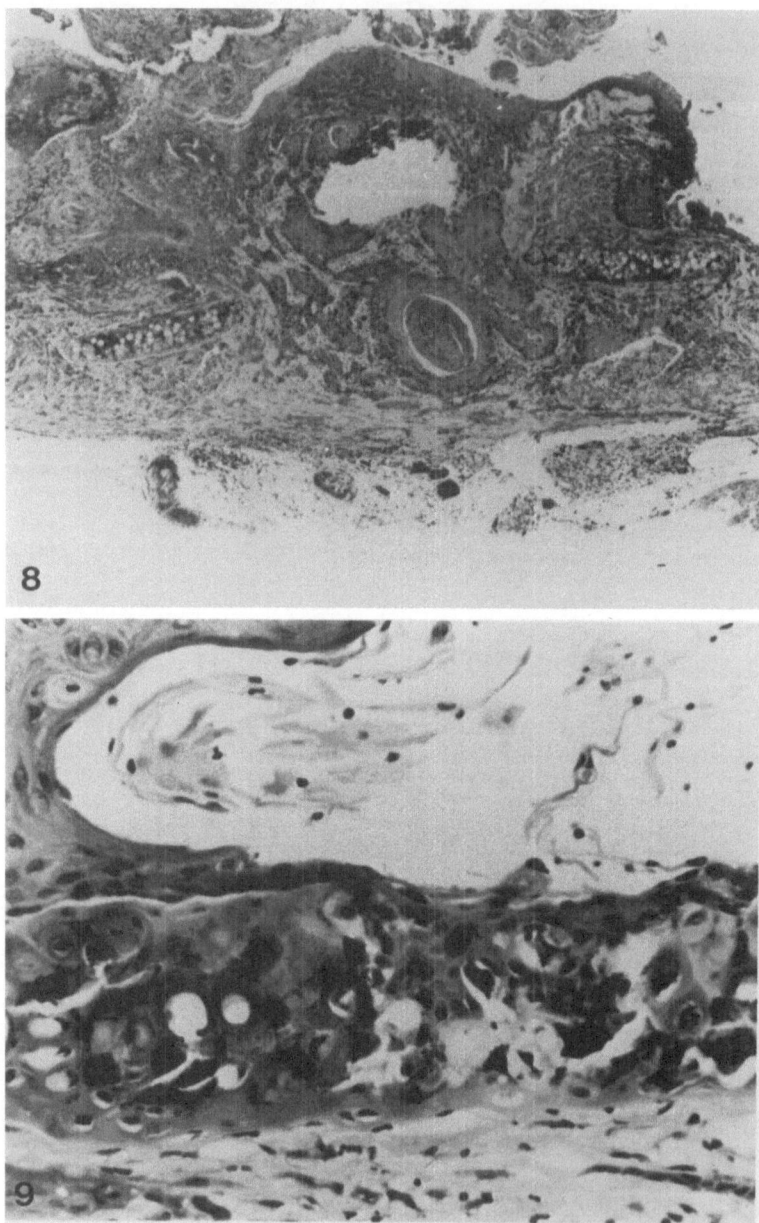

Fig. 8.   Large invasive squamous carcinoma of the trachea. HE (x 32)

Fig. 9.   Invasion of cartilage by squamous carcinoma of the trachea.
HE (x 200)

Discussion

The tumor response of hamsters treated with both BaP plus Fe_2O_3 and
NMU occurred with much reduced latency than in animals receiving only
1 of the 2 carcinogens. Comparison of the observed probability of
death with tumor for hamsters given BaP plus Fe_2O_3 and NMU in 10 consecutive weekly instillations each, with the derived probabilities
expected, based on the direct additive effect of these 2 carcinogens
given separately, indicates that there is interaction, or synergism,
in response to the 2 carcinogens. Synergism was not apparent directly
by comparison of the total incidences or number of tumors; however,
there were great differences in the mortality rates of the various
groups with consequent differences in the numbers of animals at risk.
1 animal treated with both carcinogens survived for 50 weeks, whereas
both groups treated with only 1 carcinogen had 50% of animals surviving at that time. An accurate direct comparison of tumor incidences
would require analysis by serial sacrifice.

Groups 3 to 5 all received the same total dose of each carcinogen,
yet their mortality rates differed considerably. When the total dose
of BaP plus Fe_2O_3 was administered before the start of NMU (Group 3),
average survival was longer than in the case where all (Group 4) or
some (Group 5) of the doses of BaP plus Fe_2O_3 followed doses of NMU.
It is likely that the widespread loss of ciliated and mucus-producing
epithelial cells of the upper respiratory tract caused by NMU, as seen
in this experiment and previously reported by HARRIS et al. (1973),
may be related to this effect. Clearance of BaP plus Fe_2O_3 may be considerably impaired by this altered epithelium and, thus, animals
treated with doses of NMU before doses of BaP plus Fe_2O_3 (Groups 4
and 5) may have sustained the effects (e.g., longer residence of a
larger quantity of BaP plus Fe_2O_3) of a larger effective dose of BaP
plus Fe_2O_3.

Tumor incidences with the carcinogen doses employed in this experiment
were lower than in some previous reports. SAFFIOTTI et al. (1972a) observed a tumor incidence comparable to Group 1 with the administration
of only 30 mg each of BaP plus Fe_2O_3. In an experiment comparable to
Group 1, HENRY et al. (1974) reported similar incidences and rates of
tumor observation with BaP, Fe_2O_3 and animals from the same source
as those in the present experiment. HERROLD (1970) observed a higher
tumor incidence after 10 weekly doses of 0.5 mg NMU, but the sources
of animals and NMU differed, and in her experiment, treatment was begun at 4 weeks of age.

The present experiment offers additional information regarding the
interactions of carcinogens in respiratory carcinogenesis. Much additional work remains, however, before we will begin to understand the
nature of this interaction and how it relates to human lung cancer.
This experiment also demonstrates a method for the rapid development
of malignant and premalignant lesions of the larynx and trachea in
hamsters. This property of the protocols, particularly of Groups 3
and 5, may make these useful methods for preparing hamster tracheal
tissue for the evaluation of anti-carcinogenic substances in organ
culture. Furthermore, the much reduced latency of tumors with these
treatment schedules may permit the performance of some respiratory
carcinogenesis bioassays in much shorter times. In 1 such carcinogenesis bioassay currently in progress, where hamsters received 5 mg
BaP plus 5 mg Fe_2O_3 and 0.5 mg NMU on alterating weeks for a total
of 5 doses of each, treatment of hamsters with large doses of vitamin
A has shown a protective effect on the development of respiratory tract
tumors (KAUFMAN and MADISON, unpublished observation).

218

Acknowledgements

We thank Mr. REG DAVIES and Miss JEAN GRAF for preparation of the
hand-ground mixtures of BaP plus Fe_2O_3, and Miss JUDY OBER and Mr.
STEVEN SPRINGER for technical assistance. We thank Mr. CHARLES EPPS
and Mr. WILLIAM KAUFMANN for their assistance in the evaluation of
these results and Mr. FRANK E. JACKSON for his preparation of the
photographs.

References

HARRIS, C.C., KAUFMAN, D.G., SPORN, M.B., SMITH, J.M., JACKSON, F.,
  SAFFIOTTI, U.: Ultrastructural effects of N-methyl-N-nitrosourea
  on the tracheobronchial epithelium of the Syrian golden hamster.
  Int. J. Cancer 12, 259-269 (1973).
HARRIS, C.C., SPORN, M.B., KAUFMAN, D.G., SMITH, J.M., BAKER, M.S.,
  SAFFIOTTI, U.: Acute ultrastructural effects of benzo(a)pyrene
  and ferric oxide on the hamster tracheobronchial epithelium. Cancer
  Res. 31, 1977-1989 (1971).
HENRY, M.C., KAUFMAN, D.G.: Clearance of benzo(a)pyrene from hamster
  lungs after administration of coated particles. J. nat. Cancer Inst.
  51, 1961-1964 (1973).
HENRY, M.C., PORT, C.D., KAUFMAN, D.G.: Role of particles in respira-
  tory carcinogenesis bioassay. These Proceedings, pp. 173-185.
HERROLD, K.M.: Upper respiratory tract tumors induced in Syrian hamsters by N-methyl-N-nitrosourea. Int. J. Cancer 6, 217-222 (1970).
PORT, C.D., HENRY, M.C., KAUFMAN, D.G., HARRIS, C.C., KETELS, K.V.:
  Acute changes of surface morphology of hamster tracheobronchial
  epithelium following benzo(a)pyrene and ferric oxide administration. Cancer Res. 33, 2498-2506 (1973).
SAFFIOTTI, U.: Morphology of respiratory tumors induced in Syrian
  golden hamsters. In: Morphology of experimental respiratory carcino-
  genesis (P. Nettesheim, M.G. Hanna, Jr., J.W. Deatherage, Jr., eds).
  AEC Symposium Series no. 21, pp. 245-254. Oak Ridge, Tennessee:
  U.S. Atomic Energy Commission, Division of Technical Inf. 1970.
SAFFIOTTI, U., CEFIS, F., KOLB, L.H.: A method for the experimental
  induction of bronchogenic carcinoma. Cancer Res. 28, 104-124 (1968).
SAFFIOTTI, U., MONTESANO, R., SELLAKUMAR, A.R., CEFIS, F., KAUFMAN,
  D.G.: Respiratory tract carcinogenesis in hamsters induced by
  different numbers of administrations of benzo(a)pyrene and ferric
  oxide. Cancer Res. 32, 1073-1081 (1972a).
SAFFIOTTI, U., MONTESANO, R., SELLAKUMAR, A.R., KAUFMAN, D.G.:
  Respiratory tract carcinogenesis induced in hamsters by different
  dose levels of benzo(a)pyrene and ferric oxide. J. nat. Cancer Inst.
  49, 1199-1204 (1972b).
SELLAKUMAR, A.R., MONTESANO, R., SAFFIOTTI, U., KAUFMAN, D.G.: Hamster
  respiratory carcinogenesis induced by benzo(a)pyrene and different
  dose levels of ferric oxide. J. nat. Cancer Inst. 50, 507-510 (1973).

The Effects of Particulates on Respiratory Carcinogenesis by Diethylnitrosamine

Robert L. Farrell[1] and G. W. Davis[2]

[1]Department of Veterinary Pathology, University of Georgia, Athens, GA 30602, USA
[2]Department of Veterinary Pathobiology, Ohio State University, Columbus, OH 43210, USA

ABSTRACT

It has been shown that hamsters treated with diethylnitrosamine (DEN)
develop a greater number of respiratory tract tumors when DEN treatment is followed by intratracheal instillations of ferric oxide. To
evaluate the various factors involved in carcinogenesis in the above
study, an experiment was designed to determine the effects of each
of the materials used. The objective of the experiment was to determine the effects of gelatin, saline, anesthetic, and 5 particulates*
(carbon, ferric oxide, aluminum oxide, cobalt oxide, nickel oxide)
on DEN carcinogenesis in hamsters. 15 groups (50 per group) of hamsters
were started on experiment in the same week. Subcutaneous inoculations
of DEN or saline were administered once a week for 12 weeks. The week
following the last subcutaneous inoculation intratracheal instillations
of each of the 5 particulates was begun and continued for a total of
30 weekly instillations. There were 4 control groups that received subcutaneous DEN with no subsequent particulate instillation.

In the 4 groups that received DEN and no particulates, there was a
total of 3 tumors in the nasal cavity, 1 of which was malignant. In
the 5 groups that received DEN followed by intratracheal instillation
of particulates (carbon, ferric oxide, aluminum oxide, cobalt oxide,
nickel oxide), there were 14 intranasal tumors, 9 of which were malignant. In both the DEN and the DEN + particulate groups, papillomas
developed in the larynx and trachea frequently and in the bronchi
and bronchioles occasionally. The reason for the difference in the
number and degree of anaplasia of tumors in the nasal cavity of the
DEN groups compared to the DEN + particulate groups could not be
determined.

Introduction

It has been demonstrated that diethylnitrosamine varies in its carcinogenic effect on different parts of the respiratory tract of hamsters.
The degree of reaction is directly related to dose.

In 4 groups of hamsters, each of which were inoculated subcutaneously
with diethylnitrosamine (DEN) at dose levels of 4.0, 2.0, 1.0, and
0.5 mg, respectively, MONTESANO and SAFFIOTTI (1968) demonstrated a

---

All particulates used in this study were prepared by R. DAVIES,
Illinois Institute of Technology Research Institute, Chicago.

positive dose-response correlation for tumor induction in the nasal
cavities, larynx, and trachea while the neoplastic response in the
bronchi, bronchioles and alveoli remained very low in all 4 groups.
MONTESANO and SAFFIOTTI (1968) also demonstrated that a synergistic
carcinogenic response between DEN and ferric oxide occurs in the respiratory tract of hamsters when the animals are treated subcutaneously with DEN followed by tracheal instillation of ferric oxide. This
resulted in a higher incidence of tumors than would have occurred with
DEN alone.

To evaluate the various factors involved in carcinogenesis in this
study, an experiment was designed to determine the effects of each
of the materials used. The objective of this experiment was to determine the effects of 5 particulates (carbon, ferric oxide, aluminum
oxide, cobalt oxide, nickel oxide) and, in controls, those of gelatin,
saline, and anesthetic on DEN carcinogenesis in Syrian hamsters.

Materials and Methods

15 groups of 50 (25 male, 25 female) hamsters were started on experiment in the same week (Table 1). The 750 5-week old hamsters were obtained from 1 supplier at 1 time. Subcutaneous inoculations of DEN

Table 1

Groups[a]	First 12 Weeks[b]	Next 30 Weeks
I	DEN sc	no treatment
II	DEN sc	gelatin + saline + anesthetic
III	DEN sc	saline + anesthetic
IV	DEN sc	anesthetic
V	saline sc	gelatin + saline + anesthetic
VI	DEN sc	gelatin + saline + anesthetic + carbon[d]
VII	DEN sc	gelatin + saline + anesthetic + ferric oxide
VIII	DEN sc	gelatin + saline + anesthetic + aluminum oxide
IX	DEN sc	gelatin + saline + anesthetic + cobalt oxide
X	DEN sc	gelatin + saline + anesthetic + nickel oxide
XI	saline sc	gelatin + saline + anesthetic + carbon[d]
XII	saline sc	gelatin + saline + anesthetic + ferric oxide
XIII	saline sc	gelatin + saline + anesthetic + aluminum oxide
XIV	saline sc	gelatin + saline + anesthetic + cobalt oxide
XV	saline sc	gelatin + saline + anesthetic + nickel oxide

[a] 50 hamsters per group (25 male, 25 female).
[b] Hamsters 9 weeks old at time of first injection.
[c] sc = subcutaneously.
[d] carbon = nut shell charcoal.

or saline were started when the animals were 7 weeks old. Each of the animals in 9 groups was inoculated subcutaneously once a week for 12 weeks with a solution of 0.5 mg diethylnitrosamine (DEN) in 0.25 mg sterile physiological saline (saline). Each animal received a total dose of 6 mg DEN.

Each of the animals in the 6 control groups was injected subcutaneously once a week for 12 weeks with 0.25 ml saline.

The week following the last subcutaneous (sc) inoculation, the intratracheal particulate treatments were started and continued for 30 weeks. Particulates of carbon (nut shell charcoal), ferric oxide, cobalt oxide, and nickel oxide were used in a size range of 0.5 to 1.0 μm. 2 grams of each type of particulate were mixed with 100 ml of 0.5% gelatin-in-saline. Animals were instilled intratracheally, using the technique of SAFFIOTTI et al. (1968), with 0.2 ml of the appropriate suspension according to Table 1.

The probability of a tumor being present at death was calculated using the method of KAPLAN and MEIER (1958).

Results

The mortality in hamsters following treatment with DEN and/or 1 of the 5 tracheally administered particulates is shown in Table 2. More deaths occurred during the 42 week treatment period in the DEN particulate groups than in either the DEN or particulate control groups. The mortalities were 28%, 23.5%, and 14.4%, respectively, in these 3 major groups during the treatment period. Pulmonary neoplasms (tracheal papillomas) were first detected at 23 weeks in group IX. Earlier deaths were attributed to nonneoplastic diseases, especially suppurative pneumonia and enteritis.

Final cumulative death rates during the observation period did not vary significantly among the different treatment groups.

The distribution of tumors in the 15 DEN groups is shown in Table 3. The average number of laryngeal tumors was approximately the same in the DEN + particulate groups (11.4), compared to the groups given DEN only (12). The average number of tracheal tumors was slightly less in the DEN only groups (27.75), compared to the average number of tumors in the DEN + particulate groups (30). In the 5 groups that received DEN subcutaneously plus a tracheally administered particulate, there was a greater average number of nasal tumors per group (2.6) than the average number of nasal tumors per group in the 4 groups receiving DEN only (0.75). Comparison of these same groups also demonstrated an increase in the average number of both bronchial (2.0 vs 0) and peripheral lung (5.2 vs 2.7) tumors. There were no pulmonary neoplasms in the particulate control hamsters (groups XI to XV) except for 4 benign lesions in the peripheral lung.

The tumors observed in the larynx and trachea were all squamous papillomas similar to those previously reported.

A significant number of malignant neoplasms occurred in the nasal cavity. 9 carcinomas were observed in the 5 DEN + particle groups, and 1 in DEN groups. 1 nasal papilloma was observed in each of 2 of the 4 DEN control groups. 5 papillomas were observed in the DEN +

Table 2. Mortality in hamsters treated with DEN and/or particulates

	Group (50 Animals per Group)						
Weeks Post Inoculation	I DEN sc No Treat.	II DEN sc Gel-Sal. Anes.	III DEN sc Saline Anes.	IV DEN sc Anes.	V Saline sc Gel-Sal. Anes.	VI DEN sc Gel-Sal. Anes. C	VII DEN sc Gel-Sal. Anes. Fe_2O_3
12 sc Inoculations 30 IT Instillations Total - 42 Weeks	8	17	14	12	7	25	11
3	4	3	2	4	1	4	7
8	6	4	0	2	4	2	3
13	11	2	6	12	4	5	5
18	7	4	7	8	2	5	4
23	3	8	5	3	3	1	4
28	3	6	7	1	4	6	5
33	2	5	5	0	6	0	2
38	2	1	2	2	5	2	2
43	1	0	1	2	9	0	3
48	1	0	1	2	1	0	1
53	1	0	0	1	0	0	1
58	0	0	0	1	1	0	2
63	1	0	0	0	1	0	0
68	0	0	0	0	2	0	0
	50	50	50	50	50	50	50

particle groups. Neither carcinomas nor papillomas were observed in
the saline + particle control groups (Table 3). The nasal carcinomas
were unilateral solid masses, which had replaced the turbinates (Fig.1)
and, to varying degrees, had distorted and invaded facial bones and
nasal septums (Fig. 2). In 1 animal facial bones had been destroyed
by the underlying nasal adenocarcinoma (Fig. 3). Microscopically, the
neoplasms were all carcinomas but varied in their degree of differentiation. There were 3 very undifferentiated carcinomas characterized
by irregularly arranged cords and occasional nests of cells suggesting abortive attempts at acinar formation (Fig. 4). There was a high
mitotic index and minimal stroma. 2 other carcinomas were similar except for more differentiation with recognizable acini and increased
vascularity (Fig. 5). The remaining 5 well-differentiated adeno-carcinomas consisted principally of well-developed, uniform sized acinar
structures (Fig. 6). There were occasional nests of less differentiated epithelial cells scattered among the acini.

10 bronchial neoplasms were detected only in hamsters administered
DEN + particulate (groups VI to X). 6 of these 10 neoplasms were in
hamsters injected with DEN followed by intratracheally administered
Fe_2O_3. All 10 neoplasms were bronchial papillomas with the exception
of 2 adenomas observed in group VII.

Table 2 (cont.)

Group (50 Animals per Group)							
VIII DEN sc Gel-Sal. Anes. Al_2O_3	IX DEN sc Gel-Sal. Anes. Co_3O_4	X DEN sc Gel-Sa. Anes. NiO	XI Saline sc Gel-Sal. Anes. C	XII Saline sc Gel-Sal. Anes. Fe_2O_3	XIII Saline sc Gel-Sal. Anes. Al_2O_3	XIV Saline sc Gel-Sal. Anes. Co_3O_4	XV Saline sc Gel-Sal. Anes. NiO
12	11	11	9	5	8	7	7
0	4	2	4	3	1	7	0
4	7	5	0	4	1	6	2
12	13	7	6	4	4	6	5
9	4	4	2	8	8	1	6
2	4	8	5	3	1	2	11
5	2	2	7	2	5	6	7
1	2	3	2	4	2	2	1
2	3	5	7	5	7	4	3
2	0	2	1	3	1	3	4
1	0	0	4	3	5	1	1
0	0	0	1	1	2	1	2
0	0	1	2	1	3	2	1
0	0	0	0	1	1	2	0
0	0	0	0	3	1	0	0
50	50	50	50	50	50	50	50

There were 26 peripheral neoplasms in the 5 groups receiving DEN + tracheally administered particulates. 11 similar neoplasms were detected in the 4 DEN groups and 4 neoplasms in the 5 saline-particulate groups. Of these 41 neoplasms, 37 (90%) were adenomas.

The incidence and probability of tumors in each segment of the respiratory tract is shown in Tables 4 to 9.

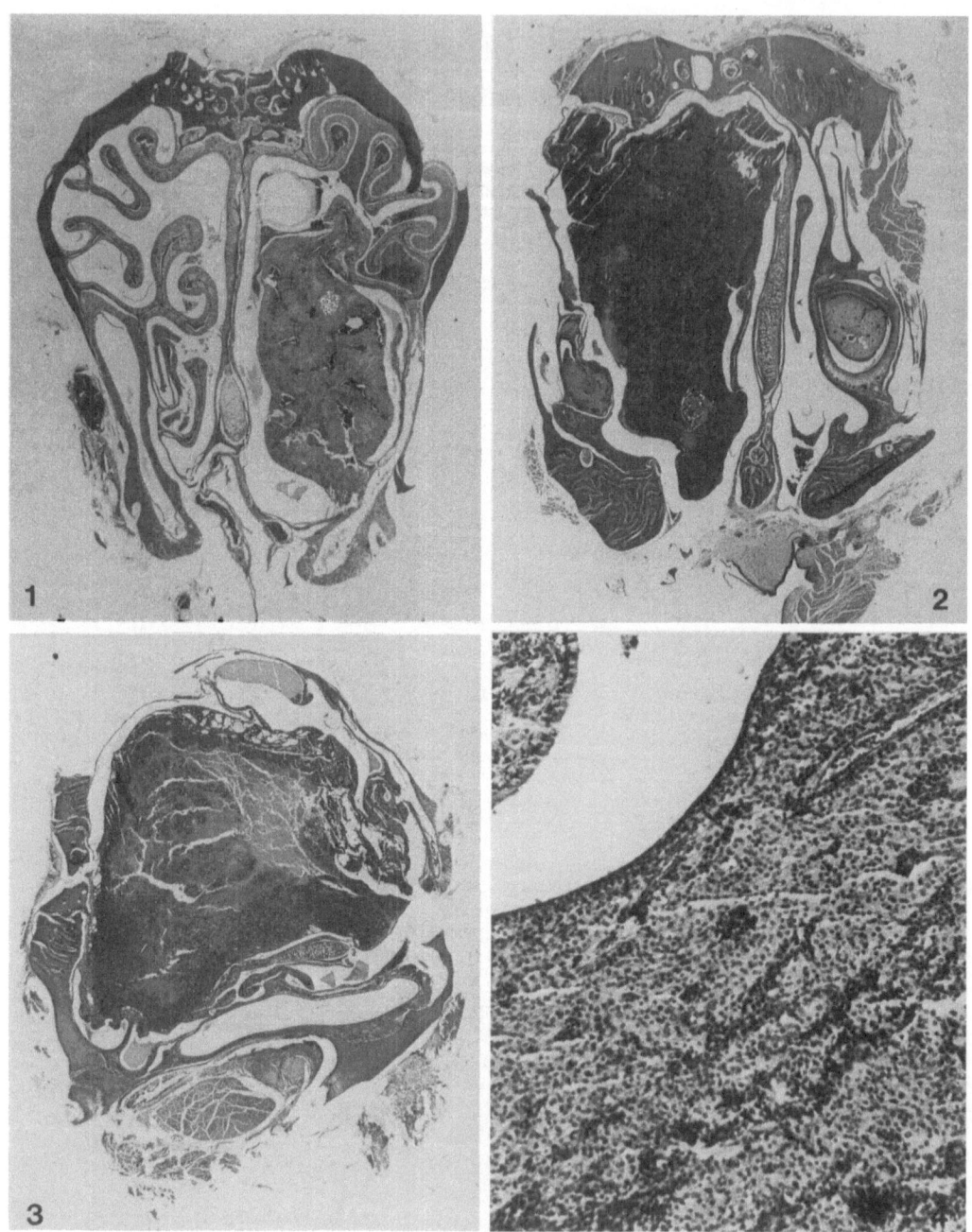

Legends see opposite page

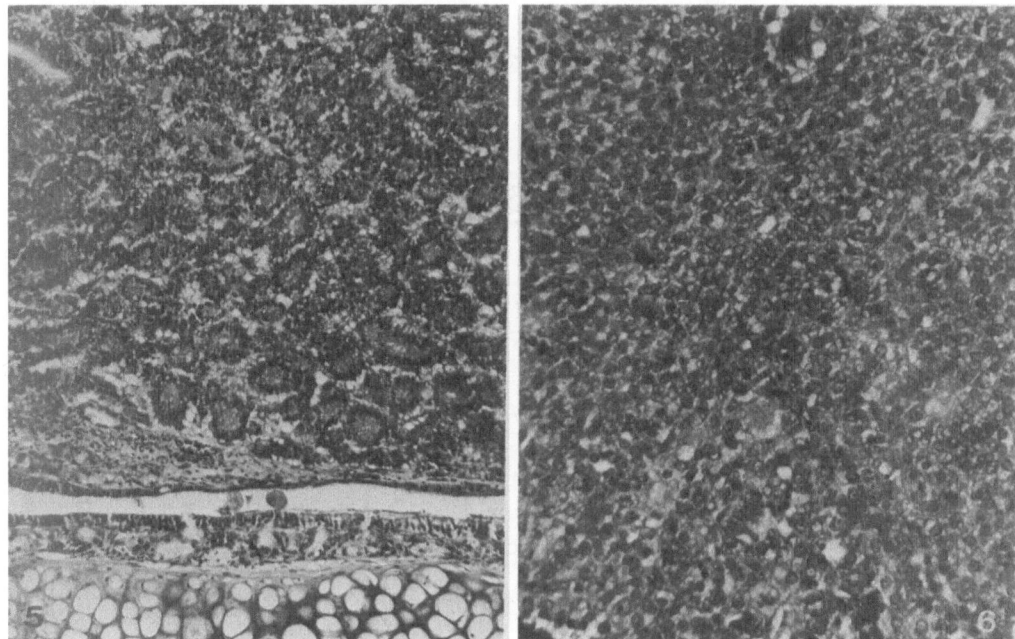

Fig. 5. Cellular detail of an adenocarcinoma from a male hamster that died at 45 weeks after the initiation of 12 weeks DEN sc inoculations followed by 30 weeks IT instillations of Fe_2O_3. The cell population is arranged in sheets of cells interrupted by partially formed acinar structures. HE (x 252)

Fig. 6. Detail from Fig. 3, illustrating 1 of the well-differentiated adenocarcinomas composed primarily of uniform sized acinar structures interrupted only by scattered nests of less differentiated epithelial cells. HE (x100)

Fig. 1. Unilateral, discrete, undifferentiated carcinoma in the nasal cavity of a female hamster that died at 47 weeks after the beginning of 12 weeks subcutaneous (sc) inoculations of diethylnitrosamine (DEN), followed by 30 weeks intratracheal (IT) instillations of NiO. HE (x 6.5)

Fig. 2. Poorly differentiated adenocarcinoma in the nasal cavity of a female hamster that died at 45 weeks after 12 weeks of sc inoculations of DEN, followed by 30 weeks IT carbon. HE (x 6.5)

Fig. 3. Adenocarcinoma in the nasal cavity of a female hamster 44 weeks after beginning treatments as described in Fig. 1. There is a marked deviation of the nasal septum and destruction of the turbinates and overlying facial bones. HE (x 6.5)

Fig. 4. Detail of Fig. 1, showing a highly cellular carcinoma and nests of epithelial cells with occasional abortive attempts at acinar formation. HE (x 100)

Table 3. Distribution of tumors in respiratory tract of hamsters treated with DEN and/or particulates[a]

Groups (50/group)	Experiment	Nasal Cavity	Larynx	Trachea	Loci of Tumors		Bronchioles	Alveoli	Other	Tumor Bearing/Total Necropsied	Percent Tumor Bearing
					Bronchi						
I	DEN + no treatment	1	13	26	0		0	0	1	31/50	62
II	DEN + GSA[b]	1	7	27	0		0	7	2(1)[c]	30/48	62
III	DEN + saline + anes.	1(1)[c]	12	29	0		1	4	0	35/48	73
IV	DEN + anes.	0	16	25	0		1	0	0	31/47	66
V	Saline + GSA	0	0	1	0		0	0	4	5/44	11
VI	DEN + GSA + C	3(3)[c]	9	26	2		0	8	1	32/47	68
VII	DEN + GSA + Fe2O3	3(2)[c]	16	34	6		1	5	0	38/46	83
VIII	DEN + GSA + Al2O3	1	8	28	1		0	4	0	32/46	70
IX	DEN + GSA + Co3O4	2(1)[c]	12	33	1		0	5	2	37/48	77
X	DEN + GSA + NiO	4(3)[c]	12	29	0		0	4	0	34/48	71
XI	Saline + GSA + C	0	0	0	0 .		0	1	3	4/50	8
XII	Saline + GSA + Fe2O3	0	0	0	0		0	1	3	3/48	6
XIII	Saline + GSA + Al2O3	0	0	0	0		0	0	1	1/47	2
XIV	Saline + GSA + Co3O4	0	0	0	0		0	2	0	2/48	4
XV	Saline + GSA + NiO	0	0	0	0		0	0	1	1/47	2

[a]All particulates, 0.5 to 1.0 μm size range.

[b]0.2 ml of 0.5% gelatin-in-saline (intratracheally) + anesthetic (Brevital sodium).

[c]Number of animals with carcinoma.

Table 4. Incidence of tumors at weeks of experiment in animals treated with DEN and/or particulate. (Probability of tumor-bearing animals)[a]

(Region of respiratory tract: nasal cavity)

Groups	Experiment	Weeks of Experiment 0-20	21-40	41-60	61-100
I	DEN[b] + no treatment	.00(0)[f]	.00(0)	.00(0)	.00(0)
II	DEN + GS[c] + A[d]	.00(0)	.00(0)	.03(1)	.03(0)
III	DEN + S[e] + A	.00(0)	.00(0)	.00(0)	.05(1)
IV	DEN + A	.00(0)	.00(0)	.00(0)	.00(0)
V	Saline + GS + A	.00(0)	.00(0)	.00(0)	.00(0)
VI	DEN + GS + A + C	.00(0)	.04(2)	.08(1)	.08(0)
VII	DEN + GS + A + Fe_2O_3	.00(0)	.02(1)	.05(1)	.05(0)
VIII	DEN + GS + A + Al_2O_3	.00(0)	.00(0)	.03(1)	.09(1)
IX	DEN + GS + A + Co_3O_4	.00(0)	.00(0)	.00(0)	.15(2)
X	DEN + GS + A + NiO	.00(0)	.00(0)	.08(3)	.08(0)
XI	Saline + GS + A + C	.00(0)	.00(0)	.00(0)	.00(0)
XII	Saline + GS + A + Fe_2O_3	.00(0)	.00(0)	.00(0)	.00(0)
XIII	Saline + GS + A + Al_2O_3	.00(0)	.00(0)	.00(0)	.00(0)
XIV	Saline + GS + A + Co_3O_4	.00(0)	.00(0)	.00(0)	.00(0)
XV	Saline + GS + A + NiO	.00(0)	.00(0)	.00(0)	.00(0)

[a] Calculated according to KAPLAN and MEIER, J. Amer. Statistical Ass. 53, 457, 1958.
[b] DEN or saline, subcutaneous.
[c] GS = 0.5% gelatin-in-saline.
[d] A = anesthesia (Brevital sodium).
[e] S = saline.
[f] Number of animals with tumors.

Table 5. Incidence of tumors at weeks of experiment in animals treated with DEN and/or particulate. (Probability of tumor-bearing animals)[a]

(Region of respiratory tract: larynx)

Groups	Experiment	Weeks of Experiment			
		0-20	21-40	41-60	60-100
I	DEN[b] + no treatment	.00(0)[f]	.00(0)	.26(11)	.36(2)
II	DEN + GS[c] + A[d]	.00(0)	.04(2)	.07(1)	.26(4)
III	DEN + S[e] + A	.00(0)	.06(3)	.18(5)	.34(4)
IV	DEN + A	.00(0)	.02(1)	.29(10)	.59(5)
V	Saline + GS + A	.00(0)	.00(0)	.00(1)	.00(0)
VI	DEN + GS + A + C	.00(0)	.09(4)	.16(2)	.44(3)
VII	DEN + GS + A + Fe_2O_3	.00(0)	.07(3)	.18(5)	.50(8)
VIII	DEN + GS + A + Al_2O_3	.00(0)	.02(1)	.14(5)	.25(2)
IX	DEN + GS + A + Co_3O_4	.00(0)	.00(0)	.18(7)	.52(5)
X	DEN + GS + A + NiO	.00(0)	.00(0)	.13(5)	.42(7)
XI	Saline + GS + A + C	.00(0)	.00(0)	.00(0)	.00(0)
XII	Saline + GS + A + Fe_2O_3	.00(0)	.00(0)	.00(0)	.00(0)
XIII	Saline + GS + A + Al_2O_3	.00(0)	.00(0)	.00(0)	.00(0)
XIV	Saline + GS + A + Co_3O_4	.00(0)	.00(0)	.00(0)	.00(0)
XV	Saline + GS + A + NiO	.00(0)	.00(0)	.00(0)	.00(0)

[a]Calculated according to KAPLAN and MEIER, J. Amer. Statistical Ass. 53, 457, 1958.

[b]DEN or saline, subcutaneous.

[c]GS = 0.5% gelatin-in-saline.

[d]A = anesthesia (Brevital sodium).

[e]S = saline.

[f]Number of animals with tumors.

Table 6. Incidence of tumors at weeks of experiment in animals
treated with DEN and/or particulate. (Probability of tumor-bearing
animals)[a]

(Region of respiratory tract: trachea)

Groups	Experiment	Weeks of Experiment			
		0-20	21-40	41-60	61-100
I	DEN[b] + no treatment	.00(0)[f]	.02(1)	.37(15)	.82(10)
II	DEN + GS[c] + A[d]	.00(0)	.06(3)	.32(9)	.83(15)
III·	DEN + S[e] + A	.00(0)	.02(1)	.32(12)	.84(16)
IV	DEN + A	.00(0)	.02(1)	.47(17)	.78(7)
V	Saline + GS + A	.00(0)	.00(0)	.02(1)	.02(0)
VI	DEN + GS + A + C	.00(0)	.13(6)	.56(13)	.90(7)
VII	DEN + GS + A + Fe_2O_3	.00(0)	.09(4)	.41(14)	.86(16)
VIII	DEN + GS + A + Al_2O_3	.00(0)	.02(1)	.42(16)	.87(11)
IX	DEN + GS + A + Co_3O_4	.00(0)	.06(3)	.54(20)	.92(10)
X	DEN + GS + A + NiO	.00(0)	.02(1)	.30(11)	.87(17)
XI	Saline + GS + A + C	.00(0)	.00(0)	.00(0)	.00(0)
XII	Saline + GS + A + Fe_2O_3	.00(0)	.00(0)	.00(0)	.00(0)
XIII	Saline + GS + A + Al_2O_3	.00(0)	.00(0)	.00(0)	.00(0)
XIV	Saline + GS + A + Co_3O_4	.00(0)	.00(0)	.00(0)	.00(0)
XV	Saline + GS + A + NiO	.00(0)	.00(0)	.00(0)	.00(0)

[a]Calculated according to KAPLAN and MEIER, J. Amer. Statistical Ass.
53, 457, 1958.
[b]DEN or saline, subcutaneous.
[c]GS = 0.5% gelatin-in-saline.
[d]A = anesthesia (Brevital sodium).
[e]S = saline.
[f]Number of animals with tumors.

Table 7. Incidence of tumors at weeks of experiment in animals treated with DEN and/or particulate. (Probability of tumor-bearing animals)[a]

(Region of respiratory tract: bronchi)

Groups	Experiment	Weeks of Experiment			
		0-20	21-40	41-60	61-100
I	DEN[b] + no treatment	.00(0)[f]	.00(0)	.00(0)	.00(0)
II	DEN + GS[c] + A[d]	.00(0)	.00(0)	.00(0)	.00(0)
III	DEN + S[e] + A	.00(0)	.00(0)	.00(0)	.00(0)
IV	DEN + A	.00(0)	.00(0)	.00(0)	.00(0)
V	Saline + GS + A	.00(0)	.00(0)	.00(0)	.00(0)
VI	DEN + GS + A + C	.00(0)	.00(0)	.08(2)	.08(0)
VII	DEN + GS + A + Fe_2O_3	.00(0)	.00(0)	.05(2)	.23(4)
VIII	DEN + GS + A + Al_2O_3	.00(0)	.00(0)	.00(0)	.07(1)
IX	DEN + GS + A + Co_3O_4	.00(0)	.00(0)	.03(1)	.03(0)
X	DEN + GS + A + NiO	.00(0)	.00(0)	.00(0)	.00(0)
XI	Saline + GS + A + C	.00(0)	.00(0)	.00(0)	.00(0)
XII	Saline + GS + A + Fe_2O_3	.00(0)	.00(0)	.00(0)	.00(0)
XIII	Saline + GS + A + Al_2O_3	.00(0)	.00(0)	.00(0)	.00(0)
XIV	Saline + GS + A + Co_3O_4	.00(0)	.00(0)	.00(0)	.00(0)
XV	Saline + GS + A + NiO	.00(0)	.00(0)	.00(0)	.00(0)

[a]Calculated according to KAPLAN and MEIER, J. Amer. Statistical Ass. 53, 457, 1958.

[b]DEN or saline, subcutaneous.

[c]GS = 0.5% gelatin-in-saline.

[d]A = anesthesia (Brevital sodium).

[e]S = saline.

[f]Number of animals with tumors.

Table 8.   Incidence of tumors at weeks of experiment in animals
treated with DEN and/or particulate. (Probability of tumor-bearing
animals)[a]

(Region of respiratory tract: bronchiole)

| Groups | Experiment | Weeks of Experiment | | | |
		0-20	21-40	41-60	61-100
I	DEN[b] + no treatment	.00(0)[f]	.00(0)	.00(0)	.00(0)
II	DEN + GS[c] + A[d]	.00(0)	.00(0)	.00(0)	.00(0)
III	DEN + S[e] + A	.00(0)	.00(0)	.03(1)	.03(0)
IV	DEN + A	.00(0)	.00(0)	.00(0)	.08(1)
V	Saline + GS + A	.00(0)	.00(0)	.00(0)	.00(0)
VI	DEN + GS + A + C	.00(0)	.00(0)	.00(0)	.00(0)
VII	DEN + GS + A + Fe_2O_3	.00(0)	.00(0)	.00(0)	.04(1)
VIII	DEN + GS + A + Al_2O_3	.00(0)	.00(0)	.00(0)	.00(0)
IX	DEN + GS + A + Co_3O_4	.00(0)	.00(0)	.00(0)	.00(0)
X	DEN + GS + A + NiO	.00(0)	.00(0)	.00(0)	.00(0)
XI	Saline + GS + A + C	.00(0)	.00(0)	.00(0)	.00(0)
XII	Saline + GS + A + Fe_2O_3	.00(0)	.00(0)	.00(0)	.00(0)
XIII	Saline + GS + A + Al_2O_3	.00(0)	.00(0)	.00(0)	.00(0)
XIV	Saline + GS + A + Co_3O_4	.00(0)	.00(0)	.00(0)	.00(0)
XV	Saline + GS + A + NiO	.00(0)	.00(0)	.00(0)	.00(0)

[a]Calculated according to KAPLAN and MEIER, J. Amer. Statistical Ass.
53, 457, 1958.
[b]DEN or saline, subcutaneous.
[c]GS = 0.5% gelatin-in-saline.
[d]A = anesthesia (Brevital sodium).
[e]S = saline.
[f]Number of animals with tumors.

Table 9. Incidence of tumors at weeks of experiment in animals treated with DEN and/or particulate. (Probability of tumor-bearing animals)[a]

(Region of respiratory tract: alveoli)

Groups	Experiment	Weeks of Experiment			
		0-20	21-40	41-60	61-100
I	DEN[b] + no treatment	.00(0)[f]	.00(0)	.00(0)	.00(0)
II	DEN + GS[c] + A[d]	.00(0)	.00(0)	.06(2)	.30(5)
III	DEN + S[e] + A	.00(0)	.02(1)	.07(2)	.11(1)
IV	DEN + A	.00(0)	.00(0)	.00(0)	.00(0)
V	Saline + GS + A	.00(0)	.00(0)	.00(0)	.00(0)
VI	DEN + GS + A + C	.00(0)	.00(0)	.15(4)	.53(4)
VII	DEN + GS + A + Fe_2O_3	.00(0)	.00(0)	.03(1)	.21(4)
VIII	DEN + GS + A + Al_2O_3	.00(0)	.00(0)	.08(3)	.14(1)
IX	DEN + GS + A + Co_3O_4	.00(0)	.00(0)	.08(3)	.23(2)
X	DEN + GS + A + NiO	.00(0)	.00(0)	.05(2)	.14(2)
XI	Saline + GS + A + C	.00(0)	.00(0)	.00(0)	.04(1)
XII	Saline + GS + A + Fe_2O_3	.00(0)	.00(0)	.02(1)	.02(0)
XIII	Saline + GS + A + Al_2O_3	.00(0)	.00(0)	.00(0)	.00(0)
XIV	Saline + GS + A + Co_3O_4	.00(0)	.00(0)	.02(1)	.07(1)
XV	Saline + GS + A + NiO	.00(0)	.00(0)	.00(0)	.00(0)

[a]Calculated according to KAPLAN and MEIER, J. Amer. Statistical Ass. 53, 457, 1958.

[b]DEN or saline, subcutaneous.

[c]GS = 0.5% gelatin-in-saline.

[d]A = anesthesia (Brevital sodium).

[e]S = saline.

[f]Number of animals with tumors.

Discussion

MONTESANO and SAFFIOTTI (1970) demonstrated an increased number of respiratory tract tumors in hamsters inoculated subcutaneously with DEN followed by instillation of ferric oxide particles. Similar results were observed in the current study using particulates of carbon, ferric oxide, aluminum oxide, cobalt oxide, and nickel oxide. There were differences in the incidence and distribution of neoplasms. Hamsters that received DEN without intratracheal particles developed fewer neoplasms of the nasal cavity and trachea than previously reported (MONTESANO and SAFFIOTTI, 1968).

The combined administration of DEN, subcutaneously followed by intratracheal instillation of particulates resulted in approximately a four-fold increase in the number of nasal neoplasms and a two-fold increase in the number of peripheral adenomas. There were no significant differences in the incidence of laryngeal or tracheal papillomas. Benign bronchial papillomas and adenomas were present in hamsters given DEN and intratracheal particulates, but not after the administration of either DEN or particulates alone. The DEN + Fe_2O_3 group accounted for 60% of the bronchial neoplasms.

A high percentage (69%) of the nasal tumors in the DEN + particulate groups were carcinomas. We have no explanation for this apparent increase in biological behavior of nasal tumors in these hamsters.

Comparison of the 5 particulate groups revealed nasal carcinomas in all but the Al_2O_3 group. There was a greater percentage of tumor bearing animals in all 5 groups, compared to the 10 control groups. The largest number of tumors was present in hamsters injected with DEN + Fe_2O_3.

These results emphasize once again the marked carcinogenic effect of even low doses of DEN on the respiratory tract of the Syrian hamster. More importantly they demonstrate that the distribution, frequency, and morphological appearance of these respiratory neoplasms can be modified by the subsequent intratracheal administration of dust particulates. Slight differences were detected among the 5 particulates assayed. The results shown support the role of the dust as not only a vehicle but a synergist in carcinogenesis of the respiratory tract.

References

KAPLAN, E.L., MEIER, P.: Nonparametric estimation from incomplete observations. J. Statist. Ass. 53, 457-481 (1958).
MONTESANO, R., SAFFIOTTI, U.: Carcinogenic response of the respiratory tract of Syrian golden hamsters to different doses of diethylnitrosamine. Cancer Res. 28, 2197-2210 (1968).
MONTESANO, R., SAFFIOTTI, U.: Synergistic effect of diethylnitrosamine (DEN) and benzo(a)pyrene (BaP) on respiratory carcinogenesis in hamsters. Proc. Amer. Ass. Cancer Res. 9, 51 (1968).
MONTESANO, R., SAFFIOTTI, U., SHUBIK, P.: The role of topical and systemic factors in experimental respiratory carcinogenesis. In: Inhalation Carcinogenesis (M.G. Hanna, Jr., P. Nettesheim, J.R. Gilbert, eds). AEC Symposium Series no. 18, Conf. 691001, pp. 353-371. Oak Ridge, Tennessee: U.S. Atomic Energy Commission, Division of Technical Inf. 1970.
SAFFIOTTI, U., CEFIS, F., KOLB, L.H.: A method for the experimental induction of bronchogenic carcinoma. Cancer Res. 28, 104-124 (1968).

Respiratory Cocarcinogenesis Studies with Ferric Oxide: A Test Case of Current Experimental Models*

Donald A. Creasia and Paul Nettesheim

Oak Ridge National Laboratory, Biology Division, Oak Ridge, TN 37830, USA

ABSTRACT

Laboratory studies conducted to date strongly suggest that ferric oxide dust can act as a cofactor in respiratory tract carcinogenesis. The available data indicate at least 2 different mechanisms by which these otherwise fairly innocuous particles might exert their effect: 1. by retarding carcinogen clearance (this applies to conditions in which the carcinogen is adsorbed to the particle surface) and 2. by causing cytopathological effects (irritation?, enhanced cell proliferation?) at the site of deposition.

These findings suggest that otherwise rather harmless particulate air contaminants might play a significant role in the pathogenesis of lung cancer.

A. Introduction

Considerable effort has been devoted to investigations designed to study the cocarcinogenic effects of various particles, notably ferric oxide dust, in respiratory carcinogenesis. It seems to me that this conference is very timely and that we should attempt to synthesize the major pieces of information derived from these studies over the last few years. Assuming that the ultimate purpose of the work conducted in the field of carcinogenesis is to contribute to cancer prevention in man, the most important question in the experimental work with ferric oxide is whether exposure to this and similar air contaminants is likely to augment the risk of people to develop lung cancer.

In the field of respiratory carcinogenesis no other chemical has been investigated for its cocarcinogenic properties as extensively as ferric oxide dust. It therefore appears appropriate to look at these investigations as a sort of model case for cocarcinogenesis studies in respiratory tract tissues. If we conclude that ferric oxide is cocarcinogenic, then we need to know why, to what degree, under what conditions, as well as what relevance our findings have to the total environment of human exposure to ferric oxide particles. If we understand some of

*Research supported jointly by the National Cancer Institute and the U.S. Atomic Energy Commission under contract with Union Carbide Corporation.

the principal mechanisms involved, we will be able to make some predictions about the likelihood of other particulate air contaminants
to have cocarcinogenic potential, which in turn will allow us to be
more selective in testing other air contaminants. The generally fragmentary information related to the cocarcinogenic effects of ferric
oxide is scattered through the literature, and the variables in experimental design, physical, and chemical characteristics of often
unknown materials, doses, analytical measurements, time scales, morphological endpoints, etc. are numerous and make comparisons difficult.
In trying to sort out the currently available data the question arises:
is ferric oxide really significant enough as an air contaminant to de-
serve that much attention? The answer is probably no. Epidemiological
studies suggest that iron ore dust is at best a weak cocarcinogen
(BOYD et al., 1970; ROUSSEL et al., 1964). However, what makes ferric
oxide an interesting, and perhaps even important, material to study
is the fact that it can serve as a prototype of a noncarcinogenic and
only weekly irritant and fibrogenic dust; in other words, relative to
other particulates such as silica and asbestos, ferric oxide would
appear to be a rather innocuous material.

To put these studies on the cocarcinogenic effects of ferric oxide into proper perspective, it seems useful to reflect briefly on the role
and significance (or assumed role and significance) of the phenomenon
of cocarcinogenesis in human neoplastic disease, and respiratory tract
cancer in particular. It appears to me that in this context the most
important task before us is not so much to prove or disprove that compound X under "appropriate" laboratory conditions exerts cocarcinogenic effects but rather to determine whether or not cocarcinogenesis
is likely to be a "real" phenomenon in man and an essential element
in the pathogenesis of some or all human neoplasms. I think it is
justifiable to state that the role of cocarcinogens and promoting
agents in the pathogenesis of lung cancer is currently unproven.
Human data on this problem are scarce. Our only clues come from epidemiological studies suggesting an augmented lung cancer risk of
smoking to asbestos workers (SELIKOFF et al., 1968), uranium miners
(SACCOMANNO et al., 1974), and perhaps iron ore miners (ROUSSEL et
al., 1964). On the other hand, one can argue that lung cancer is perhaps the best example of cocarcinogenesis in man. The idea that cocarcinogenic activity and promotion activity of tobacco smoke is
equally and perhaps more important than its initiating potency seems
to gain more and more supporters (WYNDER and HOFFMAN, 1968; VAN DUUREN
et al., 1968). The fact remains, however, that currently we do not
have adequate data to prove that the phenomenon of cocarcinogenesis
or promotion is an important factor in the pathogenesis of any of the
major neoplasms in man. Even laboratory evidence for the importance
of cocarcinogenesis and promotion to tumor induction in organs other
than the skin is scarce. The importance and practical significance
of this problem was recently re-emphasized (BOUTWELL, 1974). In his
review, "The Function and Mechanism of Promoters of Carcinogenesis",
BOUTWELL stated: "Considering the ubiquitous nature of low levels of
chemical and physical carcinogens....it is likely that most everyone
has initiated cells throughout his body.... If this is so promotion
becomes the determining factor in the appearance of a tumor and more
must be learned about the role of promoters and the identification of
promoters for other organs." With this statement in mind, we will review the work on ferric oxide cocarcinogenesis, including recent
studies from our own laboratory. Unfortunately, not all of the existing data pertinent to this topic are as yet available in the literature.

B.   Report and Interpretation of Animal Experiments

I.   Tumor Induction Studies with BaP

The original observation on the cocarcinogenic effects of ferric oxide arose out of studies (SAFFIOTTI et al., 1968) aimed at the development of an experimental model for induction of bronchogenic carcinoma. These investigators found that respiratory tract tumors could be readily induced in hamsters if the intratracheally injected carcinogen benzo(a)pyrene (BaP) was coupled to ferric oxide particles. In contrast, previous attempts to induce lung cancer with colloidal suspensions of benzo(a)pyrene had been unsuccessful (SAFFIOTTI et al., 1965). While the later studies by SAFFIOTTI et al. (1968) were not conceived and designed as cocarcinogenesis experiments, some form of cocarcinogenic action of the "inert" ferric oxide particles was obviously implied when the authors interpreted their findings: "The essential factor involved was the adequate penetration of the carcinogen into lung tissues to attain a sufficient effective dose at the target site.... It appears that in methods in which penetration of the carcinogen is impaired by mucus and ciliary barriers no effect could be exerted on the target tissue". Increasing the Fe_2O_3 to BaP ratio in such carcinogen preparations did not increase the tumorigenic activity (SAFFIOTTI et al., 1972a). Subsequent studies by other investigators with carrier-free, colloidal BaP suspensions showed either no tumor induction (KUSCHNER, 1968) or only a low tumor incidence after exorbitantly high carcinogen doses (HENRY et al., 1973). The particles in these BaP suspensions are prepared by prolonged ball milling and are mostly below 1 μm. While it seemed clear that the ferric oxide particles markedly augment the tumorigenic potency of BaP, the mechanism of this effect was not understood but was thought to be related to the carrier function of ferric oxide particles (penetration, distribution, and retention of carcinogen, see below). Important new information was added when FERON et al. (1972) reported that a respiratory tract tumor response similar though somewhat weaker to that obtained with BaP-ferric oxide could be induced with BaP crystal suspensions alone. The carcinogen suspension used contained rather large crystals of benzo(a)pyrene (about 97% above 5 μm).

Another important study (HENRY, personal communication, 1974) shows that simple addition of ferric oxide particles to benzo(a)pyrene as opposed to surface binding only slightly enhances the tumorigenicity of this polycyclic hydrocarbon. Testing several different types of particles (FARRELL et al., 1972; DAVIS and FARRELL, these Proceedings) found that adsorption of benzo(a)pyrene to different sizes of carbon particles results in a carcinogen suspension similar in tumorigenic potency to BaP-ferric oxide suspensions (particularly with the use of small carbon particles), while benzo(a)pyrene adsorbed onto aluminum oxide particles was only weakly carcinogenic. The significance of these findings with carbon and aluminum oxide particles will become apparent as we discuss data related to carcinogen clearance.

II.   Carcinogen Clearance Studies with BaP

To determine the mechanism of the enhanced carcinogenicity of BaP-ferric oxide preparations, several laboratories investigated the clearance of intratracheally injected BaP suspensions with and without ferric oxide or other carrier dusts. It was suspected that the carrier particle might markedly effect carcinogen elimination from the lung (SAFFIOTTI et al., 1968). Strict comparison of the various studies is difficult because of numerous variables such as carcinogen dose, method of preparing carcinogen suspension, method of chemical analysis, etc.; however, several common features emerge from these investigations. Colloidal BaP suspensions containing mostly small carcinogen crystals (HENRY et al., 1973) are rapidly eliminated (within hours). FERON (1972) found that BaP suspensions with large crystals (95% or more >1 μm) are cleared more slowly (within days). Benzo(a)pyrene attached to ferric oxide (SAFFIOTTI, 1970), aluminum oxide, or carbon is cleared more slowly than BaP alone not attached to carrier particles (HENRY and KAUFMAN, 1973). Addition of ferric oxide to BaP crystal suspension retards BaP clearance only slightly (SCHREIBER, 1974). The essential information on clearance and tumorigenicity of intratracheally administered BaP preparations can be summarized as follows:

1. Small BaP crystals are cleared fast and have low tumorigenicity.

2. Large BaP crystals are cleared slowly and have strong tumorigenicity.

3. BaP bound to Fe_2O_3 particles is cleared slowly and is highly tumorigenic.

4. BaP with Fe_2O_3 added is cleared slightly slower than BaP alone. The tumorigenicity is also slightly increased over that of BaP alone.

The experiments discussed thus far strongly suggest that 1 major mechanism of the Fe_2O_3 mediated enhancement of tumor response to benzo(a)pyrene is related to carcinogen clearance. Increased retention of BaP leads to an increased and protracted "effective" carcinogen dose" thus the amount of carcinogen administered is only 1 of the factors (and not necessarily the most important one) that determines effective dose per target site. However, not all of the available data are compatible with this interpretation. HENRY and KAUFMAN (1973) and FARRELL et al. (1972), conducting BaP clearance and tumorigenesis studies with BaP-aluminum oxide and BaP-carbon preparations, found that carcinogen retention and tumorigenicity do not always go hand in hand: BaP adsorbed to aluminum oxide was much less carcinogenic than BaP-ferric oxide in spite of similar carcinogen clearance rates. The tumorigenicity of BaP-carbon suspensions (carbon particles 0.5 to 1.0 μm) was similar to that of BaP-ferric oxide even though carcinogen elimination was much slower with the former. When the size of the carbon carrier particle was increased (2 to 5, 5 to 10, and 15 to 30 μm), the rate of elimination became progressively slower and the tumorigenicity of such preparations was lowered. These findings indicate that other factors such as alterations of carcinogen metabolism or lack of sufficient release of carcinogen from the carrier particle may also play a decisive role in determining the end result (i.e., tumorigenicity of carcinogen-particle mixtures).

Studies recently started in our laboratory (CREASIA and POGGENBURG, 1974, unpublished) may throw some light on the question of carcinogen release from particles and offer some explanation for the low carcinogenicity of BaP carried on large carbon particles.

Mice were intratracheally injected with microgram quantities of carbon particles labeled with [103]Ruthenium, mixed with BaP carrying carbon particles (particle size 0.5 to 1.0 μm). The elimination of the labeled carbon was measured by whole body counting and that of the BaP by chemical determination. The data of this preliminary study show that by 4 days about 50% of the carbon and about 80% of the BaP is cleared (Fig. 1). This approach allows an estimate of the rate of dissociation of the carcinogen from the carrier.

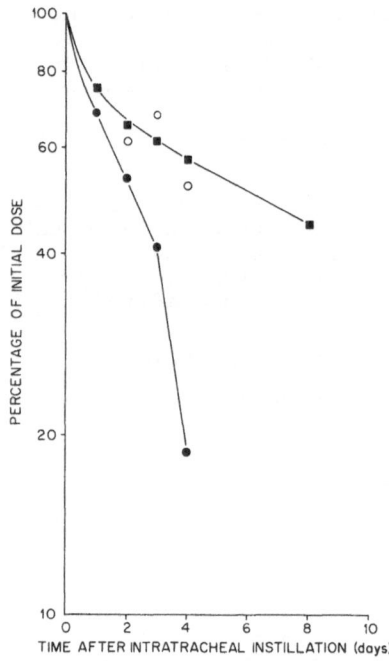

Fig. 1. Clearance of ^{103}Ru labeled carbon, BaP, and BaP coated carbon particles from the respiratory tract of mice. Squares represent clearance of ^{103}Ru labeled carbon, and closed circles represent elimination of BaP. Open circles indicate amount of ^{103}Ru labeled carbon remaining in the lungs of mice sacrificed for BaP determination

If we try to assemble the facts from the 2 or 3 pertinent studies (though this is not without hazard because of differences in experimental detail), the reason for the differences in carcinogenicity of the various carbon-BaP and BaP preparations will become obvious. The essential information is summarized in Table 1, but can be expressed more completely: Carbon is cleared very slowly (condition 1). Clearance of BaP carried on large carbon particles is essentially the same as that of carbon, i.e., almost no BaP is released from the carbon and only little BaP can come in contact with lung tissue before it is removed by physical clearance (condition 2); BaP carried on small carbon particles is cleared at a faster rate than the carrier itself, indicating that release of BaP from the particle occurs in the lung and that BaP can make contact with the tissue (condition 3); BaP (colloidal suspensions) without carrier particles is cleared very rapidly (condition 4). Conditions 2 (lack of release of BaP from carrier) and 4 (too rapid clearance of BaP) listed in Table 1 are at the opposite ends of a spectrum of conditions that disfavor delivery of an effective carcinogen dose to the target tissue.

III. Tumor Induction Studies with DEN

In the early studies with ferric oxide and benzo(a)pyrene, ferric oxide was considered to be an "inert" particle (SAFFIOTTI et al., 1968; SAFFIOTTI, 1969); however, subsequent studies have shown that ferric oxide introduced into the respiratory tract cause cell injury, increased cell proliferation, and hyperplasia (PORT et al., 1973), particularly in the peripheral airways (BOREN, 1970), and also alveolar fibrosis (Fig. 2). It is conceivable that the cytopathological effect of ferric oxide is another factor contributing to the increased carcinogenicity of the BaP-ferric oxide preparations. This notion is supported by the fact that simple addition of the ferric oxide par-

Table 1. Clearance of BaP and carbon particles

Condition	Particle	Particle size[a] (μm)	Determination in the lung	90% clearance time (min.)	Reference[b]
1	^{103}Ru-carbon	0.5-1.0	^{103}Ru-carbon	10^5	(1)
2	BaP-carbon	15 - 30	BaP	10^5	(2)
3	BaP-carbon	0.5-1.0	BaP	10^4	(1 and 2)
4	BaP	0.5-1.0	BaP	10^2	(3)

[a]Particle size refers to carrier particle.

[b]Estimates are based on data obtained by: (1) CREASIA and POGGENBURG (1974); (2) HENRY and KAUFMAN (1973); (3) HENRY et al. (1973).

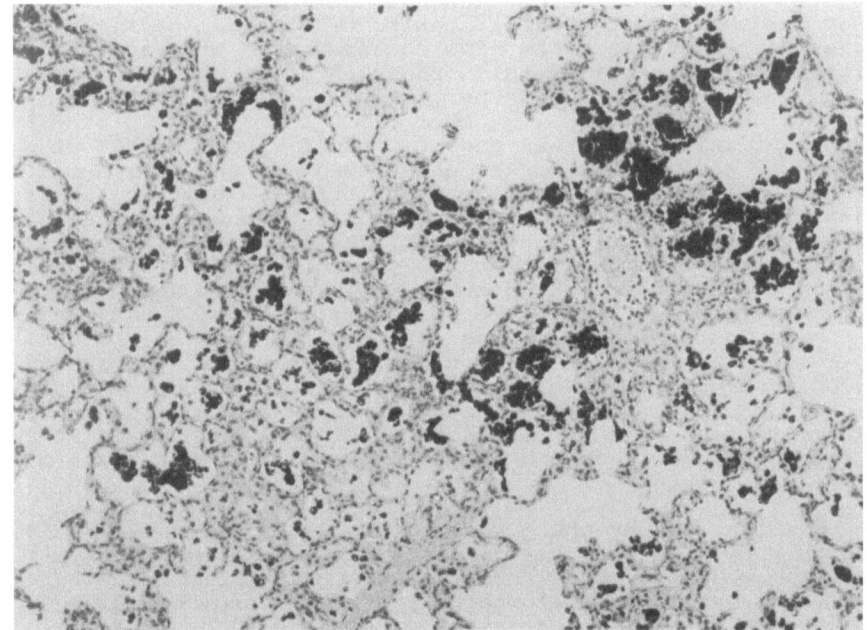

Fig. 2. Alveolar fibrosis in hamster exposed for 16 months to ferric oxide dust

ticles to the benzo(a)pyrene suspension causes some enhancement of the tumorigenicity of the polycyclic hydrocarbon, even though the elimination rate is only marginally altered (see above). Whether the irritant effect of ferric oxide is in this context of sufficient importance to explain the described effects of ferric oxide on BaP carcinogenesis is difficult to investigate in the BaP-ferric oxide tumor induction system since the 2 effects (i.e., retardation of clearance and irritation by the iron oxide particles) cannot readily be separated from each other. Another series of experiments utilizing the diethylnitrosamine (DEN) respiratory tract tumor model throws some light on this problem. In this tumor induction system the systemic carcinogen

DEN is usually given to hamsters by subcutaneous injection. Tumors
develop in all parts of the respiratory tract. (Extensive morphological
studies and dose response studies have been carried out by MONTESANO
and SAFFIOTTI (1968) with this nitrosamine.)

MONTESANO et al. (1970) reported that the peripheral lung tumor response
induced by subcutaneously injected DEN was markedly enhanced when ferric
oxide particles were repeatedly administered intratracheally, starting
at 5 weeks after the last DEN injection. The peripheral lung tumor incidence was raised from less than 10% to more than 70%. When ferric
oxide was administered prior to the DEN injections, no enhancement of
the tumor response resulted (MONTESANO, 1970a and 1970b). These findings
were in part corroborated by FERON et al. (1972), who found that intratracheal injections of DEN mixed with ferric oxide dust induced 2 to 3
times as many tumors in the bronchi and peripheral airways as DEN alone.
The histomorphology of these tumors, however, was quite different from
that seen by MONTESANO, since most of these tumors were squamoid in
appearance rather than adenomatous. FERON et al. (1972) concluded that
ferric oxide might be considered a cocarcinogen, but they also offered
an alternative explanation for the enhanced peripheral lung tumor response. They suggested that transplantation of tracheal papillomas into
the lower respiratory tract might have occurred with the repeated intratracheal instillations and that this transplantation phenomenon might
have been enhanced by ferric oxide particles.

Further pertinent information was recently added when STENBÄCK et al.
(1973a and 1973b) showed that marked enhancement of the peripheral
lung tumor response due to DEN could be achieved not only by repeated
intratracheal injection of particulates such as carbon, MgO, Fe$_2$O$_3$,
and Al$_2$O$_3$, but also by intratracheal instillation of physiological
saline. In fact, the instillation of saline produced the most marked
enhancement of the peripheral lung tumor response (from approximately
3% in controls receiving DEN only to approximately 50% in hamsters receiving DEN plus intratracheal saline injections). The experimental
design was essentially similar to that reported earlier by MONTESANO
(1970a, 1970b): the intratracheal injections were started 5 weeks
after the last DEN injection. These results threw still more doubt on
the earlier conclusion that the enhancement of the DEN lung tumor response by ferric oxide was due to the cocarcinogenicity of these particles.

We felt the issue raised by the DEN-ferric oxide experiments was important enough to warrant further investigation. In other words, if
a rather innocuous dust such as ferric oxide could promote development of pulmonary neoplasms following exposure to carcinogens, then
many other particulate air contaminants might also have to be considered as potentially serious hazards. We therefore initiated a
study to determine whether the respiratory tract tumor response induced by low levels of DEN could be affected by chronic inhalation
exposure to ferric oxide particles. Hamsters were repeatedly injected
with DEN (12 weekly injections, cumulative dose 3.0 mg). Inhalation
exposure to ferric oxide dust (40.0 mg/cubic meter) was started together with the DEN injections and continued for life. Instead of
introducing the ferric oxide into the respiratory tract by intratracheal injection, the test animals were exposed by inhalation to
avoid the possible complication of transplanting neoplastic cells
by repeated intratracheal manipulation. This approach also had the
advantage of producing data that could be more readily correlated
with the human exposure experience. The large masses of dust introduced by intratracheal injections would conceivably provoke pathological reactions that might not occur under more physiological exposure

conditions; therefore, results obtained with intratracheal injection studies might be considered somewhat of a laboratory artifact. The experimental design and the median survival time of the animals involved in these studies is summarized in Table 2. It can be seen that the median survival time was shortened in the animals receiving DEN, but was not markedly influenced by the ferric oxide exposure. That the ferric oxide particles reach the lower part of the respiratory tract was verified by a study in which the accumulation of ferric oxide particles in the lung was measured following several months of inhalation exposure to ferric oxide (the mean particle size of the ferric oxide used in this experiment was 0.11 µm). The data obtained from the chemical analysis for ferric oxide in the lungs of ferric oxide exposed hamsters are summarized in Table 3. It can be seen that a considerable amount of ferric oxide accumulates in the hamster lungs. The tumor incidence data are summarized in Table 4. Respiratory tract tumors developed only in hamsters injected with DEN, confirming previous findings that ferric oxide is not carcinogenic to hamsters. Topography and histopathology of DEN induced tumors was essentially the same as that described previously by MONTESANO and SAFFIOTTI (1968). Except for the nasal cavity, no squamous lesions or squamous cell tumors occurred anywhere in the respiratory tract. Ferric oxide exposure affected the DEN induced tumor incidence in the 3 major segments of the respiratory tract as follows: the incidence of nasal cavity tumors was reduced by ferric oxide exposure (P < .05) and the occurrence of laryngeal and tracheal tumors (papillomas) was unaffected. The incidence of peripheral lung tumors was enhanced by chronic ferric oxide exposure (P < .05). The number of tumor bearing animals as well as the total number of tumors was increased in the ferric oxide exposed group as compared to hamsters breathing clean air. Almost all of the peripheral tumors were of microscopic size and they were classified as either bronchial papillomas or as typical pulmonary adenomas (Fig. 3). We did not see the squamoid tumors described by FERON et al. (1972) and STENBÄCK et al. (1973a, 1973b), who speculated that these tumors might be derived from transplanted tracheal papillomas. All lung tumors were typical alveologenic adenomas, very similar to those seen in mice. The estimated cumulative lung tumor incidence as a function of time is given in Fig. 4. It can be seen that the tumors tended to appear earlier in the ferric oxide exposed group and that the cumulative incidence was higher in this group, even after correction for differences in mortality.

This study thus shows a mild cocarcinogenic effect of inhaled ferric oxide in lung tumor induction by a systemic carcinogen. The outcome of this experiment does not totally negate the possibility that some of the enhanced tumor response seen by the previous investigators might have been due to transplantation of laryngeal and tracheal papillomas and/or due to traumatic effects inherent in the intratracheal injection technique. Data presented here indicate that the previously observed enhancement of the DEN lung tumor response cannot be explained solely on this basis and that ferric oxide indeed has a cocarcinogenic effect in this tumor induction system. Our study also raises 2 questions: 1. what is the significance of the seemingly suppressed tumor response in the nasal cavity by ferric oxide inhalation, and 2. why does ferric oxide enhance the tumor response only in the peripheral airways and not in the larynx and trachea? While we currently have no reasonable explanation for the reduced nasal tumor incidence in ferric oxide exposed hamsters, a likely explanation for the latter question can be offered. The only site in which large amounts of ferric oxide dust accumulates in these animals is the alveoli and it is only there that chronic injury is manifest in the form of alveolar fibrosis. Large bronchi and upper airways show no indication of a hyperplastic response.

Table 2. Experimental design

| Group number | Initial number of hamsters | Exposure | | Median survival time in days |
		Carcinogen	Air contaminant	
1	135	-	-	612
2	135	DEN	-	528
3	135	-	Fe_2O_3	592
4	135	DEN	Fe_2O_3	488

Table 3. Accumulation of ferric oxide in lungs of hamsters exposed daily by inhalation

Weeks of exposure[a] to Fe_2O_3	Accumulation of Fe_2O_3 in lungs (mg/lung)
2	0.4
4	0.5
8	2.2
12	2.7
104	9.5

[a] 40 mg. Fe_2O_3/m^3, 6 hrs/day, 5 days/wk.

Table 4. Respiratory tract tumor incidence in hamsters exposed to DEN and ferric oxide

| Group | Exposure | Effective number of hamsters | Tumor incidence[a] | | |
			Nasal cavity	Larynx plus trachea	Lung plus bronchi
1	-	132	-	-	-
2	DEN	131	18	78(140)[b]	16(17)
3	Fe_2O_3	132	-	-	-
4	DEN Fe_2O_3	133	6	74(114)	27(46)

[a] Figures indicate number of tumor bearing animals.
[b] Figures in parenthesis indicate number of tumors observed.

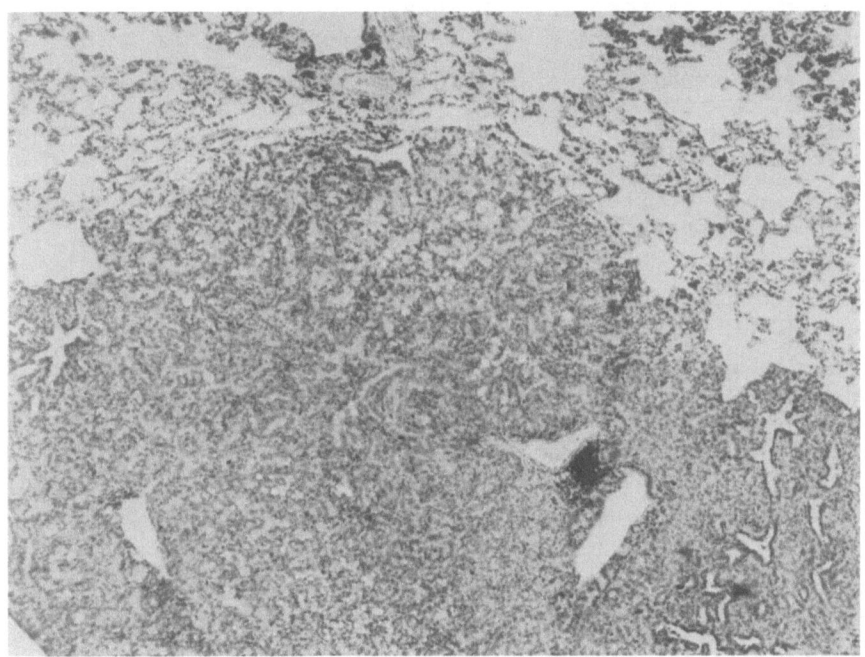

Fig. 3. Typical alveologenic tumor in lung of hamster injected with a cumulative dose of 3 mg DEN and exposed daily to ferric oxide dust

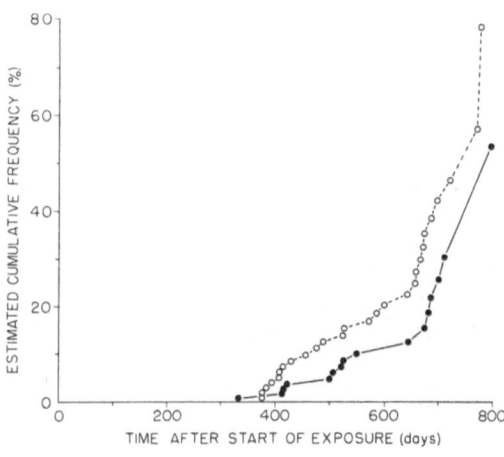

Fig. 4. Estimated cumulative frequency of lung tumors as a function of time. Open circles represent group receiving DEN plus ferric oxide. Group receiving DEN alone is represented by closed circles

References

BOREN, H. (1970), quoted by NETTESHEIM, P.: Experimental respiratory carcinogenesis studies in the Syrian golden hamster: A review. In: Prog. exp. Tumor Res. 16, 185-200 (1972).
BOUTWELL, R.K.: The function and mechanism of promoters of carcinogenesis. CRC Critical Reviews in Toxicology 2 (4), 419-443 (1974).

244

BOYD, J.T., DOLL, R., FAULDS, J.S., LEIPER, J.: Cancer of the lung in iron ore (haematite) miners. Brit. J. industr. Med. 27, 97-105 (1970).

CREASIA, D.E., POGGENBURG, J.K., Jr.: Unpublished observations, 1974.

VAN DUUREN, B.L., SIVAK, A., LANGSETH, L., GOLDSCHMIDT, B.M., SEGAL, A.: Initiators and promoters in tobacco carcinogenesis. Nat. Cancer Inst. Monogr. 28, 173-180 (1967).

HENRY, M.C.: Personal communication, 1974.

HENRY, M.C., KAUFMAN, D.G.: Clearance of benzo(a)pyrene from hamster lungs after administration on coated particles. J.N.C.I. 51, 1961-1964 (1973).

HENRY, M.C., PORT, C.D., BATES, R.R., KAUFMAN, D.G.: Respiratory tract tumors in hamsters induced by benzo(a)pyrene. Cancer Res. 33, 1585-1592 (1973).

KAPLAN, E.L., MEIER, P.: Nonparametric estimation from incomplete observations. J. Amer. Statist. Ass. 53, 457-481 (1958).

KUSCHNER, M.: The J. Burns Amberson Lecture "The causes of cancer". Amer. Rev. Resp. Dis. 98, 573-590 (1968).

MONTESANO, R.: Systemic carcinogens (N-nitroso compound) and synergistic or additive effects in respiratory carcinogenesis. Tumori 56, 335-344 (1970b).

MONTESANO, R.: Systemic respiratory carcinogenesis including synergistic effects. Oncology 4, 456-462 (1970a).

MONTESANO, R., SAFFIOTTI, U.: Carcinogenic response of the respiratory tract of Syrian golden hamsters to different doses of diethylnitrosamine. Cancer Res. 28, 2197-2210 (1968).

MONTESANO, R., SAFFIOTTI, U., SHUBIK, P.: The role of topical and systemic factors in experimental respiratory carcinogenesis. In: Inhalation Carcinogenesis (M.G. Hanna, Jr., P. Nettesheim, J.R. Gilbert, eds). AEC Symposium Series no. 18, pp. 353-371. Oak Ridge, Tennessee: U.S. Atomic Energy Commission, Division of Technical Inf. 1970.

PORT, C.D., HENRY, M.C., KAUFMAN, D.G., HARRIS, C.C., KETELS, K.V.: Acute changes in the surface morphology of hamster tracheobronchial epithelium following benzo(a)pyrene and ferric oxide administration. Cancer Res. 33, 2498-2501 (1973).

ROUSSEL, P.J., PERNOT, C., SCHOUMACHER, P., PERNOT, M., KESSLER, Y: Considerations statistiques sur le cancer bronchique du mineur de fer du bassin de Lorraine. J. Radiol. Electrol. 45, 541-546 (1964).

SACCOMANNO, G. et al.: Development of carcinoma of the lung as reflected in exfoliated cells. Cancer 33, 256 (1974).

SAFFIOTTI, U.: Experimental respiratory tract carcinogenesis. Int. Symp. of Carcinogenesis and Carcinogen Testing, Boston, Mass., 1967. Prog. exp. Tumor Res. 11, 302-333 (1969).

SAFFIOTTI, U.: Experimental respiratory tract carcinogenesis and its relation to inhalation exposures. In: Inhalation Carcinogenesis (M.G. Hanna, Jr., P. Nettesheim, J.R. Gilbert, eds). AEC Symposium Series no. 18, pp. 27-54. Oak Ridge, Tennessee: U.S. Atomic Energy Commission, Division of Technical Inf. 1970.

SAFFIOTTI, U., CEFIS, F., KOLB, L.H.: A method for the experimental induction of bronchogenic carcinoma. Cancer Res. 28, 104-124 (1968).

SAFFIOTTI, U., CEFIS, F., KOLB, L.H., SHUBIK, P.: Experimental studies of the conditions of exposure to carcinogens for lung cancer induction. J. Air Pollution Control Ass. 15, 23-25 (1965).

SAFFIOTTI, U., MONTESANO, R., SELLAKUMAR, A.R., KAUFMAN, D.G.: Respiratory tract carcinogenesis induced in hamsters by different dose levels of benzo(a)pyrene and ferric oxide. J.N.C.I. 49, 1199-1204 (1972a).

SCHREIBER, H.: Unpublished observations, 1974.

SELIKOFF, I.J., HAMMOND, E.C., CHURG, J.: Asbestos exposure, smoking and neoplasia. J. Amer. med. Ass. 204, 106-112 (1968).

STENBÄCK, F., FERRERO, A., MONTESANO, R., SHUBIK, P.: Synergistic effect of ferric oxide on dimethylnitrosamine carcinogenesis in the Syrian golden hamster. Z. Krebsforsch. 79, 31-38 (1973a).

STENBÄCK, F.G., FERRERO, A., SHUBIK, P.: Synergistic effects of diethylnitrosamine and different dusts on respiratory carcinogenesis in hamsters. Cancer Res. 33, 2209-2214 (1973b).

WYNDER, E.L., HOFFMAN, D.: Experimental Tobacco Carcinogenesis. Science 162, 862 (1968).

Induction of Pulmonary Tumors in Mice by Oral Administration of a 5-Nitrofuran Derivative

Masayoshi Kanisawa

Department of Pathology, Tokyo Metropolitan Institute of Gerontology, Tokyo, Japan

ABSTRACT

Carcinogenic action of orally treated potassium 1-methyl-7-[2-(5-nitro-2-furyl)vinyl]-4-oxo-1,4-dihydro-1,8-naphthyridine-3-carboxylate (NFN) on the lung of mice was chiefly discussed from the histogenetic point of view.

A total of 107 dd/Y mice were used, 60 animals were fed the diet containing 0.02% and later 0.01% NFN and 47 animals were fed basal diet as a control. The experiment was terminated after a course of 58 weeks and histologic and electron microscope examination were carried out on the lungs of the treated and non-treated mice.

Development of pulmonary adenoma in the treated animals was recognized 14/15 (93.3%) in males and 19/20 (95.0%) in females examined after 17 weeks, including 5 cases of pulmonary carcinoma which were classified as 3 papillary adenocarcinomas, 1 adenocarcinoma, and 1 adenoacanthoma, while control mice showed lower incidence, 10/24 (41.6%) in males and 4/21 (19.0%) in females. Sharp differences were noted in the number of lung tumors between treated and non-treated animals, 9.8 in experimental versus 2.3 in control males and 7.9 versus 1.0 in females. Regarding the histogenesis of the tumors, the results showed that most of the tumors observed both in control and experimental mice were derived from the large alveolar cell. However, some tumors induced in the experimental mice were obviously derived from bronchiolar epithelium, 1 of which was proven electronmicroscopically to be nonciliated respiratory bronchiolar cell adenoma (Clara cell adenoma) and another an adenoacanthoma.

A. Introduction

Little is known about the influence of carcinogens ingested with foods and drinks on the development of human respiratory carcinoma, although frequent exposure to such environmental conditions in modern human life is inevitable.

From experimental studies, however, such cause-effect relationship is well documented in mice, rats, hamsters, and rabbits for urethan (MOSTOFI and LARSEN, 1951), dimethyl- and diethyl-nitrosamine (DONTEN-WILL and MOHR, 1962; ZAK et al., 1960), isonicotinic acid hydrazid (MORI and YASUNO, 1959; MORI et al., 1960) and some hydrocarbons (LORENZE and STEWART, 1940, 1947; MCDONALD and WOODHOUSE, 1942).

Mice have been investigated most profoundly, though there is some question as to whether mice are suitable for an experimental model of human lung cancer, since participation of genetic factors has been established. This would be a field to be investigated, as respiratory carcinoma in man is increasing most rapidly in most countries.

This paper deals chiefly with the development of pulmonary tumors by feeding a naphthyridine derivative of 5-nitrofuran and with the histogenesis of these tumors.

B. 5-Nitrofuran Derivatives

At present 5-nitrofuran derivatives are in wide use in many countries as chemotherapeutics, as food and feed additives. Thousands of the derivatives have been synthesized by many researchers because of their potent bactericidal activity. Pronounced toxicity, however, often hinders human or domestic animal use. Recent discovery of carcinogenic 5-nitrofuran derivatives by PRICE et al. (1966) and STEIN et al. (1966) was an important finding.

Potassium 1-methyl-7-[2-(5-nitro-2-furyl)vinyl]-4-oxo-1,4-dihydro-1,8-naphthyridine-3-carboxylate (NFN), used in this study, was synthesized by NISHIGAKI et al. (1969) and its specific activity against pseudomonas confirmed by SAKATA (1970). A potent carcinogenic activity of the drug, however, was revealed by KANISAWA et al. (1974) in mice with feeding: after 38 weeks, 70% to 90% of treated animals produced squamous cell carcinoma in the forestomach epithelium, of which 50% to 70% showed extensive metastases to the regional lymph nodes, peritoneal cavity, liver, and lung. In the lung, multiple adenomas and carcinomas were induced in about 90% of the animals examined after 17 weeks.

C. Materials and Methods

A total of 107 dd/y inbred mice (Shizuoka Laboratory Animal Center), weighing about 17 g, were used, 60 animals for experimental feeding and 47 animals as controls. Commercial diet (CE-2, CLEA Japan, Inc., Tokyo) was given as a basal diet, and an experimental diet containing a certain level of NFN was also prepared by the same manufacturer according to our prescription.

Chemical structure of NFN is shown in Fig. 1 and the mode of administration with cumulative doses of the drug is indicated in Fig. 2. Intermittent feeding and reduction of the drug concentration in the course of the experiment were carried out to lessen the toxic effect.

For light microscopic observation, lung tissues were fixed in 10% formalin or Bouin's solution, embedded in paraffin, sectioned, and stained with hematoxylin and eosin. Selected blocks from several lungs were made into serial sections to examine the histogenesis of the induced tumors. Blocks of lung tissue for electron microscope were fixed in 2.0% glutaraldehyde for 2 hours and postfixed in 1.0% osmium tetroxide for 1 hour, embedded in Epon 812, and cut with an LKB Ultrotom. The sections were stained with uranyl acetate and lead citrate and examined with a Hitachi HS-9 electron microscope.

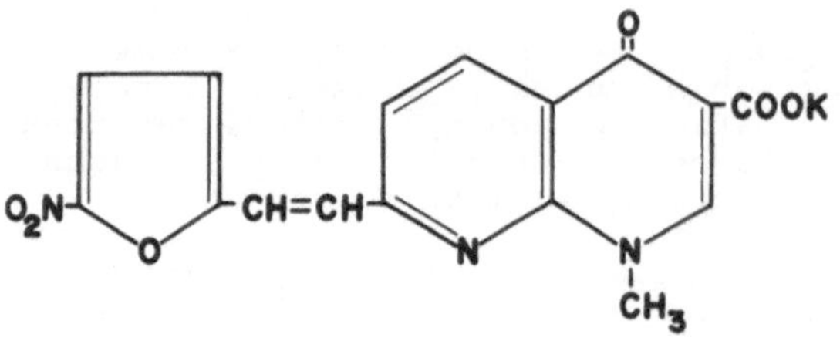

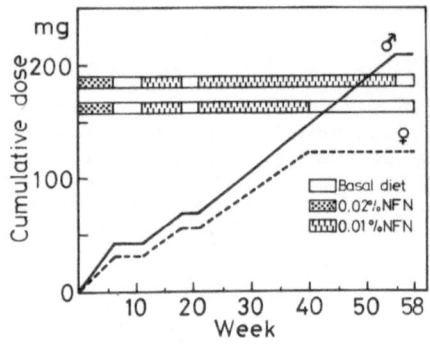

Fig. 1. Potassium-1-methyl-
7-[2-(5-nitro-2-furyl)
vinyl]-4-oxo-1,4-dihydro-
1,8-naphthyridine-3-carb-
oxylate (NFN)

Fig. 2. Mode of NFN feeding with
mean cumulative doses

D. Results

I. Incidence and Induction Time of Lung Tumors

Incidence of pulmonary adenomas and carcinomas are shown in Table 1.
Tumor induction rate in treated mice exceeded 90%. A striking difference between control and treated mice was observed in the number of
tumor nodules induced, as shown in Table 2. Female mice were much more
susceptible to NFN carcinogenicity. Induction time of tumors is shown
in Table 3. All tumors found in control mice were scored at 58 weeks,
the end of experiment.

II. Microscopic Observation

It is the purpose of this short paper to present a brief discussion
rather than a detailed description of the histological findings of
induced tumors.

NFN-induced and spontaneous tumors in control mice mostly were located
very close to the pleura and were usually smaller than a rice grain
in size, but a few nodules in the experimental group and 1 nodule in
a control mouse occupied most of a lobe of the lung (Fig. 3). Histologically, most of the tumors in control mice showed a fairly uniform
picture of loose papillary growth of small cuboidal cells, often remaining in an alveolar pattern. No cellular atypism was observed. In
the NFN-induced tumors, some nodules were not different microscopically
from those of control, but most of them consisted of closely packed
columns of cuboidal, columnar, or polygonal cells, showing moderate
atypism. In carcinoma nodules, tumor cells exhibited much packed and
solid growth with highly atypical pictures (Fig. 4), such as nuclear
hyperchromasia, increased nucleocytoplasmic ratio, anisocytosis, fre-

Table 1. Incidence of pulmonary tumors in mice fed NFN

		No. animals	Induced adenoma (No. animals)	Induced carcinoma (No. animals)
Control	Male	24	10 (41.7)%	1 (4.2)%
	Female	21	4 (19.0)	0
	Total	45	14 (31.3)	1 (2.0)
Experimental	Male	15	14 (93.3)%	2 (12.5)%
	Female	20	19 (95.0)	3 (15.0)
	Total	35	33 (94.3)	5 (14.3)

Table 2. Distribution of nodule number induced in the lungs of mice fed NFN

		Nodule number				
		1	2-5	6-10	11-	Mean no.
Control	Male	10	0	0	1	2.3
	Female	4	0	0	0	1.0
Experimental	Male	1	4	4	5	9.8
	Female	2	6	5	5	7.9

Table 3. Time-tumor incidence relationship in mice fed NFN

	Week examined							
	17-25		26-35		36-45		46-	
	Male	Fem.	Male	Fem.	Male	Fem.	Male	Fem.
No. animals	3	0	2	3	1	8	9	9
Pulmonary adenoma	3	0	2	3	1	7	8	9
Carcinoma	0	0	0	0	0	1	2	2

quent mitotic figures, invasive growth into the bronchial lumen and wall, and infiltrative growth at the periphery of the tumor. 5 induced carcinomas were classified (3 papillary adenocarcinoma, 1 adenocarcinoma, and 1 adenoacanthoma), but no metastasis was detected in any tumor.

III. Histogenesis of NFN-Induced Tumors

In most of the tumors observed in control and experimental mice, cellular origin was histologically and electron microscopically proved to be derived from the large alveolar cell, as demonstrated in Figs 5 and 6. These findings have been described repeatedly by many researchers, so I will not refer to the details here.

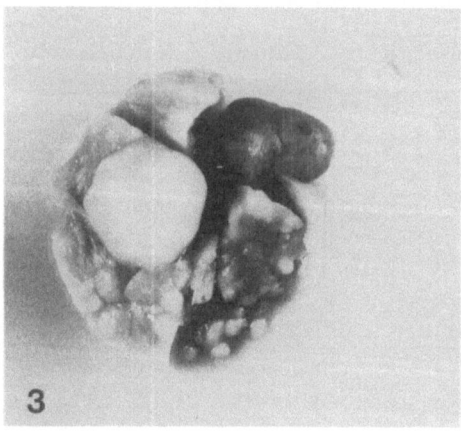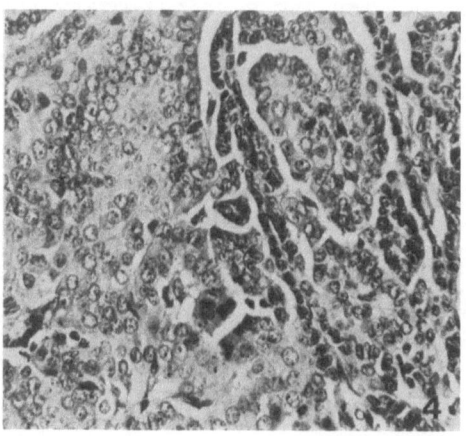

Fig. 3. Gross picture of the lung of a female mouse sacrificed at 51 weeks. A large nodule of pulmonary carcinoma and multiple small nodules are observed

Fig. 4. Photomicrograph of the large nodule shown in Fig. 3. A section of papillary growth and more packed growth of tumor cells are seen

In the present study, however, observations indicated that some tumors induced by NFN may be derived from bronchiolar epithelium. Fig. 7 shows pretumorous growth of atypical, cuboidal cells that proliferate onto the alveolar surface continuously from the epithelium of the respiratory bronchiole, where atypical cell growth is also recognizable. Since electron microscope examination was not carried out in this portion, naturally there is some difficulty in determining its precise cellular origin. However, the focus obviously located apart from the pleura. Another picture indicating possible relationship between a small adenoma nodule and bronchiolar epithelium is shown in Fig. 8. Atypical cell growth is also seen in the adjacent, bronchiolar epithelium; in addition, the characteristic vesicular feature of the cytoplasm, as shown in Fig. 5, is not recognizable in the tumor cells. Fig. 9 shows light microscopic picture of a 1 µm-thick Epon section stained with toluidine blue, a cross section of the bronchiole and its lumen filled with proliferating tumor cells. A highly magnified photograph (Fig. 10) indicates that these cells chiefly consist of multivesicular, nonciliated cells, intermingled with a few ciliated cells; 1 of them shows vacuolar degeneration. Electron microscopically, these major cells exhibited the characteristics of nonciliated bronchiolar cells (Clara cell)(Fig. 11) which contains abundant, smooth endoplasmic reticulum and specific mitochondria rich in matrix. These findings indicate that this tumor is derived from nonciliated bronchiolar epithelium.

Another evidence of bronchiolar origin is the presence of the adeno-acanthoma found in a female mouse sacrificed at 47 weeks. The greater part of the tumor shows papillary or glandular structure, lined with cylindrical or polygonal cells with acidic and slightly opaque cytoplasm; in the lumina of the glandular structure, some debris and keratin-like material are seen. Using DANE's method (1963), for pre-keratin and keratin stain, only a small portion of the material showed positive reaction. Mitotic figures were frequently observed (Fig. 12). On the other hand, some parts in the tumor showed more solid growth

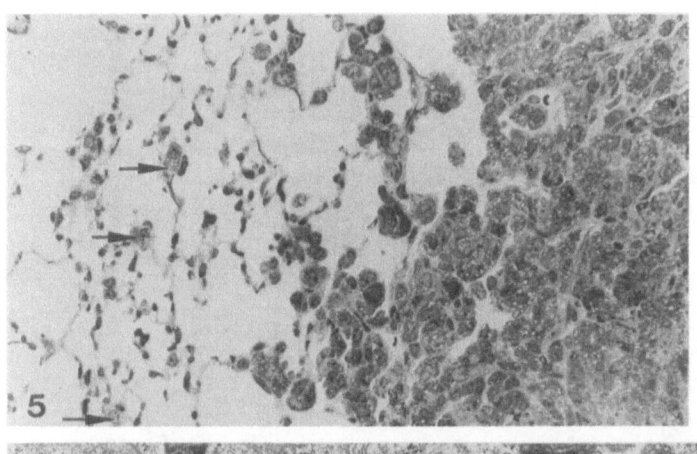

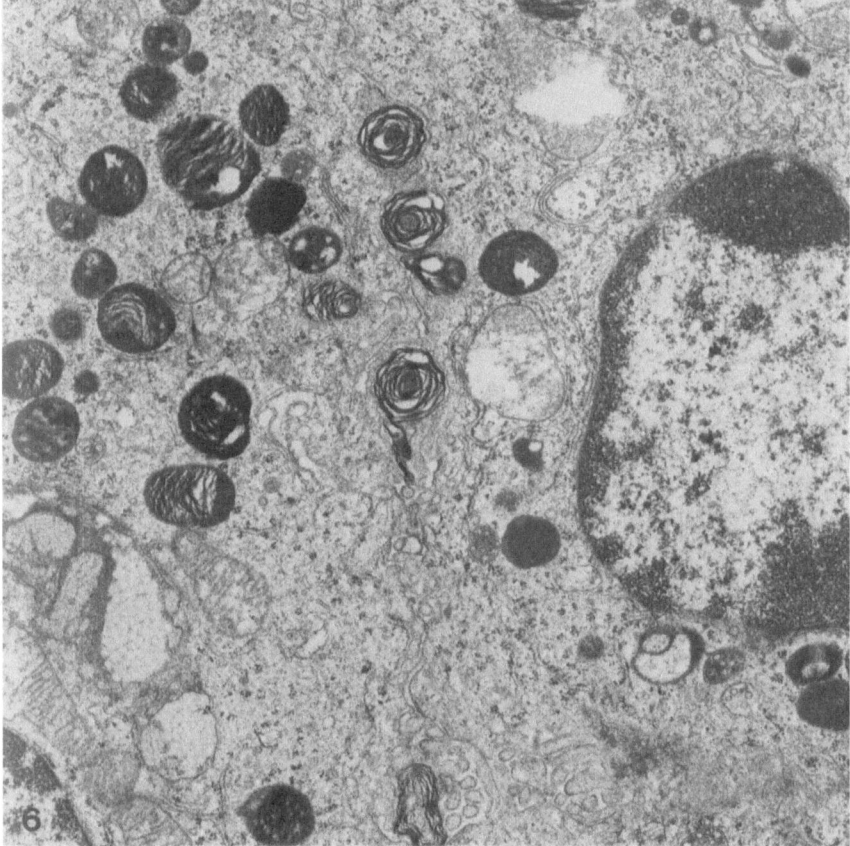

Fig. 5. Photomicrograph of the typical adenoma induced in NFN-fed mice. A close resemblance between normal large alveolar cells (arrow) and induced adenoma cells is observed. Vesiculated cytoplasm is characteristic

Fig. 6. Electron micrograph of atypical NFN-induced adenoma. Numerous cytosomes in the cytoplasm suggest this adenoma is derived from large alveolar cells

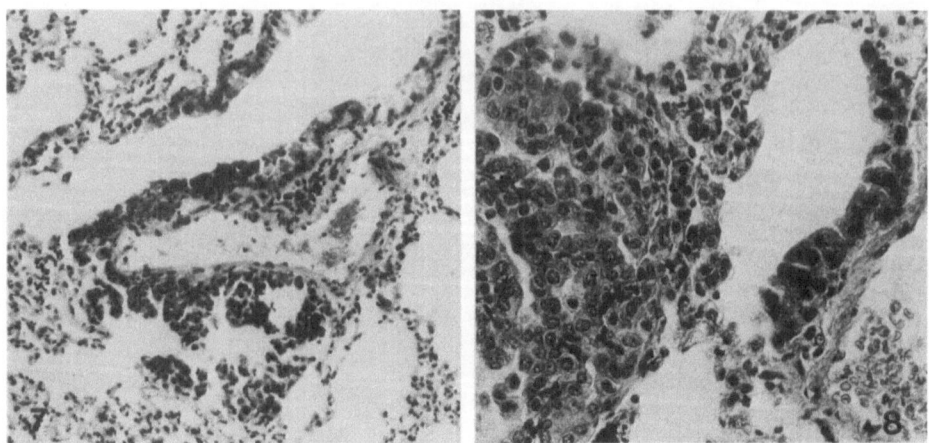

Fig. 7. Photomicrograph of a very early stage of atypical cell growth. Atypical cells proliferate onto bronchiolar epithelium and alveolar surface continuously

Fig. 8. Photomicrograph of a small adenoma nodule and respiratory bronchiole. Cellular origin of this adenoma is suspicious of bronchiolar epithelium

of spindle-shaped, basophilic cells, and in 1 area of the foci, formation of cytoplasmic bridges were observed in the intercellular spaces between the adjacent cells, as shown in Fig. 13.

Fig. 9. Light microscopic picture of 1 μm-thick section of Epon embedded material. The lumen of the respiratory bronchiole is completely occluded by atypical cells

Fig. 10. Magnified photomicrograph of Fig. 9. Most of the proliferated cells exhibit multiple vesicles in their cytoplasm, and some ciliated bronchiolar cells are degenerated

Fig. 11. Electron micrograph of Fig. 10. Nonciliated, vesiculated cells contain abundant smooth endoplasmic reticulum and specific mitochondrion with rich matrix and less cristae

253

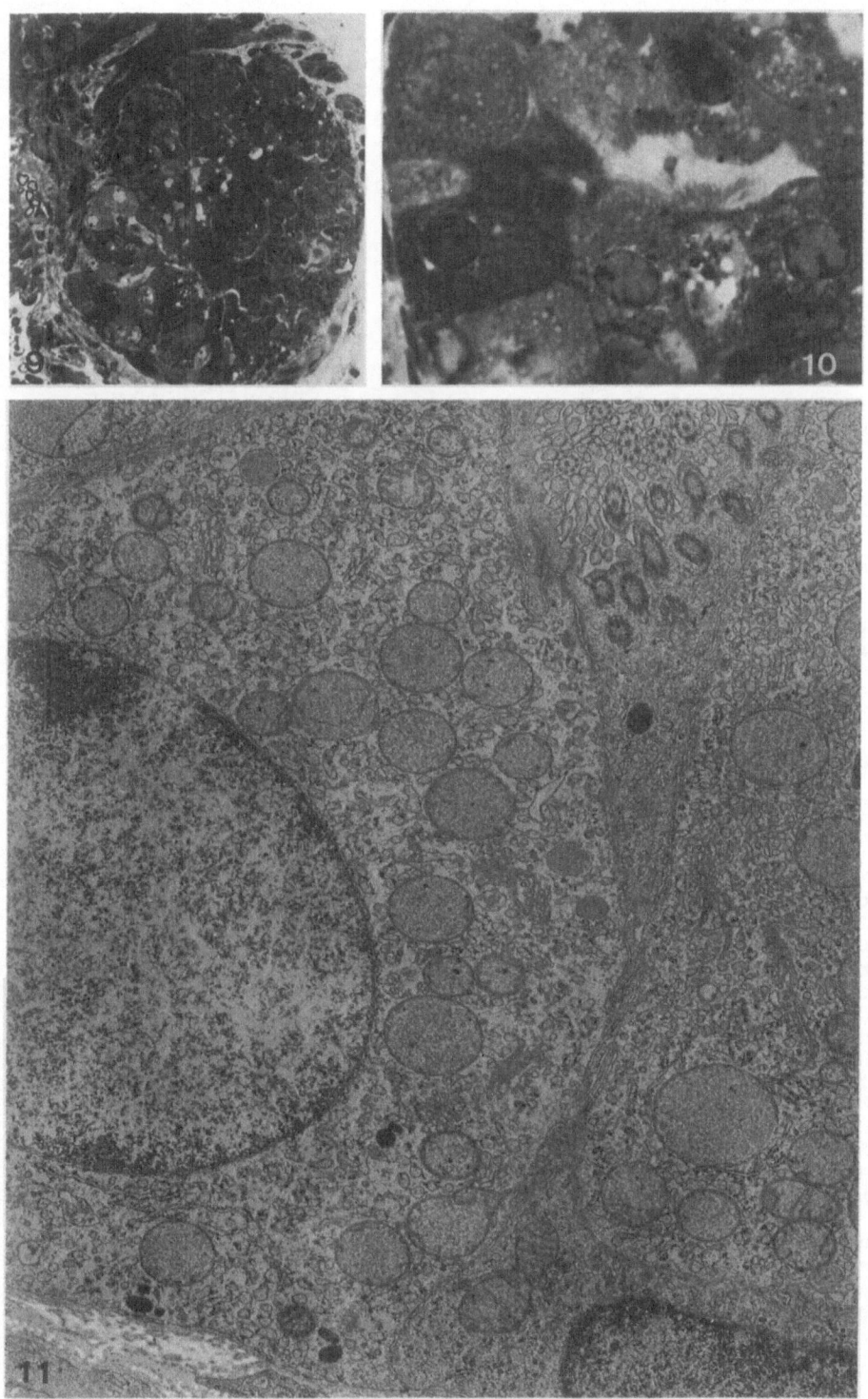

Legends see opposite page

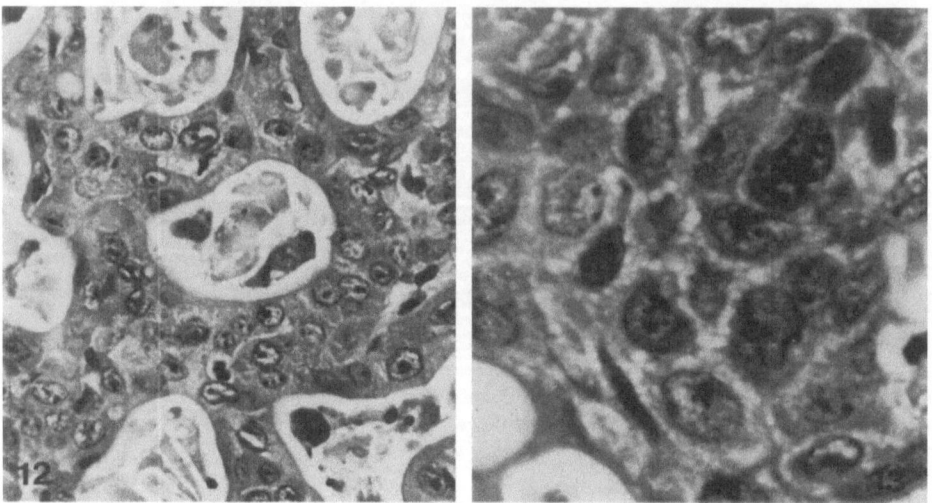

Fig. 12. Photomicrograph of adenoacanthoma induced in a male mouse (47 weeks). Lining of polygonal cells shows glandular pattern

Fig. 13. Highly magnified photomicrograph of a section of adeno-acanthoma. Basophilic, spindle-shaped or polygonal cells indicate intercellular bridge formation, but this was limited to a very narrow area

E. Discussion and Summary

Many authors have discussed the histopathogenesis of spontaneous and induced pulmonary tumors in mice. LIVINGOOD (1896), JOBLING (1910), and MAGNUS (1939) showed that spontaneous or 1,2,5,6-dibenzanthracene-induced pulmonary tumors arose from the bronchiolar epithelium. SLYE et al. (1914) and MCDONALD and WOODHOUSE (1942) concluded that pulmonary tumors in mice induced experimentally or occurring spontaneously arose either from alveolar or from bronchiolar epithelium. Most authors, however, such as TYZZER (1907), GRADY and STEWART (1940), MOSTOFI and LARSEN (1951), and CAMPBELL (1937) concluded that pulmonary tumors in mice arose from alveolar cells and were not related to the bronchiolar epithelium. KANISAWA (1962) indicated that inhalation of p-benzoquinone vapor would induce pulmonary tumors originating from the bronchiolar epithelium in A-strain mice. The present study revealed that most of the pulmonary tumors produced by NFN in dd/Y mice were derived from the large alveolar cells, although there was evidences that some tumors may be induced from the bronchiolar epithelium.

These results suggest that repeated oral ingestion of carcinogen may affect the occurrence of human lung carcinoma. Therefore, much attention should be paid to the oral route of carcinogens in research concerned with respiratory carcinogenesis.

F. Acknowledgements

The author wishes to thank Miss YORIKO SAITO and Mr. MASANORI UTSUYAMA for their valuable technical assistance.

References

CAMPBELL, J.A.: Effect of road dust "freed" from tar products upon incidence of primary lung-tumors of mice. Brit. J. exp. Path. 18, 215-223 (1937).

DANE, E.T., HERMAN, D.L.: Stain Techn. 38, 97-101, 1963. Cited in: Manual of Histologic Staining Methods of the Armed Forces Institute of Pathology (L.G. Luna, ed.), pp. 83-84. New York: McGraw-Hill 1968.

DONTENWILL, W., MOHR, U.: Carzinome des Respirationstractus nach Behandlung von Goldhamstern mit Diäthylnitrosamin. Z. Krebsforsch. 64, 305-312 (1961).

GRADY, H.G., STEWART, H.L.: Histogenesis of induced pulmonary tumors in strain A mice. Amer. J. Path. 16, 417-432 (1940).

JOBLING, J.W.: Spontaneous tumors of mouse. Monographs Rockefeller Inst. Med. Research 1, 81-119 (1910).

KANISAWA, M.: Pulmonary tumors in strain A mice induced with para-benzoquinone. Tr. Soc. Path. Jap. 51, 92-113 (1962).

KANISAWA, M., KATOH, H., AISO, K.: Carcinogenicity of potassium 1-methyl-7-[2-(5-nitro-2-furyl)vinyl]-4-oxo-1,4-dihydro-1,8-naphthyridine-3-carboxylate in ICR mice. GANN 65, 1-11 (1974).

LIVINGOOD, L.E.: Tumors in the mouse. Bull. Johns Hopk. Hosp. 7, 177-178 (1896).

LORENZ, E., STEWART, H.L.: Intestinal carcinoma and other lesions in mice following oral administration of 1,2,5,6-dibenzanthracene and 20-methylcholanthrene. J. nat. Cancer Inst. 1, 17-40 (1940).

LORENZ, E., STEWART, H.L.: Tumors of alimentary tract induced in mice by feeding olive-oil emulsions containing carcinogenic hydrocarbons. J. nat. Cancer Inst. 7, 227-238 (1947).

MAGNUS, H.A.: The experimental production of malignant papillomata of the lung in mice with 1,2,5,6-dibenzanthracene. J. Path. Bact. 49, 21-31 (1939).

MCDONALD, S., WOODHOUSE, D.L.: On the nature of mouse lung adenomata, with special reference to the effects of atmospheric dust on the incidence of these tumors. J. Path. Bact. 54, 1-12 (1942).

MORI, K., YASUNO, A.: Preliminary note on the induction of pulmonary tumors in mice by isonicotinic acid hydrazid feeding. GANN 50, 107-110 (1959).

MORI, K., YASUNO, A., MATSUMOTO, K.: Induction of pulmonary tumors in mice with isonicotinic acid hydrazid. GANN 51, 83-89 (1960).

MOSTOFI, F.K., LARSEN, C.D.: The histopathogenesis of pulmonary tumors induced in strain A mice by urethan. J. nat. Cancer Inst. 11, 1187-1221 (1951).

NISHIGAKI, S. et al.: Synthesis of 1-substituted 1,4-dihydro-7-[2-(5-nitro-2-furyl)vinyl]-4-oxo-1,8-naphthyridine derivatives. Chem. pharm. Bull. (Tokyo) 17, 1827-1831 (1969).

PRICE, J.M., MORRIS, J.E., LALICH, J.J.: Evaluation of the carcinogenic activity of 5-nitrofuran derivatives in the rat. Fed. Proc. 25, 419 (1966).

SAKATA, T.: Studies on a new introfuran derivative active against pseudomonas. Chiba Igakukai Zasshi 46, 181-187 (1970).

SLYE, M., HOLMES, H.F., WELIS, H.G.: The primary spontaneous tumors of lungs in mice. J. med. Res. 30, 417-442 (1914).

STEIN, R.J. et al.: Carcinogenic activity of nitrofurans. A histologic evaluation. Fed. Proc. 25, 291 (1966).
TYZZER, E.E.: A series of 20 spontaneous tumors in mice with accompanying pathological changes and results of inoculation of certain of
these tumors into normal mice. J. med. Res. 17, 155-197 (1907-1908).
ZAK, F.G. et al.: Renal and pulmonary tumors in rats fed dimethylnitrosamine. Cancer Res. 20, 96-99 (1960).

Surface Morphology of Tracheal Epithelium in Vitamin A Deficiency and Reversal*

Curtis D. Port[1], David W. Baxter[1], and Curtis C. Harris[2]

[1]IIT Research Institute, Chicago, IL 60616, USA
[2]Lung Cancer Branch, National Cancer Institute, Bethesda, MD 20014, USA

ABSTRACT

Vitamin A, which maintains cellular differentiation of epithelial tissues, also has an effect on metaplastic and neoplastic lesions in the respiratory tract. The surface morphology of hamster tracheal epithelium during vitamin A deficiency and during reversal upon the administration of vitamin A was studied by scanning electron microscopy. Focal squamous metaplasia of the tracheal epithelium, confined upon the upper two thirds of the ventral surface of the trachea, occurs in vitamin A deficiency. Synchronous differentiation of the epithelium with sloughing of the existing surface occurs after reversal of the deficient state. This change is rapid, occurring within 4 days of the administration of vitamin A. The SEM enabled documentation of extent distribution and surface changes in vitamin A deficiency and reversal.

A.   Introduction

The scanning electron microscope (SEM) has been widely used for morphologic studies of normal and diseased lungs (GREENWOOD and HOLLAND, 1972; GRONIOWSKI et al., 1972; HOLMA, 1969; KUHN and FINKE, 1972; NOWELL et al., 1971; WANG and THURLBECK, 1970); however, only rarely has the SEM been used specifically to study cancer of the lung (LUPULESCU and BOYD, 1972). Since morphological changes are an integral part of the neoplastic process, the SEM is a beneficial instrument for defining the process of squamous differentiation and its relationship to metaplasia and squamous carcinoma.

Adequate levels of vitamin A control the differentiation of tracheobronchial cells into mucus and ciliated cells. Deficiency of this vitamin results in the development of squamous metaplasia in tracheobronchial epithelium. Since squamous metaplasia is common to both cancer and vitamin A deficiency, it is important to ascertain any distinguishing morphological characteristics to better define the process of squamous differentiation and its relationship to carcinoma. The acute ultrastructural lesions in vitamin A deficiency (HARRIS et al., 1972) have been studied by the transmission electron microscope

---

*This work was performed in part under Contract No. NIH-NCI-72-3292, Division of Cancer Cause and Prevention, National Cancer Institute, National Institutes of Health.

258

(TEM). These studies were repeated utilizing the SEM to corroborate
and amplify the TEM results and to seek additional information.

B. Materials and Methods

Young adult Syrian golden hamsters were housed in polycarbonate cages
with filter bonnets and given a pelleted vitamin A deficient diet
(General Biochemicals, Chagrin Falls, Ohio) and sterile tap water
ad libitum. The hamsters were made deficient according to the protocol
described by HARRIS et al. (1972). Pair-fed controls were given 0.2 ml
cottonseed oil containing 200 μm of all transretinyl acetate twice
weekly. To prepare the respiratory tract for SEM examination, the
hamsters were anesthetized, the chest opened, and the lungs and trachea
removed. The trachea was cannulated to the level of the first cartilaginous ring and the lungs expanded at a pressure of 30 cm of water with
KARNOVSKY's paraformaldehyde-glutaraldehyde phosphate buffered fixative
(KARNOVSKY, 1965). Perfusion continued for at least 2 hours with the
lungs completely immersed in fixative. Upon completion of airway perfusion, the trachea was ligated and the lungs floated in fixative overnight.

The trachea and main stem bronchi were removed from the lungs, washed
in distilled water, and dehydrated with increasing concentrations of
alcohol. Amyl acetate was substituted for the alcohol and the tissue
dried by the critical point method in carbon dioxide (ANDERSON, 1951).
The dried trachea was sectioned longitudinally, cemented to a copper
or aluminum stub, coated with gold in a vacuum evaporator equipped
with a rotating turntable, and examined in a Cambridge Mark II scanning
electron microscope.

Two separate experiments were conducted. The first experiment was designed to demonstrate the surface changes resulting from vitamin A
deficiency. Deficient animals were killed at the following points:
weight plateau (90 g to 100 g at 8 weeks of age); following a 4 g to
8 g loss of body weight from peak weight; following a 10 g to 15 g
loss of body weight from peak weight; and following a 20 g to 30 g
loss of body weight from peak weight. The second experiment was designed to demonstrate the surface changes resulting from reversal of
vitamin A deficiency. Vitamin A deificient hamsters were treated with
200 μg all transretinyl acetate in cottonseen oil twice weekly starting at a loss from weight plateau of 4 g to 8 g body weight, and killed
at 1, 2, 4, 7, 14, and 21 days.

C. Results

I. Vitamin A Deficiency Study

The tracheal epithelium of deficient animals, examined at weight
plateau, showed little change upon low power examination. At higher
power, however, small focal areas of squamous metaplasia and nonciliated cell hyperplasia were present over cartilage rings in the
upper one-half to two-thirds of the ventral trachea. Few lesions, if
any, were found on the dorsal or membranous half of the trachea. In
adjacent epithelium, where the epithelium appeared normal, many
ciliated cells had shortened cilia.

The squamous metaplastic lesions began either as small circular foci
with surface cells cornifying and sloughing off (Fig. 1) or as circular to oval islands of normal appearing epithelium surrounded by
ribbons of squamous metaplastic epithelium (Fig. 2). These small
lesions progressed to larger, irregularly shaped lesions with rounded
edges and desquamating centers. Intracellular spaces between the sloughing cells were present and small fibers connecting sloughing cells to
adjacent or underlying cells were visible. These fibers were especially
prominent on the surfaces of cells from which overlying cells had recently been removed (Fig. 3). Islands of normal appearing epithelium
remained in some of these larger lesions (Fig. 4), or were separated
from underlying squamous epithelium to protrude into the tracheal
lumen attached by 1 side (Fig. 4). The epithelium adjacent to the
squamous metaplastic lesions appeared relatively normal.

Severe lesions were present in those hamsters suffering the greatest
weight loss (10 g to 20 g from peak weight). These lesions were large,
covering most of the surface of the tracheal rings (Fig. 5). Numerous
sloughing cells with wrinkled and roughened surfaces were present in
these lesions (Fig. 6).

II. Vitamin A Reversal Study

SEM examination indicated a rapid reversal of the vitamin A deficiency
with a normal epithelial surface present within 1 week from the start
of vitamin A administration. Low power examination 1 day after administration of vitamin A indicated a marked change in the epithelium.
The focal lesions visible in the deficiency study were not present
although the outline of cartilage rings was clearly visible. This
change in epithelial character was present only in the upper one-half
to two-thirds of the ventral trachea.

At higher power, the epithelium over the cartilage rings was very rough;
more normal epithelium between the rings (Fig. 7) appeared to be sloughing. Some of the epithelial cells over the cartilage rings possessed
short cilia and a lattice network on their surfaces (Figs 8 and 9) and
were interpreted as differentiating ciliated epithelial cells. In the
normal appearing epithelium between rings, the ciliated epithelial cells
possessed shortened cilia and small holes in their surfaces and were
interpreted as degenerating cells. The nonciliated epithelial cells
appeared normal (Fig. 10).

A low power view of the epithelium 2 days after the administration of
vitamin A presented findings equivalent to those seen at 1 day. However, at higher power, many of the epithelial cells on the cartilage
rings presented surfaces covered with small fibers. These structures
were interpreted, as in the vitamin A deficiency study, as connecting
fibers left when the overlying cell sloughed away. Numerous other cells
presented surfaces covered with a lattice network.

The process of cell differentiation continued until, at 4 days after
the start of vitamin A administration, a surface consisting of mainly
nonciliated cells was present (Fig. 11). The nonciliated cells possessed normal surface structure but the few ciliated cells had short cilia,
and appeared immature (Fig. 12). At 1 week after the start of vitamin
A administration, an essentially normal epithelium was present. A few
scattered focal areas of differentiating nonciliated cells were present.
The epithelia of tracheas examined at 2 and 3 weeks after the start
of vitamin A administration were normal.

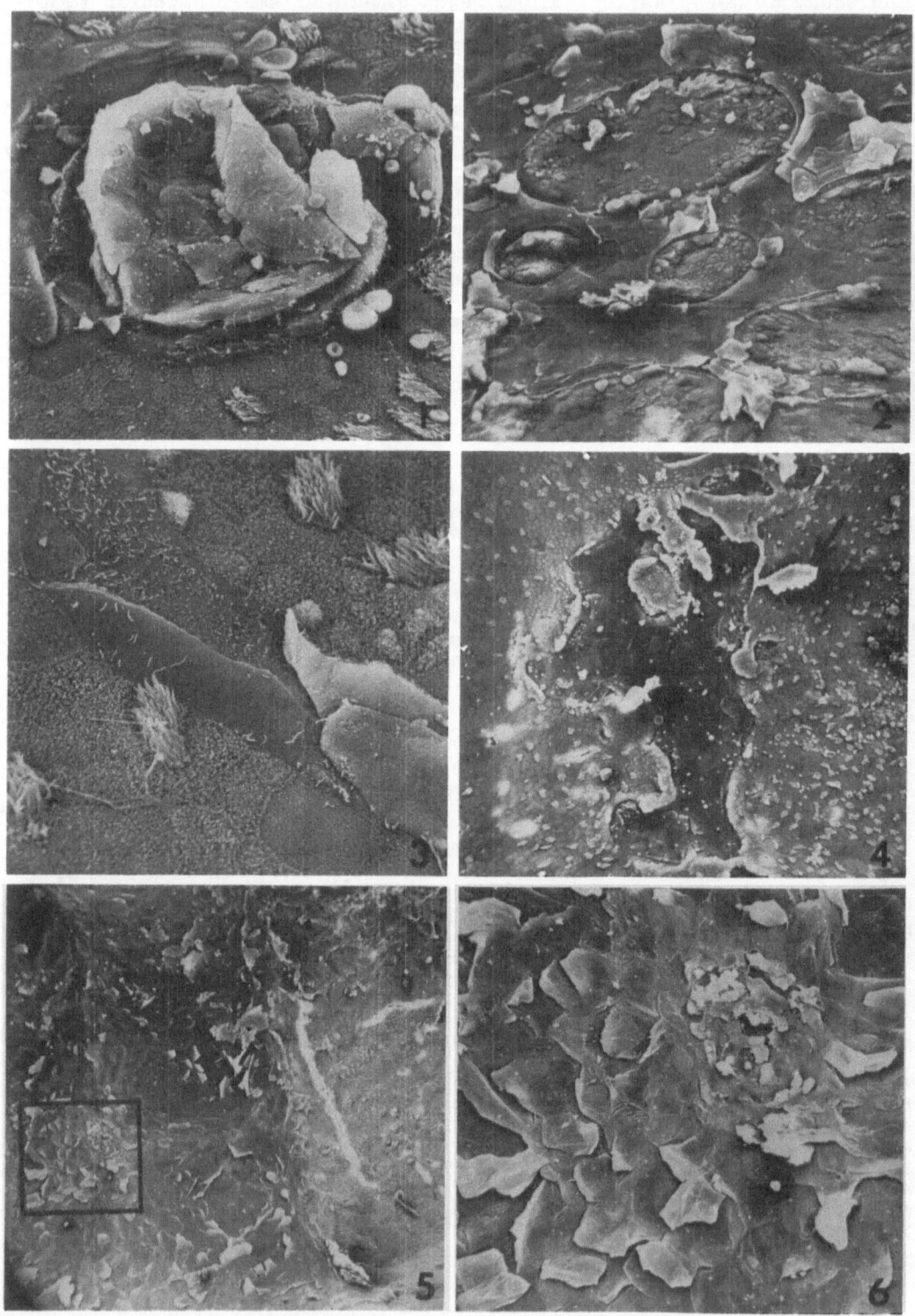

Legends see opposite page

D. Discussion

The presence of focal areas of squamous metaplasia in vitamin A deficiency and the sequential changes in their development have been documented by transmission electron microscopy (HARRIS et al., 1972). The SEM results indicate that these focal areas are located on cartilage rings in the upper one-half to two-thirds of the ventral portion of the trachea, with the dorsal or membranous half essentially unaffected. The reason for this distribution is unknown. The morphologic sequence in the formation of these focal squamous areas appears to be basal cell hyperplasia followed by squamous differentiation and sloughing of luminal cells. A similar morphologic sequence was documented by HARRIS et al. (1972). Epithelium outside of the squamous metaplastic areas appears unaffected, though slight loss of ciliated epithelial cells suggests some change.

The rapid reversal of vitamin A deficiency with corresponding change in epithelial surface, was expected upon the start of vitamin A therapy. However, the character of the epithelial change was not expected. It would be reasonable to assume that only the focal areas of squamous metaplasia would repair upon administration of vitamin A. Instead, the entire epithelial surface appears to slough and underlying basal cells start to differentiate into ciliated and nonciliated epithelial cells. In vitamin A deficiency, basal cells divide and proliferate. Differentiation does not occur and surface epithelial cells persist for a longer period of time in these areas. The exception to this occurs over the cartilage rings, where basal cells differentiate into squamous cells which subsequently slough from the luminal surface. Upon administration of vitamin A to deficient animals, a synchronous basal cell differentiation to ciliated and nonciliated cells begins, with sloughing of luminal epithelium, that is complete within 1 week.

Some differences were observed between the lesions present in this study and those observed in tracheobronchial epithelium examined by the SEM following intratracheal administration of benzo(a)pyrene (BaP) absorbed to ferric oxide (PORT, 1973). Multiple administrations of BaP and ferric oxide caused a loss of ciliated cells, epithelial hyperplasia, squamous metaplasia, and markedly abnormal protuberant cells

---

Fig. 1. Early circular to oval focus of squamous metaplasia from a vitamin A deficient hamster. Surface cells have become cornified and are sloughing. (x 495)

Fig. 2. Early focal squamous metaplasia. In contrast to that illustrated in Fig. 1, this type of focus appears as islands of normal epithelium surrounded by ribbons of cornifying squamous metaplastic epithelium. (x 190)

Fig. 3. Small fibers on the surface of a squamous cell from which an overlying cell may recently have been sloughed. (x 1260)

Fig. 4. Focal area of squamous metaplasia with remaining small island of normal appearing epithelium. To the right of the lesion, a section of epithelium has separated and is protruding into the tracheal lumen (arrow). (x 98)

Fig. 5. Severe squamous metaplasia occurring in a hamster suffering the greatest weight loss during vitamin A deficiency (10 g to 20 g from peak weight). The inset has been enlarged in Fig. 6. (x 49)

Fig. 6. Large focal area of squamous metaplasia with numerous sloughing surface cells. (x 195)

262

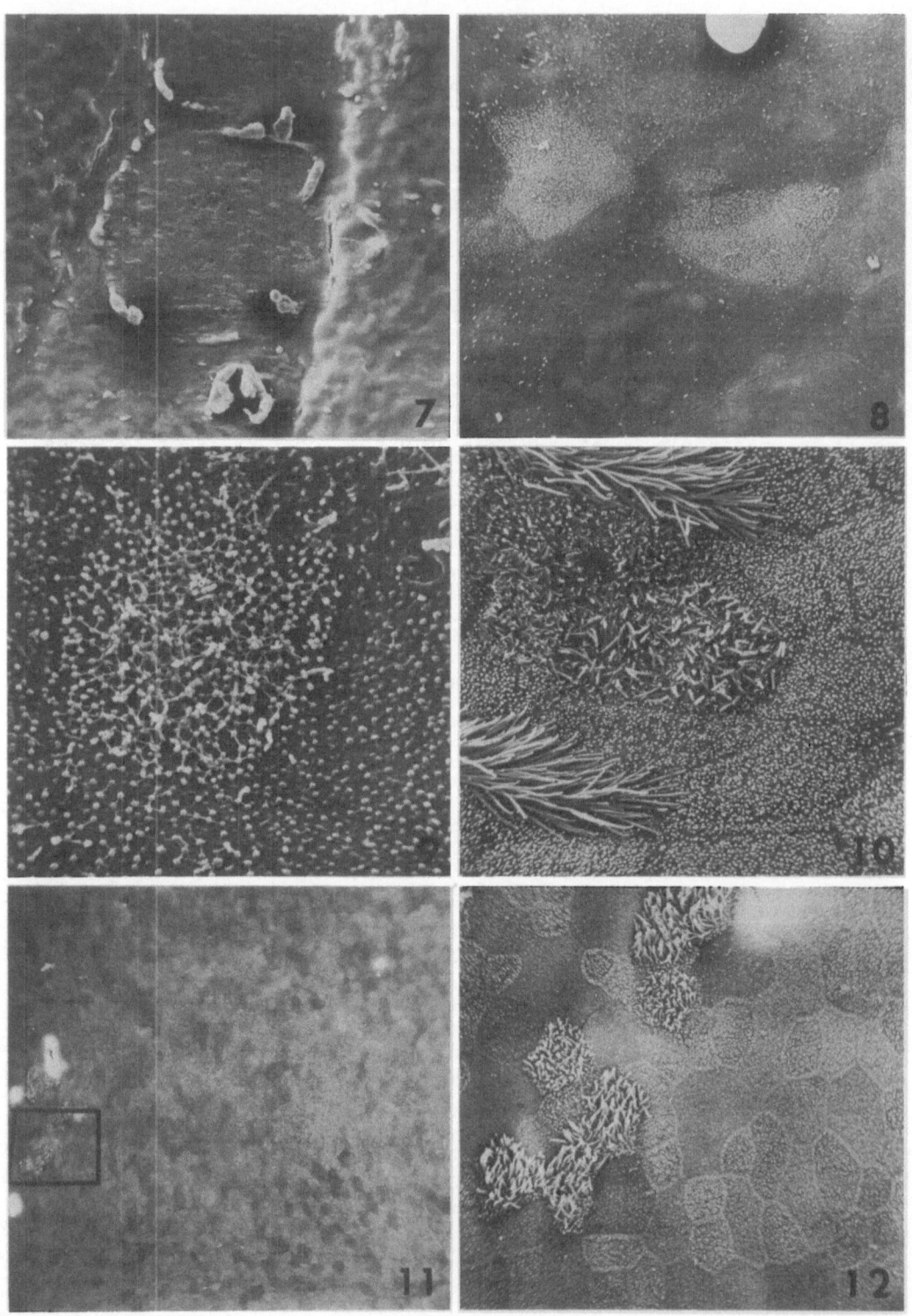

Legends see opposite page

with altered surface structure. We did not find holes representing the location of degenerated ciliated epithelial cells in the vitamin A deficiency portion of this study. The surface area which showed epithelial hyperplasia and squamous metaplasia was more extensive in the vitamin A deficiency animals, although the sloughing surface cells in regions of squamous metaplasia with extensive desquamation were indistinguishable in both studies. The large protruding abnormal cells with a variegated surface structure much like tumor cells, present in the BaP ferric oxide study, were not seen in any of the cases in the vitamin A deficiency study.

To locate and interpret the tracheal lesions seen in this study, utilizing the TEM, would be tedious and laborious. The SEM was of obvious benefit, permitting examination of all lesions without the sampling errors inherent to TEM examination. The use of the SEM to locate and identify accurately and easily tumors and preneoplastic lesions is practical and feasible.

References

ANDERSON, T.F.: Techniques for the preservation of three-dimensional structure in preparing specimens for the electron microscope. Trans. N.Y. Acad. Sci. Ser. II. 13, 130-134 (1951).
GREENWOOD, M.F., HOLLAND, P.: The mammalian respiratory tract surface. A scanning electron microscopic study. Lab. Invest. 27, 296-304 (1972).
GRONIOWSKI, J., WALSKI, M., BICZYSKO, W.: Application of scanning electron microscopy for studies of the lung parenchyma. J. Ultrastruct. Res. 38, 473-481 (1972).
HARRIS, C.C., SPORN, M.B., KAUFMAN, D.G., SMITH, J.M., JACKSON, F.E., SAFFIOTTI, U.: Histogenesis of squamous metaplasia in the hamster tracheal epithelium caused by vitamin A deficiency or benzo(a)pyrene ferric oxide. J. nat. Cancer Inst. 48, 743-761 (1972).
HOLMA, B.: Scanning electron microscopic observation of particles deposited in the lung. Arch. Environ. Hlth 18, 330-339 (1969).
KARNOVSKY, J.: A formaldehyde-gluteraldehyde fixative of high osmololity for use in electron microscopy. J. Cell Biol. 27, 137A (1965).

Fig. 7. Epithelial surface from an initially vitamin A deficient hamster 1 day after the start of vitamin A therapy. The epithelium over the rings appears rough with normal epithelium in the middle of the figure between rings. (x 94)

Fig. 8. Surface of epithelium on cartilage rings in a vitamin A treated hamster (1 day). Numerous differentiating cells are present with some presenting a lattice network on their surfaces. (x 940)

Fig. 9. Cell with short cilia and microvilli connected by a lattice network. This cell was interpreted as a differentiating ciliated epithelial cell. (x 4650)

Fig. 10. Degenerating ciliated epithelial cell in the epithelium between tracheal rings of a vitamin A treated hamster (1 day). The cell surface is visible. (x 1900)

Fig. 11. Differentiating epithelium in the trachea of an initially vitamin A dificient hamster 4 days after start of vitamin A therapy. Ciliated epithelial cells are infrequent. Inset magnified in Fig. 12. (x 180)

Fig. 12. Differentiating ciliated epithelial cells in vitamin A treated hamster. Note variation in height of cilia. (x 900)

KUHN, C., FINKE, E.H.: The topography of the pulmonary alveolus:
  Scanning electron microscopy using different fixations. J. Ultrastruct. Res. 38, 161-173 (1972).
LUPULESCU, A., BOYD, C.B.: Lung cancer: A transmission and scanning
  electron microscope study. Cancer 29, 1530-1538 (1972).
NOWELL, J.A., GILLESPIE, J.R., TYLER, W.S.: Scanning electron microscopy of chronic pulmonary emphysema: A study of the equine model.
  Proceedings of the Fourth Annual Scanning Electron Microscope Symp.,
  pp. 297-304. Chicago, Ill. 1971.
NOWELL, J.A., TYLER, W.S.: Scanning electron microscopy of the sur-
  face morphology of mammalian lungs. Amer. Rev. Resp. Dis. 103, 313-
  328 (1971).
PORT, C.D., HENRY, M.C., KAUFMAN, D.G., HARRIS, C.C., KETELS, K.V.:
  Acute changes in the surface morphology of hamster tracheobronchial
  epithelium following benzo(a)pyrene and ferric oxide administration.
  Cancer Res. 33, 2498-2506 (1973).
ROTH, J., MEYER, H.W.: Electron microscope studies in mammalian lungs
  by freeze-etching. Exp. Path. 7, 71-83 (1972).
TYLER, W.S., DELORIMIER, A.A., MANUS, A.G., NOWELL, J.A.: Surface
  morphology of hypoplastic and normal lungs from newborn lambs.
  Proceedings of Fourth Annual Scanning Electron Microscope Symp.,
  pp. 305-312. Chicago, Ill. 1971.
WANG, N., THURLBECK, W.M.: Scanning electron microscopy of the lung.
  Human Path. 1, 227-231 (1970).

Postinfluenzal Pulmonary Lesions in Vitamin A Deficient Mice*

Clayton G. Loosli, John D. Hardy, and Sherman F. Stinson

Departments of Medicine and Pathology, University of Southern California School of Medicine, Los Angeles, CA 90033, USA

ABSTRACT

There were no significant differences in lung virus growth and antibody responses in the NA, RA, and HA diet groups of mice. Epithelialization of the alveolar ducts and alveoli due to peripheral growth of regenerating bronchial epithelial cells was present in all postinfluenzal lesions regardless of diet. However, the postinfluenzal lesions in mice on an NA diet with no liver vitamin A showed extensive epithelial nodule formation with significantly more squamous metaplasia and keratinization than was seen in the lungs of mice on RA and HA diets. The importance of the vitamin A status of the mice in determining the extent of squamous metaplasia and keratinization in postinfluenzal lesions of mice was emphasized.

A. Introduction

In vitamin A deficient animals and man, the mucous membranes of the respiratory tract and other organs undergo squamous and keratinizing metaplasia (WOLBACH, 1925, 1954; WONG and BUCK, 1971). Hyperplasia and squamous metaplasia of the epithelial lining of the trachea and bronchi and epithelialization of alveoli in man have been repeatedly observed in postinfluenzal lesions since the 1918-1919 pandemic (AS-KANAZY, 1919; WINTERNITZ et al., 1920). This is true in the lungs of individuals dying of influenza A or A-prime virus infections with or without complications. Since the influenza A virus was isolated in 1933, marked antigenic shifts have occurred in virus structure, yet the pathology provoked by the A-prime viruses in man has been the same (LOOSLI, 1973c; MULDER and HERS, 1972).

The pathogenesis and pathology of experimental influenza virus infections, particularly in mice, have been studied extensively (LOOSLI, 1968). In animals given sublethal influenzal infections, the lesions in the recovered mice also show bronchial epithelial hyperplasia and metaplasia and epithelialization of alveoli similar to findings in the lungs of fatal human cases (STRAUB, 1937; LOOSLI, 1949, 1970; LOOSLI et al., 1973a).

---

*Supported in part by the Council for Tobacco Research, USA; the Howard Hughes Employees Give Once Club and the Hastings Foundation Fund of the University of Southern California.

It has been shown recently that the extent of squamous metaplasia and keratinization of the bronchial lining membranes varies with the vitamin A nutritional status of the infected animal, being significantly greater in animals in which the vitamin A content of the liver was low or absent (LOOSLI et al., 1973b). In the present study, a more reliable method, as described by MCCARTHY et al. (1952), for producing vitamin A deficiency in mice was employed.

B. Methods

Young adult white male and female (SPF) mice (CD-1 strain) were employed (Charles River Farms, Wilmington, Massachusetts, USA).

I. Production of Vitamin A Deficiency

50 female mice served as breeders. 1 male was placed with 3 females and given regular mouse chow and water ad libitum. After 10 days, the males were removed and the pregnant mice placed in individual cages. At approximately 16 days of gestation, 25 females were placed on a vitamin A deficient diet (NA) for germfree mice and rats (prepared by the Mogul Corporation, Chagrin Falls, Ohio, USA), while the remaining 25 pregnant mice were continued on a regular diet. The 2 groups were kept on the respective diets until the offspring were 3 weeks of age. They were then separated by sex. Those on the vitamin free diet were continued on it until 2 1/2 months of age. Those on a regular diet were separated into 2 groups. 1 was given a regular vitamin A test diet (RA) with heat treated casein and corn starch with 8.016 units of vitamin A/kg added (prepared by the Mogul Corporation, Chagrin Falls, Ohio, USA). The other was placed on a hypervitamin A test diet (HA) with heat treated casein and corn starch to which was added 160,000 units of vitamin A palmitate per kg (prepared by the Mogul Corporation, Chagrin Falls, Ohio, USA). Assays for vitamin A in livers of diet groups sacrificed at 4 and 10 weeks were made, employing the Carr-Price colorimetric procedure (Associated Vitamin Chemists, 1966).

II. Airborne Virus Exposure

At the time of exposure to the airborne influenza virus, the mice were approximately 10 weeks old. 90 mice from each diet group were subjected to the virus aerosol. The exposure chamber consisted of a 16 liter sterile bell jar with a capacity for 45 mice (15 from each diet group). 6 sequential exposures were carried out employing a DeVilbis Atomizer at 1 atm, using filtered compressed air. At each exposure, the mice were subjected to a sublethal cloud of 10^{-6} dilution of mouse lung suspension (10^7 EID-50) of PR8-A mouse adapted virus for 13 minutes. The details of these procedures have been published (LOOSLI et al., 1970).

After exposure, smaller groups of mice were sacrificed at close intervals of time up to 45 days. At each time interval, 2 mice were sacrificed for lung virus growth and serum antibody determinations; 3 for light (hematoxylin-azure II stain [HEA]) and electron microscopic (E.M.) study; 2 for histochemical examination employing lactate dehydrogenase (LDH) and glucose-6-phosphate dehydrogenase (Gl-6-PDH) as cell markers; and 2 for phospholipid (lecithin) determination by thin layer chromatography. The procedures cited above have been detailed in previous reports (LOOSLI et al., 1970, 1971).

C. Results

I. Vitamin A Deficiency State

The livers of each 4 mice from the NA group examined at 4 and 10 weeks after birth showed no vitamin A. Shortly before being exposed to the airborne influenza virus, a few mice from the NA group became ill, lost weight, and failed to eat. However, no outward signs of vitamin A deficiency such as nasal crusting or discharge were present. At 10 weeks, the livers of each of 4 mice from the RA and HA diet groups showed respectively 150 µg and 1025 µg of vitamin A per gram of liver.

II. Lung Virus Growth and Antibody Response

Lung virus titers were measured by the red cell hemagglutination procedure. While not carried out in this study, influenza virus cannot usually be isolated from the lungs of mice immediately after a sublethal exposure to the aerosol. However, influenza virus was present in the lungs of the 3 test groups in high titer (10^6) when examined at 3, 5, and 7 days after onset. At 11 days, the virus titers were respectively NA (10^2), RA (10^2), and HA (10^4). At 14 days, no virus was isolated from the lungs of the NA and RA mice but was present in the HA mice in titers of 10^3.

Antibody response was measured by the red cell hemagglutination inhibition procedure (LOOSLI et al., 1970). In general, there were no significant differences in antibody responses among the NA, RA, and HA diet groups. Serum antibodies were present at 7 days in titers of 1:20 and rose to 1:80 by 11 days, persisting at this level when measured at 14, 21, and 28 days. At 45 days, titers of 1:40 were present in the serum of the 3 diet groups.

III. Lecithin Content

The phospholipid (lecithin) content of unconsolidated lobes of the NA, RA, and HA groups was essentially the same at any time period up to 45 days. On the other hand, there was significantly less phospholipid in the consolidated lobes of the 3 diet groups during the same time periods, the lowest being in lungs of animals sacrificed at 7 and 11 days after onset.

IV. Pathogenesis

The bronchial air passages are lined with 2 types of cells: ciliated and nonciliated (Clara). Along the trachea and major bronchi, occasionally goblet cells can also be seen. The alveoli are lined by flattened type I and large type II granular cells. Grossly, the lungs of NA, RA, and HA mice sacrificed before and at the zero hour after exposure to the airborne influenza virus showed no abnormalities. Microscopically, in the lungs of the HA diet group, the cytoplasmic blebs of the Clara cells appeared to be more prominent than those on RA and NA diets. In the lungs of some NA mice sacrificed at 2 1/2 months, the bronchial lining cells exhibited metachromatic staining and focal proliferation. No such abnormalities were noted in the lungs of the RA and HA groups.

Following sublethal exposure to airborne virus, pulmonary lesions first could be seen grossly at 72 hours as plum-colored pinpoint areas that progressively enlarged to involve 1 or more lobes by 9 days. The consolidated lobes showed progressive atelectasis and could not be easily inflated with fixative. In this study, no differences in the gross appearance of the lungs of the NA, RA, and HA groups sacrificed from 3 to 45 days after onset could be seen.

Up to 7 days, the microscopic appearance of the influenza lesions in the lungs of the 3 diet groups of mice was generally the same. By light and electron microscopy and by histochemical staining, it could be seen that the bronchial lining cells (ciliated and nonciliated) and the types I and II pneumocytes lining the alveoli were susceptible to invasion and destruction by the virus. At 7 days, the bronchial lining membranes were reduced to a thin, flattened layer of cells. The alveolar walls were swollen and the spaces were filled with cells (primarily mononuclear), cell debris, and serous exudate.

On or about the seventh day after onset, regeneration of the bronchial lining membranes began and progressed rapidly. The regenerating epithelial cells of the 3 diet groups showed marked metaplasia and peripheral growth into the surrounding, collapsed alveolar ducts and alveoli by 11 to 12 days to form nodules.

In the lungs of mice on the HA diet, the epithelial nodules at 28 days were characterized by cyst-like spaces lined by cuboidal epithelial cells and containing mucus. No squamous metaplasia or keratinization in the epithelial nodules was seen (Fig. 1 a-d). Those on RA diets showed fewer cyst-like spaces, some alveoli being filled with syncytial masses of squamous cells, with no keratinization.

On the other hand, in the NA group, squamous metaplasia of the bronchial lining membranes could be seen as early as 7 days, and was more pronounced by 11 and 14 days. By 28 days, extensive squamous metaplasia and keratinization were present throughout the involved lobes. The 45-day postinfluenzal lesions in the NA group were similar (Fig. 2 a-d).

D. Discussion

The daily vitamin A requirements for mice vary widely according to different investigators (HOAG and DICKIE, 1966). The difficulty in producing vitamin A deficiency in mice compared to rats has been reviewed by MCCARTHY and CERECEDO (1952). They found that the procedure for placing pregnant mice on NA diets during the latter part of gestation and during the lactation period greatly hastens the depletion of vitamin A in the offspring. The presence of residual retinal and provitamins in the basic diet, particularly in casein, is considered one of the reasons for the difficulty in producing vitamin A deficiency in mice (MOORE and HOLMES, 1971).

It is now well established that the postinfluenzal epithelial nodules in the lungs of mice are bronchial epithelial cell proliferations which invade the alveolar ducts and alveolar spaces, the original linings having been destroyed by the virus (LOOSLI, 1949; LOOSLI et al., 1971, 1973a). These epithelial tumor-like growths must be differentiated from the "spontaneous" or urethane induced tumors, the origin of which is the type II granular pneumocyte (BROOKS, 1968). As these cells are susceptible to invasion and destruction by the in-

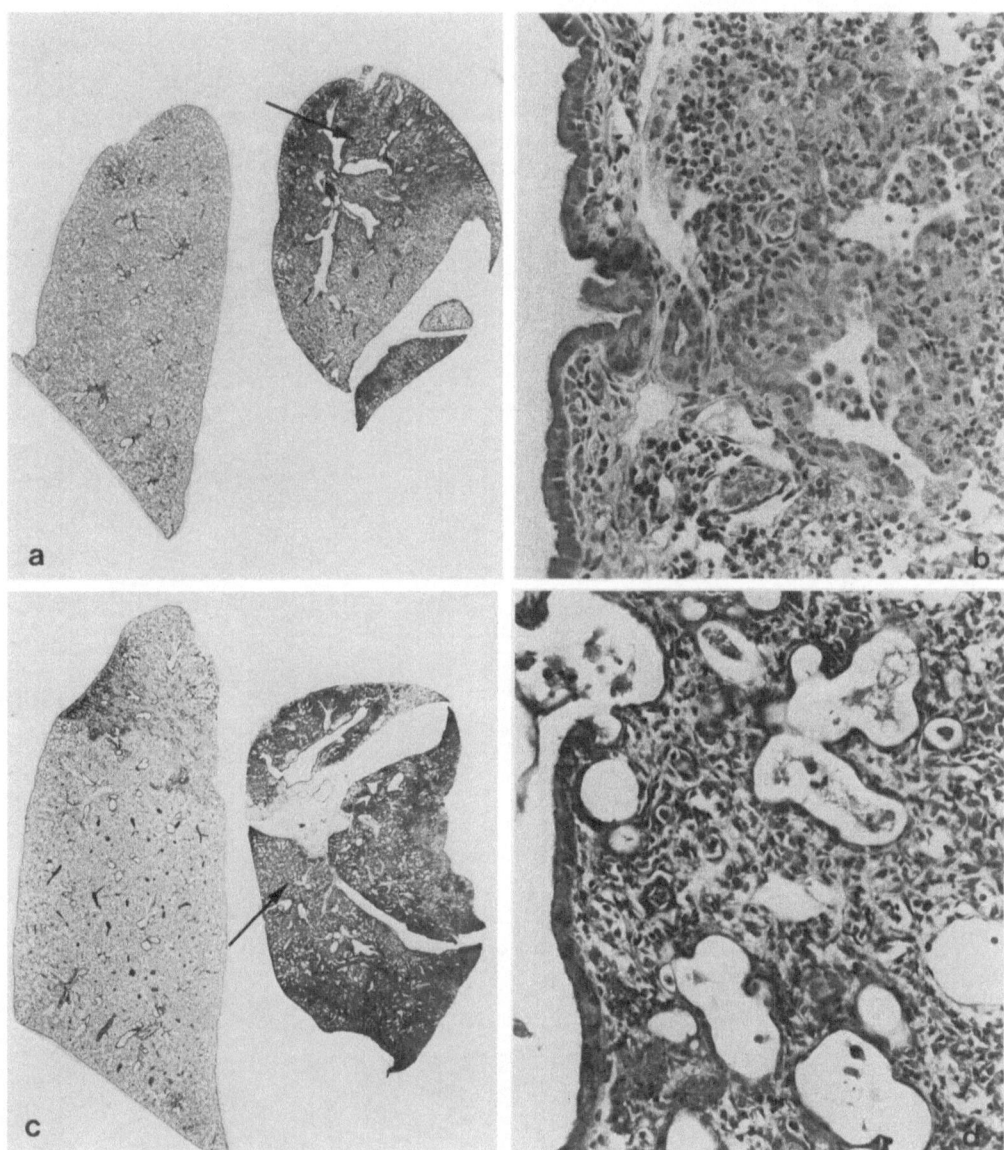

Fig. 1 a-d. Airborne influenza infections in HA mice. (a) Whole lung
section of mouse sacrificed 13 days after onset. The right upper and
lower lobes are extensively involved. HEA (x 5.3). (b) Higher power
view of area in "A" (arrow) showing regenerated bronchial epithelium
and extension of epithelium into the surrounding collapsed lungs
(x 169). (c) Whole lung of mouse sacrificed 28 days after onset. The
right upper, middle, and lower lobes, and upper part of the left lobe
are extensively involved. HEA (x 5.3). (d) Higher power view of area
in "C" (arrow) showing regenerated epithelium and cyst-like spaces
in surrounding lung tissue. (x 169)

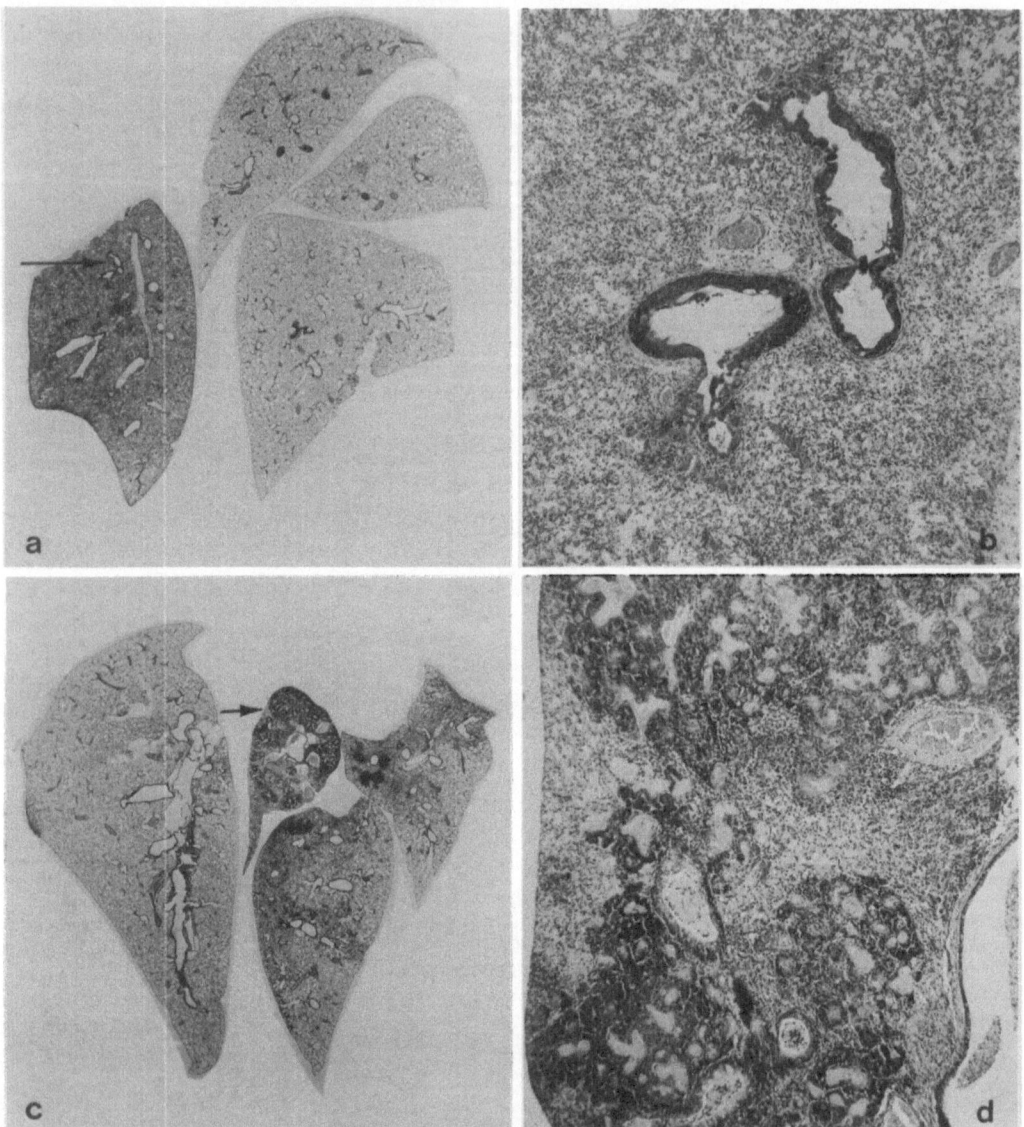

Fig. 2 a-d. Airborne influenza A infections in NA mice. (a) Whole
lung section of mouse sacrificed 13 days after onset. Left lobe shows
extensive pneumonitis. Upper part of the left lobe taken for E.M.
examination. No involvement of right upper middle or lower lobes.
HEA (x 5.3). (b) Higher power view of bronchus in "A" (arrow) showing
marked squamous metaplasia of regenerating bronchial epithelium. (x 41).
(c) Whole lung section of mouse sacrificed 28 days after onset. Essentially all of right upper lobe and focal areas in right, middle, and
lower lobes contain squamous metaplastic nodules. HEA (x 5.3). (d)
Higher power of area in "C" (arrow) showing extensive squamous metaplasia and keratinization. (x 41)

fluenza virus, this may explain why influenza virus infections appear to suppress spontaneous lung adenomas made up of type II cells (STEINER and LOOSLI, 1950; NETTESHEIM et al., 1970).

Because of the similarity of postinfluenzal lesions and squamous cell carcinoma in man, the influenza virus has been considered to be a possible carcinogenic or cocarcinogenic agent (ASKANAZY, 1919; WINTERNITZ et al., 1920). CAMPBELL (1940) studied the combined effect of influenza virus and exposure to atmospheric dusts from tarred roads on lung lesions in mice, and found that influenza virus infections had, if anything, an inhibitory effect on the development of primary lung tumors. STEINER and LOOSLI (1950) concluded that the PR8-A strain of influenza virus was a powerful growth stimulant to regenerating bronchial epithelial cells but did not induce lung tumors. Likewise, NETTESHEIM et al. (1970) concluded that the PR8-A influenza virus retarded lung tumor growth in mice exposed to whole body x-irradiation, ozonized gasoline, or chromium oxide dust. STAEMMLER et al. (1970) and FOITZIK et al. (1972) concluded respectively that sublethal intranasal instillations of PR8-A and Asian influenza viruses produce lung carcinoma in Albino mice. The tumors appearing early were mostly the squamous cell type and those appearing after 14 days were adenocarcinomas.

LEUCHTENBERGER et al. (1963) observed that atypical proliferative changes in the lungs of mice were highest in animals subjected both to cigarette smoke inhalation and influenza virus infections. KOTIN and WISELEY (1963) infected C57Bl mice with 3 different strains of influenza virus, along with continuous exposure to an aerosol of ozonized gasoline. They concluded that the combination of influenza virus exposure and hydrocarbon aerosols progressed fromthe initial proliferative response to the influenza virus through squamous metaplasia with keratinization to the development of squamous cancer, whereas exposure to influenza viruses or hydrocarbon aerosols alone did not produce squamous metaplasia or squamous cancer. On the other hand, HARRIS and NEGRONI (1967) found the tumor yield in C57Bl mice infected with influenza virus followed by exposure to aerosols of benzpyrene or cigarette smoke to be the same as when influenza virus was used alone. SCHMIDT-RUPPIN and PAPADOPULU (1972) observed that repeated infections with the PR8-A and A2 influenza viruses for 6 months, followed by application of diethylnitrosamine in the drinking water for an additional 6 months, caused a significant increase in primary lung carcinomas in mice compared to the incidence in mice drinking diethylnitrosamine alone.

This and a previous study (LOOSLI et al., 1973b) demonstrate the tremendous importance of vitamin A status in determining the histological character of the postinfluenzal lesion in mice. None of the investigators cited above who have interpreted postinfluenzal lesions alone or in combination with hydrocarbons or cigarette smoke inhalation as adenocarcinoma or squamous cell carcinoma apparently considered the vitamin A status of their mice. In this study, histological areas in the lungs of the NA, RA, and HA groups can be selected that are identical with those considered by others to be adenocarcinoma, squamous cell carcinoma, etc. The tremendous variation in the histological character of the postinfluenzal lung lesion in the mouse, depending on the vitamin A status of the animal, suggests that lesions described by others as adenocarcinoma, squamous cell carcinoma, etc., may be the natural response to the virus. While these look like adenocarcinomas and squamous cell carcinomas, in the absence of metastases, they probably should not be considered as such. The question as to whether the influenza A virus should be considered a carcinogen or cocarcinogen requires further study.

272

E. Acknowledgements

Grateful acknowledgement is given to HELGARD NIEWISCH, D.V.M., for
performing the virus isolation and serological procedures, to ERICA
STONE, M.S., for histological procedures and to SUE HERTWECK, M.S.,
for E.M. examination of tissues, and to RAIMONDA APEIKIS for assistance in preparation and typing of the manuscript.

References

ASKANAZY, M.: Über die Veränderungen der großen Luftwege besonders
   ihre Epithelmetaplasie bei der Influenza. Clb. allg. Path. path.
   Anat. 30, 443-452 (1919).
BROOKS, R.E.: Pulmonary adenoma of strain A mice: An electron micro-
   scopic study. J. nat. Cancer Inst. 41, 719-742 (1968).
CAMPBELL, J.A.: Influenza virus and the incidence of primary lung
   tumours in mice. Lancet (1940) II, 487.
Carr-Price Colorimetric Procedure: Methods of Vitamin Analysis.
   Chapter 4, Vitamin A, pp. 70-80, Associated Vitamin Chemists.
   New York: Interscience 1966.
FOITZIK, E., STAEMMLER, M., POSZICH, G.: Experimenteller Lungen-
   krebs bei weißen Mäusen nach intranasaler Infektion mit Influenza-
   Virus A2 Asia. Z. Krebsforsch. 77, 11-82 (1972).
HARRIS, R.J.C., NEGRONI, G.: Production of lung carcinomas of C57Bl
   mice exposed to a cigarette smoke and air mixture. Brit. med. J.
   4, 637-641 (1967).
HOAG, W.G., DICKIE, M.M.: Nutrition. In: Biology of the Laboratory
   Mouse (E.D. Green, ed.), 2nd ed., Chapter 5, pp. 39-43. New York:
   McGraw-Hill 1966.
KOTIN, P., WISELY, D.V.: Production of lung cancer in mice by inhala-
   tion exposure to influenza virus and aerosols of hydrocarbons. Prog.
   exp. Tumor Res. 3, 186-215 (1963).
LEUCHTENBERGER, C., LEUCHTENBERGER, R., RUCH, F., TANAKA, K., TANAKA,
   T.: Cytological and cytochemical alterations in the respiratory
   tract of mice after exposure to cigarette smoke, influenza virus,
   and both. Cancer Res. 23, 555-565 (1963).
LOOSLI, C.G.: The pathogenesis and pathology of experimental air-
   borne influenza virus A infections in mice. J. infect. Dis. 84,
   153-168 (1949).
LOOSLI, C.G.: Synergism between respiratory viruses and bacteria.
   Yale J. Biol. and Med. 40, 522-539(1968).
LOOSLI, C.G.: Influenza and the interaction of viruses and bacteria
   in respiratory infections. Medicine 52, 369-384 (1973c).
LOOSLI, C.G., BUCKLEY, R.D., HARDY, J.D., HERTWECK, M.S., HWANG KOW,
   S.-Y., SEREBRIN, R., RYAN, D.P., STINSON, S.F.: The pathogenesis
   of postinfluenzal collapse of the lungs of mice. Trans. Ass. Amer.
   Phys. 84, 182-189 (1971).
LOOSLI, C.G., BUCKLEY, R.D., HWANG KOW, S.-Y., HARDY, J.D., RYAN, D.P.,
   SEREBRIN, R., JOYCE, J.A., HERTWECK, M.S.: Experimental airborne
   influenza PR8-A infections in germfree mice. In: Germfree Research
   Biological Effect of Gnotobiotic Environments (J.B. Heneghan, ed.),
   pp. 395-404. New York, London: Academic Press 1973a.
LOOSLI, C.G., HERTWECK, M.S., HOCKWALD, R.S.: Airborne influenza
   PR8-A infections in actively immunized mice. Arch. Environ. Hlth 21,
   332-346 (1970).
LOOSLI, C.G., STINSON, S.F., HWANG KOW, S.-Y., RYAN, D.P., JOYCE, J.A.,
   HARDY, J.D., BUCKLEY, R.D.: Effect of vitamin A intake on the
   pathology of airborne influenza A virus infection. In: Airborne
   Transmission and Airborne Infection (J.F.Ph. Hers and K.C. Winkler,
   eds), pp. 248-253. Utrecht, the Netherlands: Oosthoek Publ. Co. 1973b.

MCCARTHY, P.T., CERECEDO, L.R.: Vitamin A deficiency in the mouse. J. Nutrition 46, 361-376 (1952).

MOORE, T., HOLMES, P.D.: The production of experimental vitamin A deficiency in rats and mice. Lab Animals 5, 239-250 (1971).

MULDER, J., HERS, J.F.Ph.: Influenza. Groningen: Walters Noordhoff Publ. 1972.

NETTESHEIM, P., HANNA, M.G., DOHERTY, D.G., NEWELL, R.F., HELLMAN, A.: Effects of chronic exposure to artificial smog and chromium oxide dust on the incidence of lung tumors in mice. In: Inhalation Carcinogenesis. AEC Symposium Series no. 18, pp. 305-320. Oak Ridge, Tennessee: U.S. Atomic Energy Commission, Division of Technical Inf. 1970.

SCHMIDT-RUPPIN, K.H., PAPADOPULU, G.: Zur Wirkung von Diäthylnitrosamin (DAENA) und Influenza-Viren auf die Entstehung von Lungencarcinomen bei Mäusen. Z. Krebsforsch. 77, 150-154 (1972).

STAEMMLER, M., FOITZIK, E., HEYDENREICH, M.: Influenza-Virus und Lungenkrebs im Tierversuch. Z. Krebsforsch. 74, 283-294 (1970).

STEINER, P., LOOSLI, C.G.: The effect of human influenza virus (type A) on the incidence of lung tumors in mice. Cancer Res. 10, 385-392 (1950).

STRAUB, M.: The microscopical changes in the lungs of mice infected with influenza virus. J. Path. 45, 75-78 (1937).

WINTERNITZ, M.C., WASON, I.M., MCNAMARA, F.P.: The Pathology of Influenza. New Haven, Connecticut: Yale University Press 1920.

WOLBACH, S.B., HOWE, P.R.: Tissue changes following deprivation of fat-soluble A vitamin. J. exp. Med. 42, 753-777 (1925).

WOLBACH, S.B.: Effects of vitamin A deficiency and hypervitaminosis A in animals. In: The Vitamins (W.H. Sebrell, Jr., R.S. Harris, eds), Chapter 11, pp. 106-137. New York: Academic Press 1954.

WONG, Y.-C., BUCK, R.C.: An electron microscopic study of metaplasia of the rat tracheal epithelium in vitamin A deficiency. Lab Invest. 24, 55-66 (1971).

Influenza-Virus-Induced Hyperplasia of the Respiratory Tract of the Hamster*

Curtis D. Port[1], David W. Baxter[1], David G. Kaufman[2], and Valerio Genta[2]

[1]IIT Research Institute, Chicago, IL 60616, USA
[2]Lung Cancer Branch, National Cancer Institute, Bethesda, MD 20014, USA

ABSTRACT

Hamster-adapted A/PR/8 influenza virus infection followed by a secondary insult consisting of 0.25 ml of 0.5% gelatin-saline instilled directly into the trachea causes epithelial hyperplasia of both the trachea and lung. The extent of the response is related to, and dependent upon, the time interval between virus infection and gelatin-saline administration; the optimal time interval is between 12 and 18 hr. The presence of hyperplasia was measured by ^{3}H-thymidine incorporation. Hyperplasia of the trachea is first apparent 3 days after virus infection, peaks at the fourth day, and is no longer present by the twentieth day. Hyperplasia in the lung begins 4 days after virus infection, peaks at the sixth day, and is undetectable by the twentieth day. Additional studies are in progress to determine the effect of virus-induced hyperplasia on benzo(a)pyrene-ferric oxide initiated respiratory carcinogenesis.

Introduction

Previous work at IITRI has demonstrated that intranasal administration of hamster-adapted A/PR/8 influenza virus, followed at selected intervals by an additional intratracheal insult, produces a hyperplastic bronchial and bronchiolar epithelium. The hyperplasia occurs whether the additional insult is nickel oxide, gelatin-saline, or saline, and appears to be related to the time interval between infectious challenge and administration of the insult. Markedly hyperplastic bronchial and bronchiolar epithelia, adenomatosis, pleural thickening, and an intense interstitial response were present in the lungs of hamsters upon histological examination.

The studies reported here were designed to determine the time relationship between virus infection and a secondary tracheal insult on the development of epithelial hyperplasia, which may be a facet in the expression of respiratory cancer. The objective is to test whether a maximum hyperplastic response from the virus infection with a subsequent administration of a carcinogen at the proper time leads to a high incidence of tumor. Epithelial hyperplasia can be induced by

---

*This work was performed in part under Contract No. NIH-NCI-72-3292, Division of Cancer Cause and Prevention, National Cancer Institute, National Institutes of Health.

a number of conditions, including vitamin A-deficiency, exposure to
injurious chemicals, and virus infection. There seems to be some relationship between viral infection and carcinogens. This relationship
is either direct as a cofactor, or indirect as an increase in susceptibility. Studies documenting this relationship have been published
(KOTIN, 1958, 1963; STRAUB, 1937). We hope to obtain additional data,
utilizing the hamster, and to build on this work. Such studies will
provide an animal model to investigate the concept that epithelial
proliferation may lead to an increased susceptibility to chemical carcinogenesis.

Materials and Methods

Random-bred male Syrian golden hamsters were housed in groups of 5 in
polystyrene cages with a filter bonnet (Filtex, Appleton, Wisconsin).
The animals were fed a pelleted stock diet (Rockland Mouse/Rat Diet,
Glen Ellyn, Illinois) and given bottled tap water ad libitum. Cages,
bedding, filter bonnets, and water were steam-sterilized and changed
twice a week. Temperature in the room was maintained at 24°C with a
12-hour light-dark lighting cycle.

Influenza virus, A/PR/8 strain, was adapted to hamsters by serial
passaging, with a final 20% lung suspension used for infectious
challenge. The virus was identified by use of specific A/PR/8 influenza virus antiserum obtained from the National Institutes of
Health.

Hamsters were anesthetized with dry ice (CO_2) and 0.1 ml of the 20%
lung suspension was placed on the septa between the nares. The viral
suspension was carried into the lungs upon inhalation. A single 0.2 ml
dose of gelatin-saline (0.5% gelatin) was injected intratracheally,
as a secondary insult, according to the method of SAFFIOTTI (1968),
at various time intervals after infectious challenge. Each animal received an intraperitoneal injection of 300 µCi-tritiated thymidine 1
hour before sacrifice. The lungs and trachea were removed en block
from each animal, weighed by sections, frozen, and examined for tritiated thymidine incorporation into DNA, and by autoradiography for
thymidine labeling of epithelial cells. Both trachea and lung samples
were analyzed for thymidine incorporation into DNA. Results were expressed as DPM/µg DNA.

Autoradiography of tracheal sections from animals injected with tritiated thymidine was carried out to confirm the biochemical data.
Cross-sections of trachea were fixed in s-collidine-buffered 5%
glutaraldehyde, embedded in Epon 812 containing 5% Araldite, and
sectioned with an ultramicrotome. Photomicrographs of 1 µm tracheal
sections were taken at a microscopic magnification of 32.5 X. The
negatives were enlarged 8.25 X to a total magnification of 268 X.
The epithelial length was measured at the junction of the epithelium
and connective tissue from the photographic prints, with correction
for microscopic and photographic enlargement. Labeled cells were
microscopically counted in the same area on the original tracheal
section through a 100 X oil-immersion objective lens. The results
were then expressed as mean number of labeled cells per 10,000 µm
of epithelial length ± standard error (labeling index).

Experimental Design

To determine the optimal timing for gelatin-saline administration, hamster-adapted influenza A/PR/8 virus was administered intranasally, followed by intratracheal gelatin-saline to 12 hamsters at 6, 12, 18, and 48 hours (Groups A-D). When 3 hamsters from each group were killed at 2, 6, 12, and 20 days following virus infection, the extent of tritiated thymidine incorporation was determined.

Based upon the results of this experiment, the development of hyperplasia was studied. Seven groups of 10 hamsters were given virus followed by intratracheal gelatin-saline at 18 hours. The groups were killed at 3/4, 1, 2, 3, 4, 6, and 10 days after virus. The labeling index was determined with 1/2 of the animals in each group, and thymidine incorporation was quantitated with the remaining animals. Four additional groups were added to this experiment, to better define the optimal time for gelatin-saline administration. Two of these received gelatin-saline at 12 hours after virus challenge and 2 groups received gelatin-saline at 15 hours. Animals from these groups were killed at either 2 or 6 days after virus challenge.

Results

The optimal time for the administration of gelatin-saline after virus infection was between 12 and 18 hours. The extent of thymidine-incorporation to DNA in both trachea and lung was greatest with these time intervals. Maximum incorporation occurred between 2 and 6 days after infection (Table 1). Since both 12 and 18 hours appeared to be satisfactory intervals between virus infection and the secondary intratracheal insult, 18 hours was chosen for convenience in a second experiment designed to clarify the development of the hyperplastic response.

Table 1. Virus induced hyperplasia Part 1: ^{3}H-thymidine incorporation (DPM per μg DNA, mean ± SE)

Time (hrs) of gel-saline insult after virus infection		Days after virus infection			
		2	6	12	20
Lung	6	130±75	209± 79	74±28	82±12
	12	57± 7	154(N=1)	123±33	48± 0
	18	217±64	598±492	51± 6	24± 5
	48	127±16	294±155	81± 6	66±10
	not given	58±17	173± 72	64±31	43± 3
Trachea	6	128±26	191± 32	53±23	74±26
	12	541±83	491(N=1)	68±12	65± 9
	18	504±70	192±117	50± 6	20± 3
	48	177±72	179± 50	48±15	79±16
	not given	51±10	150± 75	26±24	56±18

In this study, maximum hyperplasia occurred in the trachea at 4 days and lung at 6 days after virus infection (Fig. 1 and Table 2). The additional groups added to this study verified that the optimal time interval between virus infection and gelatin-saline insult is 12 to 18 hours. No significant effect was present at 2 days, regardless of the time of gelatin administration, and the effect at 6 days was not statistically significant when the gelatin-saline was given at 18 hours as compared to 12 or 15 hours. Of interest is the fact that the tracheal response preceded the lung response and that the maximal hyperplasia was achieved at day 4 in the trachea, versus day 6 in the lung.

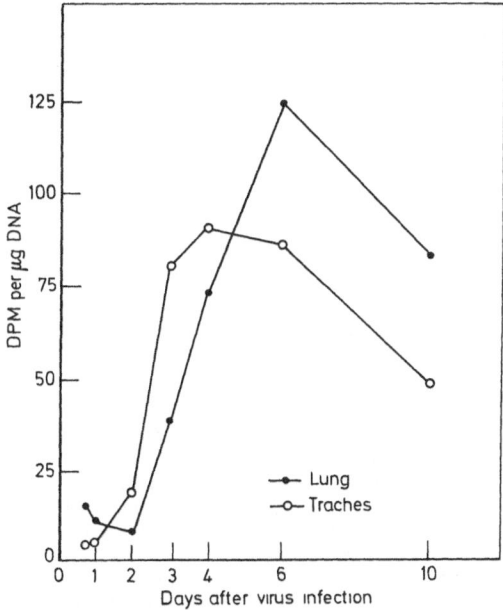

Fig. 1. ^{3}H-thymidine binding to DNA in lung and trachea

Table 2. Virus induced hyperplasia Part 2: ^{3}H-thymidine incorporation (DPM per µg DNA, mean $\pm$ SE)

Time (hrs) of gelatin-saline insult after virus infection		Days after virus infection						
		3/4	1	2	3	4	6	10
Lung	12	–	–	13$\pm$1	–	–	200$\pm$80	–
	15	–	–	9$\pm$3	–	–	212$\pm$44	–
	18[a]	15$\pm$2	11$\pm$2	8$\pm$3	38$\pm$6	73$\pm$29	124$\pm$20	83$\pm$21
Trachea	12	–	–	14$\pm$5	–	–	171$\pm$56	–
	15	–	–	12$\pm$1	–	–	71$\pm$20	–
	18[a]	4$\pm$1	5$\pm$1	18$\pm$5	80$\pm$29	90$\pm$11	86$\pm$17	48$\pm$8

[a]These data are also shown in Fig. 3.

The data for the labeling index is shown in Table 3. A rise in number
of labeled cells was present at 2 days in the trachea, with a peak
at 4 days. The results obtained by this method parallel the biochemical
data and confirm the hyperplastic response.

Table 3. Labeling index in tracheal epithelium at selected
times after virus administration

Time after virus	Labeling index[a]
18 hr	$82^{\pm}$ 13
1 day	$64^{\pm}$ 8
2 day	$219^{\pm}144$
3 day	403
4 day	$781^{\pm}253$
6 day	$577^{\pm}$ 89
10 day	176

[a]The mean $\pm$ SE are given on those groups with 3 or more animals.
Otherwise only the mean is stated.

Discussion

The effect of influenza infection on the respiratory system has been
studied by a number of investigators (LOOSLI, 1949; STEINER and LOOS-
LI, 1950; STRAUB, 1950; WAGNER, 1956). A consistent finding was a
characteristic epithelial proliferative response. KOTIN et al. (1958,
1963) expanded on this work and produced lung cancer in C57B mice by
inhalation-exposure to influenza virus and carcinogenic aerosols.
While administration of virus alone resulted in extensive epithelial
proliferation, virus and hydrocarbon aerosols produced extensive
squamous change that eventually progressed to epidermoid cancer. The
carcinoma began in the areas of epithelial proliferation. In these
studies, the carcinogen was administered over broad periods of time
in respect to the proliferative response.

Despite the documentation of the interaction between virus-induced
hyperplasia and carcinogenic hydrocarbons, little work has been accomplished to define the experimental conditions of this interaction which
results in increased tumor formation. The purpose of this study was
to establish the conditions required for a maximal epithelial response.
It was found that a virus infection plus a secondary insult is necessary; when either the virus or the insult is administered alone, the
proliferative response is minimal. The extent of the response is related to and dependent upon the time interval between virus infection
and gelatin-saline as the additional insult.

This method of inducing an epithelial response was selected because
the results are reproducible and easily obtained, and all of the
respiratory epithelia are involved. Vitamin A-deficiency and direct
exposure to dilute hydrochloric acid cause epithelial proliferation
but, with methodologies used at the present time, have produced less
well-characterized and synchronous responses.

In future studies, our intent is to examine the relationship of cell proliferation, induced by a variety of methods, to lung cancer. There is evidence that proliferating cells are more susceptible to carcinogens, and that cell proliferation after administration of a carcinogen is also involved in the expression of malignancy (CRADDOCK, 1971; FREI, 1964). The kinetics of the proliferative response in this system are such that a carcinogen can be administered before, during, or after maximal hyerplasia. A well-defined proliferative response now makes possible better experiments to investigate the relationship between epithelial proliferation and carcinogenesis. Results from any one such system will have to be compared to other means of producing hyperplasia in order to establish the generality of the relationship. In addition to potentially providing information about the mechanisms of proliferation and carcinogenesis, these same studies may help determine whether viral infection is a state of increased susceptibility to carcinogens.

Acknowledgements

The authors wish to thank Dr. CURTIS C. HARRIS of the National Cancer Institute and ELIZABETH KINGSBURY of Litton Bionetics for their assistance and cooperation in obtaining the autoradiographic data for this paper.

References

CRADDOCK, V.M.: Liver carcinomas induced in rats by single administration of dimethylnitrosamine after partial hepatectomy. J. nat. Cancer Inst. 47, 899-905 (1971).

FREI, J.V., RITCHIE, A.C.: Diurnal variation in the susceptibility of mouse epidermis to carcinogen and its relationship to DNA synthesis. J. nat. Cancer Inst. 32, 1213-1220 (1964).

KOTIN, P., FALK, H.L., MCCAMMON, C.J. III.: The experiment induction of pulmonary tumors and changes in the respiratory epithelium in C57 Black mice following their exposure to an atmosphere of ozonized gasoline. Cancer 11, 473-481 (1958).

KOTIN, P., WISELEY, D.V.: Production of lung cancer in mice by inhalation exposure to influenza virus and aerosols of hydrocarbons. Prog. exp. Tumor Res. 3, 186-215 (1963).

LOOSLI, C.G.: The pathogenesis and pathology of experimental airborne influenza A virus infection in mice. J. infect. Dis. 84, 153-168 (1949).

SAFFIOTTI, U., CEFIS, F., KOLB, L.: A method for experimental induction of bronchogenic carcinoma. Cancer Res. 28, 104 (1968).

STEINER, P.E., LOOSLI, C.G.: The effect of influenza virus (Type A) on the incidence of lung tumors in mice. Cancer Res. 10, 385-392 (1950).

STRAUB, M.: The microscopical changes in the lungs of mice infected with influenza virus. J. Path. Bact. 45, 75-78 (1937).

WAGNER, R.R.: Studies on the pathogenesis of influenzal pneumonitis. Intranasal vs. intravenous infection in mice. Yale J. Biol. Med. 28, 598-614 (1956).

Inoculation of Owl Monkeys *(Aotus trivirgatus)* with 7,12-Dimethylbenz(a)anthracene and *Herpesvirus saimiri.* Induction of Epidermoid Carcinoma in the Lung*

W. Ellis Giddens, Jr.

Regional Primate Research Center and Department of Pathology, University of Washington, Seattle, WA 98195, USA

ABSTRACT

An experiment was designed to determine whether the owl monkey is an appropriate animal model for nasopharyngeal carcinoma. 11 owl monkeys received a single IT inoculation of 170 mg DMBA. 4 weeks later, 6 treated and 6 untreated monkeys were given HVS by IT or IM routes. All but 1 HVS-infected animal died of malignant lymphoma. The mean survival time of IT-inoculated monkeys was longer than for IM-inoculated monkeys. Pretreatment with DMBA significantly increased the survival time of HVS-infected monkeys. DMBA produced nonspecific focal necrotizing bronchopneumonia in the lung, and large amounts of it were detectable throughout the experiment.

At 350 days posttreatment, 1 of 2 monkeys with detectable DMBA in their lungs developed epidermoid carcinoma of bronchial epithelium which was regenerating over the necrotic bronchial wall. There were many atypical anaplastic epithelial cells with enlarged hyperchromatic nuclei, numerous abnormal mitotic figures, and invasion of the epithelium into adjacent connective tissue and cartilage.

The owl monkey would appear to be an excellent primate model for experimental respiratory carcinogenesis.

Introduction

100% of patients with nasopharyngeal carcinoma (NPC), a very common tumor of adult Chinese people, has antibodies, usually in very high titer, against Epstein-Barr Virus (EBV)(HENLE et al., 1970). DE-THE (1972) has hypothesized that EBV may be either a passenger virus, without any etiological role, or a causative factor or cofactor, playing an etiological role in the development of NPC. In addition to the genetic predisposition of Chinese to the development of NPC (HO, 1972), various environmental factors have been suggested as essential cofactors. Smoke from cooking fires (DOBSON, 1924; CLIFFORD and BEECHER, 1964) and incense (HO, 1972) have been cited as possible cocarcinogens present in the environment. FREEMAN (according to HO, 1972) reported that smoke from a burning Chinese incense stick could induce transformation of rat embryo cells in tissue culture equivalent to that of a potent carcinogen.

---
*Supported by grant RR00166 from the National Institutes of Health, U.S. Public Health Service, and an institutional grant from the American Cancer Society.

I reasoned that perhaps chronic exposure to an irritant or carcinogen present in smoke from cooking fire or incense might produce a population of respiratory epithelial cells susceptible to malignant transformation by EBV. I designed an experiment to test this hypothesis, using the owl monkey (*Aotus trivirgatus*) as the host, 7,12-dimethylbenz (a)anthracene (DMBA) as the chemical, and *Herpesvirus saimiri* (HVS) as the virus. HVS is a lymphocytotropic herpesvirus that produces malignant lymphoma when injected intravenously or intramuscularly (IM) into owl monkeys (MELENDEZ et al., 1969; DEINHARDT, 1973). It has many similarities to EBV (EPSTEIN, 1972; FALK et al., 1972), and is currently considered the best animal model of EBV infection.

Materials and Methods

20 male and female owl monkeys, weighing 600 to 800 g each, were obtained from South America through a commercial supplier. They were caged in 6 groups of 2 to 4 each and were quarantined for 3 months. Following the method of CROCKER and NIELSEN (1966), DMBA (Lot F2A, Eastman Kodak Company, Rochester, New York 14650) was suspended in triethylene glycol (TEG)(Practical Grade, J.T. Baker Chemical Company, Phillipsburg, New Jersey 08865) to a final concentration of 340 mg/ml. The suspension was stirred constantly with a magnetic stirrer while being administered. In the inoculation procedure, each monkey was sedated with ketamine hydrochloride. 11 monkeys were each given 0.5 ml of the DMBA-TEG suspension (containing 170 mg DMBA) by intratracheal (IT) inoculation, using a disposable catheter for each monkey (Intracath intravenous placement unit, Catalog No. 3162, Deseret Pharmaceutical Company, Sandy, Utah 84070). 9 other monkeys were given IT inoculations of 0.5 ml TEG only.

4 weeks posttreatment (PT) with DMBA, 4 monkeys were injected IM and 8 IT with 10^4-10^5 tissue culture infective doses of HVS. The details of the virological aspects of the experiment will be described in detail elsewhere (GIDDENS, 1974).

The experimental design is outlined in Table 1 and was intended to provide controls for 3 variables: inoculation with DMBA, IM inoculation with HVS, and IT inoculation with HVS. Monkeys were allowed to die spontaneously if they developed tumors or other diseases. Complete necropsies were performed on each monkey. At 350 days PT, 3 DMBA-inoculated monkeys and 3 TEG-inoculated controls, all clinically normal, were euthanized and perfused intracardially with Karnovsky's fixative for light- and electron-microscopy. Simultaneously, their lungs were infused intratracheally with the same fixative at 25 cm pressure. Complete necropsies were then conducted.

Results

All monkeys given HVS by IM or IT inoculation died with malignant lymphoma, except 1 which is still alive (No. 65), and 1 (No. 66) which died from exsanguination following venipuncture. The latter is a common malady of owl monkeys, due to a coagulopathy (LOEB et al., 1974) that affects a large percentage of the species. The surviving monkey does have lymphocytes which are latently infected with HVS, and is expected to die with malignant lymphoma (GIDDENS, 1974). Mean survival time after IM inoculation with HVS was 138 days, and after IT inoculation, 213 days (Table 1). This difference had a low degree of significance (P = .082), as determined by the Mann-Whitney U test (SIEGEL, 1956). Mean survival time for monkeys previously given DMBA was 227.4 days after HVS injection; for those not given DMBA, it was 149.3 days. This was a highly significant difference (P = .015).

10 owl monkeys given DMBA and 3 control monkeys given TEG were available for histopathologic evaluation of the effects of DMBA (Table 2). 2 of the 10 DMBA-treated monkeys died from acute fibrinopurulent pneumonia due to the inoculation of the DMBA. 5 more died from other causes during the course of the experiment, and 3 DMBA-treated monkeys and the 3 controls were euthanized.

Lesions due to DMBA were found only in the lung, and did not differ significantly in HVS-infected and uninfected monkeys, except that in the former there was generally more diffuse lymphoid infiltration of the entire lung.

In all DMBA-inoculated monkeys save 1 (No. 59), there was a solitary focus of inhalation pneumonia 3 to 10 mm in diameter, usually affecting the dorsal right cardiac or diaphragmatic lobes (Fig. 1). This focus had a yellow chalky center, usually around a large bronchus, consisting almost entirely of the DMBA itself, a middle zone of necrotic and/or reactive fibrous tissue, and a peripheral zone of alveolar tissue with inflamed walls. Histopathologic changes were acute (2 to 14 days PT), subacute (118 to 295 days PT) and chronic (350 days PT) in nature (Table 2).

In acute DMBA-induced pneumonia, the crystals filled bronchial and alveolar lumens and there was severe focal and diffuse fibrinopurulent pneumonia resulting in death (Fig. 2). In subacute DMBA-induced pneumonia, the fibrinopurulent reaction was confined to that area adjacent to the DMBA crystals. Lymphoid infiltration and alveolar-lining cell hyperplasia were prominent in the zone between fibrous tissue and alveolar parenchyma, and in the center of the lesion there was complete necrosis of all pulmonary tissue. In 1 monkey (No. 66), there was beginning regeneration of bronchial epithelium.

Electron-microscopic observations revealed the presence of the DMBA crystals which were represented, as in the paraffin sections, by angular, crystal-like, clear spaces (Fig. 3). The DMBA was presumably removed by organic solvent during processing. The hyperplastic alveolar-lining cells were granular pneumocytes, and the interstitial infiltrate consisted of plasma cells, lymphocytes, and occasional neutrophils (Fig. 4).

In chronic DMBA-induced pneumonia, lesions were similar except that there was pronounced hyperplasia and squamous metaplasia of regenerating bronchial epithelium adjacent to DMBA-filled bronchi. In No. 58, intercellular bridges, sheets of keratin, and keratinization were present in the hyperplastic epithelium (Figs 5 and 6). Mitotic figures were numerous, and there were several atypical giant cells containing large hyperchromatic nuclei. In some areas, nuclei were clustered together and cell boundaries were indistinct. The basement membrane underlying the anaplastic epithelium was not intact, and several anaplastic epithelial cells were present in the underlying connective tissue. There was invasion of tumor cells into the adjacent bronchial cartilage (Figs 7 and 8). On the basis of the intercellular bridges and keratinization, the presence of many atypical anaplastic cells with enlarged hyperchromatic nuclei, and invasion of the epithelium into the adjacent

Table 1. Experimental design and survival time (days) of owl monkeys dying of malignant lymphoma after infection with *Herpesvirus saimiri* (HVS)

	No DMBA				DMBA				
	Animal no.	Cause of death	Postinfect. survival	Mean surv.	Animal no.	Cause of death	Postinfect. survival	Mean surv.	Total mean surv.
No HVS	56	EU	322	NA	58	EU	322	NA	NA
	57	EU	322	NA	59	EU	322	NA	NA
	15	EU	322	NA	60	EU	322	NA	
IM HVS	61	ML	84		71	ML	90		
	62	ML	101	92.5	72	ML	267	193.5	138.0
IT HVS	67	ML	123		63	ML	259		
	68	ML	257		64	ML	181	260	
	69	ML	168	177.7	65	alive	340		
	70	ML	163		66	EX	112[a]		213.0
Total mean survival				149.3					227.4

EU, euthanized; ML, malignant lymphoma; EX, exsanguination.
[a] Survival not included in mean values.

Table 2. Summary of histopathologic observations in monkeys examined at various intervals post-treatment (PT) with DMBA

	Animal no.	Days PT DMBA	Cause of death	Fibrinopurulent reaction	DMBA crystals	Lymphocyte infiltration	Alveolar cell hyperplasia	Bronchial metaplasia
Acute	79	2	PN	++++	++++	0	0	0
	73	14	PN	+++	++++	+	0	0
Subacute	71	118	ML	+	+++	++	++	0
	66	146	EX	++	++++	+	0	+
	64	209	ML	+	++++	++	+	0
	63	287	ML	++	++++	+	+	0
	72	295	ML	+	++	+	+	0
Chronic	58	350	EU	0	+++	++	+++	++++
	59	350	EU	0	0	0	0	0
	60	350	EU	0	++++	+++	++	+
Control	56	350	EU	0	0	0	0	0
	57	350	EU	0	0	0	0	0
	15	350	EU	0	0	0	0	0

PN, pneumonia; ML, malignant lymphoma; EX, exsanguination; EU, euthanized.

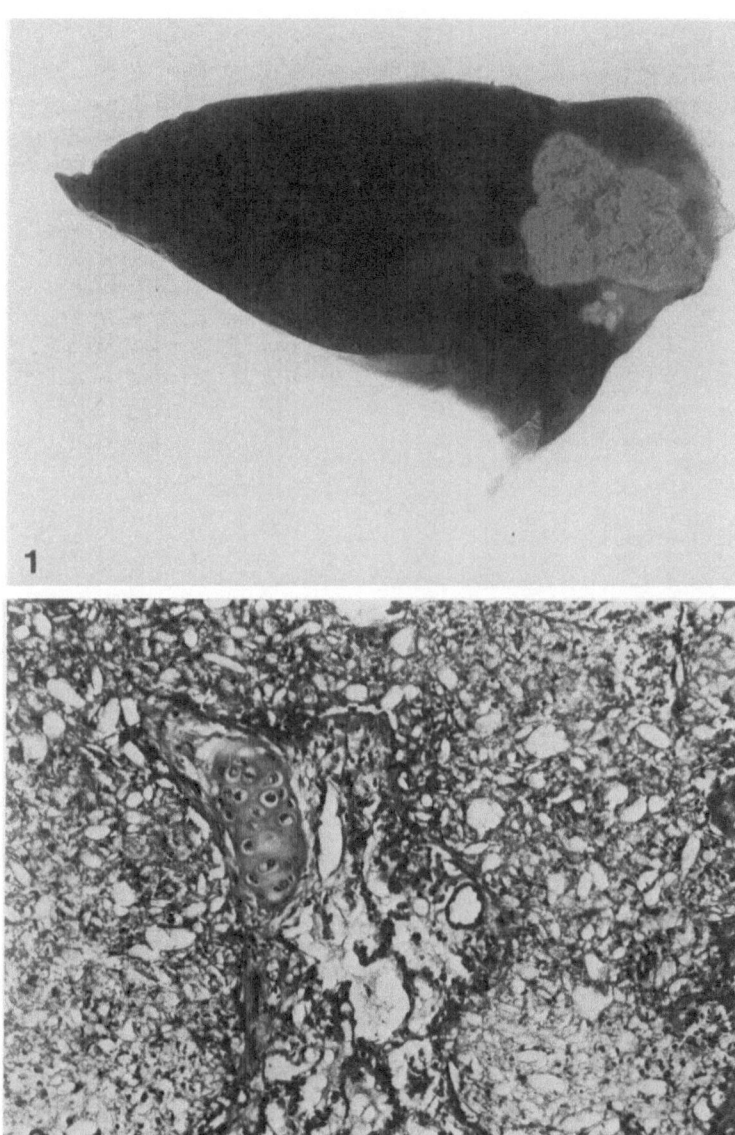

Fig. 1. Transverse section of inflated lung of monkey No. 60, 350 days PT with DMBA. Note chalky DMBA surrounded by wall of connective tissue

Fig. 2. Acute necrotizing bronchopneumonia in monkey No. 73, 14 days PT with DMBA. Numerous clefts are caused by dissolution of DMBA crystals during processing. HE x 320

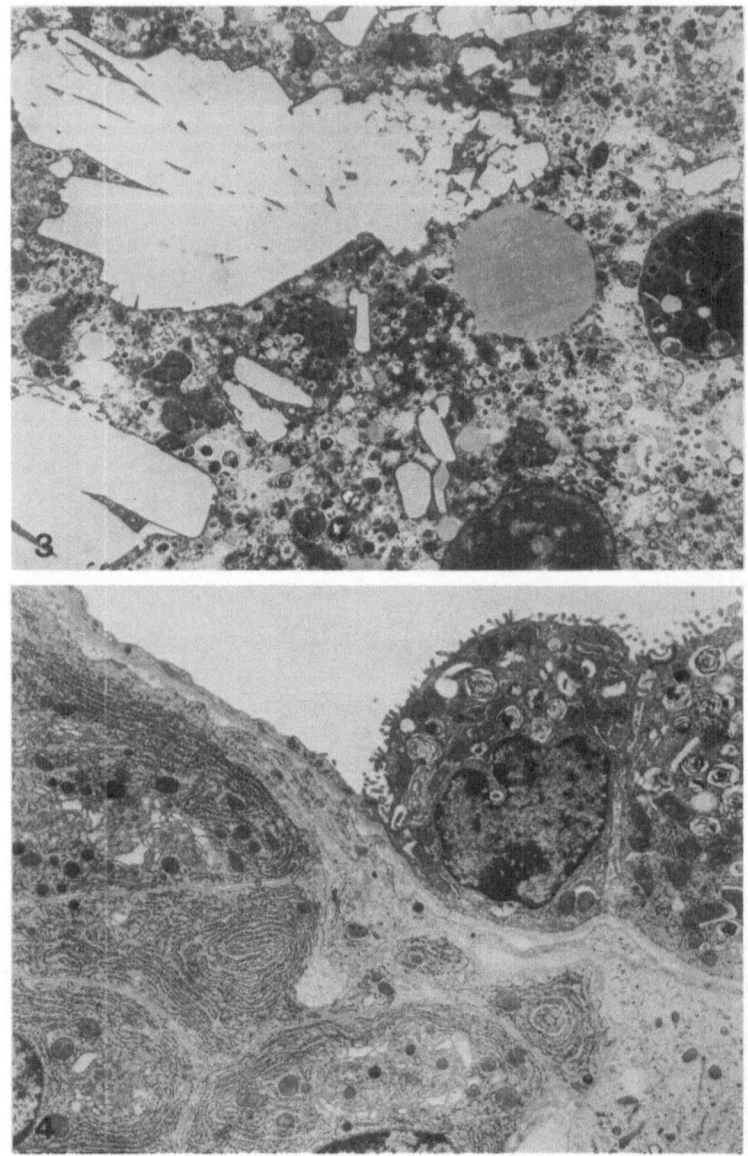

Fig. 3. Crystals of DMBA surrounded by remnants of cell organelles, nuclei, lipid droplet, and a neutrophil; monkey No. 60, 350 days PT with DMBA. Uranyl acetate and lead citrate. x 3,720

Fig. 4. Hyperplasia of granular pneumocytes and infiltrations of alveolar walls with plasma cells. Uranyl acetate and lead citrate. x 4,100

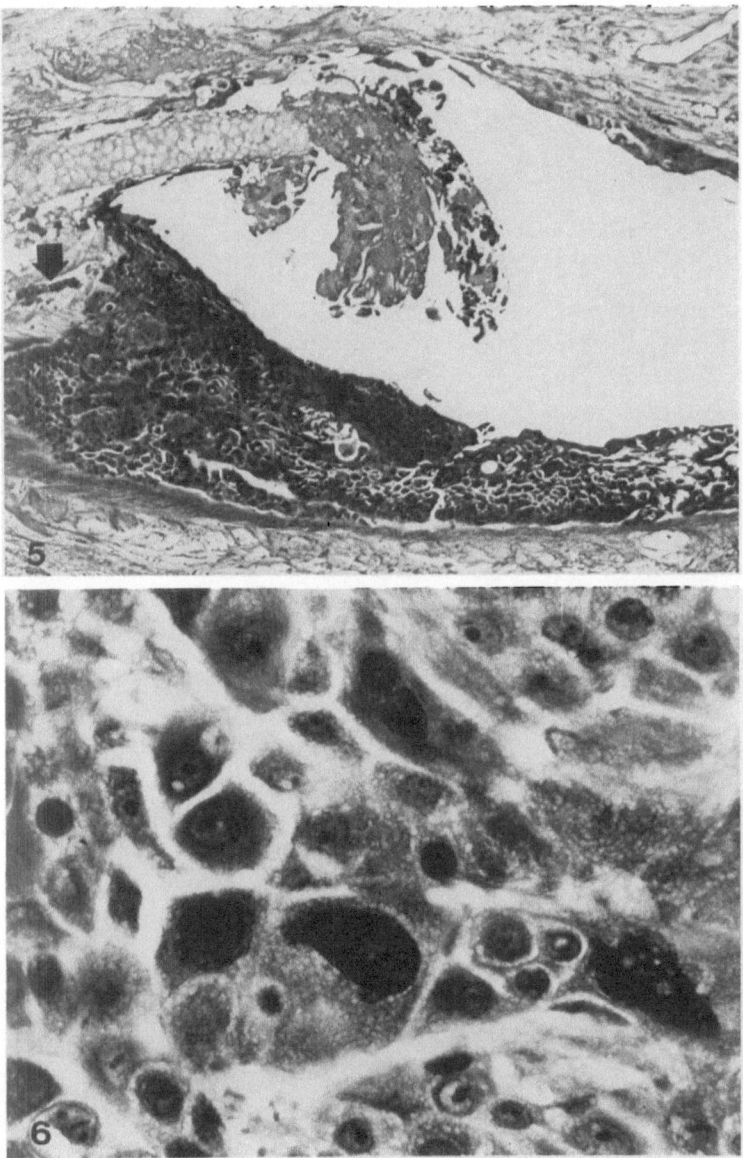

Fig. 5. Epidermoid carcinoma of bronchus adjacent to alveoli containing DMBA. The bronchial cartilage and much of the submucosal connective tissue are necrotic. Cellular and tissue debris are present in the bronchial lumen. Epithelial cells are invading the submucosa (arrows). HE x 51

Fig. 6. Intercellular bridges, cells with prominent nucleoli, and large atypical cells with hyperchromatic nuclei are present in this cluster of anaplastic epithelium. Epidermoid carcinoma. HE x 320

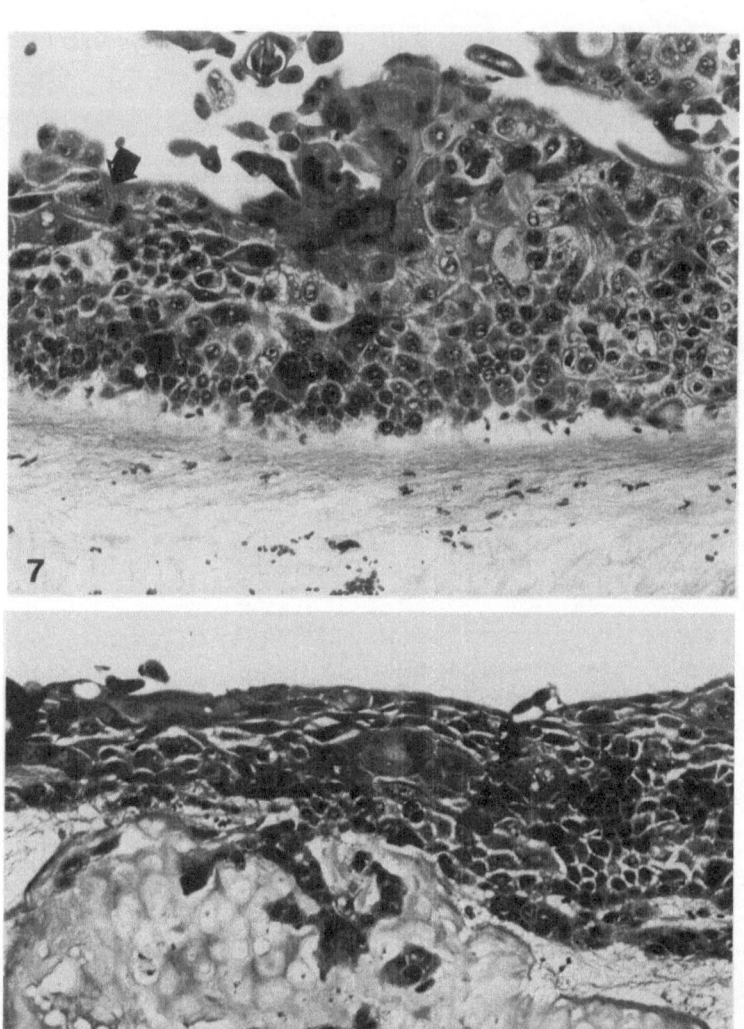

Fig. 7. Anaplastic, atypical epithelial cells. There are abnormal mitotic figures (arrow). Epidermoid carcinoma. HE x 130

Fig. 8. Invasion of carcinoma cells from epithelium down into sub-jacent bronchial cartilage. HE x 130

connective tissue and cartilage, the lesion was diagnosed as the early stage of primary epidermoid carcinoma of the lung.

Examination of frozen sections of lung fixed in Karnovsky's fixative revealed the DMBA deposits to be birefringent and to fluoresce a brilliant green when examined with ultraviolet light (mercury lamp with UG 1 exciter filter) and any barrier filter transmitting light with a wave length greater than 410 nm.

Discussion

Little is known about the biology of lung tumors in monkeys; our recent review indicates that spontaneous or induced primary lung tumors are extremely rare in nonhuman primates (GIDDENS and DILLING-HAM, 1971). I believe the epidermoid carcinoma seen in the bronchus of monkey No. 58, 350 days after a single IT inoculation of 170 mg DMBA, was invasive, even though obviously in an early stage, and that if the animal had not been sacrificed, it would eventually have died from the cancer. This cannot be proved, however, with the present data. It must be confirmed by further studies in which inoculated animals are kept for longer periods, examined frequently by ausculta-tion and radiographs, and periodically sacrificed to define the biology and pathogenesis of DMBA-induced lung cancer in monkeys.

Although CROCKER et al. (1970) induced carcinoma of the lung in pro-simians with benzo(a)pyrene, this appears to be the first example of respiratory carcinogenesis with polycyclic hydrocarbons in monkeys or higher primates. ADAMSON et al. (1970) reviewed the difficulties in inducing any kind of cancer in monkeys with polycyclic hydrocarbons. Perhaps this is a function of species-susceptibility to oncogenesis in general. Those monkeys in which cancer was induced with polycyclic hydrocarbons (*Aotus trivirgatus*, *Tamarinus nigricollis*, *Sanguinus oedipus*) are also highly susceptible to viral oncogenesis.

No model corresponding to NPC was produced in this experiment, probab-ly due to the extreme oncogenicity of HVS for the lymphoreticular system. If infected monkeys had not died of malignant lymphoma, sig-nificant differences might have been noted in the development of lung lesions in infected, versus uninfected, monkeys. Since the inception of this experiment, it has been shown that EBV will infect owl monkeys (SHOPE et al., 1973) but is not as oncogenic as HVS is. This experi-ment might profitably be repeated with EBV instead of HVS.

The highly significant increase in survival time of DMBA-inoculated monkeys which were subsequently infected with HVS is probably related to the suppressive effect DMBA has on stem cells (BALL et al., 1973). Presumably, the population of lymphocyte stem cells susceptible to transformation by HVS was decreased in number or susceptibility to oncogenesis by the administration of DMBA 4 weeks prior to inoculation with HVS.

Aside from the carcinoma in monkey No. 48, the pulmonary reaction to DMBA did not appear to differ much from that of any strong irritant which would cause a focal necrotizing lesion.

The owl monkey is susceptible to the oncogenic properties of EBV and HVS, and the data presented here indicate that it is susceptible to respiratory carcinogenesis by polycyclic hydrocarbons. It is sufficient-

ly related to humans so that many immunologic reagents of humans, e.g.,
fluorescein-labeled antihuman gamma globulin, can be used in the owl
monkey (GIDDINS, 1974). It would appear to be an excellent model for
studies on respiratory carcinogenesis.

Acknowledgement

I acknowledge the excellent technical assistance of PAT MCGUIRE, PAT
MANNING, GLEN KNITTER, and BRENDA BUTZON.

References

ADAMSON, R.H., COOPER, R.W., O'GARA, R.W.: Carcinogen-induced tumors
  in primitive primates. J. nat. Cancer Inst. 45, 555-559 (1970).
BALL, JR., HOSHIMO, S., MCCARTER, J.A.: Depressive effect of 7,12-
  dimethylbenz(a)anthracene and ionizing radiation on bone marrow
  colony-forming cells. J. nat. Cancer Inst. 51, 1491-1495 (1973).
CLIFFORD, P., BEECHER, J.L.: Nasopharyngeal cancer in Kenya. Clinical
  and environmental aspects. Brit. J. Cancer 18, 25-43 (1964).
CROCKER, T.T., CHASE, J.E., WELLS, S.A., NUNES, L.L.: Preliminary
  report on experimental carcinoma of the lung in hamsters and in a
  primate. In: Morphology of Experimental Respiratory Carcinogenesis
  (P. Nettesheim, M.G. Hanna, Jr., J.W. Deatherage, Jr., eds), pp.
  317-328. AEC Symposium Series no. 21. Oak Ridge, Tennessee: U.S.
  Atomic Energy Commission, Division of Technical Inf. 1970.
CROCKER, T.T., NIELSEN, B.I.: Effect of carcinogenic hydrocarbons
  on suckling rat trachea in living animals and in organ cultures.
  In: Lung Tumors in Animals (L. Severi, ed.), pp. 765-787. Division
  of Cancer Research, University of Perugia 1966.
DEINHARDT, F.: Herpesvirus saimiri. In: The Herpesviruses (A.S. Kaplan,
  ed.), pp. 595-626. New York: Academic Press 1973.
DE-THE, G.: Virology and immunology of nasopharyngeal carcinoma:
  present situation and outlook, a review. In: Oncogenesis and Herpes-
  viruses (P.M. Biggs, G. De-Thé, L.N. Payne, eds), pp. 275-284. Lyon,
  France: International Agency for Research on Cancer 1972.
DOBSON, W.C.: Cervical lymphosarcoma (letter to editor). Chin. med.
  J. 38, 786 (1924).
EPSTEIN, M.A.: Burkitt's lymphoma and Herpesvirus saimiri lymphoma:
  comparative aspects. In: International Symposium on Health Aspects
  of the International Movement of Animals, Scientific Publication.
  P.A.H.O. 235, 124-129 (1972).
FALK, L.A., WOLFE, L.G., HOEKSTRA, J., DEINHARDT, F.: Demonstration
  of Herpesvirus saimiri-associated antigens in peripheral lymphocytes
  from infected marmosets during in vitro cultivation. J. nat. Cancer
  Inst. 48, 523-529 (1972).
GIDDENS, W.E., Jr.: Ultrastructural observations of cultured lymphocytes from owl monkeys infected with Herpesvirus saimiri . In: Biology
  of the Owl Monkey (A. Hertig, N. Kind, eds). In preparation, 1974.
GIDDENS, W.E., Jr., DILLINGHAM, L.A.: Primary tumors of the lung in
  nonhuman primates. Literature review and report of peripheral carci-
  noid tumors of the lung in a rhesus monkey. Vet. Path. 8, 467-478
  (1971).
HENLE, W., HENLE, G., BURTIN, P., CACHIN, Y., CLIFFORD, P., DE SCHRYVER,
  A., DE THE, G., DIEHL, V., HO, H.C., KLEIN, G.: Antibodies to
  Epstein-Barr virus in nasopharyngeal carcinoma, other head and neck
  neoplasms, and control groups. J. nat. Cancer Inst. 44, 225-231 (1970).

HO, H.C.: Current knowledge of the epidemiology of nasopharyngeal carcinoma, a review. In: Oncogenesis and Herpesviruses (P.M. Biggs, G. De-Thê, L.N. Payne, eds), pp. 357-366. Lyon, France: International Agency for Research on Cancer 1972.

LOEB, W.F., CICMANEC, J., WIRKUM, M.: A coagulopathy of the owl monkey. In: Biology of the Owl Monkey (A. Hertig, N. King, eds). In preparation, 1974.

MELENDEZ, L.V., HUNT, R.D., DANIEL, M.D., GARCIA, F.G., FRASER, C.E.O.: *Herpesvirus saimiri*. II. Experimentally induced malignant lymphoma in primates. Lab. Anim. 19, 378-386 (1969).

SHOPE, T., DECHAIRO, D., MILLER, G.: Malignant lymphoma in cottontop marmosets after inoculation with Epstein-Barr virus. Proc. Nat. Acad. Sci. (Wash.) 70, 2487-2491 (1973).

SIEGEL, S.: Nonparametric Statistics for the Behavioral Sciences, pp. 116-127. New York: McGraw-Hill 1956.

Session III Bioassays of Respiratory Carcinogens in Tobacco Products

Chairman: Walter P. Dontenwill

Forschungsinstitut der Cigarettenindustrie e. V., Hamburg, W.-Germany

Review and Introductory Remarks:
Bioassays of Respiratory Carcinogens in Tobacco Products

Walter P. Dontenwill

Forschungsinstitut der Cigarettenindustrie e. V., Hamburg, W.-Germany

Up till some years ago tobacco smoke inhalation experiments with laboratory animals did not lead to tumor formation. These negative results were related to the deposition of particles in the area of the nasal passages or the deposition of too small doses of smoke constituents in the lower respiratory tract. This was one reason for carrying out again and again the testing of smoke constituents in subcutaneous tissue or on the skin.

There are questions which still can be better answered by the skin painting experiment than by the inhalation experiment, for example, when testing the different effect of cigarette smoke condensate fractions. All experiments with smoke condensate have a considerable handicap. Smoke condensate does not represent whole smoke or even fresh smoke. Aging processes of the condensate and absence of the vapor phase as well as different anatomical and functional conditions of skin and respiratory epithelium may result in alterations of the biological activity. Therefore, application of smoke condensate in the respiratory tract should be considered under the same restrictions as on mouse skin. Cigarette smoke condensate was mostly applied intratracheally in solvents (WYNDER and HOFFMANN, 1967; SCHIEVELBEIN, 1968). The stay period of smoke components in the lung plays a decisive role for carcinogenic activity and is influenced by the solvent.

When condensate was blown into the respiratory tract (DONTENWILL and MOHR, 1962) a better distribution could in fact be obtained but the effect predominantly appeared in the upper respiratory tract. When condensate was injected according to the method of BLACKLOCK (1957), STANTON et al. (1972), or YERLY and NEUKOMM (1973), mechanical effects were as important as the localization of the injected material. The bronchial rubbing manipulations described by ROCKEY and SPEER (1966) are methodically nearly comparable with the epicutaneous condensate application.

As can be assumed, these methods showed a corresponding carcinogenic effect in the treated areas. An exact dosage in all experiments was very difficult. As OTTO (1974) we produced condensate aerosols and treated rats, hamsters, and mice for their entire lifespan. In these experiments, OTTO (1974) found adenomatoid lesions and metaplastic alterations in the rat lung. A distinct carcinogenic effect could not be proved. The production of aerosol with different generators and different solvents always leads to an alteration of condensate particles, i.e., aging processes cannot be excluded and physical-chemical alterations can influence the effect to a considerable degree.

Following the experiments of MERTENS (1930), CAMPBELL (1936), LORENZ et al. (1943), and ESSENBERG (1952) and others, these problems induced numerous investigators to carry out bioassays with native smoke. These investigations were based on the following questions:

1. Is the native smoke carcinogenic when inhaled?

2. Does the activity in the subcutaneous tissue or on the skin show a comparable effect in the respiratory tract?

3. Is there a comparable dose-response relationship between results of inhalation and skin painting experiments?

It is impossible to cite all authors having been engaged with inhalation experiments. Results of experiments are summarized in several monographs (for example, WYNDER and HOFFMANN, 1967, and SCHIEVELBEIN, 1968).

In order to stimulate discussion, we include some examples to show the principles of the different inhalation methods. Our first inhalation chamber was a copy of the type described by ESSENBERG (1952) (Fig. 1). Very soon, however, we realized that the CO-concentration and the risk of CO-intoxication was a handicap of this method. The toxic effect of CO limited the dose of application. Moreover, aging processes of the smoke and the deposition of smoke particles all over the skin were a problem, as in all experiments in which the animal body is exposed to smoke in large chambers.

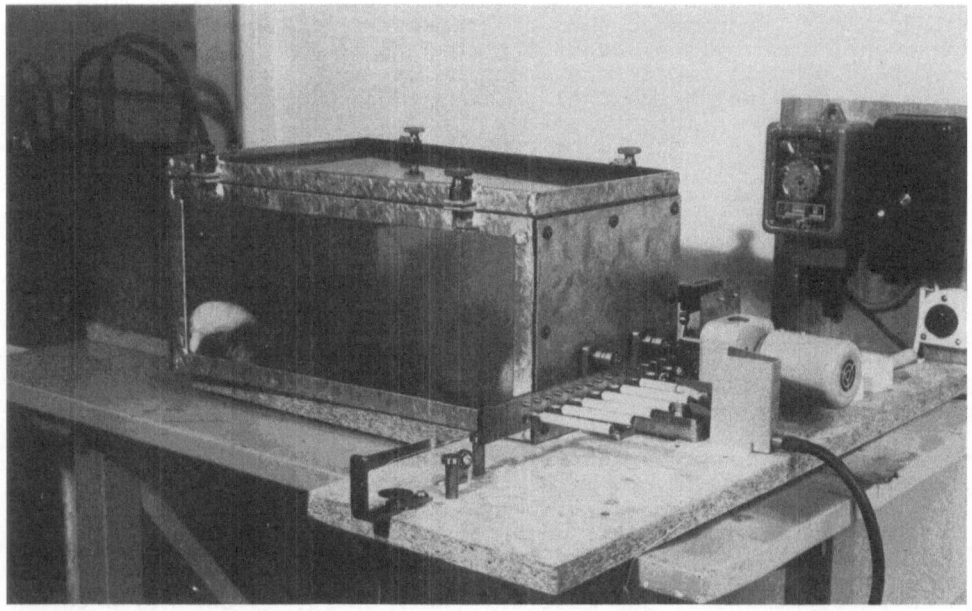

Fig. 1. Smoking machine with a large vacuum chamber designed for 10 hamsters ("closed smoking system")(DONTENWILL and MOHR, 1962)

By operative and mechanical occlusion of the nasal passages we tried to avoid nasal deposition, which is considered to be a limiting factor for the quantity of particles getting into the lower respiratory tract. This method, however, was not very successful.

In our second smoking machine (Figs 2 and 3), a so-called intermittent smoker with static smoke, the inhalation chamber was much smaller (DONTENWILL and WIEBECKE, 1966). Only the nose of the animal was exposed to smoke. With this method we tried to copy actual human smoking patterns as closely as possible: following a puff duration of 2 sec, the smoke remained in the smoking chamber for 8 sec; the puff volume was 35 ml, the smoke-to-air mixture was 1:5. In this experiment, we found severe precancerous lesions in the upper respiratory tract. One reason for changing over to other methods was the possibility of aging processes and alterations of the aerosol with this method.

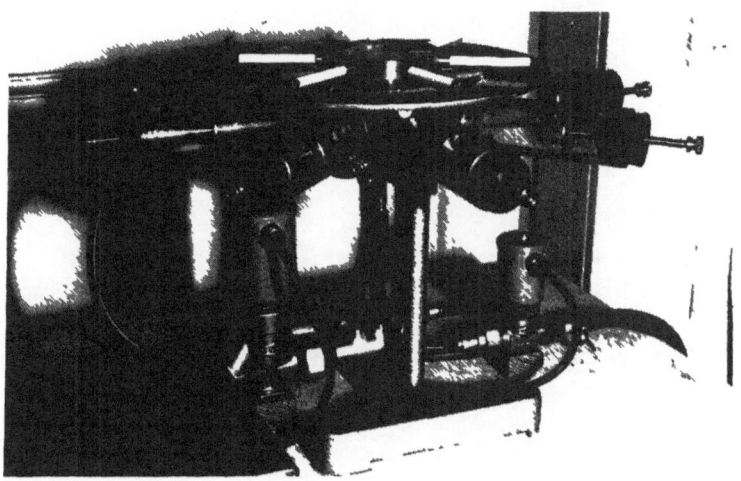

Fig. 2. Smoking machine with automatic smoke/air ventilation designed for 8 hamsters (type, DONTENWILL "closed smoking system")(DONTENWILL et al., 1966)

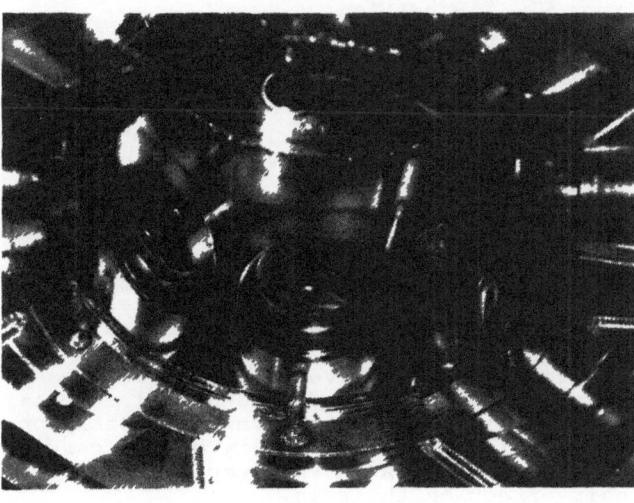

Fig. 3. Smoking chamber for the smoking machine described in Fig. 2

Our smoking machine, Hamburg II, provides a smoking cycle with conditions standardized according to human smoking habits (Figs 4 and 5).

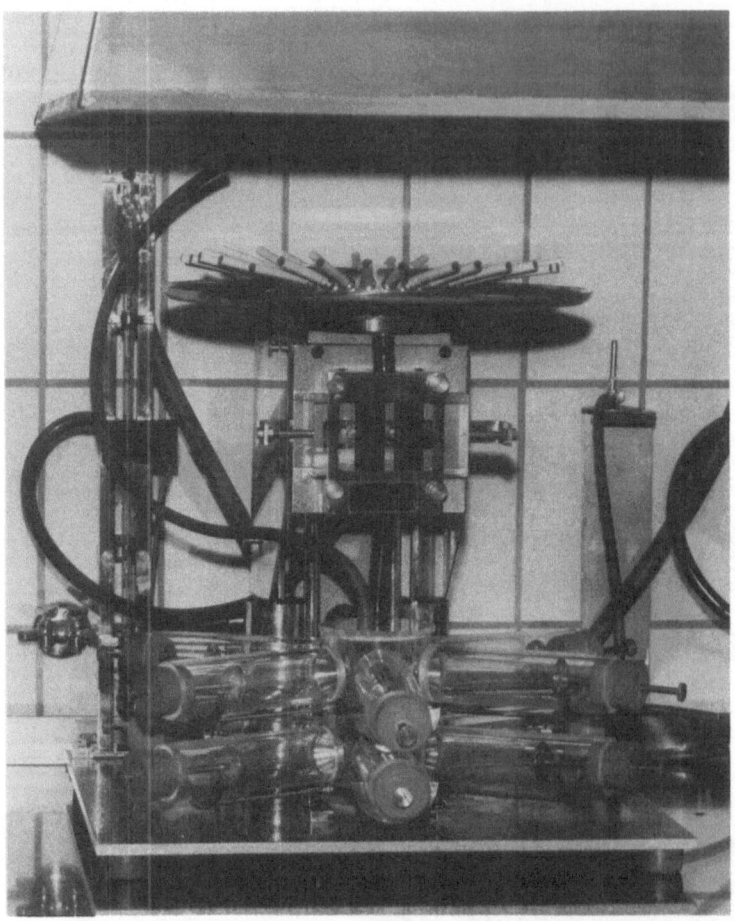

Fig. 4. Smoking machine type, Hamburg ("open smoking system"), adaptable to 10 hamsters, 10 rats, or 10 mice. The concentration of the smoke-to-air admixture is adjustable, and the puff volume is automatically controlled (RECKZEH et al., 1969)

The machine offers fresh, dynamic smoke; however, some alterations of the smoke aerosol cannot be avoided. The animals must inhale a high quantity of smoke without having a great chance of lung clearance. The guiding principle was to compare the effect of different smoke qualities in the respiratory tract. The decisive criterion in these experiments is the different tumor incidence under identical experimental conditions. We are of the opinion that these experimental conditions enable not only an evaluation of the intensity of the carcinogenic activity of different smoke qualities in the respiratory tract but also a comparison of their effect on the skin.

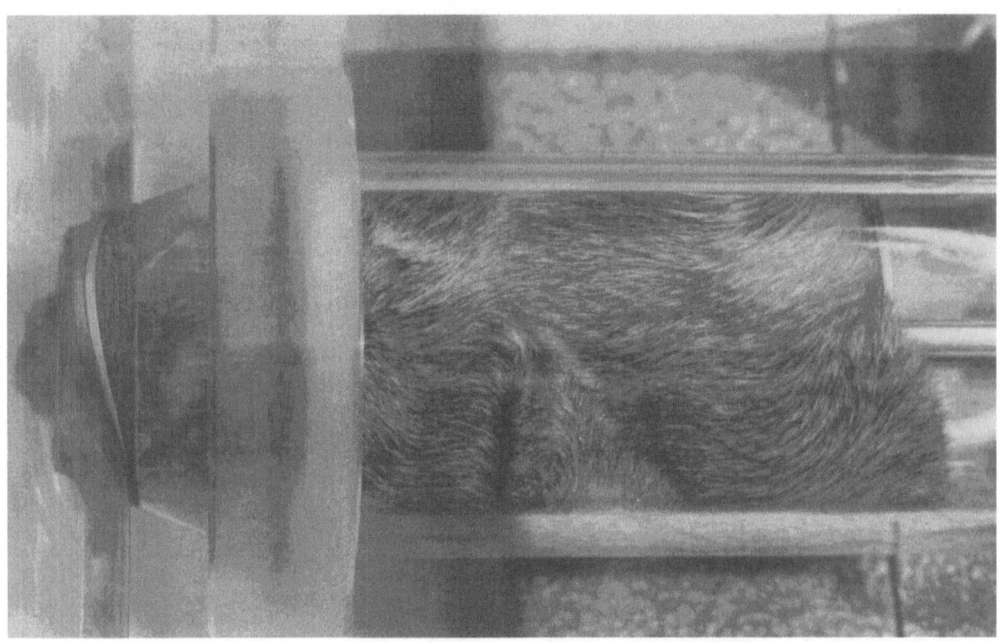

Fig. 5. Animal-holding tube of the smoking machine type, Hamburg.
Within the tube are immobilization equipment and an opening into the
smoking chamber for the nose and mouth of the hamster

The fact that in our experiments with hamsters tumors did not appear
in the lung but in the larynx is, in our opinion, not as decisive for
the basic question. However, it is desirable, and we hope possible,
that improvement of the smoking machines will provide stronger concentrations of the smoke aerosol in the lung, especially when using
animals showing a more effective aerosol distribution in the lung
than do Syrian golden hamsters. If such a method leads to a sufficient
number of tumors in the lung, a good model will have been found.

DAVIES (1974), for example, exposed rats to smoke using an intermittent
smoking machine. He found a stronger deposition of particles in the
lung and observed a low percentage of lung carcinomas in the animals.
The number of induced lung tumors was below 1% or 2%. Such a low tumor
incidence makes it difficult to compare 2 smoke qualities with different biological activity.

The method applied by HAMMOND et al. (1970) and AUERBACH et al. (1970)
is advantagous, first with regard to application of native smoke without substantial admixture of air, and second with regard to the bypass of nasal passages. A disadvantage of the experiments with dogs
is the duration of the experiment and the small number of animals per
group; findings are difficult to evaluate.

Experiments of AUERBACH et al. (1970) and our experiments (DONTENWILL,
1970; DONTENWILL et al., 1970, 1972, 1973) have mostly shown a comparable effect between inhalation and skin painting tests and a similar dose-response-relationship.

298

From the present findings it may be concluded that the inhalation experiment is a useful test for carrying out investigations on the development of safer cigarettes, i.e., it is possible to complete the experience and findings of the epicutaneous and subcutaneous experiments and to observe which changes of the product (tobacco mixture, filter tips, synthetic material, and reconstituted tobacco sheets) make the cigarettes less harmful.

References

AUERBACH, O., HAMMOND, E.C., KIRMAN, D., GARFINKEL, L.: II. Pulmonary Neoplasms. Arch. Environ. Hlth 21, 754-768 (1970).
BLACKLOCK, J.W.S.: The production of lung tumours in rats by 3,4-benzpyrene, methylcholanthrene and the condensate from cigarette tar. Brit. J. Cancer 11, 181 (1957).
CAMPBELL, J.A.: The effects of exhaust gases from internal combustion engines and of tobacco smoke upon mice, with special reference to incidence of tumours of the lung. Brit. J. exp. Path. 17, 146 (1936).
DAVIES, B.R.: Personal communication, 1974.
DONTENWILL, W.: Experimental investigations on the effects of cigarette smoke inhalation on small laboratory animals. In: Inhalation Carcinogenesis (M.G. Hanna, Jr., P. Nettesheim, J.R. Gilbert, eds). AEC Symposium Series no. 18, pp. 389-412. Oak Ridge, Tennessee: U.S. Atomic Energy Commission, Division of Technical Inf. 1970.
DONTENWILL, W., CHEVALIER, H.-J., HARKE, H.-P., KLIMISCH, H.-J., LAFRENZ, U., RECKZEH, G., FLEISCHMANN, B., KELLER, W.: Experimentelle Untersuchungen über die tumorerzeugende Wirkung von Zigarettenrauch-Kondensaten an der Mäusehaut. IV. Mitt. Z. Krebsforsch. 78, 236-264 (1972).
DONTENWILL, W., CHEVALIER, H.-J., HARKE, H.-P., LAFRENZ, U., RECKZEH, G., SCHNEIDER, B.: Investigations on the effects of chronic cigarette smoke inhalation in Syrian golden hamsters. J. nat. Cancer Inst. 51, 1781-1832 (1973).
DONTENWILL, W., ELMENHORST, H., HARKE, H.-P., RECKZEH, G., WEBER, K.-H., MISFELD, J., TIMM, J.: Experimentelle Untersuchungen über die tumorerzeugende Wirkung von Zigarettenrauch-Kondensaten an der Mäusehaut. I.-III. Mitt. Z. Krebsforsch. 73, 265-314 (1970).
DONTENWILL, W., MOHR, U.: Experimentelle Untersuchungen zum Problem der Carcinomenentstehung im Respirationstrakt. I. and II. Z. Krebsforsch. 65, 56 and 62 (1962).
DONTENWILL, W., RECKZEH, G., STADLER, L.: Inhalationsexperimente mit Zigarettenrauch. Beitr. Tabakforsch. 3, 437-447 (1966).
DONTENWILL, W., WIEBECKE, B.: Tracheal and pulmonary alteration following the inhalation of cigarette smoke by the golden hamster. In: Lung Tumours in Animals. Proc. of the Third Quadrennial Conference on Cancer, Perugia 1965, p. 519 (L. Severi, ed). Division of Cancer Res., University of Perugia 1966.
ESSENBERG, J.M.: Cigarette smoke and the incidence of primary neoplasm of the lung in the albino mouse. Science 116, 561 (1952).
HAMMOND, E.C., AUERBACH, O., KIRMAN, D., GARFINKEL, L.: Effects of cigarette smoking on dogs. Arch. Environ. Hlth 21, 740-753 (1970).
LORENZ, E., STEWART, H.L., DANIEL, J.H., NELSON, C.V.: The effect of breathing tobacco smoke on Strain A mice. Cancer Res. 3, 123 (1943).
MERTENS, V.E.: Zigarettenrauch eine Ursache des Lungenkrebses. Z. Krebsforsch. 32, 82 (1930).
OTTO, H.: Personal communication, 1974.

RECKZEH, G., RÜCKER, K., HARKE, H.-P., DONTENWILL, W.: Untersuchungen
zur Bestimmung der akuten and chronischen Toxizität von Zigarettenrauch bei passiver Berauchung von Versuchstieren. Arzneimittel-
Forsch. 2, 237-241 (1969).

ROCKEY, E.E., SPEER, F.D.: The ill effects of cigarette smoking in
dogs. Int. Surg. 46, 520 (1966).

SCHIEVELBEIN, H.: Nikotin - Pharmakologie and Toxikologie des Tabak-
rauches. Stuttgart: Georg Thieme 1968.

STANTON, M.F., MILLER, E., WRENCH, C., BLACKWELL, R.: Experimental
induction of epidermoid carcinoma in the lung of rats by cigarette
smoke condensate. J. nat. Cancer Inst. 49, 867-877 (1972).

WYNDER, E.L., HOFFMANN, D.: Tobacco and tobacco smoke. Studies in
Experimental Carcinogenesis. New York, London: Academic Press 1967.

YERLY, C., NEUKOMM, S.: Un test sensible et relativement rapide de
cancérisation du poumon de la souris. Z. Präventivmed. 18, 385-390
(1973).

A Modified Method for Locating Labeled Smoke Particles in Organs of Syrian Golden and European Hamsters

Gerd Reznik and U. Mohr

Abteilung für Experimentelle Pathologie, Medizinische Hochschule Hannover, Hannover-Kleefeld, W.-Germany

ABSTRACT

European and Syrian golden hamsters were passively exposed in a closed system to 32 puffs of labeled research cigarette smoke. All animals were trained with the smoke of unlabeled research cigarettes 21 days before the exposure to labeled smoke so that, as was demonstrated by pilot studies, the 2 hamster species could adjust themselves to the experimental conditions. Tissue samples were macerated during a 1 hour reflux-boiling in 100 ml of 20% methanolic KOH. Cambridge filters, butts, ashes and cellulose waddings which had been used to clean the suction hoods, exposure chambers and tubings were extracted with 150 ml toluene each. The additional procedures and measurements are described. The described smoking system represents a suitable model by which one can attain reproducible values regarding the effective dose of inhaled smoke particles in experimental animals.

Introduction

Chronic inhalation experiments with smoke are unsatisfactory when the total smoke dose administered throughout the experiment cannot be established. To determine where in the smoking apparatus as well as in the animal body, especially in respiratory system, the particles of the cigarette smoke are deposited, quantitative studies were under-taken by means of nonradioactive (LEWIS et al., 1972; CHEVALIER and DONTENWILL, 1972) or radioactive tracer techniques (JENKINS, Jr. et al., 1970; DONTENWILL et al., 1971; RUBIN, 1973; PAGE et al., 1973; DAVIS et al., 1973). The early investigators used various animal species, and their experimental equipment and smoking apparatuses differed markedly one from another, so that a comparison of their re-sults is somewhat difficult. Most of these experiments were performed by means of exposure chambers containing only 1 animal per exposure. The animals were brought into contact with the cigarette smoke by means of either a mask (LEWIS et al., 1972) that tightly enclosed the nose or by a collar that fixed their heads. DONTENWILL and colleagues (1971, 1973) exposed 10 Syrian golden hamsters simultaneously with the smoking machine type Hamburg. In almost all of these experiments, the animals were fixed and unable to move; in this way only their nasal apices and mouths were exposed to cigarette smoke.

To establish in which parts of the organism and smoking apparatus the smoke particles deposit, the cigarettes need to be labeled with a radioactive substance that is incorporated into the total particulate matter (TPM) of the smoke. Moreover, this substance must be chemically

and physiologically inert, should have a low volatility and must not
pyrolize. Paraffinic hydrocarbon dotriacontane-16,17-^{14}C satisfies
these conditions (RUBIN, 1973; HOUSEMAN, 1973; JENKINS et al., 1970;
DAVIS et al., 1973).

Materials and Methods

For our investigations we used research cigarettes, 60 mm long, labeled with dotriacontane-16,17-^{14}C, which had a specific activity of
55 mCi/mmol. For the first experiment, each cigarette was labeled
with 12 µCi dotriacontane dispersed in 120 µliter cyclohexane, according to the method of HOUSEMAN and HENAEGE (1973), while in the second
experiment, research cigarettes were labeled with 12.8 µCi dotriacontane. 11 male and 9 female European hamsters and 10 male and 10 female
Syrian golden hamsters were involved in the first experiment and 5
male and 4 female European hamsters and 4 male and 7 female Syrian
golden hamsters in the second experiment. All animals were 6 months
old and were daily trained for 21 days by exposure to the smoke of
unlabeled cigarettes.

For all of our experiments, a smoking machine Type RM 20/68 (Figs 1-3)
was employed. The smoking ring was equipped with 4 cigarettes (Figs
1 and 2) placed in the first, sixth, eleventh, and sixteenth holes,
thereby allowing 4 puffs of fresh air to be drawn between any 2 puffs
of smoke. During the 21 training days, the animals were daily exposed
for 10 minutes to 40 puffs of smoke and 160 puffs of fresh air. All
animal weights were weekly controlled. During the experiments with
labeled cigarettes, which were always performed on the twenty-second
day, 1 European and 1 Syrian golden hamster were alternatively exposed either in the morning or in the afternoon. In this way, the influence of probable variations in the activity of the animals caused
by a day-night cycle were excluded. The 4 labeled cigarettes were
smoked up to the eighth puff, inclusively, thus providing the animals
with 32 puffs of smoke and 128 puffs of fresh air. The exposure chambers were made of glass and had a volume of 1300 ml for the European
and 1000 ml for the Syrian golden hamster. The dead volume of the tubing connections and the cambridge filter pad was 76.8 ml. The mainstream smoke reached the exposure chamber through a 20-cm-long tube
(Figs 1-3). After it had passed through the exposure chamber, the
mainstream smoke reached a cambridge filter with a diameter of 90 mm
(Figs 1 and 2). There the resting particles of the mainstream smoke
were collected.

The combusted gas phase of the mainstream smoke was drawn by a syringe
pump (Figs 1 and 2) into the exposure chamber with a frequency of 1
puff smoke per minute per cigarette. Before each exposure, this pump
was bubbled out at a puff-volume of 35 ml Hg/2 sec. Behind the pump,
the gas phase passed over a KOH absorber (2N KOH) into 2 successive
beakers, each filled with 50 ml of scintillator liquid (Insta-Gel).
Both two-way spigots (Figs 1 and 2) placed before the high-vacuum
pump were open. This large pump drew the sidestream smoke over the
cambridge filter situated in the uppermost tapering of the suction
hood (Figs 1-3). The gas phase of the side stream of smoke was also
directed over 2N KOH to 2 beakers filled with 50 ml of scintillator
liquid. After the fourth puff of air following the last puff of smoke,
the two-way spigot at the rear exit of the exposure chamber was opened
(Figs 1-3), the spigot positioned before the high-vacuum pump (Fig. 3)
was closed, and the residual smoke in the chamber was drawn out. The

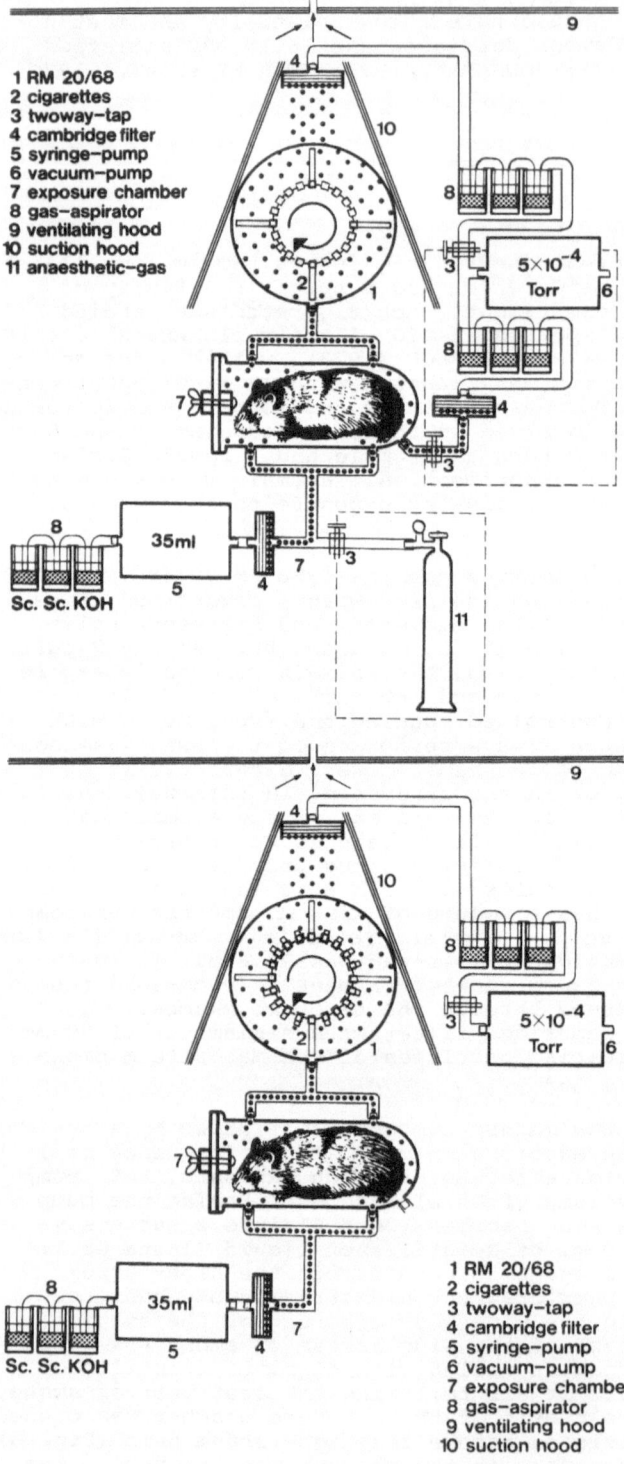

1 RM 20/68
2 cigarettes
3 twoway-tap
4 cambridge filter
5 syringe-pump
6 vacuum-pump
7 exposure chamber
8 gas-aspirator
9 ventilating hood
10 suction hood
11 anaesthetic-gas

Sc. Sc. KOH

Fig. 1. Total experimental equipment for passive smoke exposure of European and Syrian golden hamsters. Broken lines indicate appararatus for exhaust of sidestream smoke and gas for sacrificing of animals

1 RM 20/68
2 cigarettes
3 twoway-tap
4 cambridge filter
5 syringe-pump
6 vacuum-pump
7 exposure chamber
8 gas-aspirator
9 ventilating hood
10 suction hood

Fig. 2. Smoking system during the exposure time: the mainstream smoke is drawn into the animal chamber by means of a syringe pump (5), whereas the sidestream smoke is drawn over a cambridge filter by means of a vacuum pump (6)

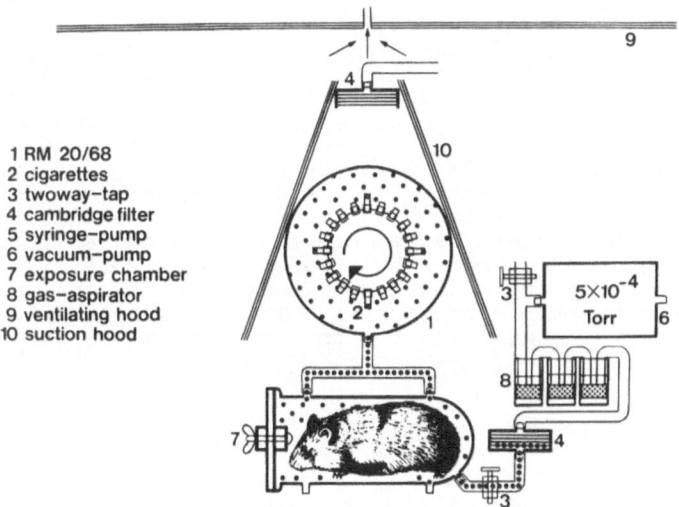

1 RM 20/68
2 cigarettes
3 twoway-tap
4 cambridge filter
5 syringe-pump
6 vacuum-pump
7 exposure chamber
8 gas-aspirator
9 ventilating hood
10 suction hood

5×10^{-4} Torr

Fig. 3. Experimental conditions at the end of the exposure: the smoke remaining in the animal chamber is exhausted after stopping of the smoking machine

residual smoke particles were collected from the chamber on the cambridge filter behind the exposure chamber (Fig. 2). Thereafter, the animal in the exposure chamber was killed with nitrous oxide (N_2O). Also from each hamster species, 1 male and 1 female were exposed to the gas phase of labeled cigarettes. During these exposures, a cambridge filter, 90 mm in diameter, was placed between the smoking machine and exposure chamber. When all experiments were completed, 1 additional male European hamster, which served as a control, was exposed to the mainstream smoke of unlabeled cigarettes in the same smoking system.

After death, all animals were immediately removed from the exposure chamber and autopsied in a vertical hanging position. Precautions were taken to avoid cross-contamination. Tissue samples were macerated during a 1-hour reflux boiling in 100 ml of 20% methanolic KOH solution. The maceration product was cooled and extracted 3 times with 50 ml toluene. The 3 extracts were mixed and of each sample, 2 aliquots were taken and counted in an Insta-Gel scintillator cocktail. Counting periods lasted 10 minutes or were regulated for proper counting statistics. An internal standard (dotriacontane-16,17-^{14}C of known quantity) was added to each sample and the data used for applying quenching corrections. A Packard Tricarb Model 455 liquid scintillation spectrometer was used for counting the samples. From the changes in the counting rates with and without internal standard, the gain in counts per minute (cpm) for samples of extremely different compositions and stainings can be determined in detail. After all samples with and without internal standard had been measured, the quenching factor of toluene was determined.

To determine the activity distribution of the entire system, the activity deposited on the smoking machine instrumentation, exposure chambers, tubings, butts, ashes, suction hood, rubber lips, and cambridge filters had to be measured. Immediately after each exposure, all cambridge filters were extracted for 3 hours with 150 ml toluene

in a soxhlet. The butts, ashes, and cellulose waddings that had been
used to clean the suction hoods, exposure chambers, and tubings were
also extracted with 150 ml toluene each. The combusted sidestream and
mainstream gas phases were absorbed in 2N KOH and Insta-Gel and ali-
quoted directly for counting.

The amount of dotricontane-16,17-^{14}C in the cigarettes was determined
by extracting each of 12 cigarettes for the first experiment and 5
cigarettes for the second experiment in 150 ml toluene and measuring
their activity by liquid scintillation counting. The degree of uniformity of the activity throughout the cigarettes was determined by
sectioning 1 cigarette of the second experiment into 11 equal portions
and conducting wet combustions on each in a Tricarb sample oxidizer
Model 306 (Packard). The mean value for the sections was 9.09 $\pm$ 0.77%.

Results

During the 21-day training period, the animals demonstrated a definite
weight loss during the first week. This weight loss decreased during
the next week, and by the end of the training period the hamsters began to regain weight; this was especially noticeable for the European
hamsters. The weight curves demonstrate that exposure to a maximal
amount of smoke, as in the present system, presents a definite stress
factor for the animals and that it takes nearly 3 weeks for them to
become accustomed to the smoke exposure. Therefore, one can assume
that after the 21 days training, the animals breath so that they inhale
maximal quantities of smoke during their exposure to labeled cigarette
smoke. Moreover, being kept in an elongated exposure chamber probably
did not stress the animals, because these rodents normally live in
tube-like burrows when in their natural habitat. The animals could
move about the exposure chambers unrestrained and thereby causing a
good mixing of the smoke throughout the chamber. It was previously
shown that the system requires about 2 minutes before the smoke is
equally distributed.

In the first experiment, the mean total of labeled dotriacontane activity of 12 cigarettes was found to be 11.26 µCi = 93.8% of 12 µCi
injected into each cigarette. In the second experiment, the cigarettes
contained 12.33 µCi = 96.34% of the injected 12.8 µCi. In Experiment 1,
the total recovery expressed as percentage of the initial loading was
70.27% for both hamster species wereas in Experiment 2 it amounted to
68.24% (Table 1). For the following calculations, all values are expressed as percentages of the total recovery which was set at 100%.
From these total recoveries after exposure of European hamsters 91.53%
and after exposure of Syrian golden hamsters 95.56% of the activity
was found in the various parts of the smoking system including mainstream and sidestream smoke and parts of the 4 cigarettes, e.g., butts
and ashes.

As can be seen in Table 2, the amount of labeled dotriacontane remaining in the butts was fairly constant (about 47% in Experiment 1 and
42% in Experiment 2 (Table 3) when expressed as a percentage of initial
loading). No differences were found between European and Syrian golden
hamsters in Experiment 1, whereas in Experiment 2 the differences between the 2 species amounted to 6%. Expressed as a percentage of the
total recovery the activity of the butts were 66% in the first and
63% in the second experiment (Tables 2 and 3). These values did not
differ between the 2 hamster species. Since all cigarettes were smoked

Table 1. Total recoveries from Experiments 1 and 2

Animals exposed		nCi	Total ^{14}C-activity as % of initial loading	nCi	^{14}C-activity as % of initial loading without animal	^{14}C-activity as % of total recovery without animal
Experiment 1						
EH ♂	$\bar{x}$	31341.97	69.64	28516.99	63.37	90.99
	s	1108.05	2.46	1086.26	2.41	
EH ♀	$\bar{x}$	32689.79	72.64	30097.62	66.88	92.07
	s	1687.41	3.75	1045.36	2.32	
SGH ♂	$\bar{x}$	31222.69	69.38	29717.69	66.03	95.18
	s	1460.72	3.25	1553.91	3.45	
SGH ♀	$\bar{x}$	31284.72	69.52	30012.22	66.69	95.93
	s	2410.78	5.36	2247.78	4.99	
Experiment 2						
EH ♂	$\bar{x}$	34849.38	70.66	31246.95	63.36	89.66
	s	2465.98	5.00	2228.98	4.52	
EH ♀	$\bar{x}$	34092.59	69.13	29967.95	60.76	87.90
	s	2729.25	5.53	3003.35	6.09	
SGH ♂	$\bar{x}$	32892.16	66.69	31669.10	64.21	96.28
	s	4091.20	8.30	3911.87	7.93	
SGH ♀	$\bar{x}$	32801.74	66.51	31022.66	62.90	94.58
	s	2220.52	4.50	2217.97	4.50	

Table 2. Total smoke distribution in Experiment 1

Smoke phase Animal	Percentage of total ^{14}C-activity added to 4 cigarettes[a]				Percentage of total recovered activity			
	EH ♂	EH ♀	SGH ♂	SGH ♀	EH ♂	EH ♀	SGH ♂	SGH ♀
Sidestream gas	0.38	0.32	0.25	0.29	0.55	0.44	0.36	0.42
Sidestream TPM	2.87	2.93	4.39	2.70	4.12	4.03	6.33	3.89
Mainstream gas	0.22	0.22	0.20	0.24	0.31	0.30	0.33	0.34
Mainstream TPM	12.47	11.48	15.61	17.27	17.92	15.82	22.52	24.86
Butt	48.57	49.20	45.35	47.83	68.07	67.79	65.42	66.94
Ash	0.03	0.03	0.02	0.02	0.05	0.04	0.03	0.03

[a]Total ^{14}C-activity extracted from whole unsmoked 4 cigarettes = 45040 NCi.

Table 3. Total smoke distribution in Experiment 2

Smoke phase Animal	Percentage of total ^{14}C-activity added to 4 cigarettes[a]				Percentage of total recovered activity			
	EH ♂	EH ♀	SGH ♂	SGH ♀	EH ♂	EH ♀	SGH ♂	SGH ♀
Sidestream gas	0.48	0.46	0.56	0.61	0.68	0.66	0.84	0.97
Sidestream TPM	5.05	4.83	6.27	6.44	7.14	6.99	9.41	10.24
Mainstream gas	0.09	0.14	0.13	0.17	0.13	0.20	0.19	0.27
Mainstream TPM	11.48	12.93	17.46	16.63	16.25	18.71	26.18	26.44
Butt	46.22	42.36	40.18	37.75	65.41	61.29	60.25	56.76
Ash	0.03	0.02	0.03	0.02	0.02	0.03	0.04	0.04

[a]Total ^{14}C-activity extracted from whole unsmoked 4 cigarettes = 49320 NCi.

to a butt length of 23 mm from a beginning length of 60 mm and since filtration might add a maximum of 10% to these uniformly loaded cigarettes, we should have theoretically found a final butt concentration of up to 50% of the original activity of the cigarette. Our results ranged between 42% in Experiment 2 and 47% in Experiment 1. JENKINS and colleagues (1970) found no filtration of labeled dotriacontane in a 20-mm butt, but DAVIS and his coworkers (1973) found about 9% of the activity to be filtered by the butt. The transfer of the activity to mainstream smoke (mainstream TPM) was directly measured for 4 animals, while for the remaining cases it was calculated by summing the amounts of activity found in the exhaust from the chamber, the chamber itself, and the tubing. These totals are listed in Tables 2 and 3 and expressed both as percentage of the initial loading and of the total recovered activity. The mean transfer of activity to mainstream TPM for the cigarettes amounted to 17% in both experiments for the European hamsters. For the Syrian golden hamster, it was 24% in Experiment 1 and 26% in Experiment 2. DAVIS and collaborators (1973) and JENKINS and coworkers (1970) reported about 20% transfer of labeled dotriacontane activity. The differences between the 2 hamster species might be explained by the fact that the larger European hamster represents a larger intercepting surface for the smoke particles and can take up more particles by its thicker fur than can the Syrian golden hamster (KMOCH and MOHR, 1974). These 2 factors cause a reduction of the mainstream TPM in both species as in our calculations, so that part of the TPM that was retained either in or on the animal was subtracted. The mainstream gas phase values expressed as percentages of the total recovered activity amounted to 0.3% in Experiment 1 (Table 2) and to 0.2% in Experiment 2 (Table 3), thus corresponding to the results of DAVIS and his coworkers (1973).

Discussion

The recovery of activity from sidestream TPM is listed in Tables 2 and 3 and demonstrates that the apparent transfer to sidestream TPM is about one-fourth that of the mainstream transfer in Experiment 1 and about one-third to one-half in Experiment 2. It has been found for a number of compounds used as tracers for TPM that the amount of tracer or activity transferred to sidestream TPM during the interpuff period exceeds that transferred to mainstream TPM by anything up to a ratio of 2:1, respectively (JENKINS et al., 1970; DAVIS et al., 1973). Under the present experimental conditions, similar results were not obtained as with an open smoking system, so it is impossible to get values comparable to those obtained from a closed system used by the aforementioned authors. Although the mainstream gas phase normally contains little or no activity, pyrolysis of the labeled dotriacontane during the interpuff smoulder period is known to result in appreciable amounts of activity being transferred to the sidestream gas phase. In both our experiments, the sidestream gas phase was found to be one-tenth the values measured for the sidestream TPM. The activity of the ashes was 0.03% the initial loading - a fact that does not coincide with the results of DAVIS and his collaborators (1973), who found no activity in the ashes. Possibly, during the present experiments, the ashes were contaminated during the interpuff phase when the smoking cigarette was in the sidestream.

Summary

In summary, the smoking system described here represents a suitable model by which one can attain reproducible values regarding the effective dose of inhaled smoke particles in experimental animals without their being stressed by coercive measures that might otherwise falsify the results.

Acknowledgements

The authors thank the British American Tobacco Company of Southhampton, England, for labeling the cigarettes in Experiment 1 and for partially supporting that experiment and the British American Tobacco Company of Hamburg, Germany, for furnishing equipment. We are very grateful to HORST SCHOSTEK and HEINZ RÖBER for their excellent technical assistance and NAOMA CRISP LINDGREN for editing the manuscript.

References

CHEVALIER, H.J., DONTENWILL, W.: Experimentelle Untersuchungen über die Ablagerung von inhalierten Partikeln im Kehlkopf von Syrischen Goldhamstern. Z. Versuchstierk. 14, 271-276 (1972).

DAVIS, B.R., HOUSEMAN, T.H., RODERICK, H.R.: The use of dotricontane-16,17-^{14}C as a marker for the deposition of cigarette smoke in the lungs of experimental animals. Beitr. Tabakforsch. 7 (3), 148-153 (1973).

DONTENWILL, W., CHEVALIER, H.J., HARKE, H.P., LAFRENZ, U., RECKZEH, G., SCHNEIDER, B.: Investigations on the effects of chronic cigarette smoke inhalation in Syrian golden hamsters. J. nat. Cancer Inst. 51, 1781-1832 (1973).

DONTENWILL, W., HARKE, H.P., BAARS, A., GOERTZ, E.: Experimentelle Untersuchungen über Aufnahme und Ablagerung von Rauchbestandteilen bei der passiven Berauchung von Goldhamstern mit Zigarettenrauch. Arzneim. Forsch. (Drug Res.) 21, 142-143 (1971).

HOUSEMAN, T.H.: Studies of cigarette smoke transfer using radioisotopically labeled tobacco constituents. Part II: The transference of radioisotopically labeled nicotine to cigarette smoke. Beitr. Tabakforsch. 7 (3), 142-147 (1973).

HOUSEMAN, T.H., HENAEGE, E.: Studies of cigarette smoke transfer using radioisotopically labeled tobacco constituents. Part I: The preparation of radioisotopically labeled cigarettes. Beitr. Tabakforsch. 7 (3), 138-141 (1973).

JENKINS, R.W., Jr., NEWMAN, R.H., CARPENTER, R.D., OSDENE, T.S.: Cigarette smoke formation studies. I. Distribution and mainstream products from added ^{14}C-dotriacontane-16,17. Beitr. Tabakforsch. 5, 295-298 (1970).

KMOCH, N., MOHR, U.: Dotriacontane-16,17-^{14}C distribution pattern in the respiratory system of 2 hamster species after passive exposure to radioactive labeled smoke. International Symposium "Experimental Respiratory Carcinogenesis and Bioassays", Seattle, Washington, USA, 23-26 June, 1974.

LEWIS, C.J., MCGEADY, J.C., WAGNER, J.R., SCHULTZ, F.J., SPEARS, A.W.: Dichlorbenzophenone as a nonradioactive tracer for cigarette smoke-gas chromatographie analysis of tracer. Amer. Rev. Resp. Dis. 106, 480-484 (1972).

MOHR, U., REZNIK, G., ECKHART, W., KMOCH, N., HAAS, H.: Distribution of labeled smoke particles in the respiratory tract of the hamster. Naturwissenschaften 61, 133-134 (1974).

PAGE, B.F.J., WOOLSGROVE, B., CHASSEAUD, L.F., BINNS, R.: Use of radioactive tracer techniques in investigations associated with cigarette smoking. Ann. occup. Hyg. 16, 409-416 (1973).

RUBIN, J.B.: A simplified method for the determination of labeled alkane hydrocarbons in mammalian tissue and blood after exposure to radiolabeled cigarette smoke. Analytical Letters 6 (5), 387-396 (1973).

Dotriacontane-16, 17-^{14}C Distribution Pattern in the Respiratory System of Two Hamster Species after Passive Exposure to Radioactive Labelled Smoke

Norbert Kmoch and U. Mohr

Abteilung für Experimentelle Pathologie, Medizinische Hochschule Hannover, Hannover-Kleefeld, W.-Germany

ABSTRACT

The quantitative and qualitative distribution of C^{14} labeled dotria-contane (DOT-C^{14}) determined by liquid scintillation counting and auto-radiography in the respiratory system, the digestive tract, liver and kidneys of Syrian golden and European hamsters, males and females, is described after they had been exposed to radioactive labeled cigarette smoke. The different DOT-C^{14} distributions are discussed in detail with special attention given to the respiratory tract, related species differences and the topographic subdivisions of apex nasi, fundus na-si, pharynx, larynx, trachea, and lungs. It is apparent that the abso-lute amount of activity in the respiratory tract related to body size of the Syrian golden hamster is greater than in the European hamster but that the percentual distribution exhibits a greater filtering ac-tion of the upper respiratory tract of Syrian golden hamster than of the European hamster so that a larger percentual amount of total in-haled particulate matter reaches the lungs. The European hamster might be a more useful model for the investigation of respiratory tract car-cinogenesis due to the possibility of a longer life time exposure and a higher sensitivity to respiratory tract carcinogens.

Introduction

The correlation between cigarette smoking and lung cancer outlined by STOCKS and CAMPBELL (1955) and STOCKS (1966) and others has stimulated the undertaking of many experimental approaches to this problem. MOSHY (1967) has compiled a review of the experimental results gained from various animal species with various methods. The difference between the incidence of lung cancer in smokers and the histologic results attained from experimental animals chronically exposed to cigarette smoke has led several investigators to recognize the necessity of dosimetric studies for smoke inhalation (HOLLAND et al., 1958; DONTEN-WILL, 1970; DONTENWILL et al., 1971; LEWIS et al., 1972; DAVIES et al., 1973; PAGE et al., 1973; MOHR et al., 1974). To determine the amount of cigarette smoke deposited in the various parts of the re-spiratory tract, radioactive labeled smoke tracers are most effective because of the increased sensitivity and specificity associated with radioisotopical analysis by means of liquid scintillation counting or autoradiography. In our studies, the labeled hydrocarbon dotriacontane was used as it distilled into the particulate phase of cigarette smoke with minimal pyrolysis (JENKINS et al., 1970) and was chemically and physiologically inert. We compared the distribution pattern of radio-active labeled smoke particles in 2 hamster species: the widely used Syrian golden hamster (DONTENWILL, 1970; DONTENWILL et al., 1971, 1973) and the European hamster (MOHR et al., 1972) - a new experimental animal used in our laboratory.

The European hamster has demonstrated a higher tumorigenic sensitivity of its respiratory tract (MOHR et al., 1972) and lives 2 to 3 times longer than the Syrian golden hamster (ZIMMERMANN, 1966) so that the possibility of a higher sensitivity is combined with a longer life span.

Materials and Methods

A description of the materials and methods, especially the exposure system, is given in detail by REZNIK and MOHR (these Proceedings). The animals were exposed in 2 seasonally different experiments, the first in autumn (Series A) and the second in spring (Series B). The distribution of the animals involved was as follows: in Series A, there were 11 male and 9 female European hamsters (EH) and 10 male and 10 female Syrian golden hamsters (SGH); in Series B, there were 5 male and 4 female European hamsters and 4 male and 7 female Syrian golden hamsters. For mean body weight and standard deviations, see Table 1. All animals were about 6 months old and were trained over a 3-week period by daily exposure to unlabeled smoke enabling better breathing under experimental conditions. During the experiment the trained animals were exposed to 32 puffs of labeled smoke, the volume being 35 ml for each 2-second puff drawn by an RM 20/68 smoking machine from 4 cigarettes.

Dotriacontane-16,17-^{14}C labeling of cigarettes was 12.0 µCi/cigarette for Series A and 12.8 µCi/cigarette for Series B. After exposure to the smoke, the animals were immediately sacrificed with nitrous oxide (N_2O) and dissected in a vertical hanging position as follows: skinning was performed by removing the tip of the nose until exposing the nasal cartillage. As shown in Fig. 1, the various parts of the respiratory tract were isolated. To avoid contamination of the nasal apex and nasal fundus, the mucosa was separated from the hard palate. The palatal mucosa, pharynx, tongue, and oesophagus were dissected in toto. The forestomach, stomach, and duodenom were taken from the digestive tract. Liver, kidney, and blood from the left ventricle were each separately investigated. The fur and feet were extracted with toluene in a soxhlet apparatus while blood was solubilized in a tissue solubilizer (TS-1,

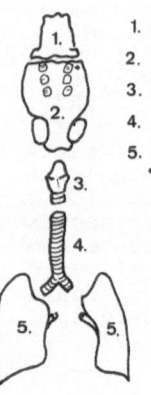

1. NASAL APEX
2. NASAL FUNDUS
3. LARYNX
4. TRACHEA
5. LUNGS
  • first molar tooth

Fig. 1. Dissection pattern for the respiratory tracts of the European and Syrian golden hamsters. The nasal apex includes the nasoturbinals and maxilloturbinals, and the nasal fundus the endoturbinals. The larynx was excised with the epiglottis and the cricoid cartilage

Table 1. Total mainstream smoke was calculated from the TPM-^{14}C found in the exposure system behind the rubber lips as well as in and on the animals. Differences between the reported number of male Syrian golden hamsters of Series A in the text and in this table are due to the death of 2 animals during the training period

| Series | Animal Species | Sex | N | Body weight (g) | | Distribution of total mainstream TPM ^{14}C-activity (nCi) | | | | | | | |
| | | | | | | Total mainstream | | Total animal | | Extrinsic[a] | | Intrinsic[b] | |
				$\bar{x}$	s	$\bar{x}$	s	$\bar{x}$	s	$\bar{x}$	s	$\bar{x}$	s
A	EH	♂	11	311	61			2,825.0	565.2	2,583.6	558.1	241.4	71.6
		♀	9	261	35	8,919.8	821.7	2,592.2	574.8	2,388.0	543.9	204.3	42.0
	SGH	♂	8	95	17			1,487.2	272.9	1,279.2	264.6	213.1	44.6
		♀	10	100	18			1,401.2	180.2	1,170.2	173.5	230.9	68.2
B	EH	♂	5	336	30			3,602.4	481.8	3,130.1	461.8	472.4	104.1
		♀	4	309	60	9,384.6	2,417.6	4,124.6	544.0	3,715.9	516.6	408.8	104.7
	SGH	♂	4	99	18			1,222.0	248.4	1,043.7	249.8	179.8	89.2
		♀	7	110	15			1,779.1	256.7	1,470.5	211.1	308.6	72.4

[a] Fur and feet.
[b] Inhaled and ingested activity.

Koch-Light Laboratories, Ltd., Buckinghamshire, England), and the
organs were boiled under reflux in methanolic KOH and extracted with
toluene. 2 identical aliquots of each organ extract were adjusted for
an optimal counting rate and measured in a liquid scintillation counter
(Model Tricarb 455, Packard). The quench factor was corrected by adding an internal standard and recounting the sample. Organ background
was determined from trained animals exposed to unlabeled smoke. For 2
animals of each species whole-body autoradiography was performed according to the method of ULLBERG (1954) and modified by PATZSCHKE (1968).
The animals were trained and exposed under the same conditions as described above, except that cigarettes were labeled with 27.0 µCi dotria-
contane/cigarette. Zero effect for liquid scintillation counting was
30 dpm including organ background. Any value twice the zero effect was
taken as valid. All research cigarettes used were radioactively marked
according to the method reported by HOUSEMAN and coworkers (1973).

Results

All the activity found in the animals was due to TPM-^{14}C, since in 4
animals exposed to the gas phase only, no activity was detected, which
agrees with the results of DAVIES and colleagues (1973). No resorption
of DOT-16,17-^{14}C took place in the respiratory tract or in the digestive
tract during exposure, since no activity was found in the blood, liver,
or kidneys by liquid scintillation counting and autoradiography. From
the values for total mainstream distribution (Table 1), it is apparent
that the activity recovered from the fur and feet - extrinsic activity -
was greater for the European hamster than for the Syrian golden hamster.
For the inhaled and ingested activity - intrinsic activity - there was
no marked difference between the animal species of Series A despite
the much lower body weight of the Syrian golden hamster. The overall
higher absolute values for Series B animals are partially due to the
somewhat greater amount of radioactivity in the cigarettes used in the
latter series. Therefore, to find seasonal differences between Series
A and B, only percentage values can be compared (Fig. 2). It is shown
that intrinsic activity in the European hamsters of Series B is almost twice as high as in Series A, whereas the intrinsic activity of
Syrian golden hamsters in Series B is not markedly different from that
in Series A. As shown in Fig. 3, where the intrinsic activities are set
at 100%, this higher intrinsic activity in European hamsters is seen
in both the respiratory tract as well as the digestive tract and cannot be due only to the slightly greater body weight of animals in Series
B but rather to possible seasonal differences in respiratory and digestive activities of this not yet completely domesticated animal. Although hormonal and metabolic seasonal differences have been reported
for this animal (KAYSER and AARON, 1938, 1950; RATHS, 1964), it is not
quite clear in what manner these factors reflect upon their breathing
and digestive patterns during smoke exposure. Comparing the European
hamster with the Syrian golden hamster in Fig. 3, more percentage of
activity was recovered from the digestive tract of Syrian golden hamsters. This was due to a much greater swallowed amount of TPM-^{14}C by
the Syrian golden hamster than by the European hamster as shown by the
absolute values for the forestomach and stomach (Table 2). This swallowed activity could have originated from the nose or mouth, but after
reviewing the autoradiographs and liquid scintillation results, we
established that the activity was displaced from the nasal pharynx into the digestive tract.

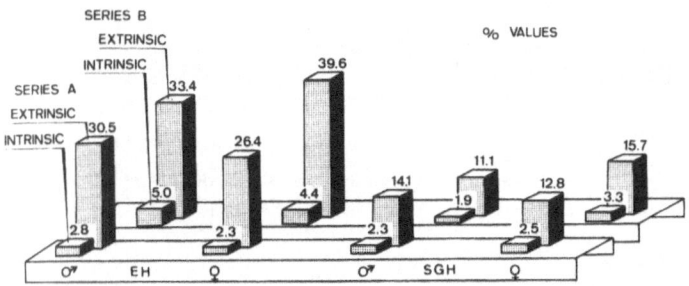

Fig. 2

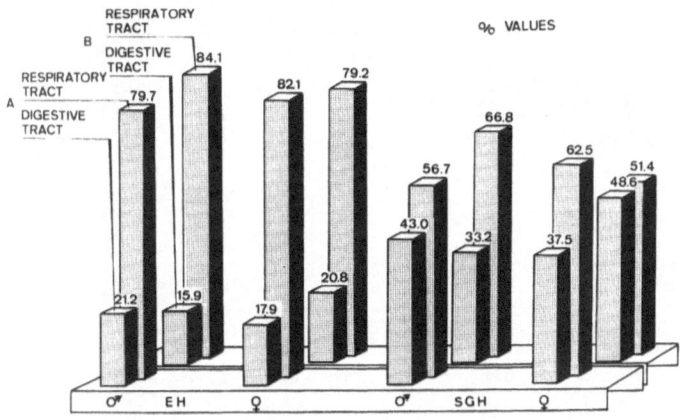

Fig. 3

Fig. 2. Columns represent the amount of TPM-^{14}C found on the animals (extrinsic) and in the animals (intrinsic) as the percentage of the total mainstream smoke, specified by animal species and sex. The front row represents Series A, the back row Series B. The absolute values of total mainstream smoke were taken from Table 1 and set at 100%. (For numbers of animals, see Tables 1 and 2)

Fig. 3. Percentage distribution of the intrinsic TPM-^{14}C activity in the respiratory tract, which includes the organs shown in Fig. 1, and in the digestive tract (pharynx, forestomach, and stomach). Total intrinsic values for each animal were set at 100% and calculated for the mean. Series, species, and sex relations are the same as in Fig. 2. (For numbers of animals, see Tables 1 and 2)

The absolute TPM-^{14}C activity of the various respiratory tract organs was summed for each sex and species and set at 100% for comparison of the respiratory tract TPM-^{14}C distribution pattern in Figs 4 (a) and (b). From these figures, the following conclusions may be drawn: 1. The amount of TPM-^{14}C activity retained in the lungs of both hamster species is high in relation to the other respiratory tract organs. This is seen in both Series A and B, indicating the reproducibility of this result. 2. Although the significance was not evaluated because of the limited number of animals, especially in Series B, there is a species difference in the distribution pattern in Series A, with a higher TPM-^{14}C activity settling in the nose, larynx, and trachea of the Syrian golden hamster.

Table 2. Distribution of the TPM-14C activity found in the animals; the duodenum irregularly exhibited values near the limit of validity (twice the zero effect) and were therefore not considered in further calculations. Differences between total activity and the sum of activity recovered from organs in the same row are due to the skewedness of the distribution of single values

Series	Animal species	Sex	N	Body weight (g)		Absolute organ values of inhaled and ingested (intrinsic) TPM-14C activity (nCi dotriacontane-16,17-14C)																
						Total		Nasal apex		Nasal fundus		Larynx		Trachea		Lungs		Pharynx[a]		Fore-stomach		Stomach	
				$\bar{x}$	s	$\bar{x}$	s	$\bar{x}$	s	$\bar{x}$	s	$\bar{x}$	s	$\bar{x}$	s	$\bar{x}$	s	$\bar{x}$	s	$\bar{x}$	s	$\bar{x}$	s
A	EH	♂	11	311	61	241.4	71.6	21.6	15.6	4.9	2.1	22.8	12.9	1.8	0.7	128.9	24.2	13.4	8.6	37.0	46.3	8.2	16.8
		♀	9	261	35	204.2	42.9	29.9	12.7	3.2	1.3	6.4	3.2	1.7	0.7	125.6	26.2	14.3	6.2	21.3	15.3	1.3	2.4
	SGH	♂	8	95	17	213.1	44.6	10.6	5.0	20.0	7.6	16.7	9.9	10.5	13.0	64.9	24.6	12.9	5.5	44.7	26.4	40.3	37.0
		♀	10	100	18	230.9	68.2	14.1	8.5	22.8	18.4	21.2	13.4	6.2	10.5	81.9	40.0	24.4	15.5	59.7	31.8	0.6	1.7
B	EH	♂	5	336	50	472.4	104.1	135.9	61.5	11.5	8.7	16.6	4.5	1.5	0.5	231.9	25.7	31.3	12.5	39.8	25.3	15.4	24.5
		♀	4	309	60	408.8	104.7	63.5	42.5	7.9	6.8	39.8	7.4	3.1	0.7	215.0	71.0	12.6	6.6	54.8	15.4	8.4	5.3
	SGH	♂	4	99	18	179.8	89.2	16.9	9.0	15.4	10.5	7.9	4.1	2.5	1.1	72.6	27.5	12.6	6.2	32.3	27.9	19.4	22.1
		♀	7	110	15	308.6	72.4	26.5	10.3	16.8	7.4	25.5	19.7	4.4	4.0	86.5	38.0	53.9	33.7	76.7	47.0	16.3	40.3

[a] Including palatum, tongue, and oesophagus.

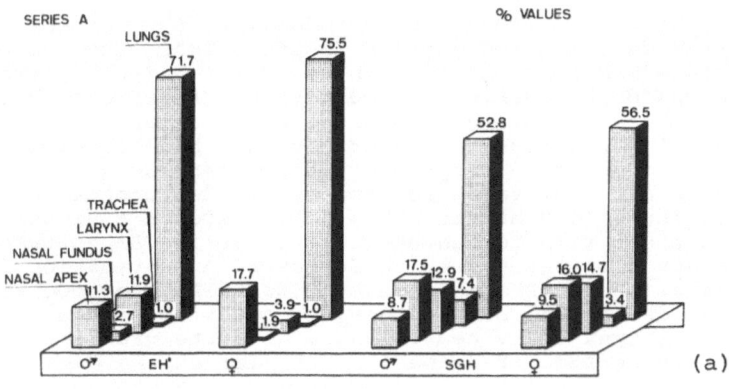

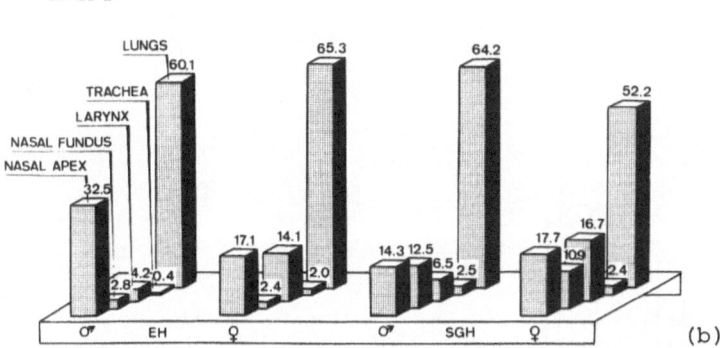

<u>Fig. 4 a and b.</u> Percentage distribution of the TPM-^{14}C activity in
the various respiratory tract organs, as shown in Fig. 1. The values
were calculated as means after setting the total respiratory tract
activity of each animal at 100%. (a) Represents the species and sex-
related values for animals in Series A, while (b) gives values for
animals in Series B. (For number of animals, see Tables 1 and 2)

Discussion

Because of differences in animal species, labeling methods, the label
itself, exposure methods, and dissection patterns, dosimetric study
results are difficult to compare. DONTENWILL and coworkers (1971) used
hexadecane-1-^{14}C as a TPM marker for Syrian golden hamsters and found
most of the activity to be in the lungs but also found a relatively
high amount in the nose, as did HOLLAND and colleagues (1958), who
used AS-74 in rabbits, and DAVIES and his collaborators (1973), who
investigated rat lungs together with trachea and larynx after exposure
to DOT-16,17-^{14}C labeled smoke. Only PAGE and colleagues (1973), using
hexadecane-1-^{14}C in mice, found more activity in the head than in the
lungs.

These and our own results indicate a high filtration action of the
nose, which seems to be extensive in very small animals (e.g., mice),
less marked in Syrian golden hamsters, and even less pronounced in

316

European hamsters. This comparison is related only to the percentage
values describing the distribution pattern in the animal. The comparison of the surface TPM concentration in various respiratory tract
organs may be more valid when deriving dose-response relations, but
this is not possible because the surface areas for the various respiratory tract organs of the European hamster have not been determined
so far. The TPM-^{14}C of the total respiratory tract per 100 g body
weight may be assumed as a raw value for comparing the European
hamster with the Syrian golden hamster (Fig. 5). There is a higher
TPM-^{14}C activity in the Syrian golden hamsters of Series A; however,
this difference is not distinctly seen in Series B. An estimation for
the surface concentration of TPM was made by DONTENWILL and coworkers
(1971) for Syrian golden hamsters; they derived a surface ratio of
0.1 : 0.6 : 1000 for larynx : trachea : lungs, with the greatest
amount of activity per surface area found in the larynx.

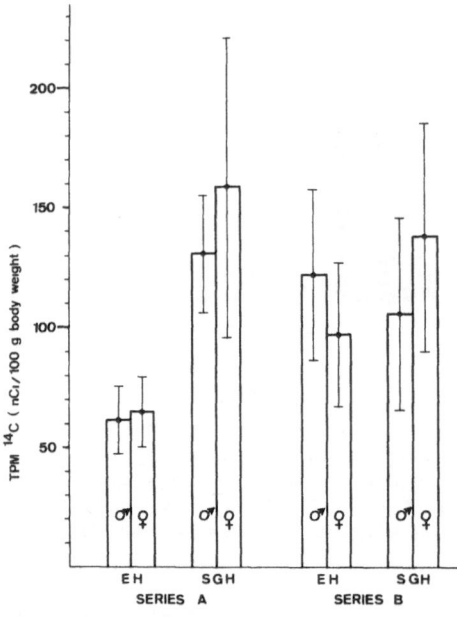

Fig. 5. Columns represent means
± standard deviations of absolute
TPM-^{14}C activity/100 g body weight,
related to series, species, and sex
of animals. (For number of animals,
see Tables 1 and 2)

In an autoradiograph of a Syrian golden hamster (Fig. 6), this surface concentration can be estimated. High TPM-^{14}C activity was found
on the lower surface of the epiglottis and the glottic region, which
corresponds to the results of CHEVALIER and DONTENWILL (1972). Homogenous distribution of TPM-^{14}C activity would facilitate the comparison of concentrations per surface unit of a definite part of the
respiratory tract, i.e., larynx or trachea. Autoradiographs indicate
that such a homogenous distribution is doubtful. The activity in the
ductus nasopharyngicus and the trachea exhibits cluster-like structures that alternate in very high and very low surface concentrations.
The paramedial part of the left lung reveals a lobulated structure,
indicating a distribution following its ramifications. Autoradiographs
of the European hamster reveal a similar picture which will be reported later in detail. Autoradiographs of the nose were difficult
to make, because these structures are difficult to keep positioned
during the cutting of a longitudinal section.

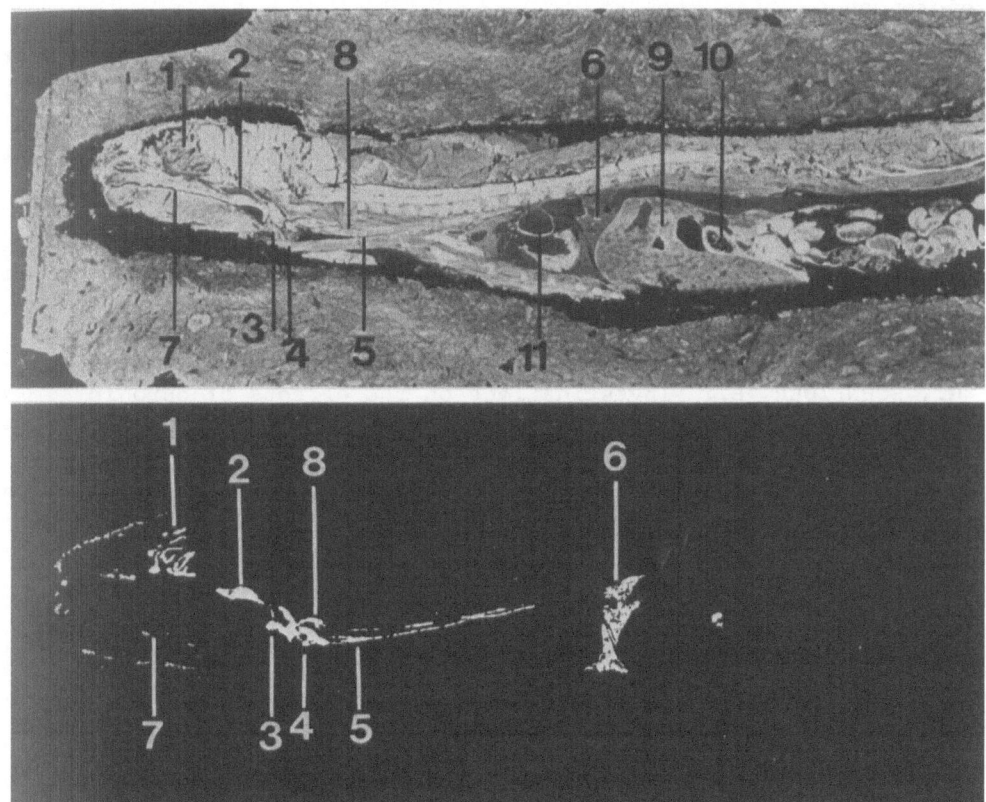

Fig. 6. Almost median longitudinal frozen section of a Syrian golden
hamster. *1* endoturbinals, *2* nasopharyngeal duct, *3* epiglottis, *4*
larynx, *5* trachea, *6* caudal part of lungs, *7* oral palate above tongue,
8 oesophagus, *9* liver, *10* stomach, and *11* hearth with great vessels.
The autoradiograph is positioned below the section

Through chronic smoke inhalation experiments it will be determined
whether the higher sensitivity of the respiratory tract of the European hamster for tumorigenic agents and/or the possibility of a
longer exposure time will result in a useful model for studies on
the effect of inhaled tobacco smoke.

Acknowledgements

The authors thank the British American Tobacco Company of Southampton,
England, for labeling the cigarettes of Series A and partially supporting the study, as well as the B.A.T. of Hamburg, Germany, for furnishing the equipment. We are also most grateful to HORST SCHOSTEK and
HEINZ RÖBER for excellent technical assistance and NAOMA CRISP LINDGREN
for editing the manuscript. KARL PATZSCHKE, M.D., of the Bayer AG corporation is acknowledged making the autoradiographs.

318

References

CHEVALIER, H.J., DONTENWILL, W.: Experimentelle Untersuchungen über die Ablagerung von inhalierten Partikeln im Kehlkopf von syrischen Goldhamstern. Z. Versuchstierk. 14, 271-276 (1972).

DAVIES, B.R., HOUSEMAN, T.H., RODERICK, H.R.: Studies of cigarette smoke transfer using radioisotopically labeled tobacco constituents. Part III: The use of dotriacontane-16,17-^{14}C as a marker for the deposition of cigarette smoke in the respiratory system of experimental animals. Beitr. Tabakf. 7, 148-153 (1973).

DONTENWILL, W.: Experimental investigations on the effect of cigarette smoke inhalation on small laboratory animals. In: Inhalation Carcinogenesis (M.G. Hanna, Jr., P. Nettesheim, J.R. Gilbert, eds). AEC Symposium Series no. 18, pp. 389-409. Oak Ridge, Tennessee: U.S. Atomic Energy Commission, Division of Technical Inf. 1970.

DONTENWILL, W., CHEVALIER, H.J., HARKE, H.P., LAFRENZ, U., RECKZEH, G., SCHNEIDER, B.: Investigations on the effects of chronic cigarette smoke inhalation in Syrian golden hamsters. J. nat. Cancer Inst. 51, 1781-1832 (1973).

DONTENWILL, W., HARKE, H.P., BAARS, A., GOERTZ, E.: Experimentelle Untersuchungen über Aufnahme und Ablagerung von Rauchbestandteilen bei der passiven Berauchung von Goldhamstern mit Zigarettenrauch. Drug Res. 21, 142-143 (1971).

HOLLAND, R.H., WILSON, R.H., MORRIS, D., MCCALL, M.S., LANZ, H.: The effect of cigarette smoke on the respiratory system of the rabbit. Cancer 11, 709-712 (1958).

HOUSEMAN, T.H., HENEAGE, E.: Studies of cigarette smoke transfer using radioisotopically labeled tobacco constituents. Part I: The preparation of radioisotopically labeled cigarettes. Beitr. Tabakforsch. 7, 138-141 (1973).

JENKINS, R.W., Jr., NEWMAN, R.H., CARPENTER, R.D., OSDENE, T.S.: Cigarette smoke formation studies. I. Distribution and mainstream products from added dotriacontane-16,17-^{14}C. Beitr. Tabakforsch. 5, 295-298 (1970).

KAYSER, C.H., AARON, M.: Cycle d'activité saisonnière des glandes endocrines chez un hibernant, le hamster (cricetus frumentarius). C.R. Soc. Biol. (Paris) 125, 225 (1938).

KAYSER, C.H., AARON, M.: Le cycle saisonnière des glandes endocrines chez les hibernants. Arch. Anat. (Strasbourg) 33, 21-40 (1950).

LEWIS, C.I., MCGEADY, J.C., WAGNER, J.R., SCHULTZ, F.J., SPEARS, A.W.: Dichlorobenzophenone as a nonradioactive tracer for cigarette smoke-gas chromatographic analysis of tracer. Amer. Rev. Resp. Dis. 106, 480-484 (1972).

MOHR, U., ALTHOFF, J., PAGE, N.: Tumors of the respiratory system induced in the common European hamster by N-diethylnitrosamine. J. nat. Cancer Inst. 49, 595-597 (1972).

MOHR, U., REZNIK, G., ECKHART, W., KMOCH, N., HAAS, H.: Distribution of labeled smoke particles in the respiratory tract of the hamster. Naturwissenschaften 61, 133-134 (1974).

MOSHY, R.J.: In: Tobacco and Tobacco Smoke (E.L. Wynder and D. Hoffmann, eds), pp. 304-310. New York, London: Academic Press 1967.

PAGE, B.F.Y., WOOLSGROVE, B., CHASSEAUD, L.F., BINNS, R.: Use of radioactive tracer technique in investigations associated with cigarette smoking. Am. Occup. Hyg. 16, 409-416 (1973).

PATZSCHKE, K.: Ganztier-Autoradiographie. Eine Methode in der Arzneimittelforschung. Münch. med. Wschr. 36, 2043-2053 (1968).

RATHS, P.: Mineralhaushalt und hormonale Aktivität im Winterschlaf. Experientia 20, 178-190 (1964).

REZNIK, G., MOHR, U.: A modified method for locating labeled smoke particles in organs of Syrian golden and European hamsters. In: These Proceedings.

STOCKS, P., CAMPBELL, J.M.: Lung cancer death rates among nonsmokers and pipe and cigarette smokers. An evaluation in relation to air pollution by benzpyrene and other substances. Brit. med. J. $\underline{2}$, 923-939 (1955).

STOCKS, P.: Recent epidemiological studies of lung cancer mortality, cigarette smoking and air pollution, with discussion of a new hypothesis of causation. Brit. J. Cancer $\underline{20}$, 595-623 (1966).

ULLBERG, S.: Studies on the distribution and fate of ^{35}S labeled benzylpenicillin in the body. Acta radiol. (Stockholm) Suppl. 118 (1954).

ZIMMERMAN, K.: In: Taschenbuch unserer wildlebenden Säugetiere, 2nd edition, p. 92. Hannover: Fackelträger 1966.

Cigarette Smoke Inhalation Studies in Inbred Syrian Hamsters*

Freddy Homburger[1], Peter Bernfeld[1], and A. B. Russfield[2]

[1]Bio-Research Consultants, Inc., Cambridge, MA 02141, USA
[2]Pathology Department, St. Vincent Hospital, Worcester, MA 01610, USA

ABSTRACT

Findings were obtained in 2 lines of inbred Syrian hamsters exposed
to cigarette smoke, and the results will be compared with those reported by DONTENWILL. The importance of the choice of animal in this
type of study will be emphasized.

Groups of 102 inbred Syrian hamsters of the BIO 87.20 and BIO 15.16
strains (Telaco, Bar Harbor, Maine) were exposed twice daily, 5 days
a week to 8 puffs from Kentucky 1R1 cigarettes of 2 second duration,
generated every minute in a Walton-Morrissey Reverse Smoker. The
smoke exposure to about 1 to 5 diluted smoke lasted 15 seconds and
was followed by a 43 seconds exposure to fresh laboratory air. 60
animals of each strain were held in cages without manipulation as
controls, and 60 additional control animals of each strain were
treated as the experimental animals, except that no cigarettes were
inserted into the machines. Histopathologic studies were performed
after 45 to 90 weeks of treatment. In hamsters exposed to smoke,
macrophage clusters containing iron pigment were seen in the pulmonary parenchyma, especially frequently and early in 87.20 hamsters.
2 tumors were found in the nasopharynges of smoke-exposed BIO 15.16
animals, 1 a fibrosarcoma and the other a cystadenoma. Dysplastic
changes were seen in the larynges after approximately 40 weeks of
smoke exposure and the total incidence of such changes in smoke-exposed animals was 40% and 13%, respectively. Incipiently invasive,
but still very small, lesions were found in the larynges of smoke-
exposed animals of each strain after approximately 80 weeks of smoking. By 90 weeks, there were microinvasive carcinomas in 19% of the
animals in the more susceptible BIO 15.16 line and 4% in the less
susceptible BIO 87.20 line. This confirms and extends the observations of DONTENWILL on laryngeal changes. Differences between the
strains used will be discussed to emphasize the effect of genetic
factors on smoke inhalation experiments.

* This investigation was supported by a contract from the Council for
Tobacco Research - U.S.A., Inc. The views expressed in this paper
are those of the authors and do not necessarily reflect the opinions
of the Council for Tobacco Research.

Introduction

Hamsters are desirable test subjects for tobacco smoke-inhalation
studies because they have a much greater resistance to toxic effects
of nicotine than rats or mice (BERNFELD and HOMBURGER, 1972). 2 strains
of inbred hamsters (BIO hamsters from Telaco, Bar Harbor, Maine) were
used in the present study in order to achieve reproducibility of results and to detect possible strain-related differences in response
to tobacco smoke.

Materials and Methods

2 strains, the BIO 87.20 and BIO 15.16, were selected for chronic
toxicity experiments. All animals weighed 108 ± 4 g at the beginning
of the chronic studies. Only males were used, housed in groups of 6
in 12 x 14 x 6.5-inch polypropylene cages. San-I-Cel, Deodor grade,
was used as bedding material. The animal room temperature was kept
between 72° and 76°F. Fluorescent bulbs were the only light source
and were automatically controlled to operate between 7:00 a.m. and
7:00 p.m. The animals received Wayne Mouse Breeder Blox and fresh
tap water ad libitum.

Modified Walton reverse smoking machines were used, as described
elsewhere (HOFFMANN and WYNDER, 1970). In these machines, air is
pushed through lighted cigarettes by applying positive pressure at
the burning end.

All animals wore well fitting, permanently-attached, felt rings around
their necks (3/16" thick, 2" outside diameter, and 5/8-3/4" inside
diameter, depending on the size of the hamster). The felt rings were
reinforced on both sides by thin, ring-shaped aluminum plates of
slightly smaller dimensions (1-7/8" outside diameter and 15/16" inside
diameter). The heads of the animals were inserted into the smoking
machine by means of these collars, so that only their heads were in
contact with the smoke. The bodies remained outside the machine, firmly restrained by the collars, thus eliminating the need to confine
the animals in tubes with attendant excessive sweating and stress.
6 animals could be exposed simultaneously to smoke inhalation. Since
the felt collars prevented the animals from grooming their eyes, these
were washed with penicillin solution on a cotton swab once a day,
5 days/week.

Only 1R1 Kentucky Reference cigarettes were used. They are produced
by, and were obtained from, the University of Kentucky, Tobacco and
Health Research Institute, Kentucky Research Foundation. Compositions
of the Reference cigarette (1R1) at 12% moisture were as follows
(ATKINSON, 1970): flue-cured lamina, 40.1%; flue-cured stem, 14.2%;
Burley lamina, 24.9%; Turkish (whole leaf), 11.6%; Maryland lamina,
1.1%; glycerine, 2.8%; invert sucrose, 5.3%.

Smoke was generated from 4 cigarettes burning simultaneously, and was
administered to the animals in a 60-second puff cycle. Each cycle consisted of a 2-second period of smoke generation followed by a 15-second
period of additional smoke exposure and a 43-second period of exposure
to fresh air.

During the 2-second period of smoke generation, 35 ml of air was pushed through each of the 4 cigarettes, yielding a total volume of 140 ml

smoke which was introduced into the 725 ml exposure chamber. A magnetic stirrer provided instant mixing. The smoke dilution factor as calculated from the physical characteristics of the machine was 725:140 or 5.2 : 1. The smoke concentration inhaled by the hamsters, uncorrected for changes due to exhaled air of the exposed animals, was therefore approximately 19.2% of that leaving the mouth-end of the cigarette. In comparison, the average concentration of smoke in the lung of a human smoker is about 0.8% (average puff volume, 35 ml; human functional residual capacity, 3.5 liters; human tidal volume, 0.7 liters).

It took the smoke less than 1 second to traverse the 6 inches between the mouth-end of the cigarette and the hamsters' heads, assuring that the hamster inhaled smoke no less fresh than that reaching the lungs of the human smoker.

Each hamster was exposed twice a day, 5 days/week, to 8 consecutive puff cycles from the Kentucky Reference cigarettes. The first through eighth puffs from the cigarettes were used, resulting in a butt length slightly longer than 30 mm. The period of exposure ranged from 45 to 100 weeks.

Cage-held control animals from each inbred line, of comparable age and initial weight, were maintained simultaneously in the same animal room and were handled in the same way as all other hamsters with regard to weekly weighing, permanently wearing felt-aluminum collars, etc., but these control hamsters did not come into contact with the smoking machines. A second control group consisted of comparable hamsters exposed to sham smoking in the machines, which were operated under standard conditions, except that no cigarettes were inserted into them. For each of the 2 lines, BIO 15.16 and BIO 87.20, 102 hamsters were exposed to smoke, 60 were exposed to sham-smoking conditions, and 60 were used as cage-held controls.

Since it was impossible to obtain all 222 hamsters required for each inbred line at the same time, animals of the proper initial age and weight were introduced into the experiment in lots of 6, staggered over a period of 37 weeks. As far as possible, 1 lot of 6 animals of each of the controls was started at the same time as 2 lots of smoke-exposed hamsters (12 animals).

Animals were exposed to smoke or to control conditions for between 75 to 100 weeks. They were sacrificed earlier when they appeared moribund, as judged by consistent weight loss or the appearance of edema. Some hamsters of all groups were also sacrificed at 45 and 60 weeks. Complete autopsies were performed. The entire respiratory tract and any other organs or tissues which appeared grossly abnormal were studied histologically. Lungs were inflated and fixed in Tellyesniczky's fluid in an apparatus especially devised by Dr. SADAMU ISHIKAWA (1972).

Results

1. Mortality: As shown in Figs 1 and 2, mortality was very low in all groups until about the 60th week of the experiment, at which time the animals had a chronological age of approximately 73 weeks. Thereafter, mortality increased rapidly in all groups, reaching 100% at about 100 weeks. Neither smoke exposure nor sham-smoking had a significant effect on mortality. There was no difference in survival between the 2 strains.

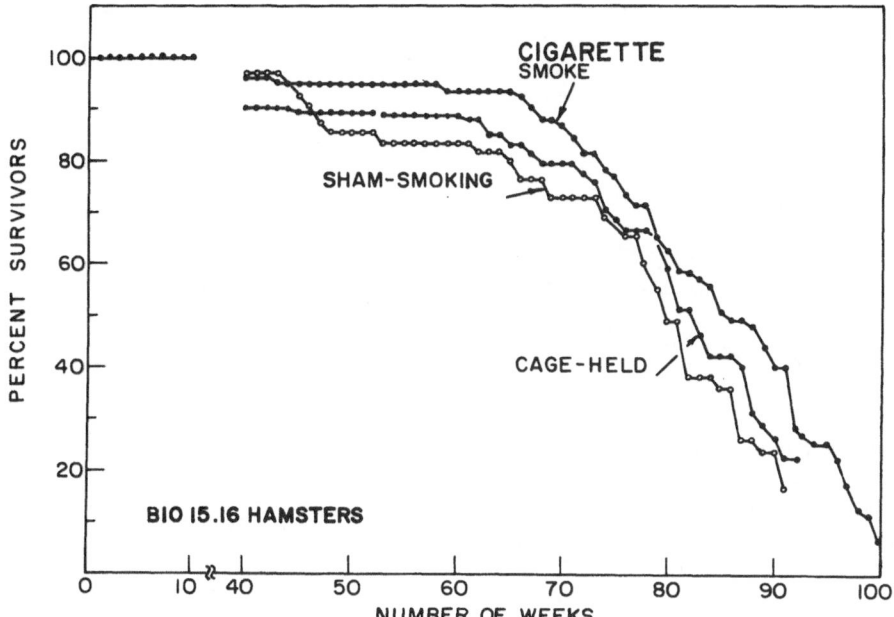

Fig. 1

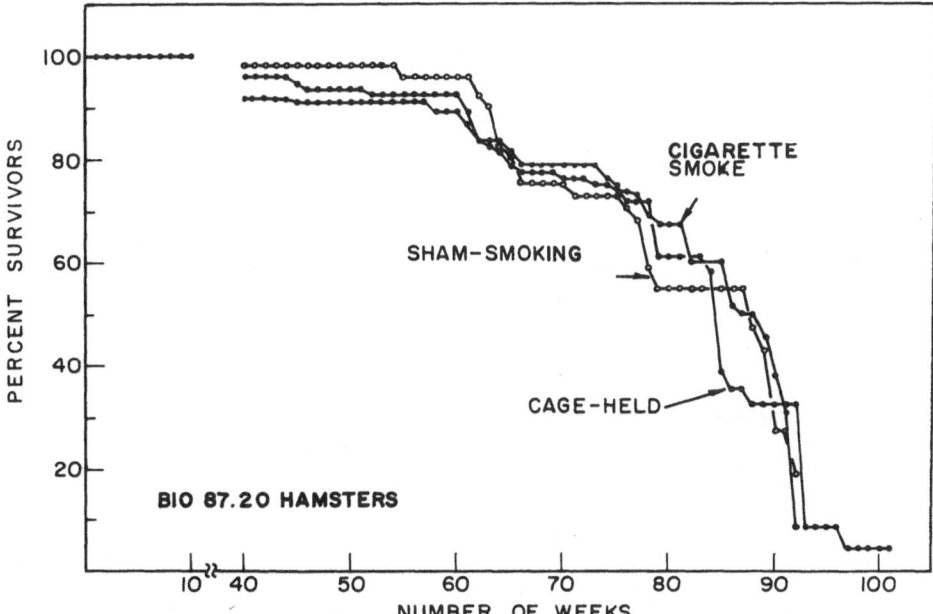

Fig. 2

2. Changes in Body Weight (Figs 3 and 4): In both lines of hamsters, individual body weights were affected by smoke inhalation and, in addition, by mere experimental manipulations, such as sham-smoking conditions and/or stress produced by the latter. Initial weight in both groups averaged 108 g. The BIO 87.20 cage-held controls attained a final weight of 144.3 g, whereas the BIO 15.16 animals attained only 125.0 g.

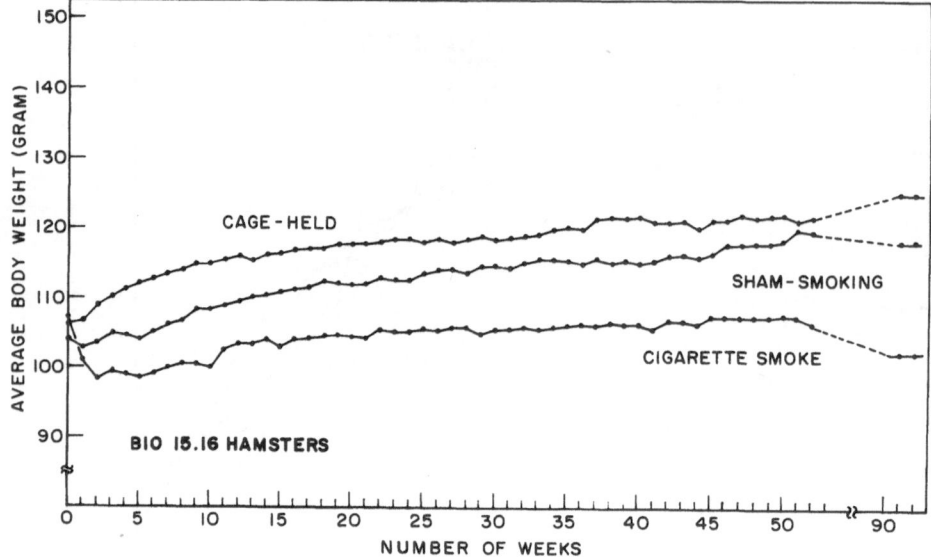

Fig. 3

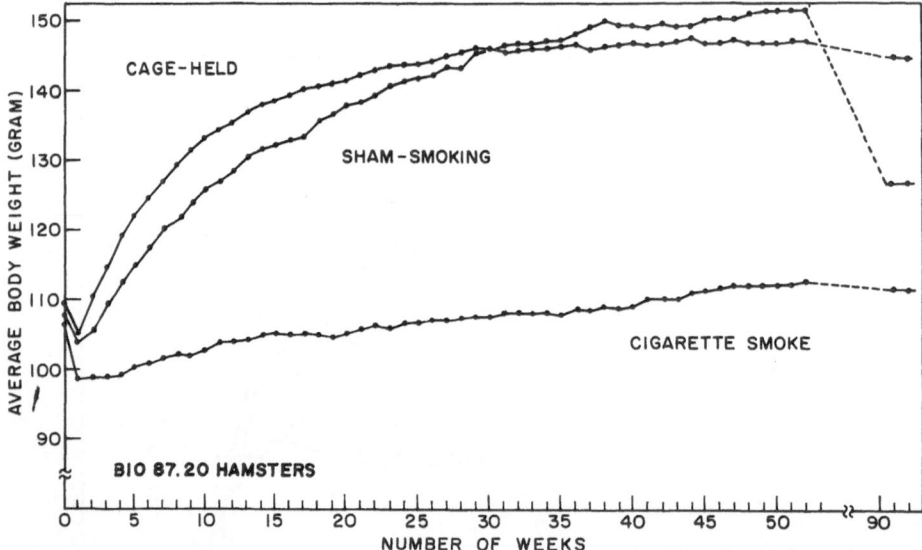

Fig. 4

Exposure to cigarette smoke reduced body weight of both inbred strains by about 10 g during the first 2 weeks of treatment. Subsequently, weights increased again, but somewhat more slowly in the BIO 15.16 than in the BIO 87.20 animals. Because of the low final weight of the cage-held BIO 15.16 hamsters, the weight difference between the controls and smoke-exposed hamsters was much less in the BIO 15.16 line than in the BIO 87.20 line. Sham-smoking produced body weights intermediate between those of the cage-held controls and the smoke-exposed animals in line BIO 15.16; it had no effect on body weight in line BIO 87.20.

It thus appears that the long-term response to smoke inhalation, i.e., the failure of the smoke-exposed animals to gain weight, was due, at least in large part, to direct effects of smoke inhalation rather than to nonspecific stress.

3. Laryngeal Lesions: By far the most important findings in this experiment occurred in the larynges (Table 1), approximately two-thirds of which were studied histologically (Figs 5-10). (The remainder were transplanted into hamster cheek pouches for an experiment which will be reported separately.) Among the smoke-exposed hamsters, only 2 out of 48 larynges in the BIO 15.16 line (4%) and 3 out of 45 from the BIO 87.20 line (7%) were regarded as histologically normal, as opposed to 68 to 90% of the larynges from the corresponding control animals. The only change seen in the control animals and sham-smoked animals was chronic inflammation.

Table 1. Laryngeal pathology

Strain	Procedure	No. of autopsies (larynx)	Numbers of animals			
			Normal	Epithelial changes	Early* invasive cancer	Small papilloma
BIO 15.16	Smoke	84 (48)	2	38	9	7
	Sham-smoke	42 (36)	27	0	0	0
	Cage-held	40 (25)	17	0	0	0
BIO 87.20	Smoke	87 (45)	3	30	2	11
	Sham-smoke	44 (30)	27	0	0	0
	Cage-held	·48 (39)	31	0	0	0

() Number of larynges histologically examined. Those not examined were transplanted. *These numbers are included among those animals with epithelial changes.

Pathological changes in the smoke-exposed hamsters were classified as follows: hyperplasia was defined as hyperplastic thickening of the squamous epithelium with acanthosis and mild nuclear dysplasia. The basal layer remained intact and fairly straight. This change was seen in 40% of the larynges of smoke-exposed BIO 15.16 hamsters and in 53% of the BIO 87.20 line, but in none of the control animals.

Epithelial hyperplasia also occurred with proliferation of the squamous epithelium in which there was a downgrowth of cells into the connective tissue, often in a reticular pattern. Nuclear dysplasia and mitotic activity tended to be more intense than in simple hyperplasia. This type of change was more frequent in BIO 15.16 animals (40%) than in the BIO 87.20 line (13%) and it was absent in the controls. In many cases of this type of change, the basal layer epidermis was clearly intact. In some, it became very irregular and apparently isolated cell clumps were seen in the connective tissue, a few suggesting lymphatic invasion. In advanced stages, this type of hyperplasia is exceedingly difficult to differentiate from early invasive carcinoma. This occurred in 18.8% of the BIO 15.16 animals and in 4% of the BIO 87.20 hamsters. It should be emphasized that no distant metastases were found in any animal. None of these tissue changes occurred in the controls.

Small squamous papillomas, similar to those occurring in some of the tracheas and bronchi, were found in the laryngeal epithelium in 24% of the BIO 87.20 and in 15% of the BIO 15.16 animals exposed to smoke. Occasionally, there was pseudoepitheliomatous downgrowth of cells at the base of papilloma.

326

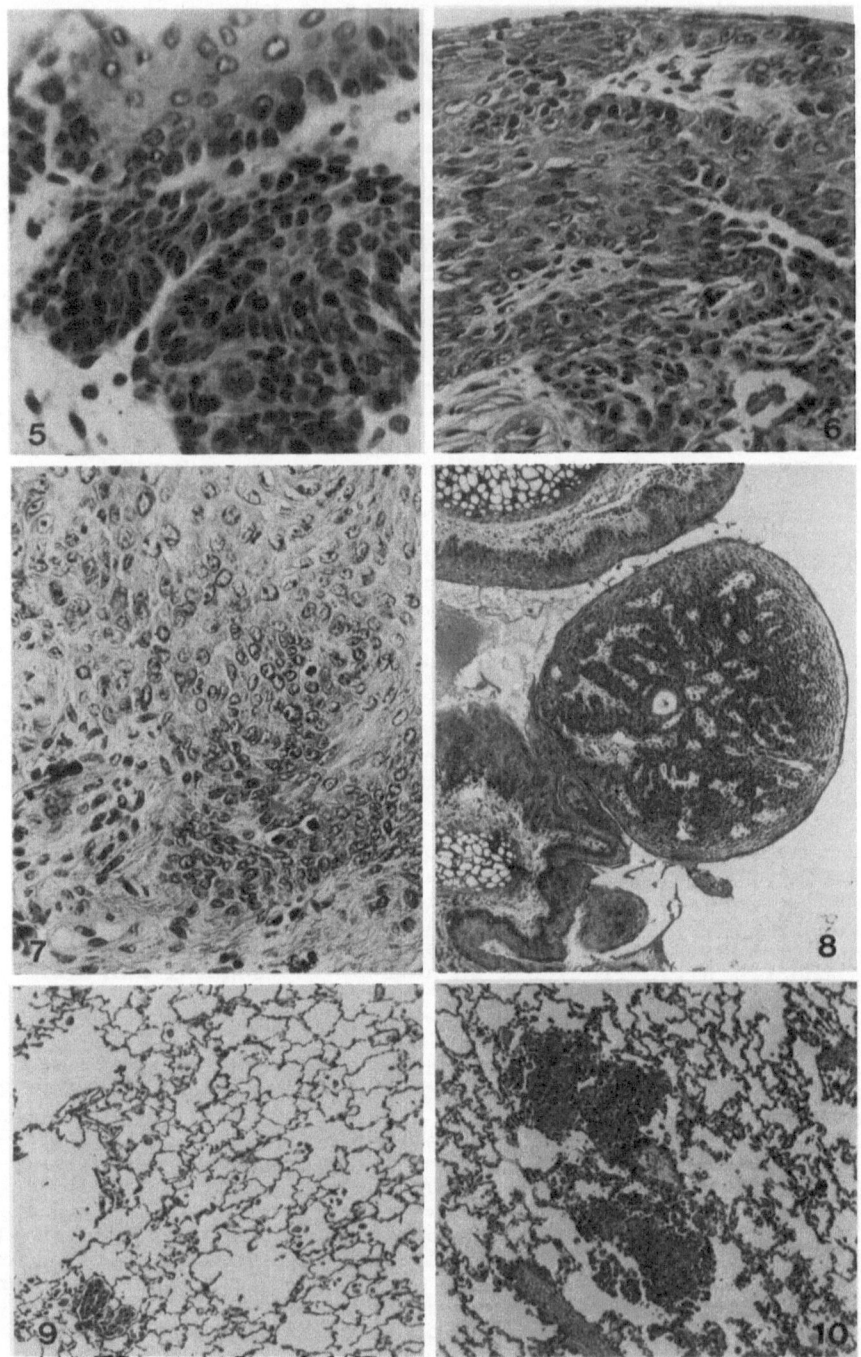

Legends see opposite page

A few larynges of smoke-exposed hamsters also showed chronic inflammation and/or squamous metaplasia of mucus glands. Chronic inflammation also occurred in a few control animals and was associated with slight epithelial thickening, but never with frank hyperplasia, pseudoepitheliomatous change, or papilloma formation. There was no significant difference between sham-smoked and cage-held controls in this respect.

4. Lung Lesions: 90% of the lungs from BIO 15.16 hamsters and all of those from the BIO 87.20 strain were examined histologically. This revealed both clear-cut strain differences and significant effects of smoke exposure.[1]

Pulmonary macrophages in both strains of hamsters can form small clumps within the alveoli. This tendency is much more pronounced in the BIO 87.20 strain than in the BIO 15.16 strain, as seen from a comparison of the cage-held control groups (44% versus 6%). It is accentuated by smoke exposure in both strains (92% versus 53%, respectively). In neither strain is the incidence of macrophage clumping affected by sham-smoking.

There were qualitative as well as quantitative differences in macrophages clumping among the various groups. In hematoxylin- and eosin-stained slides of BIO 15.16 hamster lung of all groups, and in BIO 87.20 hamster lung from the control groups, the clumps consisted of comparatively few, small, loosely-packed macrophages containing dark brown to black pigment. In lungs of smoke-exposed BIO 87.20 hamsters, the clumps were larger, more abundant, and they were composed of very large cells containing pale golden pigment. These cells were frequently mixed with polymorphonuclear leukocytes. Rare smoke-exposed BIO 87.20 hamsters which did not have such clumped macrophages in their lungs were usually those found dead of some intercurrent disease.

---

[1]The authors are grateful to Drs. STANLEY ROBBINS of Boston University and WALTER BAUER of Washington University, St. Louis, for having reviewed the histological slides of the most important laryngeal lesions.

Fig. 5. Severe epithelial hyperplasia in larynx of male BIO 87.20 hamster exposed to smoke for 78 weeks. Although some degree of basal cell orientation is retained in the upper portion of this lesion, it is disappearing in the deep portion. Note nuclear variation. Hematoxylin and eosin. X 300

Fig. 6. Severe epithelial hyperplasia in larynx of male BIO 15.16 hamster exposed to smoke for 84 weeks. Note reticular pattern of growth and complete loss of normal orientation of cells in the deepest portion of the lesion. Hematoxylin and eosin. X 190

Fig. 7. Larynx of male BIO 15.16 hamster exposed to smoke for 96 weeks. There is complete loss of normal polarity; nuclei show marked pleomorphism; 3 mitotic figures are seen. This lesion is difficult to differentiate from early invasive squamous carcinoma. Hematoxylin and eosin. X 190

Fig. 8. Large papilloma nearly occluding the larynx of a male BIO 87.20 hamster which had been exposed to smoke for 92 weeks. Hematoxylin and eosin. X 38

Fig. 9. Cluster of small macrophages in lung of male BIO 15.16 hamster exposed to smoke for 45 weeks. Hematoxylin and eosin. X 38

Fig. 10. Multiple large clusters of macrophages in lung of male BIO 87.20 hamster exposed to smoke for 45 weeks. Hematoxylin and eosin. X 38

Macrophages of both strains, both the isolated cells and those occurring in clumps, characteristically gave a positive Prussian blue reaction for iron. This was intense in the small macrophages of all BIO 15.16 animals and of the BIO 87.20 controls. It was weak in the large macrophages of smoke-exposed BIO 87.20 hamsters, which also appeared to contain yellowish iron-negative pigment. Occasional granules of black, iron-negative pigment consistent with carbon were found in a few macrophages.

Pulmonary parenchyma in both strains contained small foci of ectopic bone not associated with inflammation or other obvious disease processes. These occurred in 18% of the cage-held BIO 15.16 animals, and in 42% of the BIO 87.20's.

Sporadic lungs in both strains showed acute or chronic pneumonitis or contained metastic tumors of some sort, usually adrenal carcinoma, lymphoma, or leukemic infiltrate. There were no differences in these parameters which could be ascribed to strain or smoke exposure.

Abnormalities of the trachea and bronchi: They were comparatively rare in all groups. A few small patches of squamous metaplasia were seen in 5 to 15% of the BIO 15.16 hamsters, in which the incidence was not significantly affected by smoke exposure. In the cage-held BIO 87.20 animals, squamous metaplasia was not seen in the trachea and in only 4% of the bronchi. In smoke-exposed BIO 87.20 animals, these figures increased to 26% and 21%, respectively.

No tumors of the air passages were found in control animals of either strain. 3 benign squamous papillomas were found in smoke-exposed BIO 15.16 hamsters, all of which occurred in the trachea. 4 benign squamous papillomas were found in smoke-exposed BIO 87.20 hamsters, 2 occurring in the trachea and 2 in the main bronchus.

5. Lesions in Nasopharynx: Sections were taken through the nasopharynx and adjacent structures of the head in all groups of hamsters. Approximately half contained only normal tissues. The remainder showed a variety of pathological processes, including gingivitis, dental caries, occular inflammation with phthisis bulbi, and thromboses of orbital veins. None of these phenomena could be related to smoke exposure.

Only 2 tumors were found in the nasopharynx, both occurring in BIO 15.16 animals which had been exposed to smoke for 60 to 75 weeks. 1 was an adenoid cystic tumor, believed to have originated from mucus glands. The other was a fibrosarcoma that had produced numerous small pulmonary metastases.

6. Heart Lesions: The heart, as such, was not sectioned routinely in this experiment. However, it was included with the lungs in 20 to 25% of the animals. 25% of the cage-held control BIO 15.16 hearts showed myocardial degeneration, as compared with 17% of the BIO 87.20 hearts. This consisted of myolysis with (in the BIO 15.16 animals only) an abundant infiltration of lymphocytes. Smoke-exposure appeared to increase myocardial degeneration in both strains, especially in the BIO 15.16 animals. However, the number of animals examined was too small to permit definitive conclusions.

Mural thrombi were seen in approximately 20% of the hearts of both strains. Incidence was not affected by the experimental procedures.

Discussion

Chronic exposure to cigarette smoke produces severe hyperplastic changes in the squamous epithelium of the hamster larynx and is associated with decreased body weight. Smoke-exposure did not increase proliferative changes outside of the respiratory tract or the non-neoplastic degenerative changes characteristic of aging hamsters. (Our observations on possible smoke-related changes in the heart are presently equivocal. Further investigation would be highly desirable.)

Chronic smoke-exposure significantly reduced survival time in the previously-published DONTENWILL model; no such effect was seen in ours. This difference may be attributed to the two-fold higher carbonmonoxide concentration inhaled by DONTENWILL's hamsters than by ours. In fact, previous observations of DONTENWILL (1970, 1973), showed sustained increase in blood carboxyhemoglobin in his model, while ours produced only transient increases.

The point of greatest practical importance to emerge from our work is the demonstration of striking strain differences among various lines of hamsters with respect to susceptibility to acute toxic effects of smoke, and to hyperplastic response of the larynx to smoke (BERNFELD and HOMBURGER, 1972). Animals of the inbred BIO 15.16 line have both the highest resistance to smoke or nicotine toxicity and the greatest laryngeal susceptibility - qualities greatly increasing the sensitivity of the model. Further studies with large numbers of animals will be necessary to ascertain the significance of the laryngeal strain differences.

No tumors of the lung parenchyma following smoke exposure were observed either by DONTENWILL or by us. The slightly significant increase in adenomatoid lesions observed by DONTENWILL was not confirmed by us. In both model systems, there was an increase in so-called "smoke cells" in alveoli following smoke exposure. The observation that yellow iron-negative and also black particles occur in the macrophages suggests that the particulate phase of smoke did reach the alveolar wall to be taken up by the macrophages. Use of the 2 inbred lines in our experiment permitted the conclusion that these cells are not directly related to hyperplastic changes in the respiratory tract. They were much more abundant in the BIO 87.20 hamsters which had the lower incidence of hyperplastic lesions.

References

ATKINSON, W.O.: Production of sample cigarettes for tobacco and health research. Tobacco and Health Conference, 2, 28 (1970).
BERNFELD, P., HOMBURGER, F.: High nicotine tolerance of Syrian golden hamsters. Toxicol Appl. Pharmacol. 22, 324 (1972).
DONTENWILL, W.: Experimental investigations on the effect of cigarette smoke inhalation on small laboratory animals. In: Inhalation Carcinogenesis (M.G. Hanna, Jr., P. Nettesheim, J.R. Gilbert, eds). AEC Symposium Series no. 18, pp. 389-411. Oak Ridge, Tennessee: U.S. Atomic Energy Commission, Division of Technical Inf. 1970.
DONTENWILL, W., CHEVALIER, H.-J., HARKE, H.-P., LAFRENZ, U., RECKZEH, G., SCHNEIDER, B.: Investigations on the effects of chronic cigarette smoke inhalation in Syrian golden hamsters. J. nat. Cancer Inst. 51, 1781-1807 (1973).

HERROLD, K.M.: Induction of olfactory neuroepithelial tumors in Syrian hamsters by diethylnitrosamine. Cancer <u>17</u>, 114-121 (1964).

HOFFMANN, D., WYNDER, E.L.: Chamber development and aerosal dispersion. In: Inhalation Carcinogenesis (M.G. Hanna, Jr., P. ·Nettesheim, J.R. Gilbert, eds). AEC Symposium Series no. 18, pp. 173-189. Oak Ridge, Tennessee: U.S. Atomic Energy Commission, Division of Technical Inf. 1970.

ISHIKAWA, S.: Personal Communication 1972.

MCCORMICK, A., NICHOLSON, M.J., BAYLIS, M.A., UNDERWOOD, J.G.: Nitrosamines in cigarette smoke condensate. Nature (New Biol.) <u>244</u>, 237-238 (1973).

Tumorigenic Effect of Chronic Cigarette Smoke Inhalation on Syrian Golden Hamsters

Walter P. Dontenwill

Forschungsinstitut der Cigarettenindustrie e. V., Hamburg, W.-Germany

ABSTRACT

Results of chronic inhalation experiments on Syrian golden hamsters were reported. 3600 were used for their entire lifespans. Some animals received additional treatment with carcinogens. Experimental results demonstrated a dose-response relationship. Effects of smoke from various types of cigarettes and effects of combined smoke and carcinogen treatment were evaluated. The results were as follows: 1. Changes induced by smoke exposure - striking differences were found between experimental groups. Precancerous and cancerous alterations were observed in the larynx and depended on duration of treatment and dosage; survival times were reduced, and loss of body weight was dose dependent. 2. Effects of treatment with DMBA - the number of tumors increased in the oral cavity, pharynx, esophagus, stomach, trachea, and liver. 3. Effects of nitrosamine treatment - papillomas in the trachea and lower region of the larynx differed from those in animals exposed to smoke.

A short summary will facilitate the discussion on our smoke inhalation experiment.

Introduction

Some of the most important findings of our smoke inhalation experiment (DONTENWILL et al., 1973) will be summarized as follows:

Materials and Methods

Table 1 demonstrates the exposure methods and materials of the inhalation experiment comprising 3600 Syrian golden hamsters.

Of fundamental importance is the reproducibility of the experiment, which we confirmed in experiments with animals from different colonies. In the different colonies, inflammations of the intestines (wet tail = ileitis terminalis) and alterations in the lung (for example "adenomatoid lesions") appear in different frequencies with considerable influence on the survival time or final experimental results.

332

Table 1. Chronic inhalation experiments on Syrian golden hamsters

Group	Type of cigarette	Smoking cycle	Treatment before exposure to smoke	Number of animals ♀	Number of animals ♂
1	E$_2$ (standard cigarette)	2x30 cig. daily	500 µg DMBA in CMC injected intratracheally	80	80
2	-	Control	500 µg DMBA in CMC injected intratracheally	80	80
3	-	Control	-	100	100
K	-	Control	-	300	300
4	E$_2$ (standard cigarette)	1x30 cig. daily	-	80	80
5	E$_2$ (standard cigarette)	2x30 cig. daily	-	80	80
6	E$_2$ (standard cigarette)	3x30 cig. daily	-	80	80
7	E$_2$ (standard cigarette)	Gas-phase from 2x30 cig. daily	-	80	80
8	-	2x10 min. air daily	-	80	80
9	EN (E$_2$+8% NaNO$_3$)	2x30 cig. daily	-	80	80
10	EG$_3$ (reconst. tobacco sheet from E$_2$+6.1% NaNO$_3$ according to Gerlach-process)	2x30 cig. daily	-	80	80
11	EG$_1$ (reconst. tobacco sheet from E$_2$ according to Gerlach-process)	2x30 cig. daily	-	80	80

Table 1 continued

Group	Type of cigarette	Smoking cycle	Treatment before exposure to smoke	Number of animals	
				♀	♂
12	E_2 (standard cigarette)	2x30 cig. daily	500 µg asbestos in CMC injected intratracheally before exposure to smoke	80	80
13		Not exposed to smoke	500 µg asbestos in CMC injected intratracheally	80	80
14	"Black cigarette"=Z	2x30 cig. daily	-	80	80
15	Standard cigarette with acetate filter=A	2x30 cig. daily	-	80	80
16	Standard cigarette with cellulose filter=D	2x30 cig. daily	-	80	80
17	Standard cigarette with charcoal filter=K	2x30 cig. daily	-	80	80
18	E_2 (standard cigarette)	2x30 cig. daily	4x1 mg DENA/100 g body weight administered in 52nd and 53rd week after start of experiment	80	80
18A	-	Not exposed to smoke	4x1 mg DENA/100 g body weight administered in 52nd and 53rd week after start of experiment	45[a]	45[a]

[a]The number of animals in group 18A corresponded to the number of surviving animals in group 18 at the 52nd - 53rd week.

Results and Discussion

The dose-response-relationship is evident in various findings.

1. In the survival time: As indicated in Table 2, the mean survival time is distinctly reduced in those animals having received increased doses of smoke and in those animals having received an additional treatment of 9,10-dimethyl-1,2-benzanthracene (DMBA), when compared to the control animals.

2. In the development of body weight: Table 3 demonstrates the relationship between dose and body weight. The highest decrease in body weight is observed in the group having received the highest amount of smoke; this loss in body weight is also evident in comparison with the controls.

3. In alterations of the larynx: The optimal dose-response-relationship was achieved with a 10 minute smoke exposure twice daily (dose II).

For our classification of stages we followed the Atlas of the Armed Forces Institute of Pathology, because that classification of laryngeal alterations fully corresponds to our experiences in man and animal. Fig. 1 a-g define the classification of stages 1-6. Stages 2, 3, and 4 are, for example, classified as "facultative" precanceroses and stages 3 and 4 are compared with papillomas of the mouse skin. Stage 5 is considered an "obligatory" precancerosis because it is often difficult to differentiate this stage from preinvasive carcinomas, i.e., the so-called carcinoma *in situ*. Our classification of stage 5 is also in conformity with the above mentioned American Atlas, defining the lesions as carcinoma-like. Carcinomas are defined as those tumors showing criteria which are also the basis of diagnosis in human pathol-

Fig. 1 a-g. Laryngeal changes
(a) Normal squamous epithelium without cornification and normal cylindrical epithelium with goblet cells
(b) Stage 1: pachydermia (epithelial hyperplasia). Thickening of the stratum spinosum with a multiple of cell-layers, occurrence of cornification of the stratum corneum
(c) Stage 2: leucoplakia, thickening of the stratum spinosum, thickening of cell-layers, increased cornification of the stratum corneum, incompletely keratinized cells in the stratum corneum, moderate nuclear polymorphy and a multiple of mitoses
(d) Stage 3: verrucous leucoplakia - verrucous proliferation of the squamous epithelium with thickening of the stratum spinosum and a multiple of cell-layers. Distinct hyperkeratosis as well as dyskeratosis and beginning cell polymorphy, increase of mitoses
(e) Stage 4: papillomatous leucoplakia - distinct papillary proliferation with sharp stromal demarcation, a multiple of cell-layers, moderate nuclear polymorphy and absence of cornification
(f) Stage 5: pseudoepitheliomatous leucoplakia - strong piniform and often reticular proliferation of the squamous epithelium with increasing polymorphy, a multiple of mitoses, metaplasia and complete filling of the glandular lumen without stromal infiltration and without rupture of the basal membrane
(g) Stage 6: carcinoma - severe thickening of the proliferated epithelium with increasing nuclear polymorphy, a multiple of mitoses, proliferation into the glandular lumen and beginning of heavy stromal invasion as well as rupture through the basal membrane

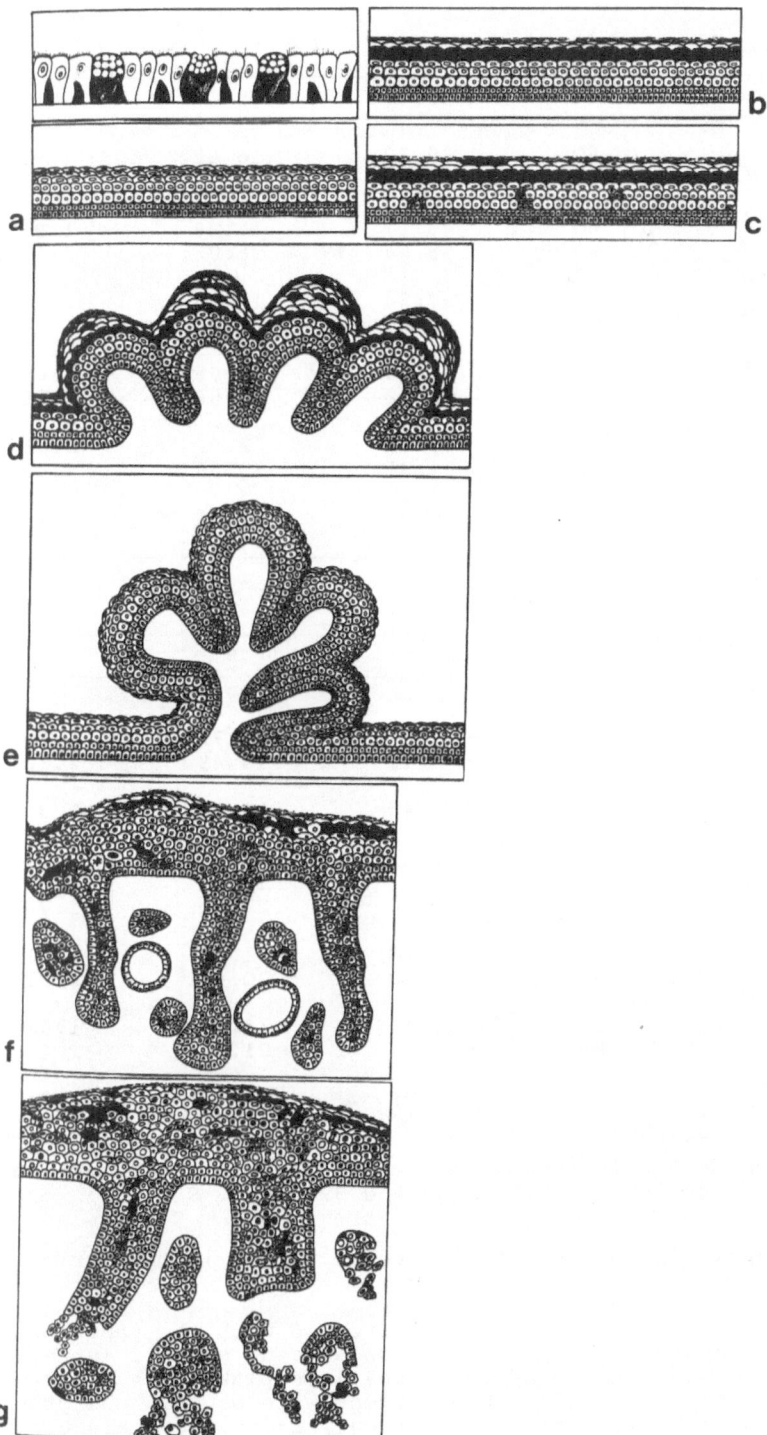

Fig. 1 a–g

Legends see opposite page

336

Table 2. Mean survival time

Group	Sex	n	$\bar{x}$	s	$s_{\bar{x}}$
DMBA +2x30 cig. E_2	♀	80	45.37	16.98	1.90
	♂	80	52.95	28.53	3.19
DMBA	♀	80	46.17	17.48	1.95
	♂	80	58.64	28.72	3.21
Control	♀	100	57.34	17.16	1.72
	♂	100	85.81	29.39	2.94
1x30 cig. E_2	♀	80	47.54	23.66	2.64
	♂	80	63.22	31.57	3.53
2x30 cig. E_2	♀	80	47.72	22.92	2.56
	♂	80	64.31	39.56	4.42
3x30 cig. E_2	♀	80	46.00	22.66	2.53
	♂	80	53.56	34.96	3.91

Table 3. Alteration of body weight

Group	Sex	n	$\bar{x}$	s	$s_{\bar{x}}$
DMBA +2x30 cig. E_2	♀				
	♂	80	− 8.64	14.72	1.65
		80	− 5.43	19.49	2.18
DMBA	♀	80	+ 6.45	21.06	2.38
	♂	80	+ 2.65	21.22	2.37
Control	♀	100	+ 7.22	18.21	1.82
	♂	100	+25.57	27.81	2.78
1x30 cig. E_2	♀	80	+ 7.00	21.59	2.41
	♂	80	+11.60	20.66	2.31
2x30 cig. E_2	♀	80	− 2.44	14.10	1.58
	♂	80	+ 1.64	21.81	2.44
3x30 cig. E_2	♀	80	− 0.01	16.42	1.84
	♂	80	− 2.40	19.47	2.18

Most pronounced reduction in body weight at the end of experiment was observed in the groups: DMBA + 2x30 cig. and 3x30 cig. E_2.

ogy. Fig. 2 a-w show findings of the laryngeal mucosa in the various stages.

In 800 control animals and in 160 animals treated with the vapor phase of the standard cigarettes, laryngeal leucoplakia of stage 1 is relatively infrequent, and stage 2 of laryngeal leucoplakia was observed only in 1 control animal. Similar observations were made in the group of animals treated with nitrosamines only: only stage 1 of laryngeal alterations was found. The group of 160 hamsters treated once with DMBA showed an exception: in 1.9% of the animals, the papillomatous stage 4 was observed (Table 4).

Table 4. Incidence of leucoplakia in control animals

I.   Incidence of leucoplakia in 800 control animals

 Stage 1: 12 cases = 1.5 %
 Stage 2: 1 case = 0.13%

II.   Incidence of leucoplakia in 160 animals exposed to vapor phase

 Stage 1: 9 cases = 5.6 %

III. Incidence of leucoplakia in 160 animals once treated with DMBA without exposure to smoke

 Stage 1: 4 cases = 2.5 %
 Stage 2: 1 case = 0.6 %
 Stage 4: 3 cases = 1.9 %

IV.   Incidence of leucoplakia in animals treated with 4x1 mg DENA/ 100 g body weight (in 52nd and 53rd week), animals not being exposed to smoke

 Stage 1: 3 cases = 3.5 %

Table 5. Relation between age to stage of leucoplakia in the larynx (males and females)

	Treatment period (weeks)	Stages						Total
		1	2	3	4	5	6	
Group 1	0 - 25	7		4	2			13
	26 - 50	16	6	13	23	11	5	74
	51 - 75	3	5	7	41	47	21	124
	76 -100			1	11	13	5	30
	>100			1	2	2	1	6
		26	11	26	79	73	32	247
	$X^2 = 82.15$			$P = 0.50$				
Group 4	0 - 25	7		1				8
	26 - 50	18	2	1	1			22
	51 - 75	17	20	25	11	5		78
	76 -100	7	11	15	7	10	1	51
	>100	2	6	8	1	3		20
		51	39	50	20	18	1	179
	$X^2 = 65.3$			$P = 0.52$				
Group 5	0 - 25	10	1	2	1			14
	26 - 50	23	9	12		1		45
	51 - 75	9	17	8	7	13	4	58
	76 -100		4	10	9	18	5	46
	>100		3	18	4	16	8	49
		42	34	50	21	48	17	212
	$X^2 = 117.2$			$P = 0.60$				
Group 6	0 - 25	7		3	2			12
	26 - 50	15	6	4	4	3		32
	51 - 75	13	11	14	13	23	4	78
	76 -100		6	15	8	20	6	55
	>100		1	4	1	3	1	10
		35	24	40	28	49	11	187
	$X^2 = 57.8$			$P = 0.48$				

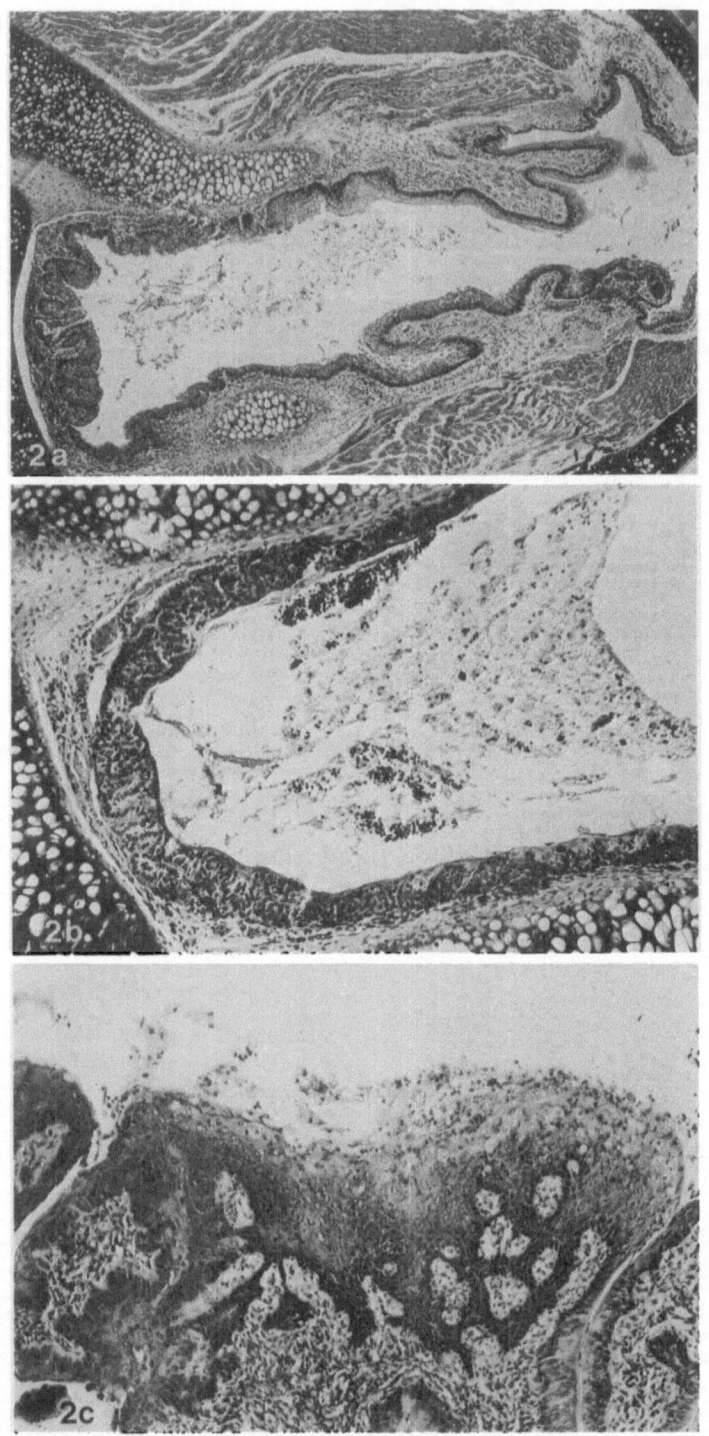

Fig. 2 a–w. (a) Pachydermia of the laryngeal mucosa (stage 1). HE x 7.50. (b) Leucoplakia of the laryngeal mucosa (stage 2). HE x 7.50. (c and d) Verrucous leucoplakia of the laryngeal mucosa (stage 3). HE x 75. (e and f) Papillary leucoplakia of the laryngeal mucosa (stage 4). HE x 7.50. (g–n) Pseudoepitheliomatous leucoplakia of the laryngeal

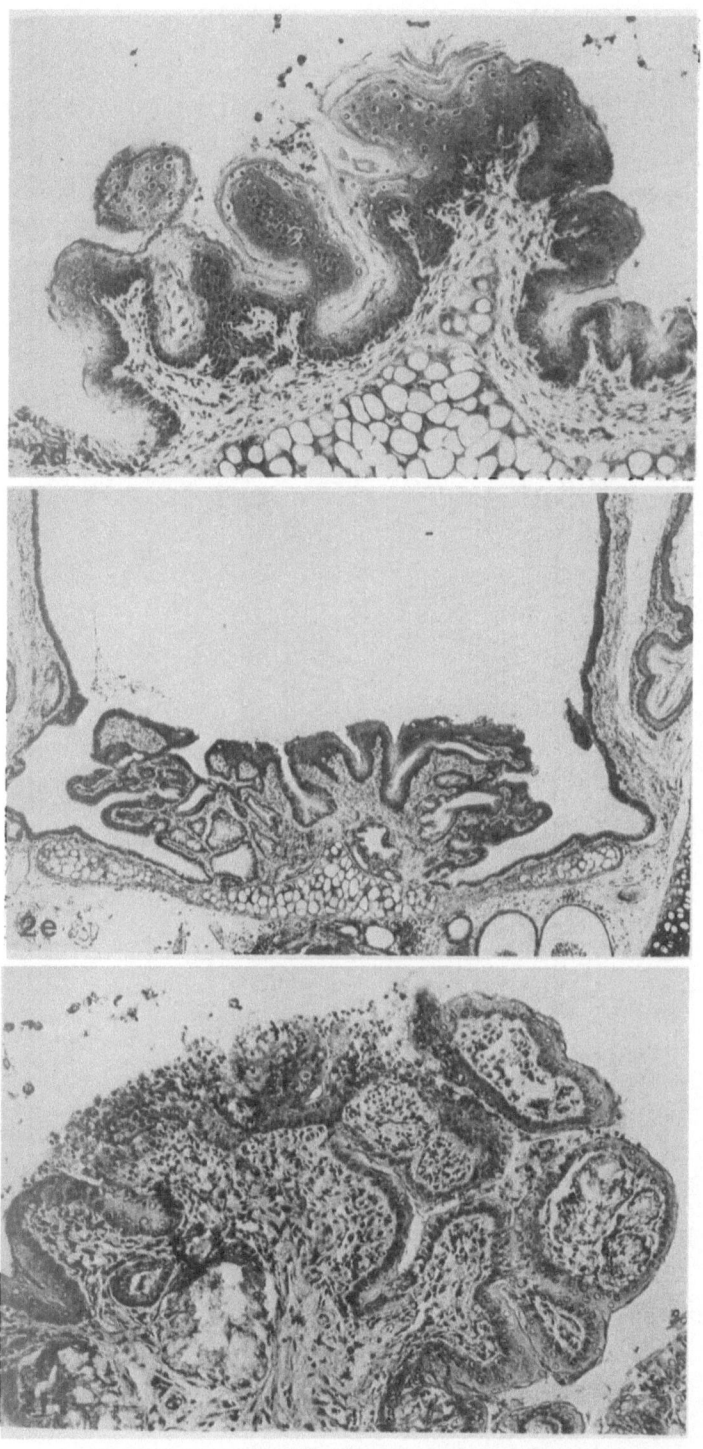

mucosa (stage 5). HE x 75, g, k-n HE x 7.50, h = magnification of g.
(o-w) Carcinoma of the laryngeal mucosa (stage 6) with various degree
of infiltration. o, t, u, w HE x 7.50; p, r, s, v HE x 75; q HE x 188;
p and q = magnification of o

340

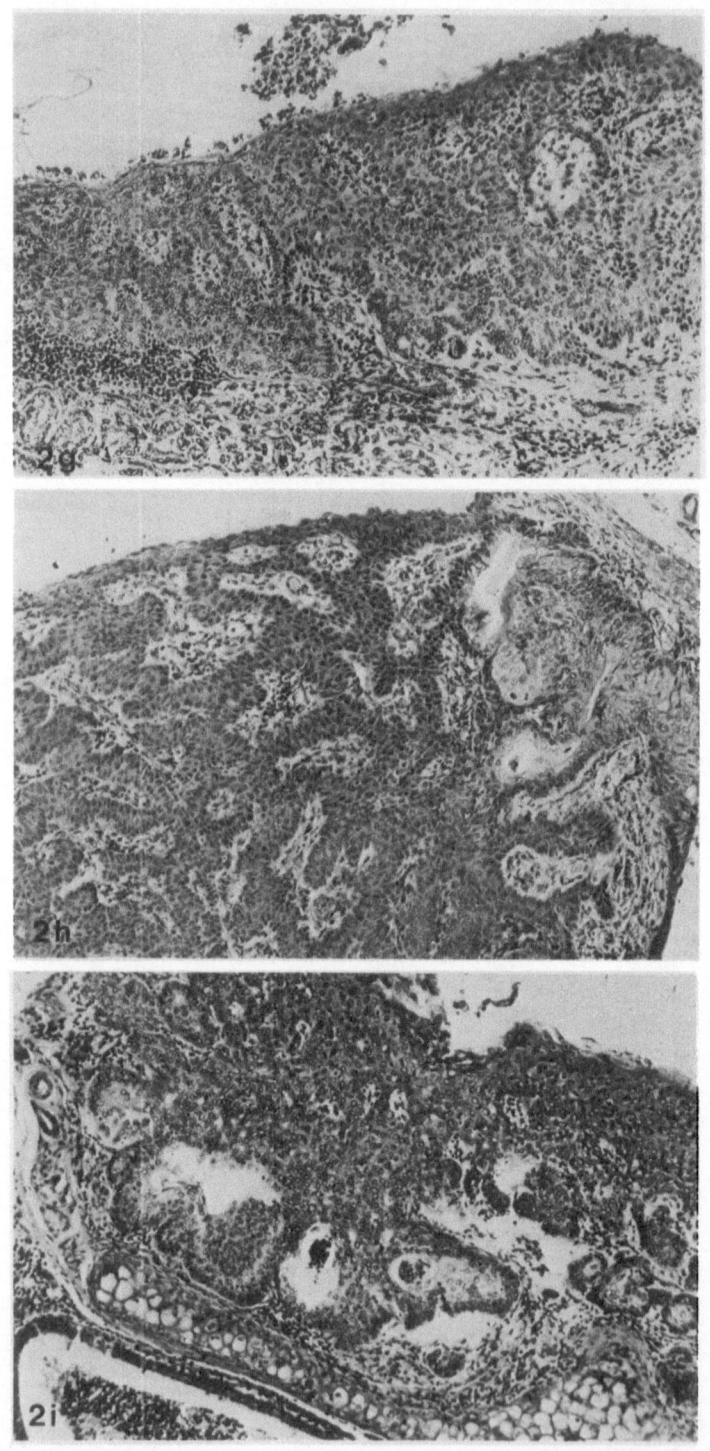

Legends see pages 338/339

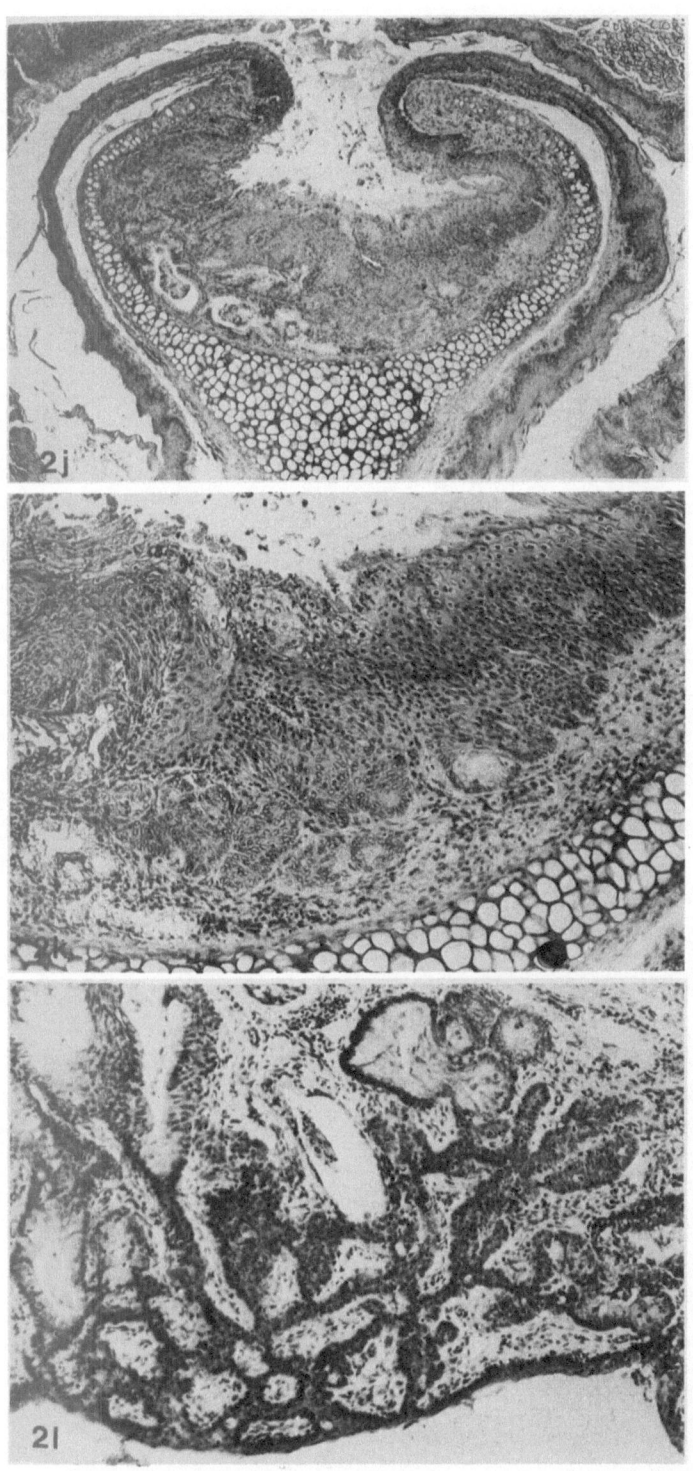

Legends see pages 338/339

342

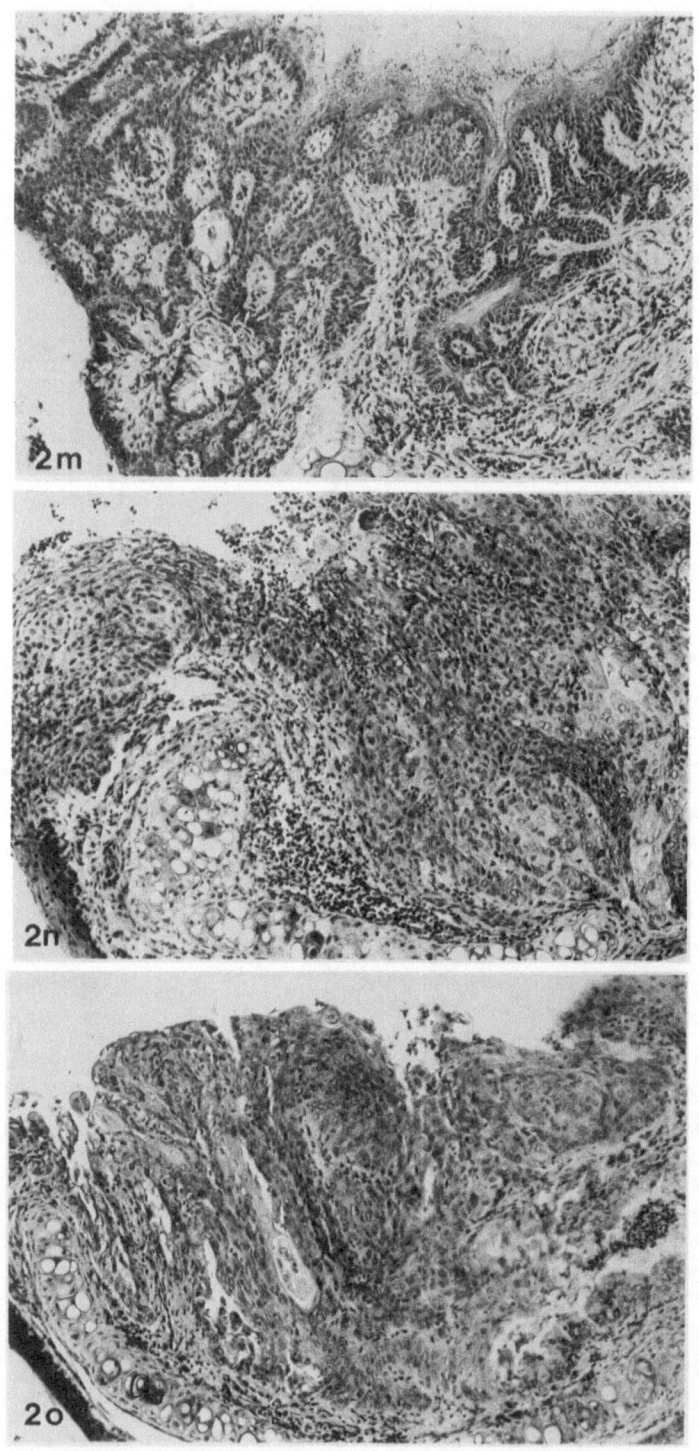

Legends see pages 338/339

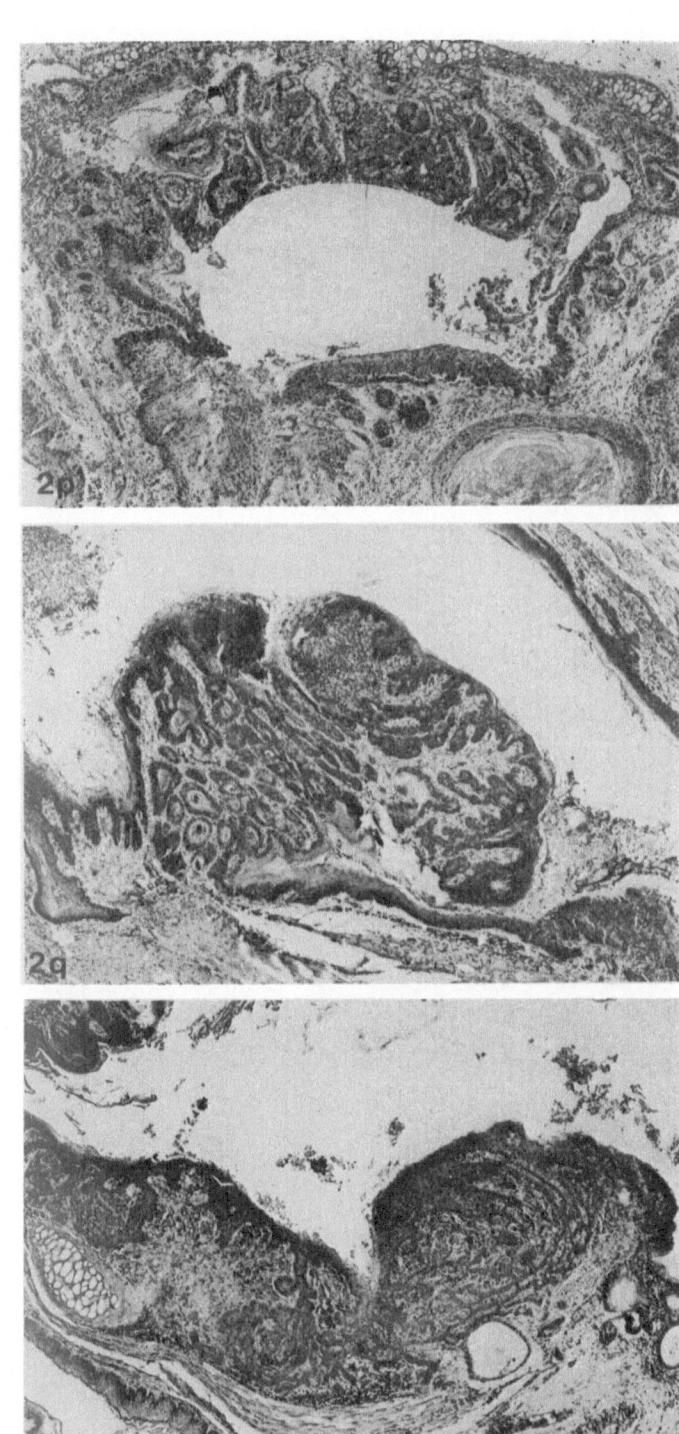

Legends see pages 338/339

344

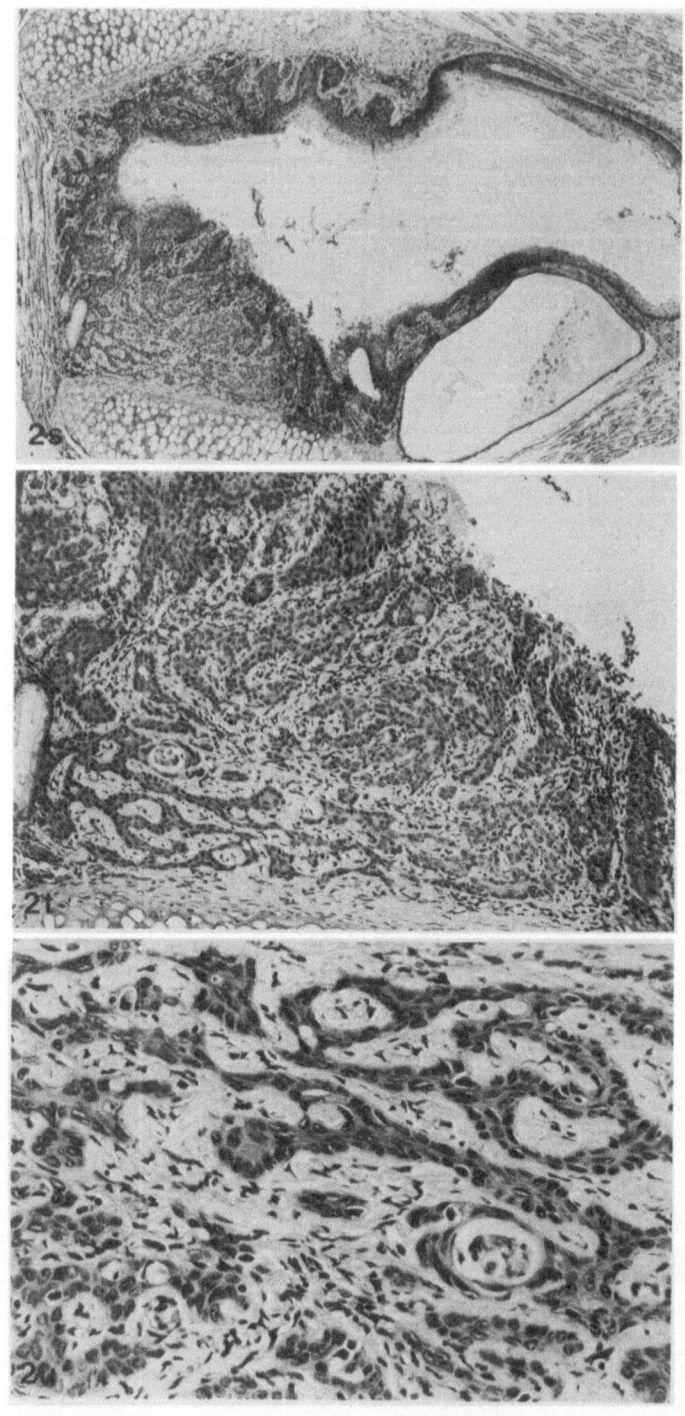

Legends see pages 338/339

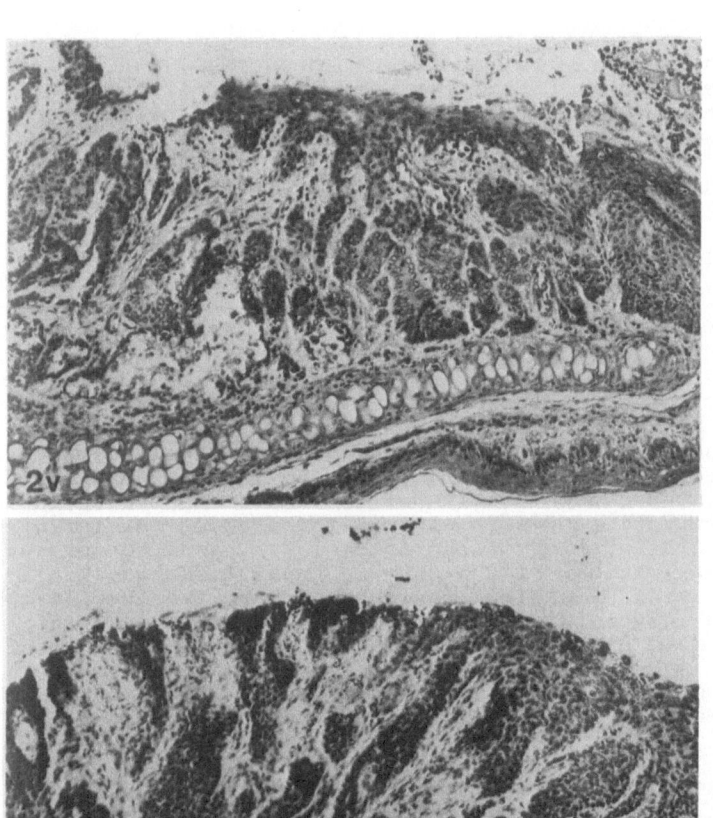

Legends see pages 338/339

HAMPERL (1973) has suggested another classification of stages: Stages
3 and 4 could have been classified as exophytic papillary proliferation
and stage 5 as endophytic atypical proliferation. This is, however,
only of academic importance.

That small carcinomas of the larynx did not infiltrate the cartilage
is not surprising. We have observed the same phenomenon during experiments in the same area following application of nitrosamines and polycyclic aromatic hydrocarbons. Also, in experiments with mice, we found
a similar behavior of tumors. The tumors induced on the ear by benzo(a)
pyrene did not show any infiltration into the cartilage.

The various stages of laryngeal alterations appear in a specific dose-
time sequence. Table 5 demonstrates this relationship, with additional
information about the time of appearance, e.g. stages 5 and 6, which in
group 1 appeared distinctly earlier than, for instance, in the comparable group 5. Even at this point, the more-than-additive effect of
the smoke is apparent, i.e. the effect cannot be explained only as the
summation of the effects of smoke exposure (dose II = 2 x 10 min) and
DMBA.

In general, animals that died early or animals that received cigarettes with lower activity have a greater tendency to stages of lower classification, e.g., stages 2 to 4. Cigarettes with lower activity clearly produce at a less frequent rate the stages of higher classification, e.g., stage 5 and stage 6 (carcinomas). Table 6 distinctly demonstrates the difference of stages within the groups. In order to offer a clear overall picture, we have summarized the most important findings in Table 7. It is evident that using $NaNO_3$ as additive or using reconstituted tobacco sheets or filters reduced condensate and thereby alterations, especially the incidence of stage 5 and 6 (cancer) in the larynx. This is also true for the "black cigarette", which showed a very low condensate yield due to the mixture used in this experiment. A significant reduction of the biological effect is also demonstrated by consideration of the different number of puffs and the period of smoke exposure. These results should inspire and influence our future work to enable production of a less harmful cigarette.

The very rare appearance of lung carcinomas - there was only 1 case following the combined treatment of DMBA and smoke - may be explained by the methodically induced accumulation of the smoke components in the larynx. The concentration of particles in the area of the larynx is obviously due to an alteration of the aerosol flow and, to some extent, due to nasal respiration. Fig. 3 shows a typical squamous cell carcinoma. Mucus-secreting bronchial adenomas, as described by SAFFIOTTI (1970), were observed only in 2 animals in group 2 (DMBA) and 1 in group 5 (dose II of smoke exposure)(Fig. 4).

Table 8 portrays the more-than-additive effect of the combined treatment with DMBA and smoke in comparison to treatment with DMBA alone or with smoke alone (dose II).

We consider this as a confirmation of results of many epicutaneous tests which show that some factors effect carcinogenesis in such a way that they are interpreted as cocarcinogenic. According to the findings obtained, DMBA seems to attack the same areas of the respiratory tract as smoke particles; this may lead to the conclusion that in the total effect, great importance should be attributed to the polycyclic aromatic hydrocarbons of the smoke.

The effect of combined treatment with smoke and diethylnitrosamine (DENA) was surprising. We intentionally did not administer the nitrosamine at the beginning, because the animal mortality rate following initial treatment in earlier experiments was too high, due to a high incidence of papillomas in the respiratory tract. The following results should be emphasized in connection with the question on the "effect of nitrosamines":

1. The additional nitrosamine effect does not enhance the "smoke effect" (Table 9).

2. Following nitrosamine application, papillomas of a different morphological structure and localization in the larynx occurred than following smoke exposure alone (Fig. 5 a and b).

3. Cigarettes treated with a high dose of sodium nitrate showed no findings explicable as nitrosamine effect as it can be found in bronchi and trachea in animals treated with DENA and DMBA (Table 10).

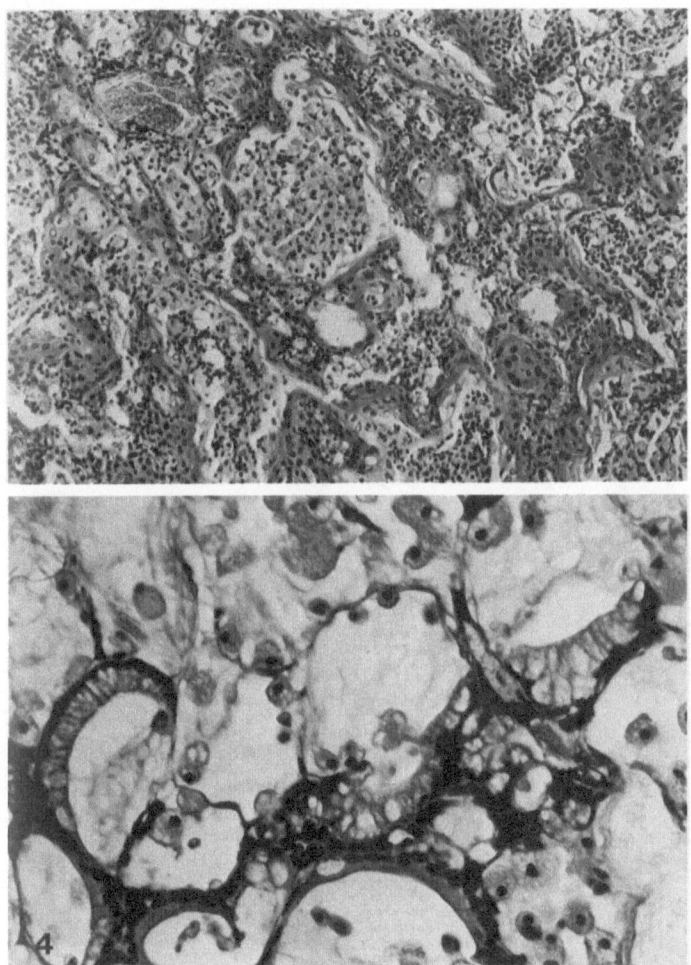

Fig. 3. Squamous cell carcinoma of the lung. HE x 75
Fig. 4. Mucus-producing adenoma of the bronchus. HE x 188

Table 6. Incidence of leucoplakia and carcinoma in the larynx (males and females)

Group		Stages 1		2		3
Control	K	1.0%	K	0.2%	K	0.0%
DMBA+ standard cig./II	1	16.3%	1	6.9%	1	16.3%
DMBA	2	2.5%	2	0.6%	2	0.0%
Control	3	3.0%	3	0.0%	3	0.0%
Standard cig./I	4	31.9%	4	24.4%	4	31.3%
Standard cig./II	5	26.3%	5	21.3%	5	31.3%
Standard cig./III	6	21.9%	6	15.0%	6	25.0%
Vapor phase of standard cig./II	7	5.6%	7	0.0%	7	0.0%
Fresh air (Placebo)	8	3.1%	8	0.0%	8	0.0%
Standard cig./II + $NaNO_3$	9	15.6%	9	10.6%	9	26.9%
Reconst.tobacco sheet/II+$NaNO_3$	10	15.0%	10	8.1%	10	33.8%
Reconst.tobacco sheet/II	11	14.4%	11	11.3%	11	33.8%
Standard cig./II + asbestos	12	6.3%	12	3.1%	12*	78.1%
Asbestos	13	0.0%	13	0.0%	13	0.0%
"Black cig."/II	14	10.0%	14	20.6%	14	66.9%
Standard cig./II with acetate filter	15	6.3%	15	18.1%	15	68.1%
Standard cig./II with cellulose filter	16	10.0%	16	15.6%	16	63.7%
Standard cig./II with charcoal filter	17	8.1%	17	6.9%	17	68.8%
Standard cig./II + DENA	18	12.5%	18	7.5%	18	68.1%
DENA	18A	3.5%	18A	0.0%	18A	0.0%

Table 6 (cont.)

Group		Stages 4		5		6
Control	K	0.0%	K	0.0%	K	0.0%
DMBA+ standard cig./II	1	49.4%	1	45.6%	1	20.0%
DMBA	2	1.9%	2	0.0%	2	0.0%
Control	3	0.0%	3	0.0%	3	0.0%
Standard cig./I	4	12.5%	4	11.3%	4	0.6%
Standard cig./II	5	13.1%	5	30.0%	5	10.6%
Standard cig./III	6	17.5%	6	30.6%	6	6.9%
Vapor phase of standard cig./II	7	0.0%	7	0.0%	7	0.0%
Fresh air (Placebo)	8	0.0%	8	0.0%	8	0.0%
Standard cig./II + NaNO$_3$	9	23.1%	9	15.6%	9	2.5%
Reconst.tobacco sheet/II+NaNO$_3$	10	31.3%	10	14.4%	10	1.3%
Reconst.tobacco sheet/II	11	21.9%	11	11.9%	11	0.0%
Standard cig./II + asbestos	12	15.6%	12	28.8%	12	7.5%
Asbestos	13	0.0%	13	0.0%	13	0.0%
"Black cig."/II	14	4.4%	14	10.0%	14	1.3%
Standard cig./II with acetate filter	15	9.4%	15	13.1%	15	0.6%
Standard cig./II with cellulose filter	16	6.3%	16	11.9%	16	2.5%
Standard cig./II with charcoal filter	17	11.3%	17	25.0%	17	2.5%
Standard cig./II + DENA	18	20.0%	18	13.8%	18	1.3%
DENA	18A	0.0%	18A	0.0%	18A	0.0%

Table 7. Laryngeal changes in groups exposed to the same dose levels of smoke (30 cigarettes twice a day)(male and female animals)

Type of cigarette	Group	Number of puffs	Time-factor	Smoke condensate (dry) mg	Condensate factor	Larynx Stage 5	Larynx Stage 6
2 x 30 cig. E_2	5	10	1.0	33.7	1.0	30.0%	10.6%
2 x 30 cig. EN	9	9	0.9	22.4	0.66	15.6%	2.5%
2 x 30 cig. EG_3	10	6	0.6	20.8	0.62	14.4%	1.25%
2 x 30 cig. EG_1	11	7	0.7	27.3	0.81	11.9%	0.0%
2 x 30 cig. A	15	10	1.0	23.5	0.70	13.1%	0.62%
2 x 30 cig. D	16	11	1.1	22.7	0.67	11.9%	2.5%
2 x 30 cig. K	17	10	1.0	26.2	0.79	25.0%	2.5%
2 x 30 cig. Z	14	8	0.8	20.9	0.62	10.0%	1.25%

Table 8. Overadditive effect of tobacco smoke inhalation and initial DMBA treatment (males and females)

	Stage 5	Stage 6
Initial dose with DMBA and smoke exposure 2x30 cig. daily (= dose level II)	45.6%	20.0%
Initial dose with DMBA in CMC intratracheally	0.0%	0.0%
Smoke exposure 2x30 cig. daily (= dose level II)	30.0%	10.6%

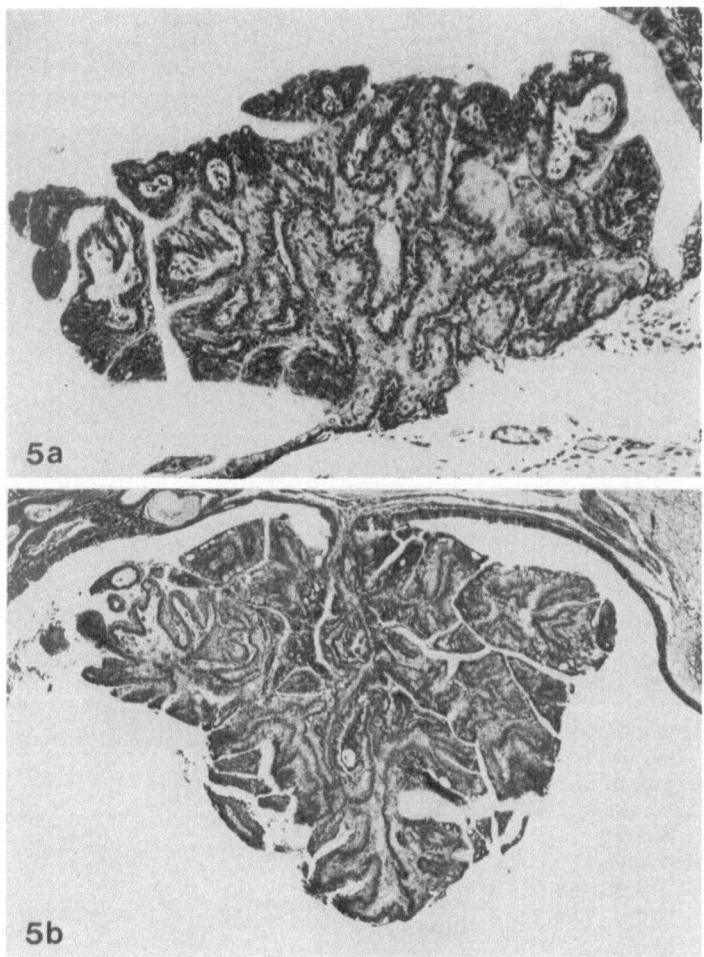

Fig. 5 a and b. Papilloma of the lower section of the larynx
(group 18 = DENA and smoke). HE x 7.50

The following Tables (11-15) illustrate which lesions are caused by
treatment with DMBA or DENA. There are some findings that have no
relationship to the treatment. For example, there is no evident relationship between treatment and induction of tumors in the soft
tissue and subcutaneous tissue of the skin (Table 16), in the nasal
cavity (Table 17), and in the urinary bladder. Only 1 bladder carcinoma appeared in the group 18A; the animals of this group were treated
with DENA. The incidence of adrenal tumors (Table 18) was age-dependent, and the distribution of sexes with regard to tumor types was
very different

The method reported is, in our opinion, suitable for comparing different smoke qualities as to their biological activity. Moreover, it
gives us information about the cigarettes and enables, to select less
harmful cigarettes, which is the main goal of our investigations.

Table 9. Incidence of papillomas in distal part of larynx

Treatment	No.	Value	Treatment	No.	Value
Control	K	-	Reconst. tobacco sheet II + $NaNO_3$	10	-
DMBA+ standard cig./II	1	-	Reconst. tobacco sheet/II	11	-
DMBA	2	-	Standard cig./II + asbestos	12	-
Control	3	-			
Standard cig./I	4	-	Asbestos	13	-
Standard cig./II	5	-	"Black cig."/II	14	-
Standard cig./III	6	-	Standard cig./II with acetate filter	15	-
Vapor phase of standard cig./II	7	-	Standard cig./II with cellulose filter	16	-
Fresh air (Placebo)	8	-	Standard cig./II with charcoal filter	17	-
Standard cig./II +$NaNO_3$	9	-	Standard cig./II + DENA	18	♀ 2.5% ♂23.75%
			DENA	18A	♀11.1% ♂22.2%

Table 10. Incidence of bronchial and tracheal papillomas

Treatment	No.	Value	Treatment	No.	Value
Control	K	-	Reconst. tobacco sheet II + $NaNO_3$	10	-
DMBA+ standard cig./II	1	♀ 3.75% ♂ 3.75%	Reconst. tobacco sheet/II	11	-
DMBA	2	♂ 6.25%	Standard cig./II + asbestos	12	-
Control	3	-			
Standard cig./I	4	-	Asbestos	13	-
Standard cig./II	5	-	"Black cig."/II	14	-
Standard cig./III	6	-	Standard cig./II with acetate filter	15	-
Vapor phase of standard cig./II	7	-	Standard cig./II with cellulose filter	16	-
Fresh air (Placebo)	8	-	Standard cig./II with charcoal filter	17	-
Standard cig./II +$NaNO_3$	9	-	Standard cig./II + DENA	18	♀10.0% ♂28.75%
			DENA	18A	♀ 2.22% ♂27.5%

Table 11. Incidence of pharyngeal papillomas

Control	K ♂	0.33%	Reconst.tobacco sheet II + NaNO$_3$	10	-
DMBA+ standard cig./II	1	♀ 32.5% ♂ 13.75%	Reconst.tobacco sheet/II	11	-
DMBA	2	♀ 33.75% ♂ 22.5%	Standard cig./II + asbestos	12	-
Control	3 ♂	1.0%			
Standard cig./I	4	-	Asbestos	13	-
Standard cig./II	5 ♂	1.25%	"Black cig."/II	14	-
Standard cig./III	6 ♀	2.5%	Standard cig./II with acetate filter	15	-
Vapor phase of standard cig./II	7	-	Standard cig./II with cellulose filter	16	-
Fresh air (Placebo)	8	-	Standard cig./II with charcoal filter	17 ♂	1.25%
Standard cig./II +NaNO$_3$	9	-	Standard cig./II + DENA	18 ♂	1.25%
			DENA	18A	-

Table 12. Incidence of papillomas in the oral cavity

Control	K	-	Reconst.tobacco sheet II + NaNO$_3$	10	-
DMBA+ standard cig./II	1	♀ 7.5% ♂ 5.0%	Reconst.tobacco sheet/II	11 ♂	1.25%
DMBA	2	♀ 5.0% ♂ 8.75%	Standard cig./II + asbestos	12 ♂	1.25%
Control	3 ♂	1.0%			
Standard cig./I	4	-	Asbestos	13	-
Standard cig./II	5	-	"Black cig."/II	14 ♂	1.25%
Standard cig./III	6	-	Standard cig./II with acetate filter	15	-
Vapor phase of standard cig./II	7	-	Standard cig./II with cellulose filter	16	-
Fresh air (Placebo)	8	-	Standard cig./II with charcoal filter	17	-
Standard cig./II +NaNO$_3$	9	-	Standard cig./II + DENA	18 ♂	1.25%
			DENA	18A ♀	1.25%

Table 13. Incidence of papillomas and carcinomas (female / male)

	Esophagus- papillomas		Stomach- papillomas		Stomach- carcinomas	
Control	K	-	K	4.5%	K	0.2%
DMBA+ standard cig./II	1	5.0%	1	68.1%	1	3.1%
DMBA	2	2.5%	2	73.8%	2	2.5%
Control	3	-	3	7.0%	3	0.5%
Standard cig./I	4	-	4	4.4%	4	-
Standard cig./II	5	-	5	5.0%	5	-
Standard cig./III	6	-	6	6.3%	6	-
Vapor phase of standard cig./II	7	-	7	8.1%	7	-
Fresh air (Placebo)	8	-	8	4.4%	8	-
Standard cig./II +NaNO$_3$	9	-	9	5.0%	9	-
Reconst.tobacco sheet II + NaNO$_3$	10	-	10	3.1%	10	0.6%
Reconst.tobacco sheet/II	11	-	11	3.1%	11	0.6%
Standard cig./II + asbestos	12	-	12	11.9%	12	1.3%
Asbestos	13	-	13	5.6%	13	0.6%
"Black cig."/II	14	-	14	5.6%	14	0.6%
Standard cig./II with acetate filter	15	-	15	8.1%	15	-
Standard cig./II with cellulose filter	16	-	16	4.4%	16	-
Standard cig./II with charcoal filter	17	-	17	5.6%	17	0.6%
Standard cig./II + DENA	18	-	18	4.4%	18	-
DENA	18A	-	18A	4.7%	18A	-

Table 14. Liver tumors

Group	K	1	2	3	4	5	6	7	8	9	10	11	12	13	14	15	16	17	18	18A
Sex	♀♂	♀♂	♀♂	♀♂	♀♂	♀♂	♀♂	♀♂	♀♂	♀♂	♀♂	♀♂	♀♂	♀♂	♀♂	♀♂	♀♂	♀♂	♀♂	♀♂
Liver cell carcinoma			1									1								
Carcinoma of the bile duct	1			1	1															
Haemangio-endothelioma	1	1	1																	
Haemangioma	1	1	1	1										1	1					
Adenoma of the bile duct						1							2							

Table 15. Tumors of the haematopoietic and lymphoreticular system

Group	1	2	3	4	5	6	7	8	9	10	11	12	13	14	15	16	17	18	18A
Leukemia myeloic	1	1																	
Leukemia lymphatic		2		2	1												1		
Lymphosarcoma Type I	3	1	2		2	1		1	2		2		1				1		2
Lymphosarcoma Type II	3	3	3		2	2	2			1	1	1					2		2
Lymphosarcoma Type III			2		1		1		1	1					1				
Plasmocytoma		1	3	2				1	1	1		1	1	1	1	1	1		2
Myelosarcoma	1																		
Total number	8	8	10	4	6	3	3	2	4	3	3	2	2	1	2	2	6	–	6
Mean induction Periods (weeks)	41.4	57.9	103.1	77.5	98.3	76.0	85.7	76.0	76.8	104.3	77.7	108.5	68.5	86.0	68.0	79.0	77.0	–	75.3

Table 16. Tumors in skin, soft tissue, and subcutaneous tissue

Group	K ♂	K ♀	1 ♂	1 ♀	2 ♂	2 ♀	3 ♂	3 ♀	4 ♂	4 ♀	5 ♂	5 ♀	6 ♂	6 ♀	7 ♂	7 ♀	8 ♂	8 ♀	9 ♂	9 ♀	10 ♂	10 ♀	11 ♂	11 ♀	12 ♂	12 ♀	13 ♂	13 ♀	14 ♂	14 ♀	15 ♂	15 ♀	16 ♂	16 ♀	17 ♂	17 ♀	18 ♂	18 ♀	18A ♂	18A ♀
Fibrosarcoma	1				1																				1						1				1					
Round-cell sarcoma									1																															
Polymorph. sarcoma		1					1								1																									1
Osteoblast. sarcoma																		1	1								1													
Haemangio-endothelioma																																1								
Spindle-cell sarcoma	1																																							
Melanosarcoma (eye)		1																																						
Melanoma (eye)		1																																						
Melanoma (skin)					1	1																																		
Melanosarcoma (skin)					1															1																				
Basalioma																						1																		
Squamous cell carc. (skin)					1																																			
Cystaden.papill.					1																																			
Papilloma																						1																		

Total = 15 sarcomas and 1 carcinoma
         2 sarcomas

Table 17. Incidence of adenomas in the nasal cavity

Control	K ♂ 0.67%		Reconst.tobacco sheet II + NaNO$_3$	10	–
DMBA+ standard cig./II	1 ♂ 1.25%		Reconst.tobacco sheet/II	11	–
DMBA	2	–	Standard cig./II + asbestos	12 ♀ 1.25%	
Control	3 ♂ 1.0%				
Standard cig./I	4 ♂ 1.25%		Asbestos	13	–
Standard cig./II	5 ♂ 2.5%		"Black cig."/II	14 ♂ 1.25%	
Standard cig./III	6	–	Standard cig./II with acetate filter	15 ♂ 1.25%	
Vapor phase of standard cig./II	7	–	Standard cig./II with cellulose filter	16 ♂ 1.25%	
Fresh air (Placebo)	8	–	Standard cig./II with charcoal filter	17 ♂ 1.25%	
Standard cig./II + NaNO$_3$	9	–	Standard cig./II + DENA	18 ♂ 3.75%	
			DENA	18A	–

Table 18.   Incidence of adrenal tumors (female / male)

Group	"Spindle-Cell"		"Round-Cell"		Carcinoma	
Control	K	3.7%	K	12.2%	K	0.3%
DMBA+ standard cig./II	1	-	1	8.1%	1	-
DMBA	2	3.1%	2	11.9%	2	-
Control	3	5.0%	3	21.0%	3	1.0%
Standard cig./I	4	4.4%	4	10.0%	4	0.6%
Standard cig./II	5	6.9%	5	6.9%	5	-
Standard cig./III	6	1.9%	6	6.3%	6	-
Vapor phase of standard cig./II	7	5.6%	7	8.8%	7	-
Fresh air (Placebo)	8	5.0%	8	13.8%	8	-
Standard cig./II + NaNO$_3$	9	5.6%	9	11.3%	9	-
Reconst.tobacco sheet II + NaNO$_3$	10	1.9%	10	9.4%	10	-
Reconst.tobacco sheet/II	11	4.4%	11	10.6%	11	-
Standard cig./II + asbestos	12	5.0%	12	12.5%	12	-
Asbestos	13	6.9%	13	18.1%	13	-
"Black cig."/II	14	3.1%	14	10.6%	14	-
Standard cig./II with acetate filter	15	4.4%	15	13.8%	15	-
Standard cig./II with cellulose filter	16	5.6%	16	7.5%	16	-
Standard cig./II with charcoal filter	17	4.4%	17	10.6%	17	0.6%
Standard cig./II + DENA	18	6.9%	18	10.0%	18	-
DENA	18A	2.4%	18A	11.8%	18A	-

References

Atlas of Tumor Pathology. (Eds. Ash, J.E., Beck, M.R., Wilkens, J.D., Washington, D.C.). Armed Forces Inst. Pathol. sect. IV, fasc. 12-13, 1964.

DONTENWILL, W., CHEVALIER, H.-J., HARKE, H.-P., LAFRENZ, U., RECKZEH, G., SCHNEIDER, B.: Investigations on the effect of chronic cigarette smoke inhalation on Syrian golden hamsters. J. nat. Cancer Inst. 51, 1781-1832 (1973).

HAMPERL, H.: Personal Communication 1973.

SAFFIOTTI, U.: Experimental respiratory tract carcinogenesis and its relation to inhalation exposures. In: Inhalation Carcinogenesis (M.G. Hanna, Jr., P. Nettesheim, J.R. Gilbert, eds). AEC Symposium Series no. 18, pp. 27-54. Oak Ridge, Tennessee: U.S. Atomic Energy Commission, Division of Technical Inf. 1970.

Effect of Chronic Exposure to Cigarette Smoke on Tumor Incidence in the Syrian Golden Hamster

Alfred P. Wehner, Robert H. Busch, and Richard J. Olson

Biology Department, Battelle, Pacific Northwest Laboratories, Richland, WA 99352, USA

ABSTRACT

A group of 51 male Syrian golden hamsters received lifespan exposures to cigarette smoke in Hamburg II type smoking machines for 10 minutes 3 times per day, 5 days per week. An additional group of 51 hamsters served as controls and received sham exposures only. At death, lungs, trachea, larynx, liver, kidneys, and tissues showing gross lesion, were histopathologically examined.

The smoke-exposed hamsters had a significantly higher incidence of the following lesions than the controls:

Total number of tumors	= 28% versus 6% ($p < 0.05$)
Malignant tumors	= 18% versus 2% ($p < 0.05$)
Epithelial lesions of the larynx	= 22% versus 0% ($p < 0.01$)

The increased tumor incidence in the smoke-exposed hamsters is not necessarily a direct effect of the exposures to cigarette smoke, but might be explained by the significantly longer mean lifespan of 19.6 months of the smoke-exposed group as compared to 15.3 months for the controls.

Introduction

The results reported in this paper are part of a larger research program in which we investigated the cocarcinogenicity of inhaled chrysotile asbestos, cobalt oxide (CoO) and nickel oxide (NiO), respectively, and cigarette smoke in hamsters. In this paper, the effect of lifespan exposure to cigarette smoke on tumor incidence in the Syrian golden hamster is described.

Methods

A group of 51 male Syrian golden hamsters (*Mesocricetus auratus*, random-bred ENG:ELA strain, Engle's Laboratory Animals, Inc., Farmersburg, Indiana) received 10-minute exposures to cigarette smoke in modified Hamburg II smoking machines (Fig. 1) 3 times per day, 5 days per week, for the duration of their natural lifespan. At the age of 2 months, the hamsters were gradually introduced to the smoke exposure regimen over a period of 2 weeks. Smoke exposures took place at 8:30 a.m., 11:30 a.m., and 9 p.m. This schedule was necessitated by the desire

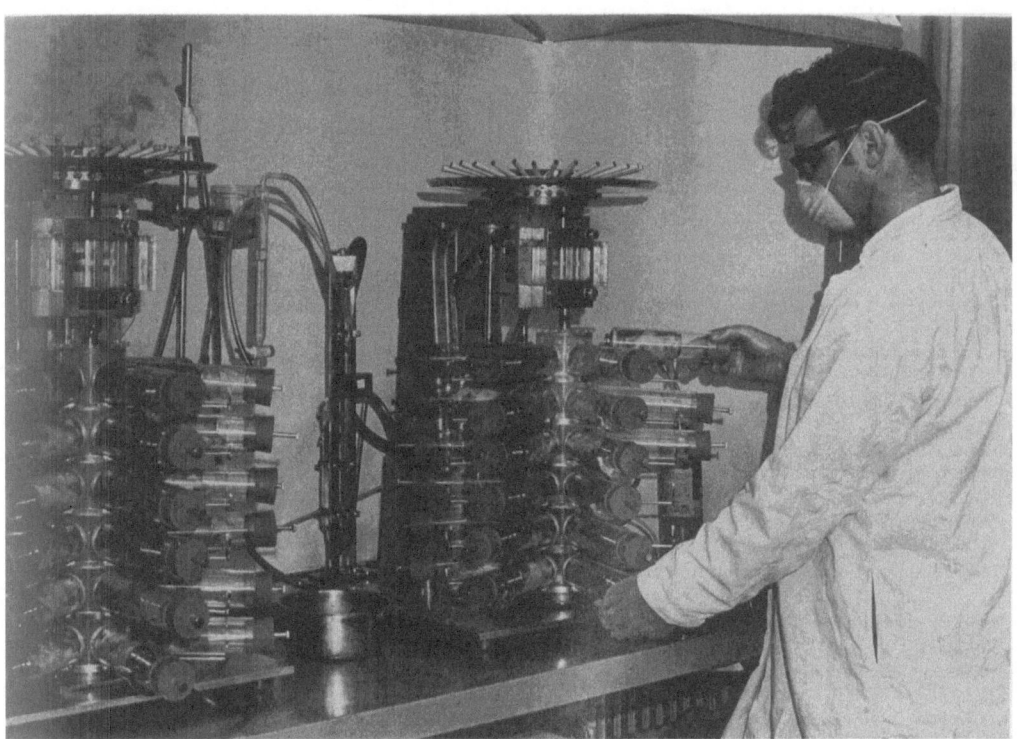

Fig. 1. Modified Hamburg II type smoking machines

to expose these hamsters to cigarette smoke at the same intervals and
at the same times of day as the hamsters of the cocarcinogenicity study.
The latter animals received a 7-hour dust exposure between the second
and third daily smoke exposure.

An additional group of 51 hamsters served as controls and received
sham exposures to simulate the stress of handling and confinement in
the restraining tubes of the smoking machine experienced by the smoke-
exposed animals.

The original Hamburg II smoking machine, developed and described by
DONTENWILL et al. (1967), can accommodate 2 tiers of 5 rodents each,
providing a total capacity of 10 rodents. By increasing the height of
the smoke exposure chamber from 13 to 41 cm, we increased its capacity
to 6 tiers of 5 rodents each, i.e., 30 rodents. This modification did
not affect the smoke dilution. There was no concentration gradient of
particulate matter in the chamber, and there was no difference in
carboxyhemoglobin (COHb) levels of hamsters which had been exposed to
cigarette smoke at different tier levels. To equalize any differences
which might have occurred in the quality of the cigarette smoke due
to its different age at the different tier levels, the position of the
animals in the smoke exposure chambers was rotated from exposure to
exposure. The age difference of the smoke between tier 1 and tier 6
was approximately 6 seconds, which probably resulted in decreased
levels of some free radicals in the cigarette smoke (personal communication with Dr. V.D. TUGHAN, British Council for Tobacco Research).

Briefly, the Hamburg II smoking machine operates as follows: the smoking head of the machine is loaded with 30 cigarettes. During the smoking process, the head turns 12 degrees after a 2-second puff on the cigarette in front of the draw port, advancing the next cigarette to the draw port. Each of the 30 cigarettes is thus drawn on once for 2 seconds every minute at a selected puff volume of 35 ml. The smoke produced in this manner is considered standard for smoke inhalation experiments. On the way to the smoke exposure chamber, the smoke is diluted with ambient air at a selected ratio of 1:7. At each smoking period, the animals receive a continuous nose-only exposure of approximately 10 minutes duration.

3 hours were allowed between the first and the second smoke exposure for the COHb levels to recede from approximately 24% immediately after smoking to levels (~8%) closer to those of the controls (~4%).

We used University of Kentucky 1R1 research cigarettes which were smoked to a butt length of 30 mm. Under these conditions, the smoke contained approximately 30 mg tar and 2.2 mg nicotine per cigarette (BENNER, 1970). For more detailed information on analysis and production of the 1R1 cigarette, reference is made to the literature (BENNER, 1970; ATKINSON, 1970).

The hamsters had access to food and water ad libitum, with the exception of the smoke- or sham-smoke periods, during which they were kept in the animal-restraining tubes of the Hamburg II smoking machines. Except for the brief periods of exposure or sham exposure to cigarette smoke, the animals were maintained in individual 150 cm^2 compartments of stainless steel wire cages. When not exposed or sham-exposed to cigarette smoke, the hamsters were kept on standard cage racks. Body weights were taken every 2 weeks during the growth period of the hamsters and every 4 weeks thereafter.

Moribund animals were sacrificed. At sacrifice or death, the body weight was taken and a detailed necropsy was performed on each animal. Lung, trachea, larynx, heart with sections of the aorta, liver, kidneys, spleen, bladder, skinned head, and tissues showing gross lesions, were fixed in 10% neutral-buffered formalin. Histopathologic examination was made of hematoxylin and eosin-stained paraffin sections. Occasionally, tissues were examined electron-microscopically.

All findings were recorded and standardized to match NCI data evaluation forms.

Results

Table 1 summarizes type and incidence of tumors in both hamster groups. The total number of tumors, as well as the incidence of malignant tumors, was significantly higher ($p < 0.05$) in the smoke-exposed group than in the sham-exposed controls. However, no primary lung cancer was found in the smoke-exposed animals.

The first lung lesion appearing in the smoke-exposed group was interstitial pneumonitis, characterized by infiltration of alveolar septa by neutrophils and mononuclear-type chronic inflammatory cells (Fig. 2). Emphysema appeared as a component of the response, the degree of emphysema showing considerable variation from area to area within the lungs of individual hamsters, and also from hamster to hamster. Generally, the change appeared to be more severe in animals which had

363

Table 1. Type and incidence of tumors[a]

Tumor type	Smoke-exposed group		Sham-exposed controls		Comments
	Number	%	Number	%	
Malignant					
Reticulum cell sarcoma	5	10	0	0	
Carcinoma	2	4	0	0	
Lymphosarcoma	1	2	0	0	
Leukemia	1	2	0	0	
Plasma cell tumor	0	0	1	2	
Subtotal	9	18	1	2	(p < 0.05)
Benign					
Adrenal cortex adenoma	4	8	0	0	
Lung adenoma	0	0	1	2	
Other adenomas	0	0	1	2	
Papillomas	1	2	0	0	
Subtotal	5	10	2	4	
Total	14	28	3	6	(p < 0.05)

[a]Multiple tumors of the same type in 1 animal are listed as 1 tumor.

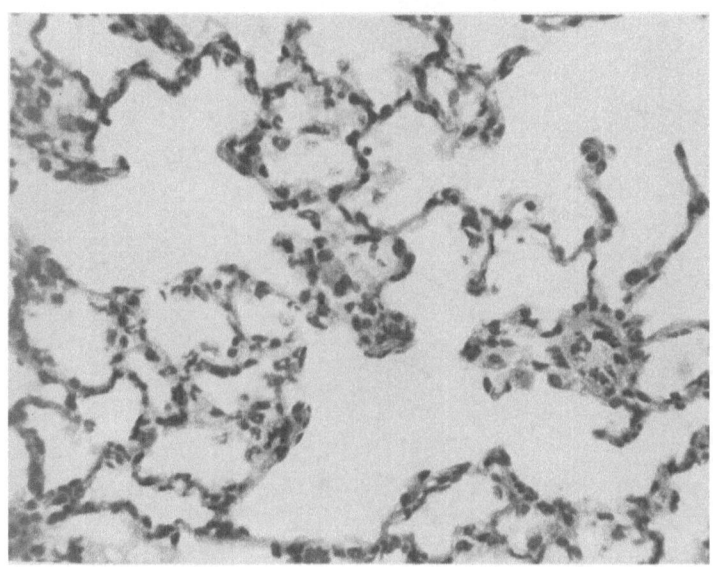

Fig. 2. Lung section of hamster No. S1B/8, showing interstitial pneumonitis characterized by infiltration of alveolar septa by neutrophils and mononuclear type chronic inflammatory cells. The animal had received a total of 434 smoke exposures. Age at death 10 months. HE x 300

received longer exposures. Increased numbers of macrophages with characteristic brown pigment were also present in the lungs of this group (Fig. 3). An alveolar macrophage from a sham-treated control hamster is shown in Fig. 4. Bronchiolization of alveolar epithelium appeared in several animals dying after 15 or more months of smoke exposure (Fig. 5).

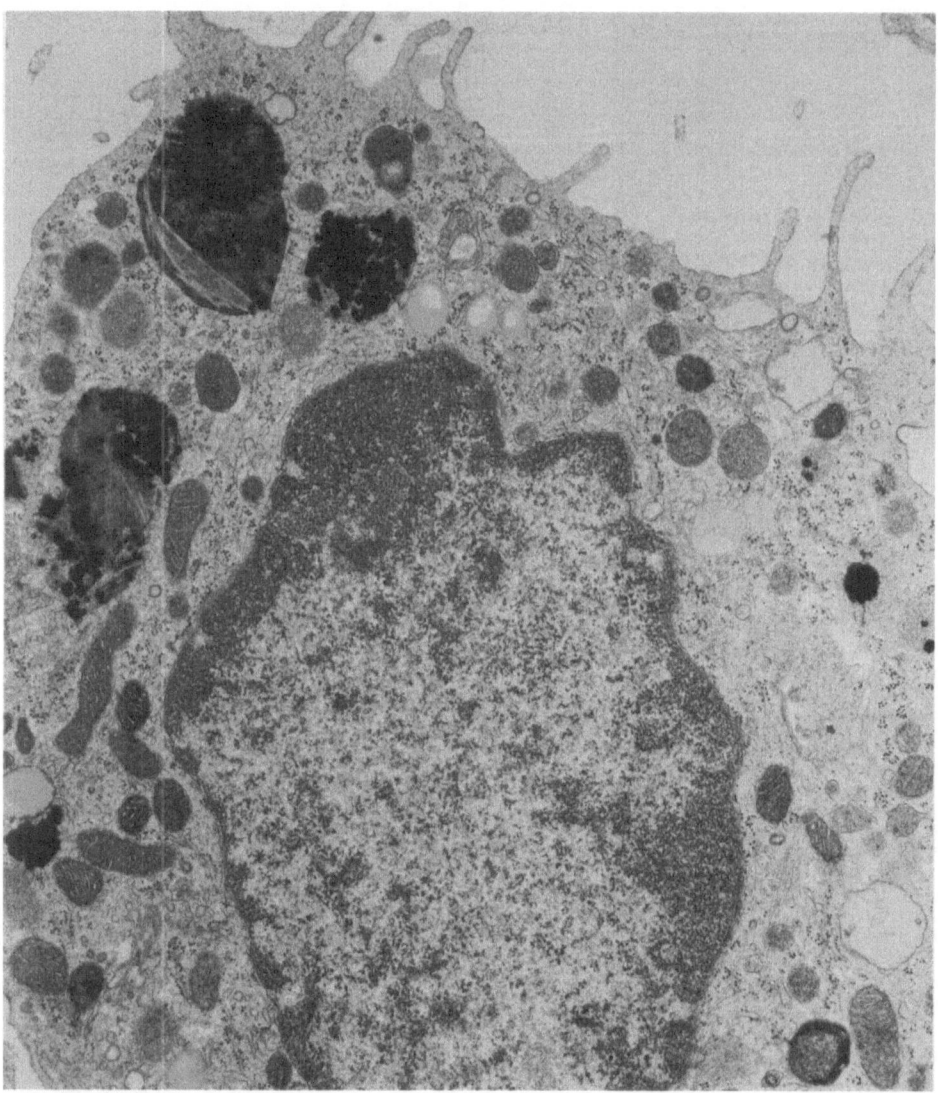

Fig. 3. Electron micrograph of an alveolar macrophage in hamster No. S2B/17 (1209 smoke exposures) showing large, dense inclusion bodies, probably lysosomes, which contain many particles, probably derived from cigarette smoke. x 18,200

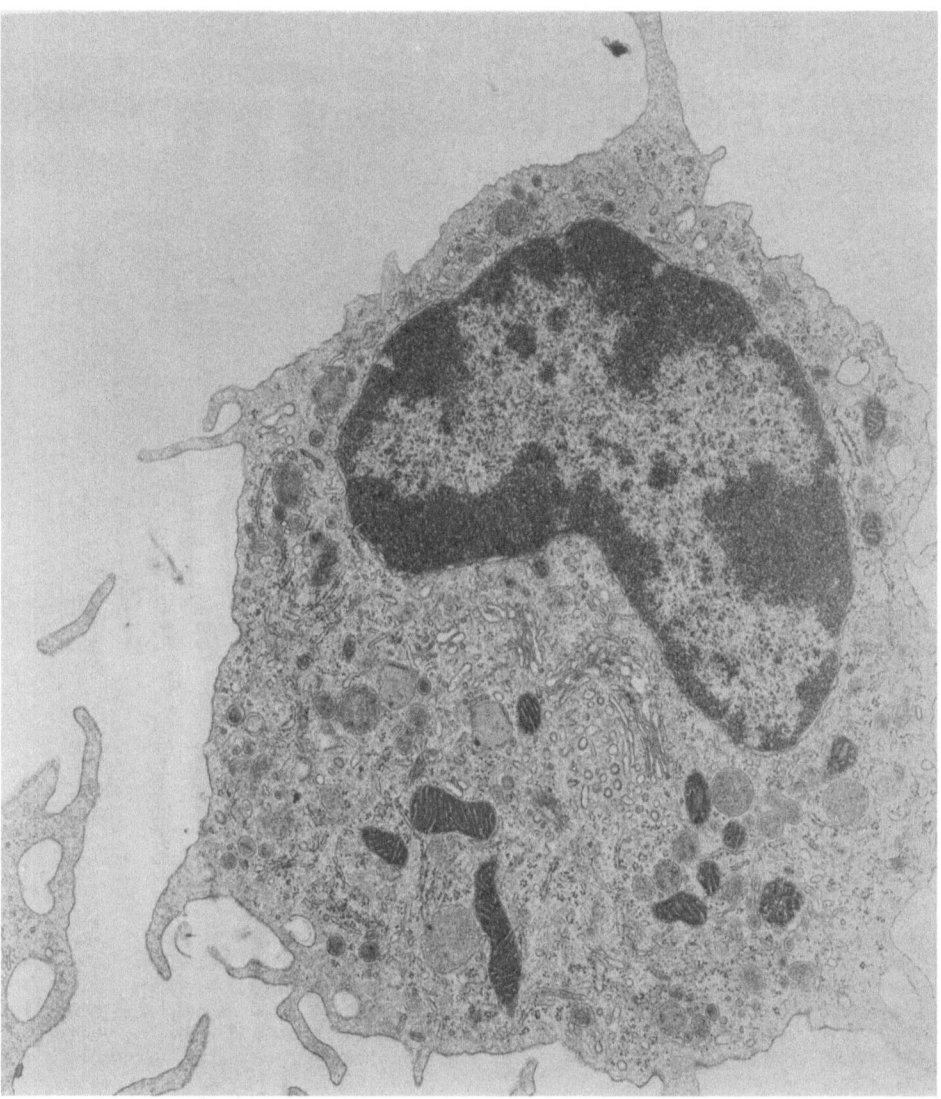

Fig. 4. Electron micrograph of an alveolar macrophage in the lung of sham-treated control hamster No. 6B/3, having received 1188 sham smoke exposures. x 14,000

Laryngeal changes in the smoke-exposed group ranged from inflammatory conditions with growth abnormalities of the epithelium to squamous papilloma formation. The abnormalities consisted of hyperkeratosis and acanthosis with varying degrees of nuclear change. Generally, the process appeared to be in the direction of loss of differentiation. There was a highly significant increase ($p < 0.01$) in epithelial lesions of the larynx in this group (22%) as compared to the control group (0%).

366

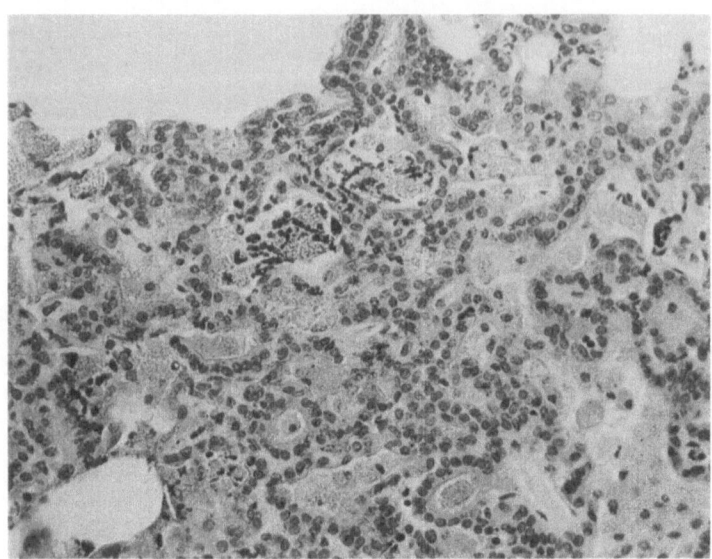

Fig. 5.   Lung section of hamster No. S1B/14, showing bronchiolization
of alveolar epithelium. The animal had received a total of 1052 smoke
exposures. Age at death 20 1/2 months. HE x 192

Parenthetically, the incidence of centrilobular necrosis of the liver
was also significantly higher (p < 0.05) in the smoke-exposed group
(14%) than in the controls (0%).

Discussion

The increased tumor incidence in the smoke-exposed hamsters is not
necessarily a direct effect of the exposures to cigarette smoke, but
might be explained by the significantly longer mean lifespan of 19.6
months of the smoke-exposed group, as compared to 15.3 months for the
controls. How many more tumors might have developed in the controls
if their mean lifespan had been 4.3 months longer remains a matter of
speculation.

Certainly the most surprising result of our experiments was the fact
that the smoke-exposed animals outlived the controls by a significant
margin. Factors contributing to this phenomenon might be the significantly lower mean body weight of the smoke-exposed group (124 g) as
compared to the controls (161 g), and a significantly delayed onset
of amyloidosis in the smoke-exposed animals, as will be described in
a different publication. Keeping animals on a restricted diet can result in a significant increase in lifespan. BERG and SIMMS (1961),
for example, reported that rats whose food intake was restricted by
33% and 46% had a significantly increased lifespan and a significant
delay in the onset of such diseases as tumors and cardiac, renal,
and vascular lesions. The reference to a significant delay in the
onset of disease is of particular interest in the light of our finding of delayed onset of amyloidosis in the smoke-exposed hamsters.
Since the extent of the amyloid deposits appeared sufficiently severe
to cause or contribute to death, the onset of amyloidosis obviously
could have affected the lifespan of our hamsters.

The relative difference in mean body weight between our smoke-exposed hamsters and the controls, and some of our histopathologic findings, are in agreement with DONTENWILL's results. However, our survival data differ from those reported by him (1970) and by RECKZEH et al. (1969). These investigators also used Hamburg II smoking machines and an exposure regimen for their Syrian golden hamsters which was very similar to ours. Yet DONTENWILL reported that of 146 hamsters, only 93 (64%) survived smoke exposure for more than 10 months. Survival data for controls, if any, were not given. By comparison, 90% of our smoke-exposed hamsters were alive after 10 months of smoke exposure. RECKZEH et al., using the same experimental procedures, quoted an "LD$_{50}$" of 39 weeks for an unspecified number of hamsters. The LD$_{50}$ for the unspecified number of controls was "greater than 52 weeks". Median survival was 90 weeks for our smoke-exposed group and 73 weeks for our controls. While the median survival times for the control groups appear to be in fairly good agreement, as far as can be told from the statement "greater than 52 weeks", the results in the smoke-exposed groups are diametrically opposed. In DONTENWILL's and RECKZEH's experiments, exposure to cigarette smoke resulted in markedly decreased survival times, while in ours it resulted in significantly increased survival times.

We have no explanation at this time for the discrepancy between the results of DONTENWILL and RECKZEH et al., and our findings. There were several differences in our experimental procedures and theirs that we are aware of, including the use of a different cigarette, a different feed, and a different hamster strain; our use of a slightly modified smoking machine; and a rest period of 8 1/2 hours instead of 3 hours between the second and third smoke exposure. The histopathologic changes in the respiratory tract of our smoke-exposed group are similar to those described by DONTENWILL (1970), with the significant difference that his hamsters eventually showed a progression of their laryngeal lesions to "obligatorily precancerous states" and, in 1 case, to an early invasive carcinoma.

Whether a 10-minute exposure to diluted smoke 3 times during a 24-hour day, 5 days per week instead of 7 days, simulates the insult in the hamster which is experienced by the lung of, say, a 2-pack-a-day human smoker appears rather questionable. The rationale behind this statement is that (a) human smokers smoke 7 days per week; and (b) a recuperation period of 2 days after 5 smoking days, (i.e., almost 30% exposure-free time, with the remaining 70% allowing for only 3 10-minute exposures per 24-hour day), might provide sufficient time for the repair of lesions which may have been induced by the smoke exposure, or at least prevent them from developing into malignancies. How much this factor might have contributed to the lack of significant malignant tumor development in the respiratory system of our smoke-exposed hamsters is a matter of speculation until further studies with more smoke exposures per day and a 7-day/week exposure regimen have been conducted.

Acknowledgement

This investigation was conducted under National Cancer Institute contract PH 43-68-1372.

For technical assistance in the conduct of the experiments we are
indebted to Messrs. EDWARD M. MILLIMAN, J. DAVID BURRUS, HERMAN O.
MYERS, THOMAS K. ANDREWS, and JOHN K. STRIKWERDA.

We acknowledge with thanks the contributions of our colleague Dr.
JAMES C. HAMPTON in the field of electron microscopy.

References

ATKINSON, W.O.: Production of sample cigarettes for tobacco and
    health research. In: Proc. Tobacco and Health Conference, Lexington,
    Kentucky, February 24/25, 1970, Conference Report 2, U. of Kentucky
    Tobacco and Health Research Institute, pp. 28-30.
BENNER, J.F.: Tentative summary of leaf and smoke analysis of the
    University of Kentucky reference and alkaloid series cigarettes.
    In: Proc. Tobacco and Health Conference, Lexington, Kentucky,
    Febuary 24/25, 1970, Conference Report 2, U. of Kentucky Tobacco
    and Health Research Institute, pp. 30-32.
BERG, B.N., SIMMS, H.S.: Nutrition and longevity in the rat. J.
    Nutrition $\underline{74}$, 23-32 (1961).
DONTENWILL, W., RECKZEH, G., STADLER, L.: Berauchungsapparatur für
    Laboratoriumstiere. Beitr. Tabakforsch. $\underline{4}$, 45-49 (1967).
DONTENWILL, W.: Experimental investigations on the effect of cigarette
    smoke inhalation on small laboratory animals. In: Inhalation Carcino-
    genesis (M.G. Hanna, Jr., P. Nettesheim, J.R. Gilbert, eds), pp.
    389-409. (Conf.-691001) National Technical Information Service,
    Springfield, Virginia 1970.
RECKZEH, R., RÜCKER, K., HARKE, H.P., DONTENWILL, W.: Untersuchungen
    zur Bestimmung der akuten und chronischen Toxizität von Cigaretten-
    rauch bei passiver Berauchung von Versuchstieren. Arzneimittel-
    Forsch. (Drug Res.) $\underline{19}$, 237-241.

Carcinogenicity of Inhaled Cigarette Smoke in the NMU-Pretreated Hamster Larynx

Eberhard Karbe and Kari Köster

Battelle-Institut e. V., Frankfurt/Main, W.-Germany

ABSTRACT

122 1-month-old Syrian golden hamsters were pretreated intratracheally with NMU (N-methyl-N-nitroso-urea) using various dosages and methods.

After the pretreatment period of 1 month, half of the animals in each of the 7 groups were exposed 5 days per week for 6 months to diluted cigarette smoke. The other half of the animals were also put in the inhalation tubes, but not exposed to smoke. An additional 36 animals, not pretreated with NMU, were used as controls, half of which were exposed to smoke for 6 months.

A grading system of epithelial changes in the larynx was established that included hyperplastic and metaplastic lesions (grades 1 to 3), severe endophytic proliferations and carcinoma *in situ* (grade 4), and epidermoid carcinomas (grade 5).

6 out of 43 NMU-pretreated and smoke-exposed hamsters had epidermoid carcinomas (grade 5), whereas only 2 out of 41 NMU-treated hamsters not exposed to smoke had lesions of this type. The corresponding numbers of animals with grade-4 lesions were 11 and 2, respectively. Thus, the inhalation of smoke increased the incidence of grade-4 and grade-5 lesions in NMU-initiated hamsters about 4-fold. No such lesions were observed in the 36 control animals.

The intratracheal instillation of NMU in hamsters appears to be a suitable method of examining the tumor-enhancing effect of inhaled cigarette smoke for experimental purposes. Such a NMU treatment may lead to a new bioassay for weak particulate carcinogens or cocarcinogens.

A. Introduction

Various investigators (DONTENWILL et al., 1972; WYNDER and HOFFMANN, 1969) and our own unpublished experiments have shown that tobacco smoke condensate promotes tumor development when applied repeatedly to the skin of mice after a single pretreatment with a low dose of a chemical carcinogen, such as 7,12-dimethylbenz(a)anthracene (DMBA). This information suggests that inhaled tobacco smoke might cause similar respiratory carcinogenesis.

Long-term inhalation of cigarette smoke in Syrian hamsters leads to the formation of precancerous and cancerous epidermoid lesions develop-

ing from the laryngeal epithelium (DONTENWILL, 1969, 1974). Intratracheal application of NMU (HERROLD, 1970) in Syrian hamsters
causes the same type of lesion in the respiratory tract, especially
in the larynx, but the lesions develop earlier and more frequently
than after cigarette smoke inhalation. To investigate the tumor-promoting activity of cigarette smoke, we decided to use NMU as an initiator by the intratracheal route in Syrian hamsters, followed by inhalation of cigarette smoke.

B. Materials and Methods

I. Experimental Animals

Male Syrian hamsters (*Mesocricetus auratus*) 3 to 4 weeks old were used.
They had a mean body weight of 45 g on arrival at the laboratory; the
animals were bred by Seeboth, Frankfurt.

The hamsters were kept individually in Makrolon cages, type II, at a
constant room temperature of 22°C to 23°C; they were fed on pelleted
Altromin hamster feed (not fortified) and water ad libitum. The NMU
was applied after an accommodation period of 10 days.

II. Application of the Initiator

Pretreatment for a period of 4 weeks started when the animals were
about 5 weeks old. The carcinogenic compound used was N-methyl-N-
nitroso-urea (NMU)[1], of which a fresh solution was prepared each
day and a new ampule opened each week. The NMU was used as a 1% solution either in a physiological salt solution (0.9% aqueous NaCl) or
in a buffer solution (isotonic phosphate buffer, pH 6.0, 1/15 m).

The application scheme for NMU in the various experimental groups is
shown in Table 1. For the tracheal application of NMU solution or the
solvents, animals were anaesthesized using Brevimytal-sodium[2] (0.3 ml/
50 g body weight) or Ketanest[3] (0.15 ml/50 g body weight) and were
fixed to an inclined operating table.

The solutions were instilled by means of a bulb-headed probe. The
larynges of the animals in group 2 were freed from mucus by means of
swabs before NMU was applied. The NMU solutions were applied 4 or 8
times (Table 1). During the week following pretreatment the hamsters
were acclimatized by placing them into the tubes of the smoking machine
during short time periods without exposing them to smoke.

III. Inhalation

After the pretreatment period, the hamsters within the individual
groups were subdivided into groups to be exposed and those not to be
exposed to smoke. Since some of the animals died during the application period, the number of animals was smaller when the inhalation

---

[1] Glass ampules containing 1 g NMU under nitrogen (Schuchardt, Munich).

[2] Brevimytal-sodium, 1% solution (Eli Lilly GmbH, Giessen).

[3] Ketanest, 50 mg/ml (Parke-Davis, Munich).

Table 1. Pretreatment of larynges in experimental groups

Experimental group	Total number of animals	Single dose of NMU (µl)	NMU concentration (%)	Solvent for NMU	Number of applications	Total dose of NMU (mg)	Method of application
1	26	36	1	0.9% aqueous NaCl	8	2.88	instillation into trachea
2	26	36	1	isotonic phosphate buffer	8	2.88	larynx cleaned instillation into trachea
3	26	36	1	isotonic phosphate buffer	8	2.88	instillation into trachea
4	22	9	1	isotonic phosphate buffer	8	0.72	instillation into trachea
5	22	9	1	isotonic phosphate buffer	4	0.36	instillation into trachea
6	22	-	-	isotonic phosphate buffer	8	-	instillation into trachea
7	20	-	-	-	-	-	-

experiments started than at the beginning of the pretreatment period (Tables 1 and 2).

The inhalation exposure, which extended over a period of 26.5 weeks, was undertaken using the Borgwaldt smoking machine (type Hamburg II).

With the puff volume adjusted at 35 ml, this machine takes a 35-ml puff of 2 seconds duration from each cigarette per minute. The rotating head holds 30 cigarettes, so that the first and successive puffs are drawn on each of the 30 cigarettes in turn to provide a fresh supply of dilute smoke (1 + 7) every 2 seconds to the exposure chamber. Usually 10 hamsters were exposed at a time. The cigarettes used for the production of smoke were all of the same type and were manufactured from a flue-cured tobacco blend. Each cigarette yielded 9 puffs.

The animals were exposed to smoke 5 days a week. Exposure started with the first puff from each of 30 cigarettes on the first day. The number of puffs taken on the set of cigarettes was gradually increased, so that 9 puffs of a total set of 30 cigarettes were offered from the seventh exposure day onward, 18 puffs (2 sets) from the third exposure week, and 27 puffs (3 sets) during the second half of the exposure period.

The control hamsters not exposed to smoke were also put into tubes for comparable time periods, but were not connected to the smoking machine.

IV. Postmortem and Histological Examinations

After the inhalation period of 26.5 weeks, all hamsters still alive were killed by means of carbon dioxide. The following organs or parts of the body were taken from the animals and fixed in a 10% formalin solution: larynx, trachea, lung, stomach, brain, and head. From each of the larynges, embedded in paraffin, every fourth transverse section was prepared for microscopic investigation by staining with haematoxylin-eosin: about 60 sections per larynx. From the other respiratory organs, 4 sections were taken from the trachea and 3 sections from each of the 6 lobes of the lung.

Animals that were found to be moribund during the inhalation period were also killed by means of carbon dioxide, and in addition to the organs listed above, any other organs found to have pathological changes were taken for examination. Animals found dead during the inhalation period were investigated accordingly.

C. Results

I. Weights and Mortality Rate

The hamsters were weighed once every week. At the beginning of the experiment the mean body weights of all groups were about the same. Toward the end of the NMU pretreatment period, animals lost weight in the higher dose groups; this NMU effect was dose-dependent.

In the course of the inhalation period, a marked difference in weight was observed between smoke-exposed animals and their controls within

Table 2. Lesions of grades 4 and 5 and papillomas found in pharynx

Experimental group	Animals exposed to smoke			Animals not exposed to smoke		
	Initial number of hamsters	Number of hamsters with grade 4 and 5 lesions	Number of hamsters with papillomas	Initial number of hamsters	Number of hamsters with grade 4 and 5 lesions	Number of hamsters with papillomas
1	8	1	–	7	–	3
2	9	2	–	9	1	3
3	10	2	–	9	–	3
4	8	2	1	8	2	3
5	8	1	1	8	–	3
6	8	–	–	8	–	–
7	10	–	–	10	–	–
Total number	61	8	2	59	3	15

the individual groups, i.e., the smoke-exposed animals generally weighed
less. This difference became still more pronounced as inhalation continued. During the inhalation period, the mean weight of most groups
was similar for smoke-exposed animals and, at a higher level, for their
controls, which means that early differences due to the pretreatment
were compensated. The mortality rate was raised in all hamsters receiving NMU.

II.   Histopathological Investigations

All the sections prepared from the larynges, tracheas, and lungs of
the 122 experimental animals that had died during the inhalation period
or had been killed at the end were evaluated histopathologically. For
classifying the epithelial changes, the most severe lesions observed
in the laryngeal mucosa was used. In most cases, this was located
around the plica vocalis or at the anterior floor of the larynx. The
tissue changes were less severe in the posterior portion of the larynx.
The changes in the larynx were classified according to the grading
system described below.

1.   Grading of Laryngeal Epithelial Lesions

Grade 0

Definition: Hyperplasia or no change.
Explanation: The normal epithelium of an untreated hamster represents
a squamous stratified epithelium in the anterior of the larynx, while
ciliated respiratory epithelium is found in the posterior region. In
general, the laryngeal squamous epithelium does not form keratin except for the most anterior portion. Epithelial hyperplasia leads to
an increase in the number of cell layers and to a thickening of the
epithelium which is observed best in areas where respiratory epithelium is present. Metaplasia is not included in grade 0.

Grade 1

Definition: Metaplastic epithelium with stratum spinosum and various
degrees of keratin formation.
Explanation: Metaplasia refers to the change of the ciliated respiratory epithelium to stratified squamous epithelium. The term "metaplasia" is used independent of the size of the affected area.

Grade 2

Definition: Parakeratosis characterized by nuclei in stratum corneum.
Explanation: In most cases parakeratosis is confined to small areas
of the larynx; the parakeratotic nuclei must be present in groups
(Fig. 1). The number of the parakeratotic cell layers is not considered.

Grade 3

Definition: Endophytic growth with cellular differentiation with or
without parakeratosis.
Explanation: Epithelial endophytic growth with cellular differentiation normally does not occur in the hamster larynx as it does in the
skin (Fig. 2). It may be considered as an increased activity of the
epithelium, similar to that observed in purely inflammatory processes.
A possibly artificial wrinkling should not be mistaken for the formation of very small epithelial sprouts.

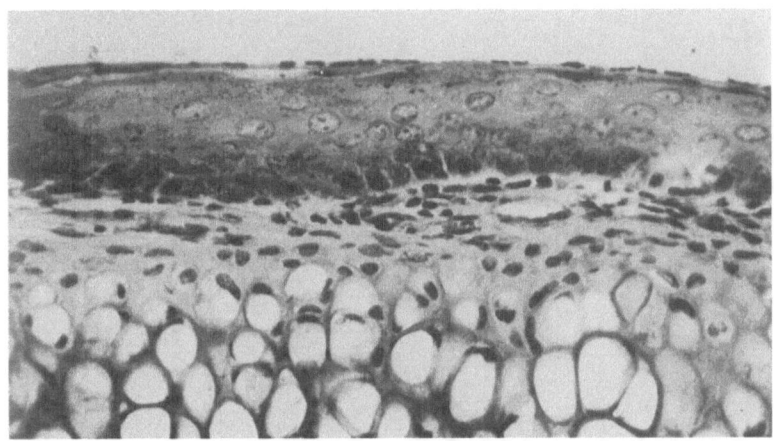

Fig. 1. Grade 2: Posterior portion of hamster larynx pretreated with 2.88 mg NMU in saline and subsequently not exposed to smoke. Parakeratosis. Group 1, week 27 (x 280)

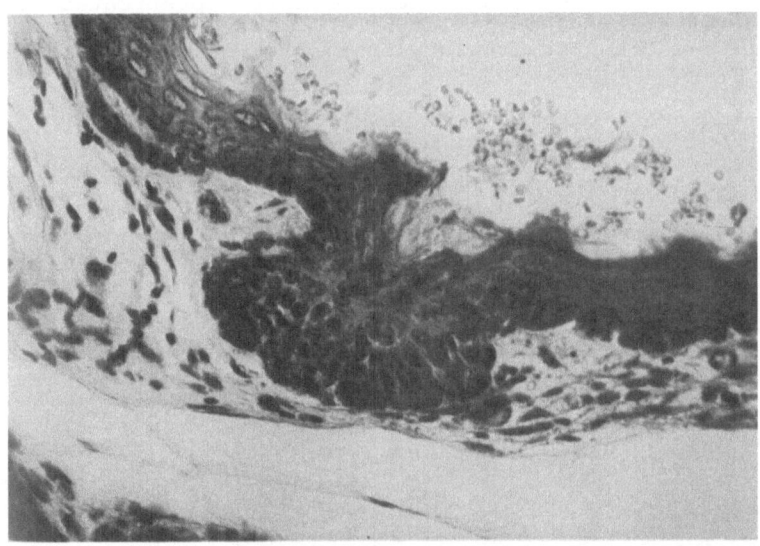

Fig. 2. Grade 3: Anterior portion of hamster larynx pretreated with 2.88 mg NMU in buffer and subsequently exposed to smoke. Endophytic growth with cellular differentiation. Group 3, week 27 (x 280)

Grade 4

Definition: Epithelial endophytic growth with lack of cellular differentiation.
Explanation: In this category, basal cells do not differentiate readily to form a stratum spinosum within endophytic sprouts or elsewhere (Fig. 3). Slender sprouts do not permit the recognition of differentiation for lack of space; if such slender sprouts are relatively long, the lesion is also classified as grade 4, because this constitutes the most severe type of proliferation (Fig. 4).

376

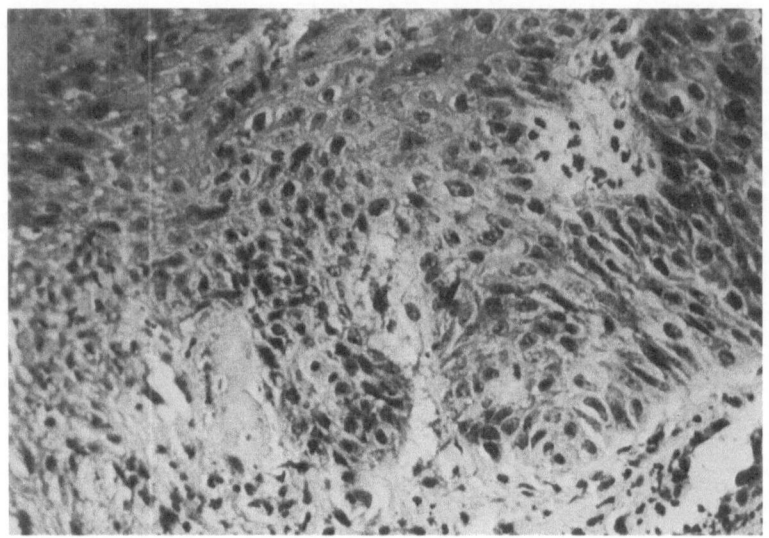

Fig. 3. Grade 4: Posterior portion of hamster larynx pretreated with
2.88 mg NMU in buffer after cleaning larynx and subsequently exposed
to smoke. Epithelial endophytic growth with lack of cellular differentiation. Group 2, week 27 (x 280)

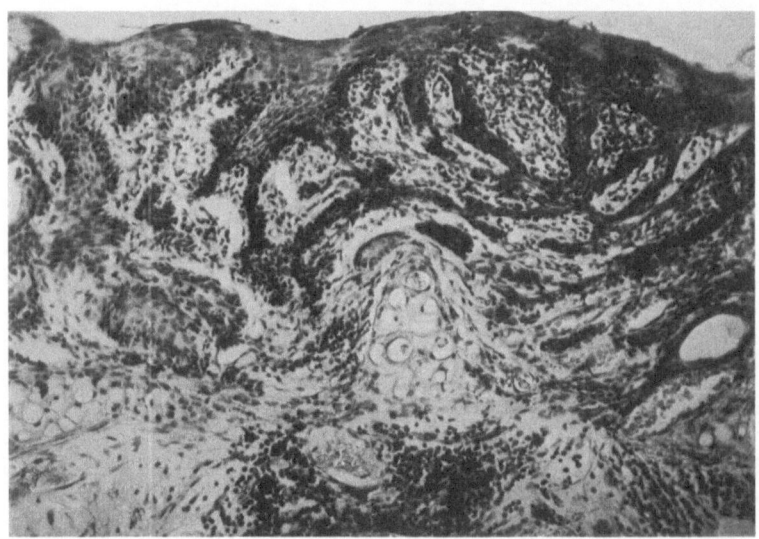

Fig. 4. Grade 4: Anterior portion of hamster larynx pretreated with
2.88 mg NMU in buffer and subsequently exposed to smoke. Epithelial
endophytic growth with long slender sprouts. Group 3, week 27 (x 112)

Grade 5

Definition: Epidermoid carcinoma.
Explanation: Tumor cells invade into the connective tissue while penetrating the basal membrane. Keratinisation, however moderate, is usually observed (Figs 5 and 6).

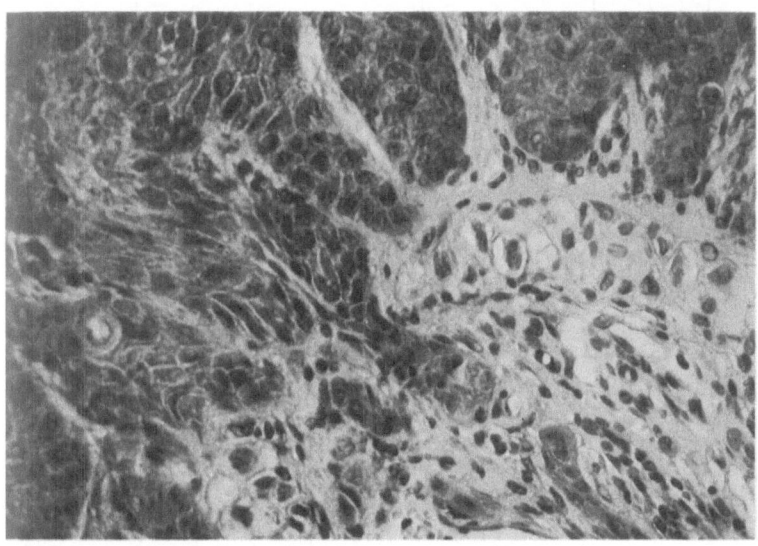

Fig. 5. Grade 5: Anterior portion of hamster larynx pretreated with
0.72 mg NMU in buffer and subsequently not exposed to smoke. Epidermoid
carcinoma infiltrating area of epiglottic cartilage. Group 4, week 27
(x 280)

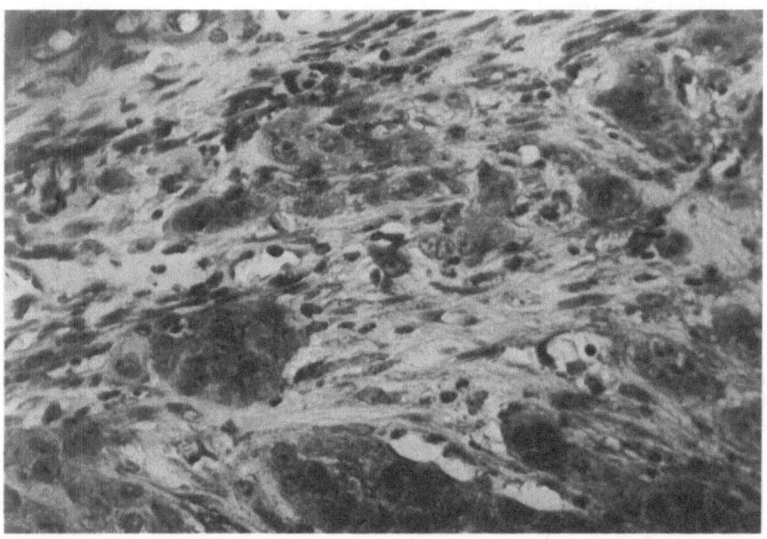

Fig. 6. Grade 5: Posterior portion of hamster larynx pretreated with
2.88 mg NMU in buffer after cleaning larynx and subsequently exposed
to smoke. Epidermoid carcinoma with polymorphous tumor cells in submucosal tissue. Group 2, week 14 (x 280)

378

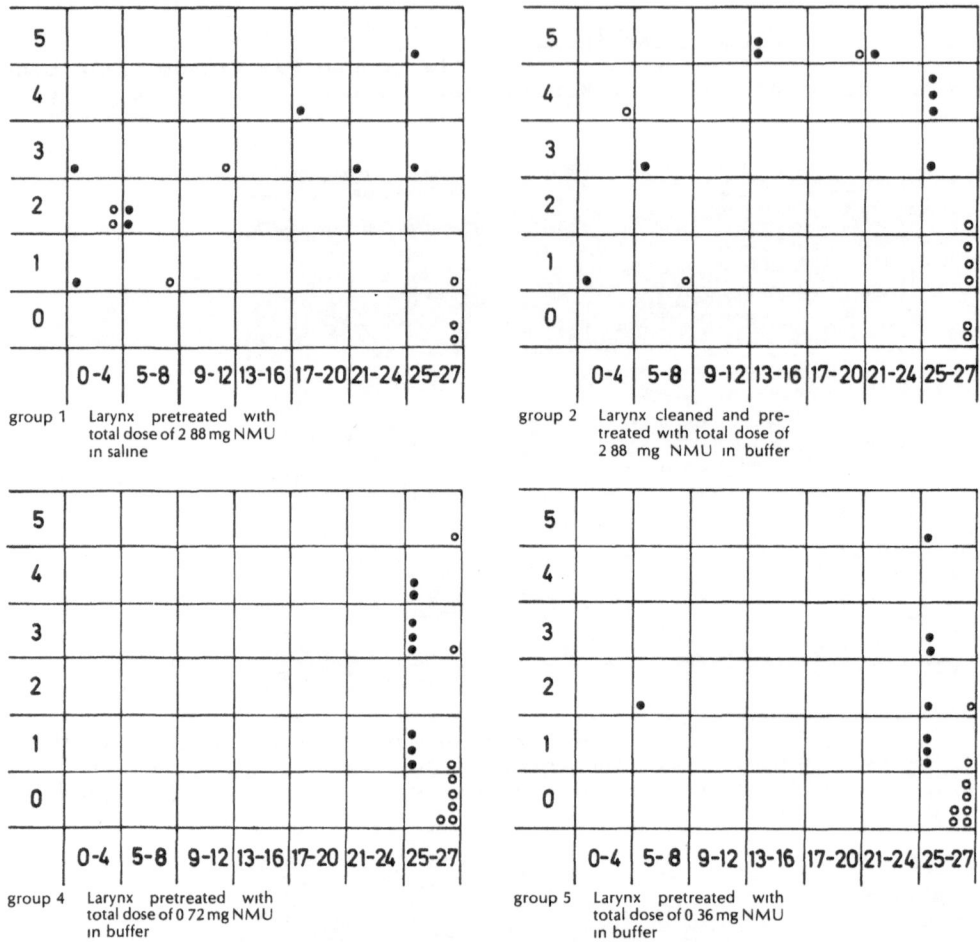

group 1   Larynx pretreated with
          total dose of 2 88 mg NMU
          in saline

group 2   Larynx cleaned and pre-
          treated with total dose of
          2 88 mg NMU in buffer

group 4   Larynx pretreated with
          total dose of 0 72 mg NMU
          in buffer

group 5   Larynx pretreated with
          total dose of 0 36 mg NMU
          in buffer

The results of the classification of the laryngeal lesions of all
animals are shown in Fig. 7 for each experimental group separately.

2. Pharyngeal Lesions

In the histological preparation of the larynx, parts of the pharynx
(small sections of pharynx respiratorius, trachynx, and vestibulum
oesophagi) were cut and evaluated. There is normally a squamous epithelium in this area, so that squamous metaplasia cannot be observed.
More severe lesions were similar to those in the larynx and classified as grade 4 or grade 5 (Table 2). In addition, papillomas were
frequently found on the outside of the epiglottis (Table 2).

The epidermoid carcinoma of the larynx had infiltrated the surrounding
tissues to such an extent that in 6 of the 8 affected animals, the
tumor was present in the adjacent pharynx too (Table 3). In all cases
the larynx was more severely involved than the pharynx, and there was
no animal with a carcinoma in the pharynx not involving the larynx.

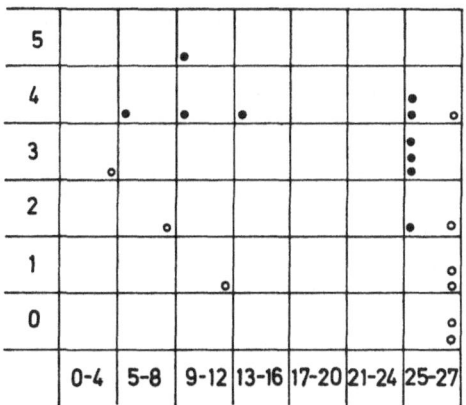

group 3 Larynx pretreated with
total dose of 2 88 mg NMU
in buffer

Fig. 7. Classification of
laryngeal lesions (grades 0
to 5) in hamsters related to
their time of death (inhalation weeks 0 to 27). Hamsters
exposed to smoke = ●, hamsters
not exposed to smoke = o

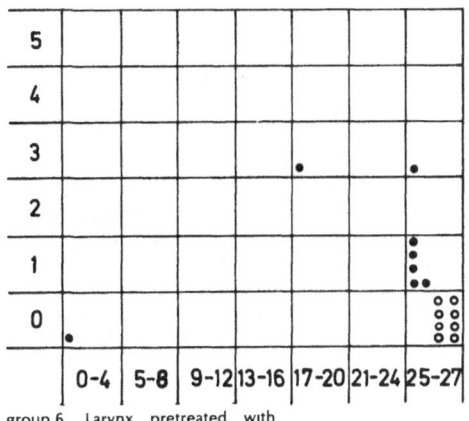

group 6 Larynx pretreated with
buffer (control group)

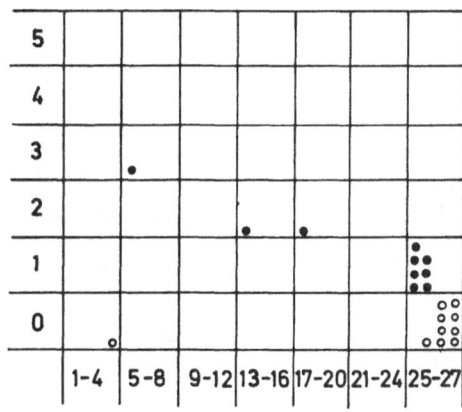

group 7 Larynx not pretreated
(control group)

3. Lung and Stomach Lesions

Apart from inflammatory reactions, no changes - especially no neoplastic changes - were found in the tracheas and lungs of any of the
hamsters. Pseudoadenomatoid lung lesions were found in all groups,
whether exposed to smoke or not, and were considered a spontaneous
condition (CHEVALIER and DONTENWILL, 1971).

Outside the route of inhalation no tumors were found, except for
papilloma in the anterior stomach of a smoke-exposed animal in group
2.

Table 3. Number of animals with epidermoid carcinomas in both larynx
and pharynx

Experimental group	Smoke-exposed animals with lesions		Animals not exposed to smoke with lesions	
	in larynx	in larynx and pharynx	in larynx	in larynx and pharynx
1	1	-	-	-
2	3	2	1	1
3	1	1	-	-
4	-	-	1	1
5	1	1	-	-
6	-	-	-	-
7	-	-	-	-
Total number	6	4	2	2

D. Discussion

The outstanding result of this experiment was that, within 6 months,
6 out of 43 pretreated hamsters exposed to smoke developed epidermoid
carcinomas in the larynx (grade 5), while only 2 out of 41 pretreated
hamsters not exposed to smoke had tumors of this type. In addition,
among the smoke-exposed animals 11 had what one may call precancerous
lesions (grade 4); these lesions were observed only in 2 hamsters not
exposed to smoke. These 2 most advanced types of lesions (grades 4
and 5) were not observed among 18 animals exposed to smoke only and
appear to be extremely rare in untreated animals (DONTENWILL et al.,
1973).

These data indicate that the combined treatment with NMU and inhaled
smoke leads to an overadditive carcinogenic effect. Long-term inhalation experiments demonstrate (DONTENWILL, 1969) that tobacco smoke
alone will eventually lead to grade-5 lesions in a small proportion
of the animals. Obviously, tobacco smoke has the properties of a
comparatively weak but complete carcinogen. Therefore, the overadditive effect observed could be explained as a result of potentiating activities of the carcinogens used (syncarcinogenesis). However,
the overadditive carcinogenic effect could be explained also by a promoting activity of smoke components (cocarcinogens).

No matter which interpretation is used, it is obvious that NMU pretreatment enhances the effect of tobacco smoke markedly with respect
to the severity and time of occurrence of laryngeal precancerous and
cancerous lesions in hamsters. It appears that hamsters pretreated
with NMU are well suited to be used in experiments designed to test
especially this overadditive effect of tobacco smoke.

In such a bioassay system, NMU treatment on its own should produce
a minor incidence of laryngeal lesions, but following the inhalation
of tobacco smoke the incidence should be high. Considering grade-4
and -5 lesions, the ratio between smoke-exposed and nonexposed hamsters in the various experimental groups was 2:0 (group 1), 6:2
(group 2), 6:1 (group 3), 2:1 (group 4), and 1:0 (group 5). From

these results, it appears that group 3 met the above objectives most closely.

Initially an attempt was made to grade laryngeal lesions according to the system published by DONTENWILL (1969). Since it was rather difficult to assign various types of lesions to one of the grades proposed by him, a grading system was developed on the basis of the lesions observed in this experiment. It was not difficult to establish a system that takes account of the progression of the lesions, but it was not possible to name the various grades by clearly defined terms used in histopathology. No attempt was made to correlate the various grades observed in hamsters to lesions seen in the human respiratory tract.

6 animals had epidermoid carcinomas that involved both the laryngeal and the adjacent pharyngeal epithelium (Table 3), and it was not possible to decide where the lesion had started. On the basis of the observations outlined below it was assumed that at least the majority of these 6 carcinomas had arisen in the larynx: first, the tumors had spread more extensively in the larynx and, second, isolated grade-5 lesions were not seen in the hypopharynx and, third, the incidence of animals with grade-4 lesions (precursors of grade-5 lesions) in the hypopharynx was lower than in the larynx (5:13).

The incidence of grade-4 or -5 lesions in the pharynx of hamsters was higher in animals exposed to smoke (8 out of 43) than in those not exposed to smoke (3 out of 41). This difference (Table 2) parallels that observed with regard to animals with grade-4 and -5 lesions in the larynx (17 out of 43; 4 out of 41); thus it appears that tobacco smoke enhanced the development of these lesions in both locations.

In addition to grade-4 and -5 lesions, NMU induced the formation of papillomas in the pharynx (Table 2). The incidence of animals affected with these lesions was remarkably lower in smoke-exposed groups (2 out of 43 animals) compared to groups not exposed to smoke (15 out of 41 animals), which corresponds with the results obtained by DON-TENWILL (1973) using DMBA and cigarette smoke.

It is of interest to note that papillomas were not induced in the hamster larynx by NMU, smoke, or both, whereas they develop after diethylnitrosamine treatment (MONTESANO and SAFFIOTTI, 1968). The pharyngeal papillomas observed in this experiment were small and do not appear to interfere with the development of a bioassay for weak carcinogens or promoters in the hamster larynx.

The method used in this experiment appears suitable for the development of a new bioassay for inhaled cocarcinogens or weak carcinogens such as cigarette smoke.

References

CHEVALIER, H.J., DONTENWILL, W.: Zur formalen Genese der Pseudo-adenomatose (adenomatoid lesions) der Lunge beim Syrischen Gold-hamster. Z. Versuchstierkunde 13, 38-50 (1971).
DONTENWILL, W.: Experimental investigations on the effect of cigarette smoke inhalation on small laboratory animals (M.G. Hanna, Jr., P. Nettesheim, J.R. Gilbert, eds), pp. 389-409. In: Inhalation Carcino-genesis. (Conf.-691001). National Technical Information Service, Springfield, Virginia 1970.

DONTENWILL, W., CHEVALIER, H.J., KLIMISCH, H.J., LAWRENZ, U., RECK-
ZEH, G.: Experimentelle Untersuchungen über die tumorerzeugende
Wirkung von Zigarettenrauch-Kondensaten an der Mäusehaut. Z. Krebs-
forsch. 78, 236-264 (1972).

DONTENWILL, W., CHEVALIER, H.J., HARKE, H.-P., LAWRENZ, U., RECKZEH,
G.: Spontantumoren des syrischen Goldhamsters. Z. Krebsforsch. 80,
127-158 (1973).

DONTENWILL, W.: Tumorigenic effect of chronic cigarette smoke inhalation on Syrian golden hamsters. These Proceedings 1974.

HERROLD, K.: Upper respiratory tract tumors induced in Syrian hamsters
by N-methyl-N-nitrosourea. Int. J. Cancer 6, 217-222 (1970).

MONTESANO, SAFFIOTTI, U.: Carcinogenic response of the respiratory
tract of Syrian golden hamsters to different doses of Diethylnitrosamine. Cancer Res. 28, 2197-2210 (1968).

WYNDER, E.L., HOFFMANN, D.: A study of tobacco carcinogenesis. X.
Tumor promoting activity. Cancer 24, 289-301 (1969).

Validity of the Sebaceous Gland Test and the Hyperplasia Test for the Prediction of the Carcinogenicity of Cigarette Smoke Condensates and Their Fractions

Philippe Lazar[1] and Ivan Chouroulinkov[2]

[1]Unité de Recheres Statistiques de l'Institut National de la Santé et de la Recherche Mèdicale, Villejuif, France
[2]Laboratoire d'Etude des Effets Pathologiques du Tabac de l'Institut de Recherches Scientifiques sur le Cancer, Villejuif, France

ABSTRACT

Short-term tests involving estimation of the suppression of sebaceous glands and the extent of hyperplasia of the mouse skin can be used as screening tests to detect the potential carcinogenicity of some fractions of cigarette smoke condensates or to measure the relative activity of different condensates. It is shown that the correlation between carcinogenicity and a positive response in short-term tests is significant for several families of chemicals, and that there is also a highly significant correlation between the promoting activity of a set of tested condensates or fractions of condensates and the level of their response to short-term tests.

A. Introduction

Since the systematic survey of BOCK and MUND (1958), it is recognized that a great number of carcinogenic substances, especially among the polycyclic aromatic hydrocarbons (PAH), can destroy part or all of the sebaceous glands of the mouse within a few days after application to the skin, at the dose level used for long-term experiments (Table 1). In addition, the same substances usually provoke cutaneous hyperplasia under the same experimental conditions (GUERIN and CUZIN, 1961). Whether these phenomena, and especially the latter phenomenon, play an effective role in tumorigenesis is controversial (VAN DUUREN et al., 1973). Our aim is to discuss whether these early manifestations of the activity of carcinogenic substances may be used as screening tests either to detect the potential carcinogenicity of some fractions of cigarette smoke condensates (CSC) or to measure the relative activity of different CSC (CHOUROULINKOV et al., 1969).

B. Extension of the Short-Term Tests to Different Families of Chemicals

Taking into account our ignorance of the nature of all of the substances responsible for CSC carcinogenicity, the first logical question to seek an answer to is the following: Is the correlation between carcinogenicity and a positive response to short-term tests significant only for the families of substancces studied in the first surveys and especially PAH?

Table 1. Activity of compounds in short-term tests

(Taken from BOCK and MUND, 1958)

| Compound category | Number substances applied | Sebaceous gland test activity | | |
		Strong	Weak	No activity
Strong skin carcinogens	9	67 %	33 %	0%
Weak, doubtful, incomplete carcinogens	25	24 %	24 %	52%
Not carcinogenic substances	67	1.5%	7.5%	91%

(Taken from GUERIN and CUZIN, 1961)

| Compound category | Number substances applied | Sebaceous gland test activity | | | Hyperplasia test | | |
		Strong	Weak	No activity	Strong	Weak	No activity
Carcinogens	13	62%	23%	15%	15%	70%	15%
Not carcinogenic substances	13	0%	30%	70%	0%	30%	70%

We have conducted 3 studies to partially answer this question. The first study was a comparative test of the short- and long-term activities of 6 isomeric dimethylbenzacridines (Table 2). Our results showed that the 3 chemicals that were the most carcinogenic were also the most active in short-term tests (LIBERMANN et al., 1968a).

In the second study, we tested the short-term activities of 5 potent promoters: 1-fluoro-2,4 dinitrobenzene (DNFB), anthralin, cantharidin, croton oil, 12-O-tetra-decanoyl-phorbol-13-acetate (TPA)(LIBERMANN et al., 1968b), and of 1 nonpromoting substance similar to DNFB, N^6-(2,4-dinitrophenyl)-1-lysine (DNPL). The 5 promoters were strong hyperplasiants. 4 of them destroyed a great proportion of the sebaceous glands. DNPL was no more active in short-term tests than it was in long-term experiments (Table 3).

In the third study, we studied the tumor promoting activity of colchicine - 1 of the "exceptions" to the correlation - and of 6 derivatives of this substance: 2 active and 4 inactive in short-term tests. We found a weak promoting activity of the first 2 substances and no such activity for the 4 other (Table 4). Colchicine had been itself reported by BOCK et al. (1966) to be a slight promoter.

From this first series of experiments, we may conclude that the correlation between short- and long-term activities concern a great number of substances not only from 1 definite chemical family, and therefore we wonder whether this correlation is not mainly related to tumor-promoting activity of these substances. The following discussion then

Table 2. Sebaceous gland test and hyperplasia test showing responses
to 6 isomeric dimethylbenzacridines

Substances (5 mg/ml)	Short-term tests		Carcinogenicity[a]	
	Sebaceous gland test[b] (%)	Hyperplasia test[c] (%)	Epithelioma index	Sarcoma index
7,10-dimethyl-benz(c)acridine	100	184	56	69
7,9 -dimethyl-benz(c)acridine	89	155	81	41
7,11-dimethyl-benz(c)acridine	82	38	14	42
9,12-dimethyl-benz(a)acridine	17	21	11	0
8,12-dimethyl-benz(a)acridine	40	5	-	5
10,12-dimethyl-benz(a)acridine	40	18	-	3.5

[a]Data taken from IBALL and LACASSAGNE et al.
[b]Suppression rate with regard to controls.
[c]Increasing rate with regard to controls.

Table 3. Sebaceous gland test and hyperplasia test showing responses
to 5 promoters and 1 control substance

Substances	Dose (mg/ml)	Sebaceous gland test[a] (%)	Hyperplasia test[b] (%)
1-fluoro-2,4-dinitrobenzene (DNFB)	0.004	0	165
N^6-(2,4-dinitrophenyl)-1-lysine (DNPL) (nonpromoter control of DNFB)	10	0	0
Anthralin	5	72	311
Cantharidine	1	94	92
Croton oil	6	59	337
12-O-tetradecanoyl-phorbol-13-acetate (TPA)	0.1	77	223

[a]Suppression rate with regard to controls.
[b]Increasing rate with regard to controls.

logically concerns 1. the procedure and properties of short-term tests
applied to CSC, and 2. the correlation between the short-term responses
and the promoting activities of CSC and condensate fractions.

C. Test Procedures for CSC

All of the CSC and fractions studied were prepared by the laboratories
of the French Service d'Exploitation Industrielles des Tabac et Allumettes (SEITA). 2 doses of a 25% to 46% solution of CSC in acetone
or methanol are usually tested. For each dose, 20 albino mice receive
a dorsal application of 1/20 ml of the solution on days 1, 3, and 5.

Table 4. Sebaceous gland test and hyperplasia test showing responses to and promoting activity of colchicine and 6 derivatives

Substances	Short-term tests			Promotion tests[c]		
	Short-term test dose (mg/ml)	Sebaceous gland test[a] (%)	Hyperplasia test[b] (%)	Surviving mice at first tumor	Tumor-bearing mice	Epithelioma-bearing mice
Colchicine	5	45	153	35	0	0
Thiocolchicine	1.6	100	311	36	3	1
Desacethylthiocolchicine (base)	5	45	105	37	1	1
Colchicoside	5	0	0	35	0	0
Thiocolchicoside	10	0	4	39	0	0
Trimethylcholchicinic acid		0	0	34	0	0
Hydroxymethylcolchicine	10	0	0	33	0	0
Croton oil	6	59	337	32	18	11

[a] Suppression rate with regard to controls.
[b] Increasing rate with regard to controls.
[c] Initiation with 150 µg DMBA. Promotion by 2 applications of 50 µg per week.

The mice are sacrificed on day 8. For each mouse, the total number x of sebaceous gland and the mean thickness y of the epidermis are determined for a set of 12 microscopic fields "blindy" chosen (LAZAR et al., 1963). The following calculations are made (to linearize the dose-effect relationship and to get absolute indexes).

I. Sebaceous Gland Test

1. Calculate for each dose

$$\frac{\sqrt{x}}{\sqrt{x_C}}$$

where $\sqrt{x}$ is the average square root of the number of sebaceous glands of a treated mouse and $\sqrt{x_C}$ the same quantity for the control group.

2. Draw the dose-effect relationship and determine the ED 50 (dose destroying in the average half of the glands).

3. Take as an index of activity on the sebaceous glands g = 1/ED 50.

II. Hyperplasia Test

1. Calculate

$$\frac{\overline{\log y}}{\overline{\log y_C}}$$

where $\overline{\log y}$ is the average of the logarithm of the mean thickness of the epidermis of a treated mouse and $\overline{\log y_C}$ is the same quantity for the control group.

2. Draw the dose-effect relationship and determine the ED 220 (dose multiplying the thickness of the epidermis by 2.2). This particular ED has been chosen because it is equal, in the average, to the mean ED 50 for the sebaceous gland test.

3. Take as an index of activity in the hyperplasia test h = 1/ED 220.

Fig. 1. illustrates this procedure, and Fig. 2 shows the strong correlation existing between the 2 tests carried out on 848 condensates and 344 fractions or mixtures of fractions. The coefficients of correlation are respectively r = 0.68 for the condensates and r = 0.73 for the fractions. It is interesting to notice, by comparison with the diagonal line, that the CSC activity was more apparent in the hyperplasia test and the activity of fractions was more apparent in the sebaceous gland test.

D. Correlation between Short-Term Physical and Chemical Measurements

For 834 condensates, we obtained from SEITA their dry weight, their alcaloid content, and their phenol content. These 3 measures were significantly correlated to both indexes of activity in the short-term tests, and Table 5 shows that these correlations remain significant if one takes into account the 3 measurements together in a multiple regression. The response in short-term tests is then partially "explained" by these physical and chemical data - but only partial-

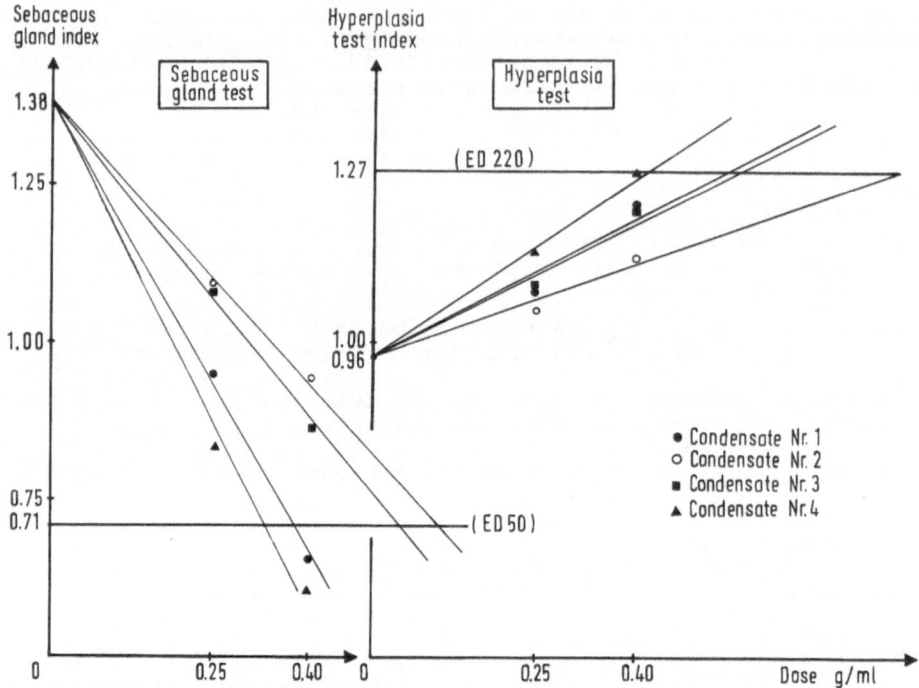

Fig. 1. Dose-response relationships for sebaceous gland test and hyperplasia test

ly, since the correlation between the hyperplasia and the sebaceous gland test remains highly significant after taking into account the 3 mentioned variables.

E.   The Correlation between Short-Term Tests and Promoting Activity

27 CSC and fractions were studied in long-term tests (promotion after an initiation with 100 µg of 7,12-dimethylbenz(a)anthracene (DMBA) in acetone) in 5 successive experiments. To take into account the un-avoidable heterogeneity among experiments, we only studied the rela-tive potencies of the CSC or fractions to the most potent of them in each experiment. Fig. 3 shows the observed correlations between short-term and long-term results. The coefficients of correlation between the sebaceous gland test or the hyperplasia test activities and pro-motion activity are respectively $r = 0.72$ and $r = 0.74$; these results are highly significant (the value of the level of significance p is mentioned in Fig. 3).

One particularly interesting feature is the additional correlation between the dry weight of condensate per cigarette and the intrinsic promoting activity of these CSC: the more a cigarette produces con-densate, the more this condensate is active. Let us recall that the same result was observed in short-term tests. On the contrary, there is no significant correlation between the alcaloid or phenol content of the CSC and their promoting activity, even though such a correla-

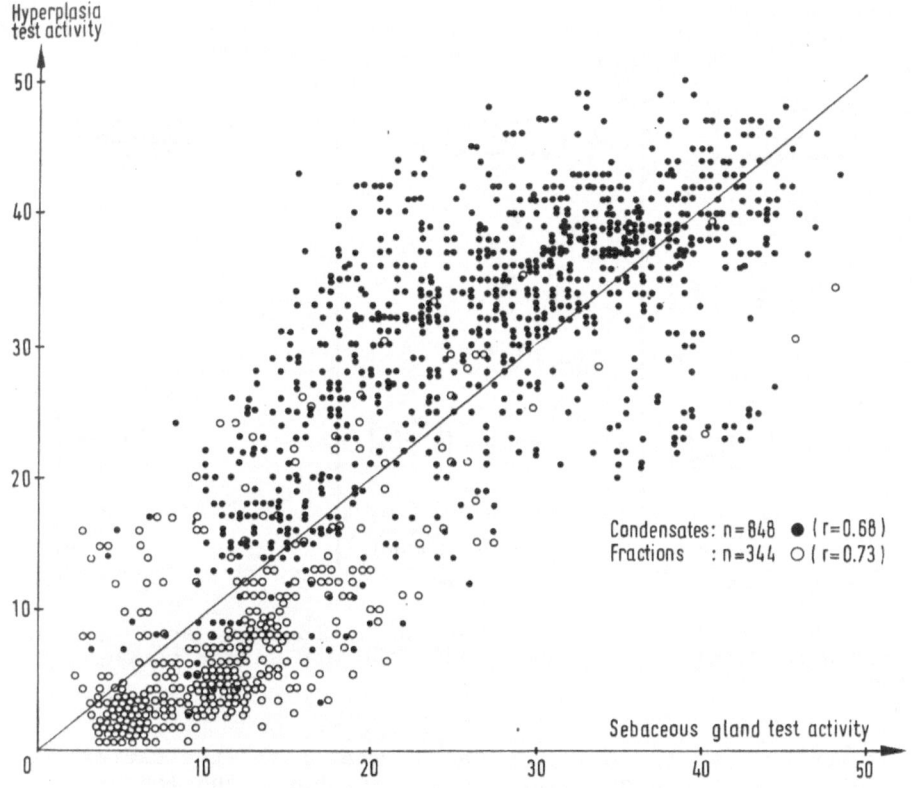

Fig. 2. Correlation between sebaceous gland test and·hyperplasia test

Table 5. Multiple regression of short-term tests on dry weight of the condensates and their alcaloid and phenol contents (n = 834 condensates)

	Dry Weight (per cigarette)	Alcaloid Content (per gram of dry condensate)	Phenol Content (per gram of dry condensate)
Mean	23.0 mg/cig	71 mg/g	5.7 mg/g
Partial correlation with sebaceous gland test activity	0.07[a]	0.38[d]	0.55[d]
Partial correlation with hyperplasia test activity	0.10[b]	0.14[c]	0.53[c]

Correlation between sebaceous gland test and hyperplasia test activities:

Simple correlation . . . . 0.69[d]

Correlation after taking into account dry weight and alcaloid and phenol content . . . . 0.43[d]

Legend:

[a]:p = 5%,   [b]:p = 1%,   [c]:p = 1°/oo,   [d]:p = 1°/ooo.

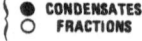

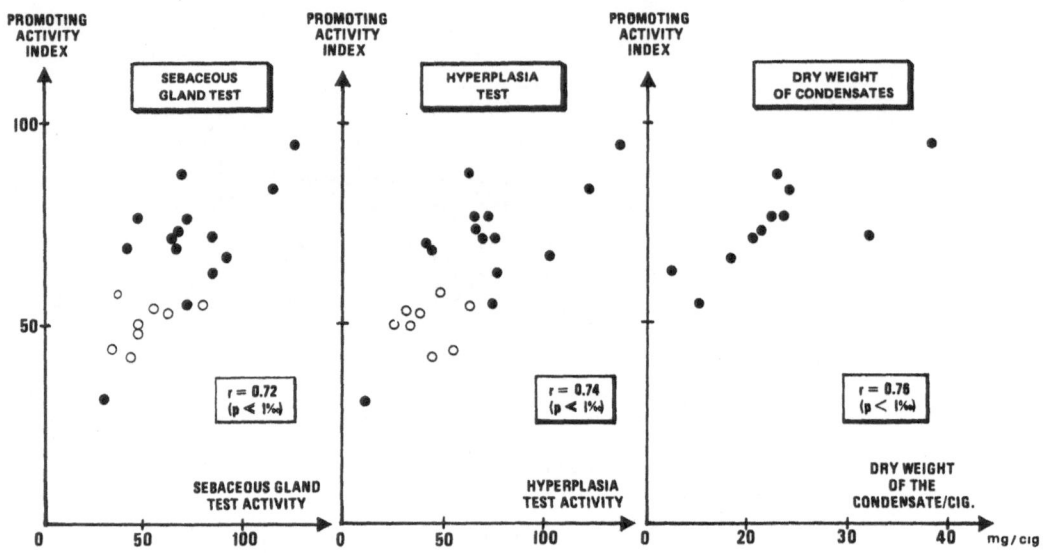

<u>Fig. 3.</u> Correlation between long-term promotion test activity and sebaceous gland test, hyperplasia test, and dry weight of the condensates

tion was observed with short-term tests. Therefore, the latter correlation cannot explain the correlation between short- and long-term test results.

The relatively small number of CSC tested, both in long-term and short-term tests, does not allow obtaining a precise <u>relative</u> value to predict the promoting activity from the results of the sebaceous gland test and the hyperplasia test. Nevertheless, it seems that, mainly for CSC, the results of the hyperplasia test correlate slightly better with the promoting activity than those for the sebaceous gland test. Further studies, on a greater number of CSC and fractions, are necessary to give more accurate results, and in particular to state precisely the weight to give to the dry weight of condensate per cigarette in the prediction of its long-term activity. Currently, short-term tests appear to be rather good screening procedures to get a first <u>quantitative</u> estimation of the promoting activity of a CSC or a fraction, and then to be a valuable tool either to guide the fractionation of tobacco toward a better understanding of its carcinogenicity (IZARD et al., 1974; LAZAR et al., 1974) or to appreciate the effects of modifications introduced into the manufacture of cigarettes in order to try to make them less harmful.

References

BOCK, F.G., MUND, R.: A survey of compounds for activity in the suppression of mouse sebaceous glands. Cancer Res. 18, 887-892 (1958).

BOCK, F.G., MYERS, H.K., FOX, H.W.: Tumor-promoting activity of compounds of interest in the laboratory. Proc. Amer. Ass. Cancer Res. 7, 7 (1966).

CHOUROULINKOV, I., LAZAR, P., IZARD, C., LIBERMANN, C., GUERIN, M.: Sebaceous gland and hyperplasia tests as screening methods for tobacco tar carcinogenesis. J. nat. Cancer Inst. 42, 981-985 (1969).

VAN DUUREN, B.L., SIVAK, A., SEGAL, A., SEIDMAN, I., KATZ, C.: Dose response studies with a pure tumor-promoting agent, phorbol myristate acetate. Cancer Res. 33, 2166-2170 (1973).

GUERIN, M., CUZIN, J.: Tests cutanés chez la souris pour déterminer l'activité carcinogène des goudrons de fumée de cigarette. Bull. Ass. franç. Cancer 48, 112-121 (1961).

IBALL, J.: The relative potency of carcinogenic compounds. Amer. J. Cancer 35, 188-190 (1939).

IZARD, C., MOREE-TESTA, P., CHOUROULINKOV, I., LAZAR, P., LIBERMANN, C.: Fractionation of cigarette smoke condensate for carcinogenic bioassays. Biomedecine 20, 206-213 (1974).

LACASSAGNE, A., BUU-HOI, N.P., DAUDEL, R., ZAJDELA, F.: The relation between carcinogenic activity and the physical and chemical properties of angular benzacridines. Adv. Cancer Res. 4, 315-369 (1956).

LAZAR, P., LIBERMANN, C. CHOUROULINKOV, I., GUERIN, M.: Tests sur la peau de souris pour la détermination des activités carcinogènes. Bull. Ass. franç. Cancer 50, 567-577 (1963).

LAZAR, P., CHOUROULINKOV, I., IZARD, C., MOREE-TESTA, P., HEMON, D.: Bioassays of carcinogenicity after fractionation of cigarette smoke condensate. Biomedecine 20, 214-222 (1974).

LIBERMANN, C., LAZAR, P., CHOUROULINKOV, I., GUERIN, M.: Efficacité des tests courts cutanés pour le classement selon leur pouvoir carcinogène des benzacridines angulaires. C.R. Soc. Biol. (Paris) 162, 835-838 (1968a).

LIBERMANN, C., LAZAR, P., CHOUROULINKOV, I., GUERIN, M.: Response of an active component of croton oil to short-term tests of carcinogenicity. Nature 217, 563-569 (1968b).

Squamous Carcinoma of the Lung from Cigarette Smoke Condensate in Implanted Beeswax Pellets

Mearl F. Stanton, Maxwell W. Layard, and Eliza Miller

Laboratory of Pathology and Biometry Branch, National Cancer Institute, National Institutes of Health, Bethesda, MD 20014, USA

ABSTRACT

A simple method of inducing carcinomas of the lung in rats has been employed to examine the mechanism of pulmonary carcinogenesis by cigarette smoke condensate (CSC). The method consists of injecting directly into the surgically exposed lung a heated mixture of beeswax and tricaprylin to which CSC or its components has been added. During the subsequent 2 years, a progressive series of metaplastic and neoplastic epithelial changes occur at the surface of the solidified pellet which, because of their focal nature, can be examined in detail and compared quantitatively. Final crude incidence rates for squamous cell carcinoma of the lung ranged from 14% to 34% when doses of a refined heptane soluble fraction were employed at levels of 12 mg to 72 mg. Preliminary response to the neutral fraction of CSC and a primary subfraction indicate that the highest carcinogenic potential resides with the neutral polynuclear aromatic hydrocarbons. Both the highly polar subfraction of the neutrals and the weak acid fraction are also active at proportions compatible with response on mouse skin painting experiments.

Previous reports indicate that carcinogenic polycyclic hydrocarbons or cigarette smoke condensate (CSC) mixed with heated beeswax and injected directly into the lungs of rats induce a progressive series of metaplastic and neoplastic lesions in regenerative bronchiolar epithelium that surrounds the carcinogen-incorporated wax pellet (STANTON et al., 1969, 1972; HIRANO et al., 1974). This report is both a follow-up on the preliminary report of our first experiments with CSC and an initial report on results with several fractions of CSC that have shown significant carcinogenic activity when applied to the skin of mice.

Materials and Methods

We are particularly indebted to Dr. F.G. BOCK, Roswell Park Memorial Institute, Buffalo, New York, and Drs. A.P. SWAIN, J.E. COOPER, and R.L. STEDMAN of the Eastern Utilization Research Division, U.S. Department of Agriculture, Philadelphia, for providing the CSC and the selected fractions at -60°C. Their preparation and employment in mouse skin painting experiments have been described previously, and these references should be consulted in detail for the best idea of their content and activity (SWAIN et al., 1969a, 1969b; BOCK et al., 1969, 1970). Briefly, the heptane soluble fraction (HSF) is the one-third by volume of CSC that can be separated from acetone-dissolved CSC with excess heptane. It contains virtually all of the nonpolar components of CSC, and by weight is approximately 4 times more effective than CSC in mouse skin carcinogenesis. The 4 more defined fractions of CSC were prepared by a different method. These consisted of the ether-soluble weak acid fraction (F_8) and the neutral fraction (F_{15}), which were separated from CSC by solvent partitioning (SWAIN et al., 1969a), and 2 of the subfractions of the neutral fraction after chromatography on silicic acid and elution with select solvents to yield a series of subfractions of increasing polarity (SWAIN et al., 1969b). The 2 subfractions tested were those designated F_{26} and F_{43} that were shown to yield significant response on mouse skin. Subfraction F_{26} is the partition of the neutral fraction not eluted from silicic acid by petroleum ether, diethyl ether, or benzene, but eluted by methanol and soluble in aqueous methanol when distributed between petroleum ether and 90% aqueous methanol. It is the most polar of the subfractions from the neutral fraction. Subfraction 43 of the neutral fraction consists of the combined partitions F_{19}, F_{20}, and F_{22} (SWAIN et al., 1969b) that contain essentially all of the polynuclear aromatic hydrocarbons eluted from silicic acid.

Finally, we tested fraction 53 which represents a recombination of the acidic fraction (F_8) with the 2 active subfractions (F_{26} and F_{43}) of the neutral fraction at their recoverable proportions. Fraction 53 presumably contains all of the separate fractions with skin activity, including the tumor-promoting agents, in proportion to their concentration in CSC. All fractions were tested and compared with crude CSC (designated F_1) in weighed quantities proportional to their content in CSC. The F_8 fraction was tested at 1/10 the weight of CSC (F_1), the F_{15} fraction at 1/6, the F_{26} fraction at 1/60, the F_{43} fraction at 1/40, and the F_{53} fraction, representing $F_8 + F_{26} + F_{43}$, at 1/7 the weight of F_1. Crude CSC (F_1) was tested at levels of 72, 24, 6, and 1.2 mg in 0.1 ml beeswax pellets, and each fraction was tested by using doses comparable to their concentration in CSC at these 4 dose levels.

The method of administering the materials in heated beeswax has also been described (STANTON et al., 1972; HIRANO et al., 1974). Briefly, each of the CSC components was weighed in quantities sufficient to make 1 to 5 ml of CSC-wax mixture. So that half the volume of all pellets was beeswax and consequently of similar consistency, tricaprylin was added to the weighed samples of low dose levels to yield half the final colume. Tricaprylin was omitted from all samples containing 48 or 72 mg, since the fraction alone occupied approximately 1/2 to 3/4 the final volume. Purified USP beeswax, heated to 76°C, was then added to make up the total volume, so that half the volume of each low dose sample was beeswax and the remaining half was the appropriate fraction of CSC and tricaprylin. Since beeswax made up only 1/4 the final volume of pellets containing 72 mg of CSC, the resultant pellets were less solid in consistency. After thorough mixing, the preparations were sealed and stored at 0°C until used.

The rats were 12- to 15-week-old pen-bred females of Osborne-Mendel, pathogen-free stock, that were randomly distributed in groups of 50 to 120 for each test. Open thoracotomies were performed under diethyl ether anesthesia. By direct visualization, the lower third of the left lung was injected with either 0.05 ml or 0.1 ml of the reheated (76°C) wax-condensate mixture employing a heated 0.25-ml syringe with a short-beveled, 20-gauge needle, 6 mm long. Postoperative mortality was less

394

than 5%. Some rats were killed at quarterly intervals of the year following treatment, but most were permitted to survive between 116 and 119 weeks, at which time rats on the highest doses had been reduced in number to less than 10%. At death, all rats were necropsied and tissues from the pellet site and all other gross lesions were examined histologically. A variety of neoplasms were observed in the older rats, but no differences in site or frequencies from that of controls could be detected. For brevity, remarks are confined to the lesions that developed at the pellet site.

Results

Morphology: The injected beeswax infiltrated the lung parenchyma, generally entrapped several secondary bronchioles, and formed a roughly spherical solid deposit at body temperature. Histopathological changes in response to the sequestered beeswax were confined to the surviving tissue immediately surrounding the periphery of the beeswax deposit. These changes previously characterized (STANTON et al., 1972) seemed to represent progressive alterations that can be designated types O through IV. Type O, characteristic of tissue surrounding pellets containing either beeswax and tricaprylin alone or combined with noncarcinogenic polycyclic hydrocarbons, consisted of reactive granulation tissue with abundant phagocytic giant cells that with time became sequestered in a thin margin of scar tissue about the pellet (Fig. 1). This type of response was noted in more than 98% of cases in which pellets containing no carcinogen were used.

The rare exception in the control groups had foci of squamous metaplasia characteristic of lesions designated type I. Type I lesions consisted of replacement of granulomatous tissue at the surface of the pellet by a thin, usually contiguous, layer of keratinized, metaplastic, squamous epithelium. In many cases, this could be traced to juxtaposed bronchioles from which it was presumably derived (Fig. 2). With time, extensive keratinization and apparent growth of this epithelium resulted in cystic lesions several centimeters in diameter which sometimes resembled inverted papillomatous growth.

If in addition there was evidence of extension of the epithelium into adjacent lung parenchyma with loss of a contiguous basement membrane and disorientation of the cells, we designated the lesions type II (Fig. 3). Type II lesions presumably represent early or occult neoplasms in most cases. However, since this cannot be determined with certainty, they have been separated from the overt neoplasms.

Overt squamous cell carcinomas have been designated type III lesions (Fig. 4). Differentiation as stratified squamous epithelium was often well defined in these neoplasms, but additionally they showed evidence of cellular dysplasia, tissue invasion, and either local or distant metastases. Lesions in which the diagnosis of carcinoma was equivocal were designated type II. Spontaneous carcinomas have not been observed in the lungs of this strain of rat by us or other observers at NIH.

Distinct, but not entirely separate from the differentiated squamous cell carcinomas, were neoplasms composed largely of invasive pleomorphic to spindle-shaped anaplastic cells. These tumors were derived from tissues immediately adjacent to the pellet, and in many cases the undifferentiated cells seemed to merge with poorly differentiated squamous cells at the pellet surface. However, because the tissue of

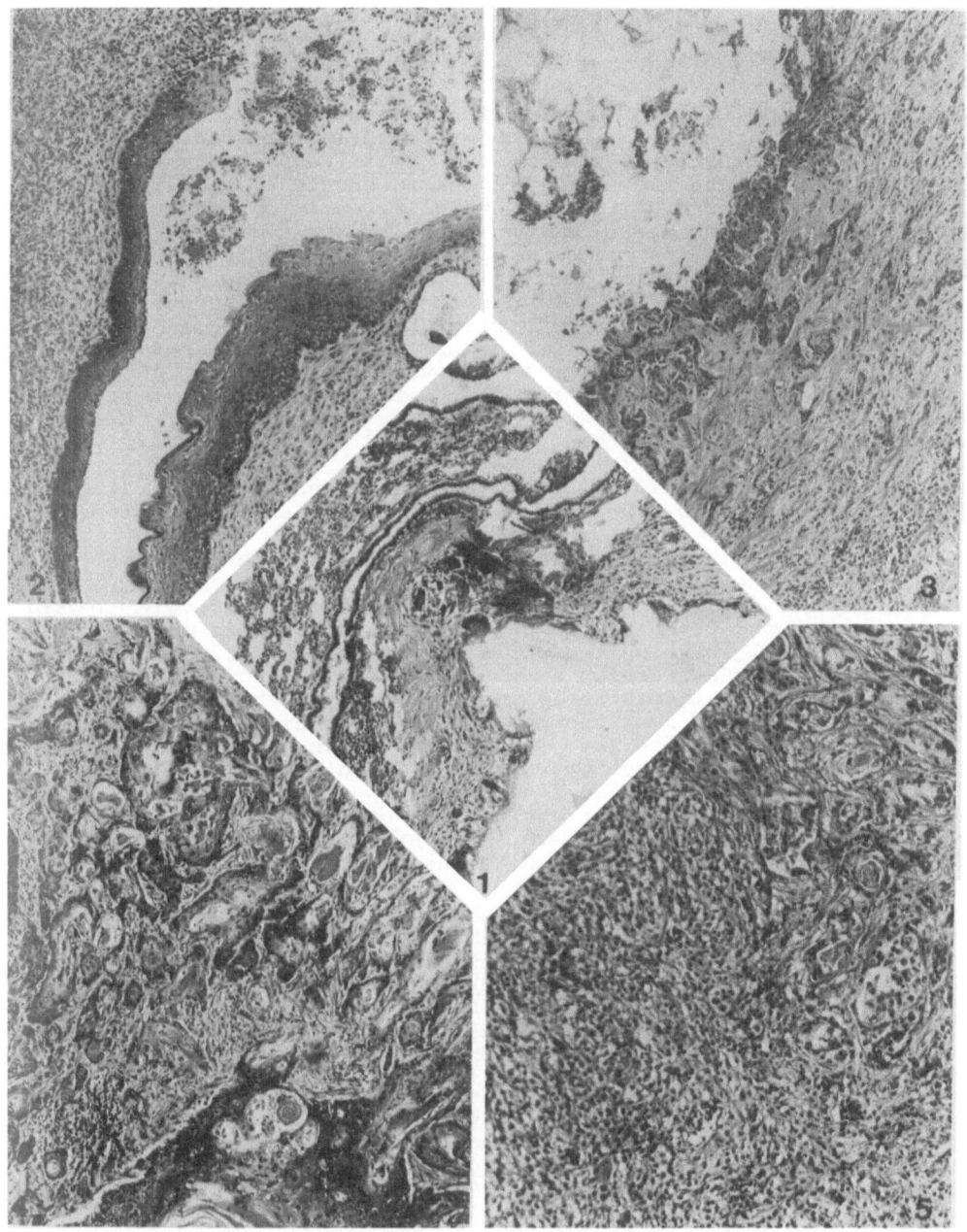

Fig. 1.   Type O lesion. Typical granulomatous response to beeswax or beeswax incorporated with noncarcinogenic compounds (x 75)

Fig. 2.   Type I lesion. Well-differentiated keratinizing squamous epithelium forming margin between wax pellet and pulmonary tissue (x 75)

Fig. 3.   Type II lesion. Note local extension of disoriented squamous epithelium beyond the epithelial lining of the pellet (x 75)

Fig. 4.   Type III lesion. Overt squamous cell carcinoma (x 113)

Fig. 5.   Type IV lesion. Undifferentiated neoplasm; note merger of undifferentiated cells with keratinizing squamous epithelium (x 113)

origin of these neoplasms could have been either epithelium, mesenchyme or both, they were given the separate designation, type IV (Fig. 5).

Comparative Studies: 3 groups of experiments have been done. The final result of the first group on which we reported previously (STANTON et al., 1972) is illustrated in Fig. 6. Cumulative frequencies of the 5 types of lesions are listed at 17-week intervals so that the effect of differences in mortality rate can be taken into account. In all of the experiments, the death rate at each interval was relatively high. This was frequently the result of pneumonia, in lungs compromised by progressively enlarging lesions at the pellet site. However, overt neoplastic lesions did not become evident until the second year. Deaths during the second year were primarily the result of progressively growing lesions at the pellet site, but neoplasms in unrelated organs caused some deaths. During the second year the frequency of neoplasms at the pellet site increased rapidly, with final yields ranging from 14% at the 12-mg level to 34% at the 48-mg level. Notably, these doses are equivalent to the tar content of 1 to 3 cigarettes.

The most significant difference in incidence and rate of neoplastic development seemed to depend on pellet size rather than on dose. Both the 0.05-ml pellets containing 24 mg HSF and the 0.10-ml pellets containing 48 mg HSF had equivalent levels of approximately 50% HSF. Nevertheless, the 0.1-ml pellets yielded significantly more neoplasms presumably because of the greater amount of tissue directly exposed. Dose-response relationships in pellets of similar size were not as clearly evident. The single experiment with crude CSC yielded no less tumors than the HSF fraction at the same dose, although the latter is reported to be significantly more effective than CSC in the induction of skin tumors of the mouse. Furthermore, only insignificant differences in incidence and distribution of the lesions could be detected between HSF doses of 48 and 72 mg in 0.1-ml pellets. The trend of the higher dose level to fewer types II and III lesions may have resulted from the lower ratio of wax to HSF and consequent softer consistency of the 72-mg pellets. However, this small variation in incidence is more probably related to the relatively small difference in the 2 doses employed.

To determine whether a dose-response curve could be established, a supplemental series of 3 experiments was done at levels of 1.2, 6, and 24 mg HSF in 0.1-ml pellets. These experiments are not through the second year, but in Fig. 7 the preliminary data coupled with that of the pertinent original experiments indicate that such a curve quite likely will be obtained. Since this graph was drawn, 2 carcinomas have developed ın the 24-mg dose group. In these 3 supplemental low dose groups, a substantial number of rats were killed at 17 weeks to determine the time at which type I and type II lesions develop. The 17-week data from dose levels of 6 and 24 mg illustrate observations more fully developed in studies with pellets containing 3-methylcholanthrene (MC) or benzo(a)pyrene (HIRANO et al., 1974). Namely, the frequency of squamous metaplasia (type I lesions) is related to dose, but it is a response that develops only within the first several weeks after treatment. In further short-term experiments recently completed with high and low doses of CSC and benzo(a)pyrene, we have found that type I lesions occur within 2 weeks at frequencies comparable to the combined frequencies of types I through IV lesions at later dates. For each experiment, the ratio of type O lesions to type I lesions remains relatively constant after the first few weeks until the more progressive lesions occur; the ratio of type O lesions to the eventual sum of lesions types I through IV is similar. Subsequently, the carcinomas

397

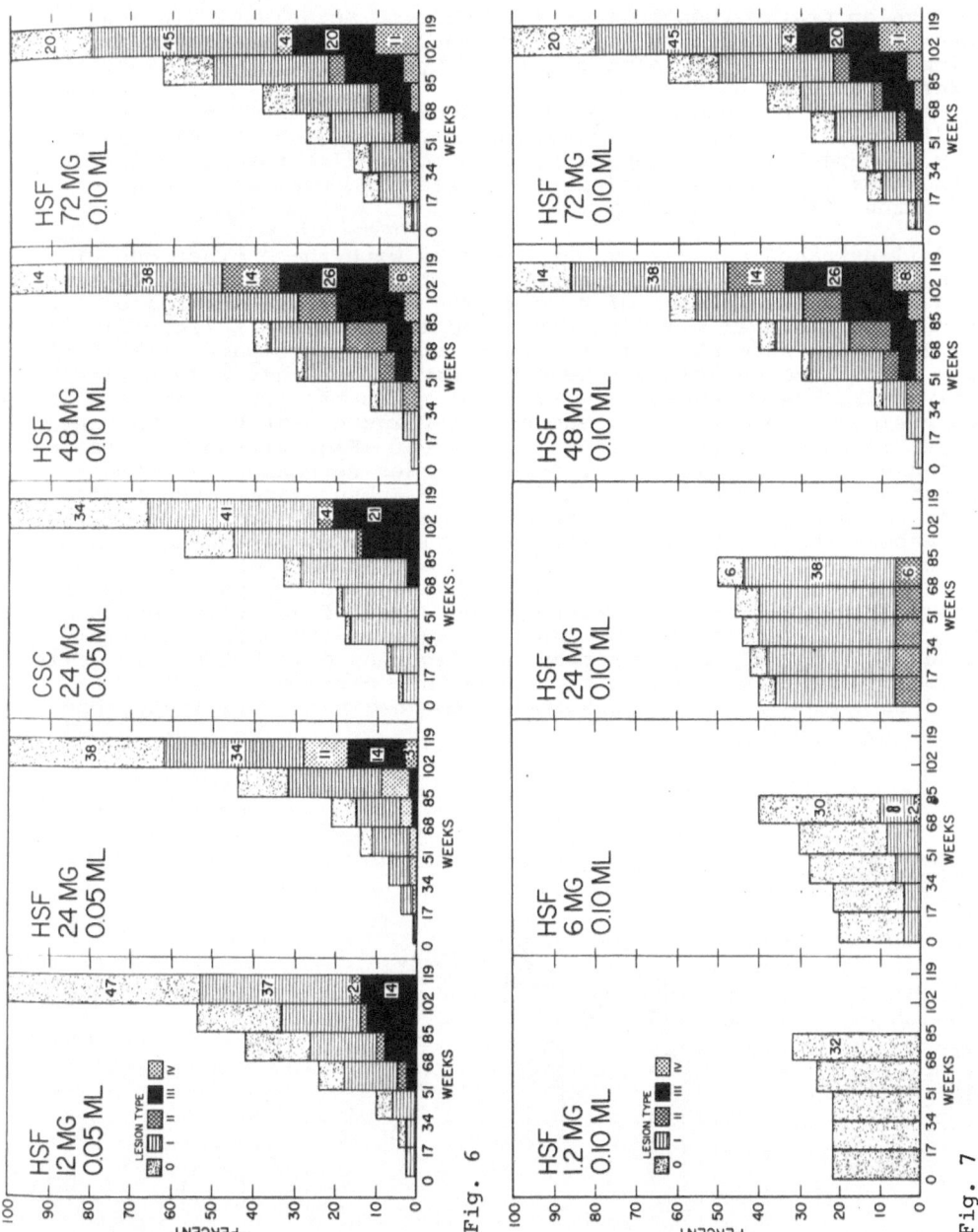

Fig. 6. Cumulative response and distribution of the 5 types of lesions after use of 4 different doses of the heptane-soluble fraction of CSC and the single intermediate level of CSC

Fig. 7. Cumulative response and distribution of the 5 types of lesions at 5 graded levels of HSF. Most of the rats in the first 3 groups were killed 17 weeks after treatment; response beyond the 85th week is not yet available

398

that develop probably do so from this pool of metaplastic lesions at
frequencies and rates also related to dose, but not in direct proportion to the frequency of the initial type I lesion. For example,
a moderate dose of MC yielded as high an incidence of type I lesions
as a high dose, but the incidence of carcinomas after 2 years was
significantly lower at the moderate dose. Hence, a high initial frequency of type I lesions cannot be used to predict the later incidence
of carcinomas. This observation is pertinent to what we have accomplished thus far with the CSC fractions.

Fig. 8 illustrates our preliminary results with the 4 fractions of
CSC in 0.1-ml pellets. The data were obtained from groups of 10 rats
killed at 17 weeks in each of 4 dose groups. Although several of the
rats had lesions that might be early neoplasms (type II lesions), it
would be unwarranted at this time to do more than compare lesions that
showed a positive metaplastic response with those that were entirely
negative. The crude condensate (F_1) from which the fractions were derived yielded a dose-related response that was compatible with that
noted at 17 weeks in the previous experiment (Fig. 6). Both the acidic
(F_8) and neutral fraction (F_{15}) showed lesser response, with the
greatest activity in the neutral fraction. Subsequently, the subfraction of the neutral fraction that contained the polynuclear aromatic
hydrocarbons (F_{43}) retained activity equal to that of the total neutral
fraction, although activity was also present at high dose levels of
F_{26}. The recombined acidic fraction with the 2 active partitions of
the neutral fraction did not restore the level of activity demonstrated by the crude condensate nor enhance the activity obtained simply
with subfraction 43. From our previous experience with the polycyclic
carcinogens, it is reasonable to assume that carcinomas will be
limited to a proportion of rats that responded before 17 weeks, but

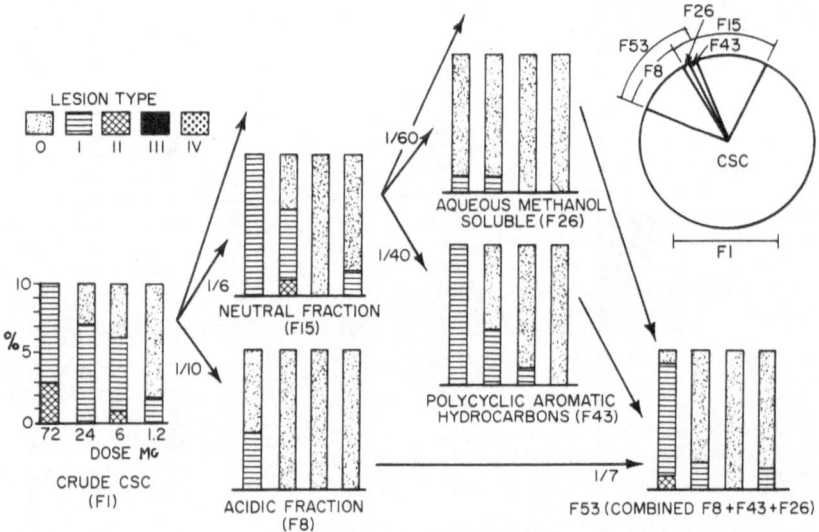

Fig. 8. Response at 17 weeks to 6 different combinations of frac-
tionated CSC. The proportion of each fraction in crude CSC is indicated graphically and numerically. The bars in each graph represent
response to doses proportional to that fraction of the dose noted
under crude CSC

the final incidence of carcinomas cannot be predicted by this early sampling. Nevertheless, it seems evident that a detectable potential for neoplasia is carried by these 4 fractions and that this potential is distributed in the fractions in proportions compatible with what might be expected on the skin.

Discussion

The advantages and disadvantages of examining pulmonary carcinogenesis by this method have been stated previously (STANTON et al., 1972; HIRANO et al., 1974). In a sense, our initial attempts to explore the effects of CSC and its fractions are simply confirmation of observations by BLACKLOCK (1957) and BLACKLOCK et al. (1962). Hopefully, observations on response in the lung will reinforce those on cutaneous carcinogenesis with CSC, so that data from both sites can be extrapolated to that of the human lung. In this regard, the preliminary response to the CSC fractions appears promising. However, we must emphasize that these are preliminary results and that repetition and reproduction of the final results are essential before the methods can be considered a valid means of assaying the carcinogenic potential of the various components of CSC. The opportunity to focus observations on a limited area of pulmonary tissue that is exposed directly over a long period of time to a remarkably small amount of CSC has obvious advantages as a bioassay procedure. Further, study of the changes that lead to cancer may offer particular opportunities for understanding the mechanisms involved. Carcinogenesis at the pellet site with both polycyclic carcinogens and CSC seems to progress through at least 2 phases of development, i.e., a prompt, dose-related, all-or-none conversion of regenerating bronchiolar epithelium to keratinizing squamous epithelium and more delayed time-dose dependent transformation of the metaplastic epithelium to squamous cell carcinoma. It is of course tempting to relate these changes to those observed in epidermal carcinogenesis in the mouse. From data on skin application of the various CSC fractions used in these experiments, we know that those fractions that retain the polynuclear aromatic hydrocarbons, i.e., fractions 15 and 43 as well as the recombined F_{53} and whole CSC, are the most capable of acting as complete carcinogens (BOCK, 1972; BOCK et al., 1962, 1969, 1970, 1972). On the other hand, fraction 8, which contains weak acids such as the phenols and fatty acids, and fraction 26, which contains the most polar substances in the neutral fraction, are only weakly carcinogenic unless preceded by a subthreshold initiating dose of 7,12-dimethylbenz(a)anthracene. BOCK (1972) and BOCK et al. (1972) have evidence that more refined fractions similar to F_8 and F_{26} act only as tumor promoters. Since on the skin, squamous hyperplasia is a response associated with promoting agents, it might be assumed that the squamous metaplasia noted so promptly at the pellet site might also indicate the presence of simple promoters that require initiation and prolonged reinforcement for carcinogenesis. Such determinations should be possible by altering the content of the pellets or by altering the rate of release of the pellet components. In this regard, it would be important to know the release rates from the pellets of various components of CSC. Such factors may be critical to induction of cancer at the pellet site or, for that matter, for the induction of cancer in man from deposition of CSC in the respiratory tract.

References

BLACKLOCK, J.W.S.: The production of lung tumours in rats with 3:4
  benzpyrene, methylcholanthrene and the condensate from cigarette
  smoke. Brit. J. Cancer <u>11</u>, 181-191 (1957).
BLACKLOCK, J.W.S., BURGEN, J.G.: The carcinogenic effects of various
  fractions of cigarette condensate. Brit. J. Cancer <u>16</u>, 453-459 (1962).
BOCK, F.G.: Tumor promoters in tobacco and cigarette smoke condensate.
  J. nat. Cancer Inst. <u>48</u>, 1849-1853 (1972).
BOCK, F.G., MOORE, G.E., DOWD, J.E., CLARK, P.C.: Carcinogenic activ-
  ity of cigarette smoke condensate. JAMA <u>181</u>, 668-673 (1962).
BOCK, F.G., SWAIN, A.P., STEDMAN, R.L.: Bioassay of major fractions
  of cigarette condensate by an accelerated technic. Cancer
  Res. <u>29</u>, 584-587 (1969).
BOCK, F.G., SWAIN, A.P., STEDMAN, R.L.: Composition studies on tobacco
  XLl. Carcinogenesis assay of subfractions of the neutral fraction
  of cigarette smoke condensate. J. nat. Cancer Inst. <u>44</u>, 1305-1310
  (1970).
BOCK, F.G., SWAIN, A.P., STEDMAN, R.L.: Carcinogenesis assay of subfractions of cigarette smoke condensate prepared by solvent-separa-
  tion of the neutral fraction. J. nat. Cancer Inst. <u>49</u>, 477-483 (1972).
HIRANO, T., STANTON, M.F., LAYARD, M.: Quantitative carcinogenic
  response of the lungs of rats to methylcholanthrene-laden beeswax
  pellets. J. nat. Cancer Inst. <u>52</u>, in press.
STANTON, M.F., BLACKWELL, R., MILLER, E.: Experimental pulmonary
  carcinogenesis with asbestos. Amer. ind. Hyg. Ass. <u>30</u>, 236-244
  (1969).
STANTON, M.F., MILLER, E., WRENCH, C., BLACKWELL, R.: Experimental
  induction of epidermoid carcinoma in the lungs of rats by cigarette
  smoke condensate. J. nat. Cancer Inst. <u>49</u>, 867-877 (1972).
SWAIN, A.P., COOPER, J.E., STEDMAN, R.L.: Large-scale fractionation
  of cigarette smoke condensate for chemical and biological investigations. Cancer Res. <u>29</u>, 579-583 (1969a).
SWAIN, A.P., COOPER, J.E., STEDMAN, R.L., BOCK, F.G.: Composition
  studies on tobacco. XL. Large-scale fractionation of the neutrals
  of cigarette smoke condensate for bioassay using adsorption chromatography and solvent partitioning. Beitr. Tabakforsch. <u>5</u>, 97-103
  (1969b).

Session IV   Radiation Carcinogenesis and Bioassays

Chairman: James F. Park

Biology Department, Battelle-Northwest, Richland, WA, USA

Radiation Carcinogenesis. Introductory Remarks

James F. Park

Biology Department, Battelle-Northwest, Richland, WA, USA

Summary

Nuclear energy is expected to provide a large fraction of the future electrical energy requirements of the world. The projected health risk of nuclear energy, compared to other electrical energy sources, is currently of much concern. The health risk concerning lung cancer is particularly important. Uranium miners have an excess of lung cancer attributed to cigarette smoking and inhalation of uranium mine air contaminants, including radon and its alpha-emitting decay products and uranium ore dust. Animal studies reported at this symposium confirmed that inhalation of radon and its daughter products alone may cause lung cancer. Experiments to evaluate the role of other uranium air contaminants and cigarette smoking in the carcinogenic process are now in progress. Future nuclear reactor fuels will contain several other alpha-emitting radionuclides. Although these radionuclides have not yet been shown to be carcinogenic in people, papers in this symposium report that inhalation of alpha-emitting radionuclides (^{239}Pu, ^{238}Pu, ^{244}Am, ^{241}Am, and ^{210}Pu) cause dose-related increased incidence of lung cancer in experimental animals. These studies are providing data necessary to assess the risk of lung cancer related to nuclear energy and to evaluate the role of radiation related to the overall lung cancer related health problem.

The Effects of Inhaled Uranium Mine Air Contaminants in Beagle Dogs

Ronald E. Filipy, Bruce O. Stuart, R. F. Palmer, H. A. Ragan, and
P. L. Hackett

Biology Department, Battelle, Pacific Northwest Laboratories, Richland, WA 99352, USA

ABSTRACT

The high incidence of lung cancer among uranium miners of the Colorado
plateau is a matter of national concern in a period of increasing demand for uranium ore. These miners are exposed to a variety of inhalation hazards, including radon daughters, uranium ore dust, and
cigarette smoking, that may cause or contribute to respiratory tract
pathology. Over 98% of the miners developing lung cancer have had
histories of cigarette smoking.

In order to determine the combined or separate roles of radon daughters
and cigarette smoking in the development of lung cancer and other
respiratory tract pathology, groups of 20 dogs each received daily
life span exposures to 4 hours of 600 Working Levels of radon daughters with ore dust, and/or cigarette smoking over 16 hours per day,
7 days per week, or both; control dogs received sham smoking. After
4 years of exposure, respiratory tract pathology included macrophage
accumulation, septal fibrosis, epithelial hyperplasia, endothelial
proliferation, vesicular and bullous emphysema, and extensive epithelial changes involving squamous metaplasia with atypical nuclei. These
effects were primarily related to exposure to radon daughters' and
uranium ore dust, with and without cigarette smoke.

Introduction

The high incidence of lung cancer among uranium miners of the Colorado
plateau is of national concern in a period of increasing demand for
uranium ore. These miners are exposed to a variety of inhalation hazards, including radon daughters, uranium ore dust, diesel engine exhaust, and blasting gases. Also, many of the miners are cigarette
smokers or have smoked cigarettes in the past.

An increased prevalence of pulmonary fibrosis, pneumoconiosis, and
emphysema has been found among the underground uranium miners (ARCHER
et al., 1964). WAGONER et al. (1965) reported a six-fold higher incidence of lung cancer among the uramium miners of the Colorado plateau. By April 1973, the total known cases of respiratory cancer
among uranium miners had reached 235 (ARCHER, personal communication,
1973).

The role of cigarette smoking in the induction of lung cancer among
the miners is still unresolved. The report by WAGONER et al. (1965)
indicated that in 60 of the 62 cases of lung cancer among the miners,

there was a history of cigarette smoking. ARCHER et al. (1973) have recently reevaluated all available histories of uranium miners developing lung cancer and concluded that cigarette smoking acts as a promoter in the induction of these lung cancers. It was found that 98.4% of the lung cancer patients had histories of cigarette smoking.

Since 1968, research designed to evaluate the carcinogenic or cocarcinogenic effects of uranium mine air contaminants in rodents and beagle dogs has been in progress at Battelle-Northwest Laboratories. The principal objectives of the experiments are to determine the biological effects of daily exposures to known levels of the uranium mine air contaminants and cigarette smoke, separately and together.

Materials and Methods

The design of the experiments using the beagle dog, a relatively long-lived laboratory animal, is shown in Table 1. Each treatment group originally contained 20 2-year old dogs with 9 dogs sham exposed for experimental controls.

Table 1. Experimental design

Group	Number of animals	Exposure regimen
1	20	600 WL[a] radon daughters with uranium ore dust (carnotite, 18 mg/m^3), plus sham smoking
2	20	Cigarette smoke[b] plus 600 WL[a] radon daughters with uranium ore dust (carnotite, 18 mg/m^3)
3	20	Cigarette smoke[b]
4	9	Controls, with sham smoking

[a]Working Level: any combination of short-lived radon daughters in 1 liter of air that will result in the ultimate emission of 1.3×10^5 MeV of alpha energy from radioactive decay.

[b]10 cigarettes per day over a 16 hour period, 7 days per week.

The dogs of groups 1 and 2 are exposed, head only, to an atmosphere containing uranium ore dust and radon daughters for 4 hours daily, 5 days per week. The dogs of groups 2 and 3 are administered cigarette smoke, by means of a specially designed mask, from 10 cigarettes daily over a 16 hour period, 7 days per week. Dogs of group 1, as well as the control dogs, are subjected to sham smoking (i.e., unlighted cigarettes). Cigarette smoking by the dogs consists of inhaling (puffing) through a cigarette at each tenth breath after 9 breaths of fresh air. Cigarettes used are the University of Kentucky Research Cigarette, 1R1. The radon daughter, uranium ore dust, and cigarette exposure system were described in detail in a report by STUART (1970).

Measurements of ore dust concentration and radon daughter levels as well as condensation nuclei levels in the exposure chambers are made twice daily. Periodic samples are taken from the chambers for determination of aerosol size spectra of the aerosolized ore dust and for fractions of unattached radon daughters. Concentrations of uranium ore dust average 17.9 ± 0.3 (standard error of the mean) mg/m^3, and show mass median diameters ranging from 0.6 μm to 2.1 μm with geometric standard deviations of 1.8 to 2.6. Condensation nuclei counts range from 68,000 to 210,000 per cm^3 in the chambers as compared to 2,000 to 12,000 per cm^3 in laboratory air. Unattached fractions of RaA are on the order of a percent or less. Unattached percentages of RaB and RaC are only fractions of RaA levels.

Blood carboxyhemoglobin levels before (1.9% to 2.2% HbCO) and after smoking 10 cigarettes (4.7% to 5.3% HbCO) are determined on a semiannual basis as an index of depositon of the gaseous components of cigarette smoke. Other cigarette smoke dosimetric parameters include blood nicotine (200 to 600 nanograms per ml of blood) and blood thiocyanate concentrations (~40 micromoles per liter). These values for carboxyhemoglobin, nicotine, and thiocyanate are similar to those reported for human smokers (RAMSEY, 1967; MADDOX, 1974; PETTIGREW and FELL, 1972). Cigarette smoke particulate deposition studies using carbon-14 labeled dotriacontane spiked cigarettes indicate ~30% of the label available for inhalation is deposited in the lungs of the dogs.

Minute volumes, tidal volumes, and respiratory rates are measured monthly on each dog. At such time that a dog exhibits respiratory insufficiency or other indications of imminent death, it is euthanized by anaesthesia and subsequent venous exsanguination. A gross necropsy is performed, organs are weighed and fixed, and samples are selected for histopathologic examination. In the cases of the dogs in the control, sham smoking group, or those exposed to cigarette smoke only, periodic sacrifices are scheduled so that pathologic data is available for comparison with that from dogs of the first 2 groups exposed to radon daughters with uranium ore dust plus smoking or sham smoking.

Results

Exposures of the beagle dogs to radon daughters, uranium ore dust, and cigarette smoke have been in progress for approximately 4 1/2 years. The smoking patterns by individual dogs and by groups of dogs are determined periodically according to the number of puffs and the time required to smoke several cigarettes. Although the mean time required to smoke a cigarette has changed very little, significantly increased numbers of puffs per cigarette are being taken by dogs receiving cigarette smoke plus radon daughters with uranium ore dust (group 2). The mean number of sham smoking puffs over a predetermined test period taken by dogs receiving daily exposures to radon daughters with uranium ore dust (group 1) have also shown a significant increase. There has been no significant increase in the number of puffs per cigarette with the dogs smoking cigarettes only (group 3) or with the control dogs (group 4). The increasing number of puffs per cigarette with dogs of groups 1 and 2 is due to elevated respiratory rates in many of those dogs. Mean minute volumes of each of the exposed groups have not differed significantly from those of the control dogs, but respiratory rates of the dogs of groups 1 and 2 (radon daughters with uranium ore dust with smoking or sham smoking) are considerably elevated. There is a wide variation between values for dogs within each of the 2 radon daughters with uranium ore exposed groups; some animals have rates of 100 to 120 respirations per minute with severe respira-

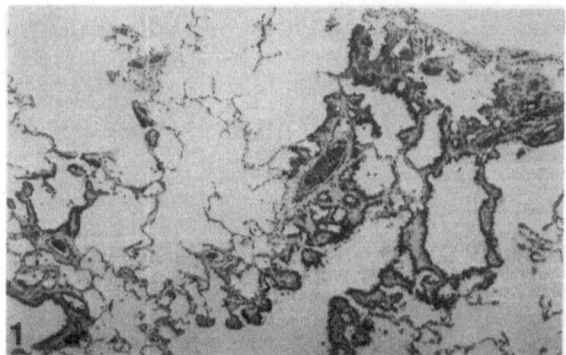

Fig. 1. Subpleural inter-stitial fibrosis with al-veolar epithelium metaplasia from the lung of a dog after 49 months of cigarette smok-ing. HE (x 120)

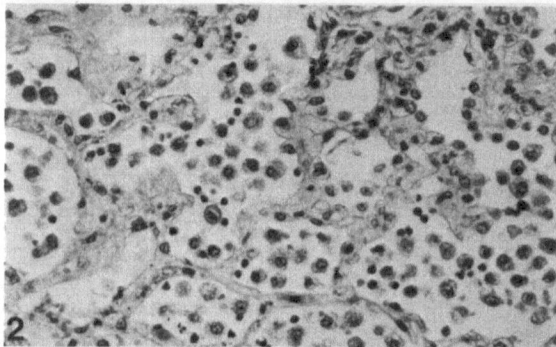

Fig. 2. Numerous alveolar macrophages in a section from the lung of a dog ex-posed to radon daughters with uranium ore dust and cigarette smoke for 48 months. HE (x 240)

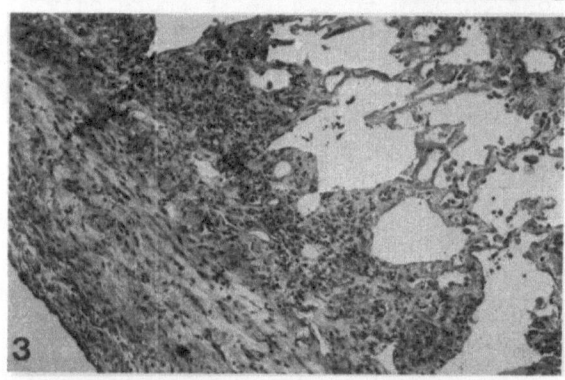

Fig. 3. Pleural thickening, peripheral alveolar septal fibrosis, and emphysematous vesicles in the lung of a dog after 47 months exposure to radon daughters with uranium ore dust. HE (x 60)

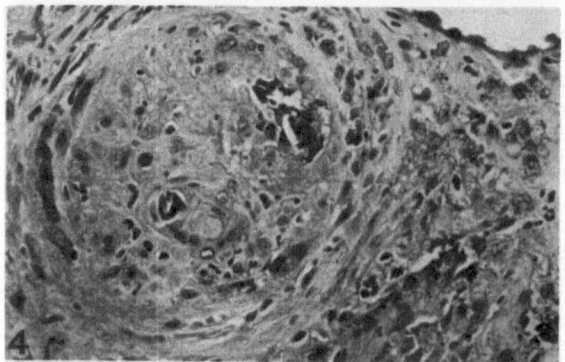

Fig. 4. An arteriole nearly completely occluded by endo-thelial cell hyperplasia and fibrosis of the vessel wall. The section is from the lung of a dog exposed to radon daughters with uranium ore dust for 47 months.
HE (x 300)

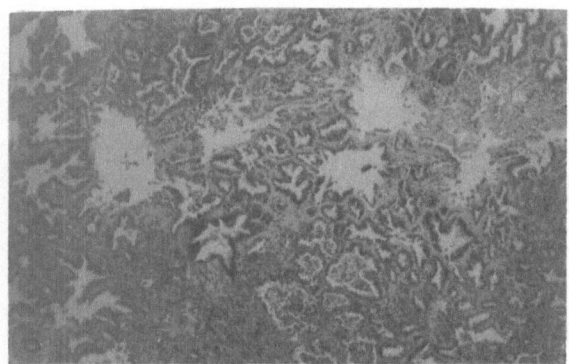

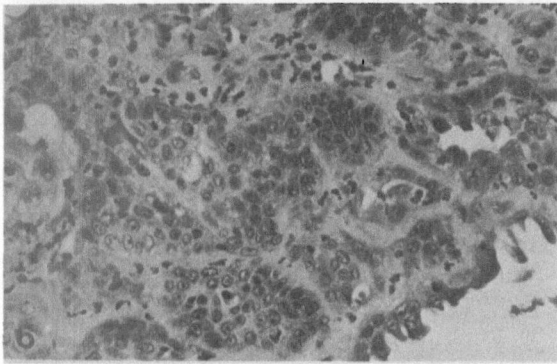

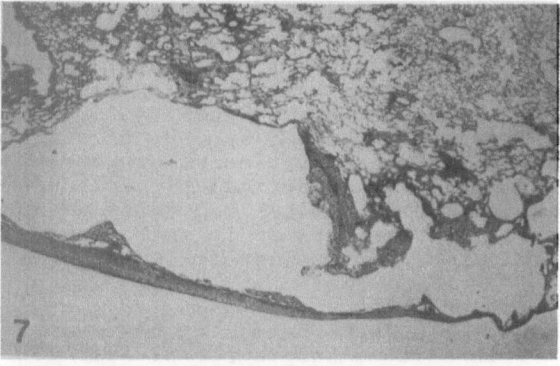

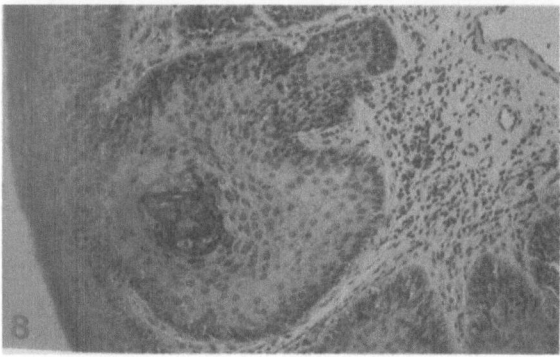

Fig. 5. Adenomatous hyper-plasia of the alveolar epi-thelium in the lung of a dog exposed to radon daughters with uranium ore dust and cigarette smoke for 32 months. HE (x 48)

Fig. 6. Squamous metaplasia of the alveolar epithelium in the lung of a dog after 46 months exposure to radon daughters with uranium ore dust. HE (x 240)

Fig. 7. Bullous emphysema in the lung of a dog after 48 months exposure to radon daughters with uranium ore dust and cigarette smoke. HE (x 14.4)

Fig. 8. Pseudoepithelio-matous hyperplasia of the epithelium in the nasal turbinates of a dog ex-posed to radon daughters with uranium ore dust and cigarette smoke for 53 months. HE (x 60)

tory insufficiency characterized by anoxemia and hypoxemia immediately perior to sacrifice.

Scheduled sacrifice of 1 dog from each group after 8 months exposure showed minimally detectable changes in the lung, with the more severe changes in the radon daughters with uranium ore exposed group. After 52 months of exposure, a dog from the control sham smoke group (group 4), and after 49 months a dog from the cigarette smoke group (group 3), were sacrificed for histopathologic examination and comparison with 12 dogs euthanized when death was imminent due to respiratory insufficiency after 21 to 52 months of exposure to radon daughters with uranium ore dust plus smoking or sham smoking.

Only minimal lesions were present in the lungs of the control dog. They consisted of a few small foci of subpleural interstitial fibrosis with slight pleural thickening and slight alveolar epithelial hyperplasia at the foci. Generally, the lungs and upper respiratory tract of this dog were normal.

The dog exposed to cigarette smoke only for 49 months had slight to moderate vesicular emphysema and scattered foci of subpleural interstitial fibrosis with associated alveolar epithelial hyperplasia and metaplasia (Fig. 1). The latter lesion was more severe and in more numerous foci in this dog than in the previously mentioned control dog. Slight squamous metaplasia of tracheal epithelium near the tracheal bifurcation was also observed and the tracheobronchial lymph nodes contained numerous histiocytes filled with a brown pigment associated with inhalation of tobacco smoke. Grossly, the lungs of this animal appeared quite normal except for some small areas of brownish discoloration.

The respiratory tracts of dogs from groups 1 and 2 (radon daughters and uranium ore dust with or without cigarette smoking) contain marked similar pathologic changes. Some examples of the types of changes observed in dogs of these 2 groups are illustrated in Figs 2 through 8. All lungs of dogs from these 2 groups contain large numbers of alveolar macrophages incorporating a pigment identified as uranium ore dust (Fig. 2). In all cases, there is a considerable accumulation of the macrophages around bronchi, bronchioles, and small blood vessels and, in many cases, this accumulation has produced a chronic inflammatory response characterized by infiltration of mononuclear cells into the area.

A remarkable feature of the lungs of dogs from these 2 groups was the pleural thickening and septal fibrosis of subpleural alveoli with accompanying chronic subpleural inflammation. This pleural thickening is visible grossly as relatively large, yellow-white patches of the outer surfaces of the lungs. The histologic aspect of the lesion is shown in Fig. 3. Numerous small blood vessels at the periphery of the lung lobes were found to be nearly occluded by fibrosis of the vascular walls, endothelial proliferation, or both (Fig. 4).

Varying degrees of adenomatous proliferation or cuboidal metaplasia of the alveolar epithelium was also present in the lungs of the dogs from groups 1 and 2, and an example of that lesion is shown in Fig. 5. The size of the involved areas varies from small foci adjacent to small bronchioles to large areas of a lung section 2 cm to 3 cm in diameter. In many cases, a progression from cubiodal metaplasia to squamous metaplasia of the alveolar epithelium may be observed. In sections of lungs from some of the dogs, numerous foci of alveolar epithelial squamous metaplasia, such as that shown in Fig. 6, have been observed. Atypical nuclei were noted in these lesions although no invasion of adjacent tissues was present.

Pulmonary emphysema is evident in all of the recently sacrificed dogs of groups 1 and 2. Varying degrees of vesicular emphysema have been observed in lungs of dogs exposed for as few as 9 months. After 4 years of exposure, however, several cases of bullous emphysema have been observed. These changes are visible grossly as large, soft elevations on the pleural surface, and an example of the microscopic appearance is shown in Fig. 7. The lesion appears sooner and with greater severity in the lungs of dogs of group 2 (radon daughters and uranium ore dust plus cigarette smoking), but 1 case was recently found in a dog from group 1 (radon daughters, uranium ore dust, and sham smoking) after 52 months of exposure.

Fig. 8 is a photomicrograph of a lesion found in the nasal turbinates of a dog exposed to' radon daughters and uranium ore dust with cigarette smoking for 53 months. The change is a pseudoepitheliomatous proliferation with some disorientation of cells of the basal layer. It was observed grossly as a 1 cm area of thickened epithelium with an irregular surface approximately 3 cm posterior to the external nares.

Discussion

The pulmonary lesions in the dogs exposed to radon daughters and uranium ore dust were a combination of radiation pneumonitis due to the inhalation of radon daughters and uranium ore pneumoconiosis due to the inhalation of uranium ore dust. Pulmonary neoplastic lesions have not been observed in dogs of any of the groups although potential pre-neoplastic lesions such as those shown in Figs 5 and 6 were frequent observations. Previous experience with hamsters exposed to the same air contaminants and with dogs exposed to plutonium by inhalation suggest that these lesions precede pulmonary neoplasia.

PERRAUD et al. (1972) and CHAMEAUD et al. (these Proceedings) have induced tumors in rats using essentially the same inhaled uranium mine air contaminants as were used in this study with dogs. Their exposure regimen, however, was different in that they exposed rats to ore dust or cerium hydroxide for a short time at the beginning of the experiment. Subsequent exposure to a very high concentration of radon daughters for a relatively short period of time (3 to 4 months) was then followed by a cessation of all exposures. They reported a high incidence of lung tumors in the rats appearing from 12 to 24 months after the beginning of exposure. The levels of exposure used in our study were considerably lower than theirs and delivered over the life-time of the dogs.

Because of the small number of cigarette smoke only exposed dogs sacrificed since the beginning of the experiment (2 dogs over 4 1/2 years), little can be said about the effects of cigarette smoke exposure in these dogs. However, the lack of severe lesions in the lungs of dogs exposed to cigarette smoke only is in contrast to the results reported by AUERBACH et al. (1970). They reported lung tumors and emphysema in dogs after slightly more than 2 years of exposure to cigarette smoke. The method of exposure was considerably different from that used in this study: they administered the smoke by means of a tracheal stoma.

410

Presumably, that method allows a high concentration of smoke to reach the lungs.

Exposures of the surviving dogs in all groups are continuing, with periodic sacrifice of dogs from the cigarette smoke only and sham smoked control groups, for comparison with dogs from the radon daughters with uranium ore and radon daughters with uranium ore plus cigarette smoke exposed groups.

Acknowledgement

This paper is based on research performed under United States Atomic Energy Commission Contract AT(45-1)-1830 and the National Institute of Environmental Health Sciences, Department of Health, Education and Welfare.

References

ARCHER, V.E. (Chief): Epidemiology Unit, Western Area Occupational Health Laboratory, National Institute for Occupational Safety and Health, Salt Lake City, Utah. Personal communication, April 1973.

ARCHER, V.E., CARROLL, B.E., BRINTON, H.P., SACCOMANNO, G.: Radiological Health and Safety in Nuclear Materials Mining and Milling. Vienna, Austria, 1963, Vol. 1, 21-36, International Atomic Energy, Vienna, Austria 1964.

ARCHER, V.E., WAGONER, J.K., LUNDIN, F.E., Jr.: Uranium mining and cigarette smoking effects on man. J. occup. Med. 15, 204-211 (1973).

AUERBACH, O., HAMMOND, E.C., KIRMAN, D., GARFINKEL, L.: Effects of cigarette smoking on dogs II. Pulmonary neoplasms. Arch. Environ. Hlth 21, 754-768 (1970).

CHAMEAUD, J., PERRAUD, R., LAFUMA, J., MASSE, R., PRADEL, J.: Lesions and lung cancers induced in rats by inhaled Radon 222 at various equilibriums with radon daughters. In: Symposium on Experimental Respiratory Carcinogenesis and Bioassays. Seattle, Wash. 1974.

MADDOX, W.L.: Oak Ridge National Laboratory, Oak Ridge, Tennessee. Personal communication, January 1974.

PALMER, R.F., CASE, A.C., STUART, B.O.: Battelle, Pacific Northwest Laboratories, Richland, Washington. Personal communication, April 1974.

PERRAUD, R., CHAMEAUD, J., LAFUMA, J., MASSE, R., CHRETIEN, J.: Cancer broncho-pulmonaire experimental du rat par inhalation de radon. Comparaison avec les aspects histologiques des cancers humains. J. Franc. Med. Chir. Thorac. 26, 25-41 (1972). (Also available as translation: BNWL-tr-85).

PETTIGREW, A.R., FELL, G.S.: Simplified colorimetric determination of thiocyanate in biological fluids, and its application to investigation of the toxic amblyopias. Clin. Chem. 18, 996-1000 (1972).

RAMSEY, J.M.: Carboxyhemoglobinemia in parking garage employees. Arch. Environ. Hlth 15, 580-583 (1967).

STUART, B.O., WILLARD, D.H., HOWARD, E.B.: Uranium mine air contaminants in dogs and hamsters. In: Inhalation Carcinogenesis (M.G. Hanna, P. Nettesheim, J.R. Gilbert, eds), p. 413. (CONF-691001) National Technical Inf. Service, Springfield, Virginia 1970.

WAGONER, J.K., ARCHER, V.E., LUNDIN, F.E., Jr.: Radiation as the cause of lung cancer among uranium miners. New Engl. J. Med. 273, 181-188 (1965).

Lesions and Lung Cancers Induced in Rats by Inhaled Radon 222 at Various Equilibriums with Radon Daughters

J. Chameaud[1], R. Perraud[1], J. LaFuma[2], R. Masse[2], and J. Pradel[2]

[1]Service Médical, Commissariat, à l'Energie Atomique, Razes, Frances
[2]Commissariat à l'Energie Atomique, Département de Protection Sanitaire, Fontenay-aux-Roses, France

ABSTRACT

To investigate the dose-effect relationships, rats were exposed to several dose levels of radon at different levels of equilibrium with radon decay products, after inhalation of stable cerium hydroxide, and in combination with uranium ore dust.

Lung cancers were induced with exposures ranging from 500 Working Level Months (WLM) to 14,000 WLM. Exposures of 3,000 WLM to 9,000 WLM delivered over 300 to 500 hours during a 3- to 4-month period, produced the highest incidence of tumors (50%). The cancers appeared from the 12th to the 24th month after the beginning of exposure. Above 14,000 WLM, the animals died due to pulmonary fibrosis by the 12th month and the cancers may not have had time to develop. At the lowest dose (500 WLM), the first cancers appeared in the 24th month. They appeared earlier as the dose was increased. The lesions appeared in the following chronological order: metaplasia, adenomatous lesions, adenomas, and cancers. Several malignant tumor types were observed, including epidermoid carcinomas, bronchiolar-adenocarcinomas, and bronchiolo-alveolar adenocarcinomas. All tumor types were sometimes seen in the same animal.

Exposure to stable cerium hydroxide prior to radon exposure shortened the induction time of the tumors by 2 to 3 months. Uranium ore dust appeared to have little influence on the tumorigenic process. The incidence of lesions was related to total exposure time, expressed as cumulative WLM. The different equilibrium levels of radon and radon decay products had no specific effect.

These studies confirmed that radon and its decay products alone can induce tumors in rats, and they provided experimental evidence supporting the epidemiological data that exposure to radon and its decay products contributes to the etiology of lung cancer in uranium miners.

Introduction

The etiology of lung cancer in uranium miners based on clinical (BAIR, 1970; LORENZ, 1944) and epidemiological data (Federal Radiation Council, 1968; WAGONER et al., 1965; SACCOMANNO, 1969; SEVC et al., 1971; SNIHS, no date) is not clear. In previous experiments, we induced lung cancer in rats by inhalation of radon and its decay products associated with inhalation of stable cerium and uranium ore dust. Later, we induced lung cancer in rats which had inhaled radon and its decay products alone (PERRAUD et al., 1970, 1972; CHAMEAUD et al., 1971). Lung cancers were induced in rats which were unlikely to develop cancers spontaneously (KUSCHNER and LASKIN, 1970). These studies provided experimental evidence that lung cancer could be induced by inhalation of radon and its decay products alone.

In addition to its relevance for investigating the etiology of lung cancer in uranium mines, this animal model has several advantages for lung cancer research. Radon is easy to handle, and the duration and concentration of the inhalation can be easily controlled. The distribution of radon and its decay products in the lung is very homogeneous. Because of the short half-lives of these radionuclides, the radiation-exposure of the lung is essentially terminated at the completion of the exposure of the animal, allowing more accurate estimation and control of the dose received by the lungs than in most other animal lung cancer models.

This paper describes current experiments investigating the dose-effect relationships of radon at different equilibriums with radon decay products, at various concentrations, associated with dust and without dust, and using several exposure regimens.

Materials and Methods

Until 1972, an inhalation apparatus composed of 2 parts was used: the part in which radon was generated and the part in which it was inhaled. Radon was obtained from very rich ore containing about 25% uranium, ground to a fine powder, and spread out on superposed trays in a hermetically-sealed steel container. Air passed through the trays and carried along the radon which was given off continuously. The radon generator was connected to a room containing 1 or 2 airtight Plexiglas animal inhalation chambers by 2 pipes that made a closed circuit with the radon generator. A pump placed on one of the pipes circulated the radon-charged air. Under these conditions, the equilibrium of radon with radon decay products was about 30%, and the radon concentration was 7.5×10^{-7} curie/liter. When a filter and an electrostatic purifying apparatus was placed on the radon circuit at the entrance of each inhalation chamber, radon equilibrium with its decay products was about 1%. The inhalation chambers contained a maximum of 100 animals which could be exposed for about 5 hours at a time.

With this apparatus, we could neither use many animals nor obtain radon equilibrium with its decay products exceeding 30%. Therefore, we built a new apparatus (BLONDEAU et al., no date), which has been used since early 1973. In this apparatus, radon comes from 2 stainless steel tanks placed underground, whose total volume is 10 m^3. They contain 57 barrels full of radium-rich lead sulphate, each containing 2 curies of radium. A system of pipes connects the tanks to a container of 1 m^3, which in turn is connected to 2 metal inhalation chambers of 10 m^3 (Fig. 1). The required quantity of radon is first drawn into the 1 m^3 container, where a centrifugal ventilator distributes the radon of the container into either or both inhalation chambers. When the inhalation exposure period is over, a fan clears the chambers of all radon. Each chamber can contain 300 rats for 4 hours. By adding oxygen, the exposure can last as long as 16 hours.

Using this apparatus, daily exposures were performed with a maximum radon concentration of 1.25 µCi/l and 100% equilibrium with radon de-

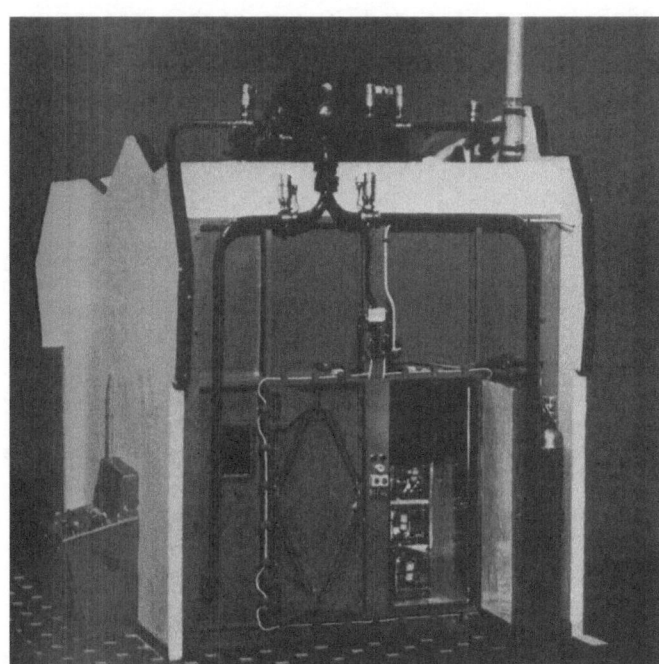

Fig. 1. 2 10 m³ in-
halation chambers.
The right door is
open, showing animal
cages

cay products. Radon levels were measured several times during each
exposure period, and radon decay product levels were measured periodically. For the lower doses with filtered radon, the fractional equilibrium levels of radon decay products were about: fA = 0.042, fB =
0.0066, fC = 0.004, for 0.75 µCi/l of Rn. The total exposure to radon
and its decay products varied from 50 to 600 hours, delivered over a
period of 1 to 10 months.

In 2 experiments, rats were exposed to either stable cerium hydroxide
or to uranium ore dust, as well as to radon with radon decay products.
In 1 experiment, animals were exposed to aerosols of stable cerium
hydroxide in a single period before exposures to radon and radon decay products; 0.5 to 1 mg of cerium hydroxide was deposited in the
lungs. In the other experiment, animals were exposed to uranium ore
dust (15% uranium, 130 mg/m³ for a total of 51 5-hour periods) and
to radon and radon decay products on alternate days. The chamber for
dust inhalation is that used by the Centre de Researches des Charbon-
nages de France (LE BOUFFANT, 1971). It operates at a slight negative
pressure and the dust concentration is maintained by an automatic
control system.

Male Sprague-Dawley S.P.F. rats were used in these studies. The lungs
of the rats were observed for lesions after spontaneous death; or
after sacrifice because their health seemed seriously impaired or
because they had suddenly lost weight; or, according to some protocols,
at various periods after the beginning of exposure(from the 6th to
the 24th month). The rats were anesthetized with Nembutal, then killed
by cutting the abdominal vessels. The lungs were perfused with saline,
then taken out of the thoracic cavity, fixed by intratracheal injection of Duboscq Brazil's fixing solution, and stored in bottles filled
with the same solution. After a few days, the whole lungs were cut in
a sagittal plane to allow a better penetration of the fixing solution.

The cut lungs were imbedded in paraffin and 20 μm-thick sections were prepared and observed for macroscopic lesions. Then 5 μm sections were made, stained with Hemalun-Phloxine-Saffran Alcyan Green and examined microscopically. Special stainings were made when necessary.

Results

A total of about 800 rats was used in these studies. All of the lungs have been examined macroscopically and about 400 lungs were examined microscopically. In the course of the studies, we found 250 benign or malignant tumors, as shown in Figs 2-4.

The alterations induced by long-time inhalation of high levels of radon included large areas of diffuse interstitial pneumonia with formation of hyaline membranes. There was severe fibrosis of inter-alveolar septae surrounding the capillaries. Death generally occurred after a few weeks or a few months.

When the cumulative dose was lower, the animals lived longer and lesions appeared that can be divided, for clarity, into 4 kinds (SHABAD and PYLEV, 1970; HOWARD, 1970). All 4 kinds appeared to be related to time-since-exposure:

I.   Metaplasia

1.   Bronchiolar metaplasia consisted of large columnar cells, with basal nuclei, light-colored protoplasms, often ciliated and generally found at the bronchiolo-alveolar junction and in the neighbouring alveoli.

2.   Alveolar metaplasia was composed of cuboidal cells, all similar, with darker protoplasms, generally developed in the peripheral parts of the lungs.

II.   Adenomatous Lesions

There were 2 main types, depending on the kind of metaplasia they represented. They formed areas of variable size, never very dense, in which the alveolar septum, covered with one or several layers of cells, was easily recognizable.

III.   Adenoma

These were round-shaped tumors made of cells, often clustered together, in which the seriously-damaged alveolar septum could be seen only after special staining.

IV.   Malignant Tumors

Several different types were observed, the main ones being:

1. Epidermoid carcinomas which were not always clearly differentiated and were often keratinized or necrosed (Fig. 3). They occasionally extended into the mediastinal cavity, producing complex epithelio-sarcoma-like tumors.

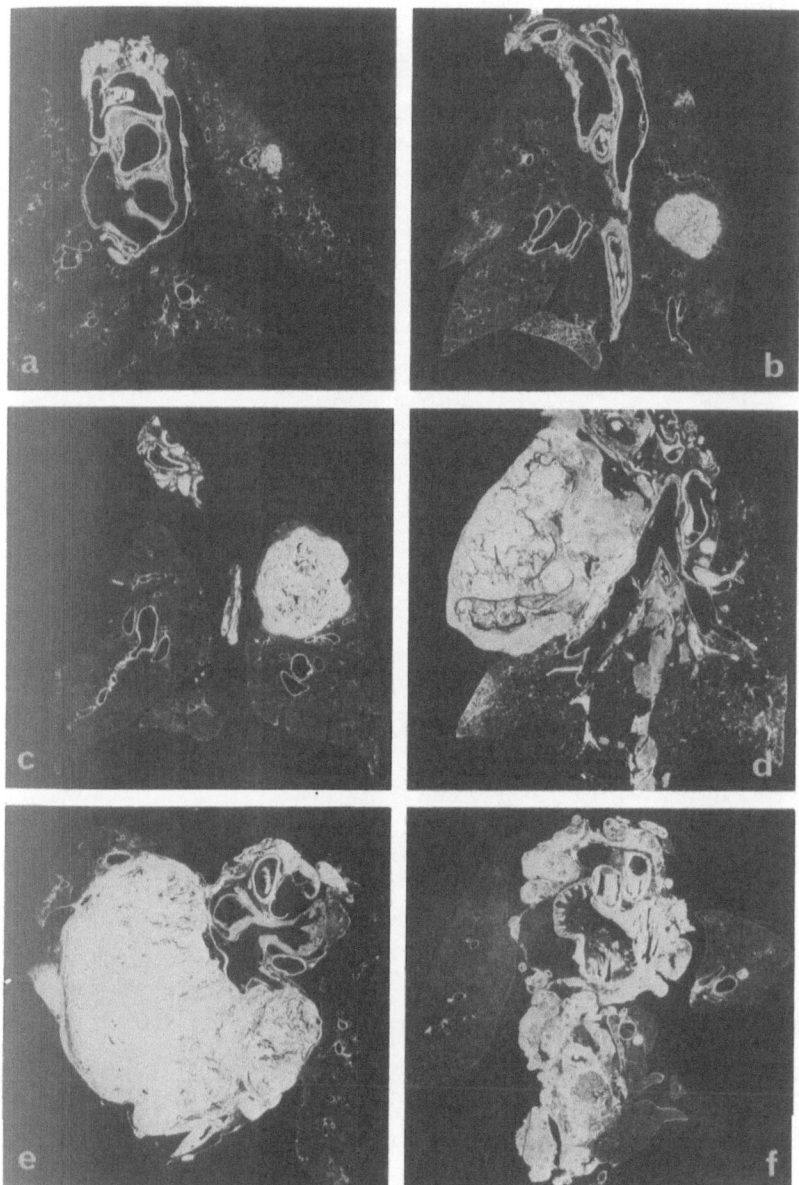

Fig. 2 a-f. Tumors induced by radon. (a) Adenoma; (b) large adenoma becoming malignant; (c) epidermoid carcinoma; (d) large epidermoid carcinoma with necrotized areas; (e) large bronchiolo-alveolar adenocarcinoma; (f) bronchiolo-alveolar adenocarcinoma invading the mediastinum

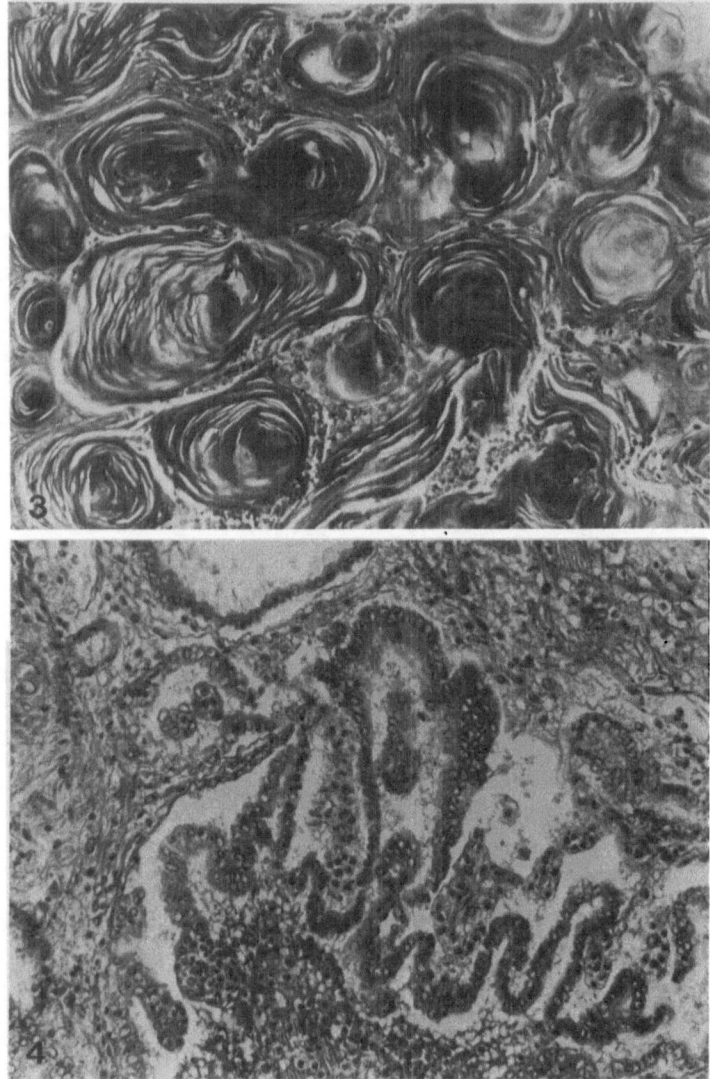

Fig. 3. Epidermoid carcinoma. Hematoxylin phloxine safranin, alcian blue (x 200)

Fig. 4. Bronchiolo-alveolar adenocarcinoma. Hematoxylin phloxine safranin, alcian blue (x 200)

2. Bronchiolar adenocarcinomas which were sometimes mucus-producing

These 2 types of tumor often invaded a whole lung lobe, or even several lobes. Their malignancy was obvious because of the numerous cellular anomalies and high number of mitosis. On the other hand, they remained limited to the lungs for a long time and were seldom metastatic.

3. Bronchiolo-alveolar adenocarcinomas in which the cells seemed to be normal and identical, with very little mitosis. The initial

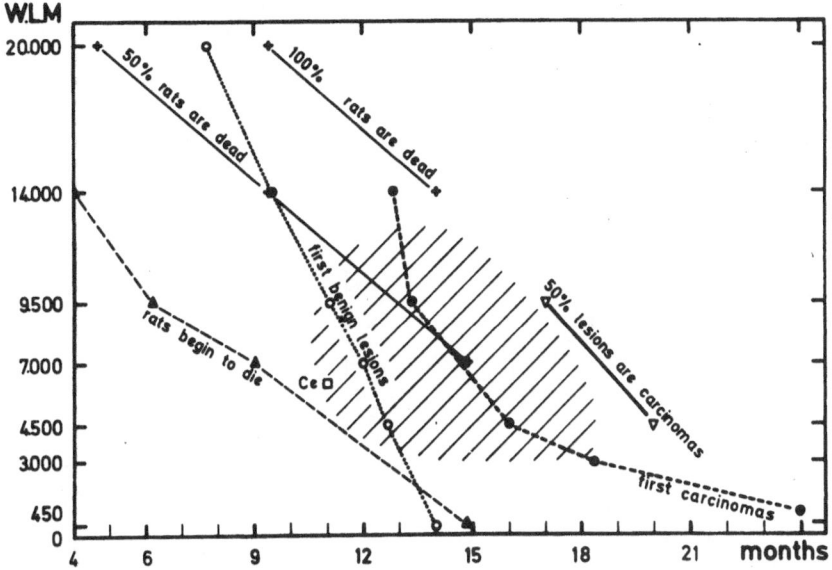

Fig. 5. The biological effects of the exposure of male Sprague-Dawley. SPF rats to radon and radon decay products exposures expressed as WLM. Cross-latched area represents the radon exposures producing a high incidence of lung cancer

lung lesion was often very small and, to find it, the entire lung had to be sectioned. However, frequently there was a significant invasion of the mediastinum, diaphragm, and thoracic wall associated with an extensive stromal reaction (Fig. 4).

Obviously, there was a whole range of intermediary lesions difficult to classify in one or another of the above categories. It was not always easy to differentiate some adnomatous lesions from carcinoma, and some adenomas showed malignant-looking characteristics (SACCOMANNO et al., 1970). There were tumors with combinations of epidermoid carcinoma and bronchiolar adenocarcinoma. Epidermoid and bronchiolo-alveolar carcinomas were found in the same animal and sometimes in the same lung. Although we found a rather large number of malignant tumors, there were very few distant metastases. Nevertheless, vessels were often invaded by the neoplasms.

Table 1 summarizes the results of these experiments.

Discussion

In Fig. 5, we chose points corresponding to the average time-of-appearance of the first 3 or 4 benign or malignant tumors. We did not take into consideration the metaplasias because, except at lower doses, they seemed to appear at random times. Lung cancers were induced in rats with doses from 500 WLM to 14,000 WLM. These cancers appeared from the 12th to 24th month after the beginning of exposure. The optimum cancer-inducing dose was from 3,000 to 9,000 WLM, delivered in 300 or 500 hours of exposure during a 3- or 4-month period.

Table 1. Lung tumors induced in rats by inhaled radon

Exposure group	Number of rats	Median survival (days)	Animals with lung tumors				
			All lung tumors	Adenoma	Epidermoid carcinoma	Bronchiolo-alveolar adenocarcinoma	"Mixed" carcinoma
Control	200	>720	0				
21,000 WLM[a]	100	180	0				
14,000 WLM[b]	50	265	4	2	1	1	
9,600 WLM[c]	20	343	18	2	8	5	3
7,000 WLM[d]	50	485	15	6	4	5	
4,500 WLM[e]	40	in progress	11	2	4	5	
3,000 WLM[f]	40	in progress	5	1	2	2	
500 WLM[g]	92	450	9	7	1	1	
Cerium hydroxide[h]	10	>720	0				
Cerium hydroxide plus 6,000 WLM[i]	12	364	10	3	5	2	
Uranium ore dust[j]	10	498	0				
Uranium ore dust plus 9,600 WLM[k]	20	443	17	3	5	9	

a) Exposure regimen 4 hrs per day for 75 days. Radon and radon decay product equilibrium 100%.
b) Exposure regimen 4 hrs per day for 50 days. Radon and radon decay product equilibrium 100%.
c) Exposure regimen 5 hrs per day for 96 days. Radon and radon decay product equilibrium 20% to 30%.
d) Exposure regimen 4 hrs per day for 25 days. Radon and radon decay product equilibrium 100%.
e) Exposure regimen 5 hrs per day for 60 days. Radon and radon decay product equilibrium 20% to 30%.
f) Exposure regimen 5 hrs per day for 40 days. Radon and radon decay product equilibrium 20% to 30%.
g) Exposure regimen 5 hrs per day for 115 days. Radon and radon decay product equilibrium 1%.
h) Without radon.
i) Exposure regimen 5 hrs per day for 108 days. Radon and radon decay product equilibrium 20% to 30%.
j) Without radon.
k) Exposure regimen 5 hrs per day for 96 days. Radon and radon decay product equilibrium 20% to 30%.

Above 14,000 WLM, benign tumors appeared; but since all animals died in the 12th month, the cancers may not have had time enough to develop. The rats seldom died of infection or other cancerous complications, but rather of fibrosis of the interalveolar walls.

At lower doses (500 WLM), the first cancers were found only in the 24th month. They appeared earlier as the dose was increased. The earlier the first cancers appeared, the greater the number of cancers induced (over 50% of the lesions observed in some dose groups). Once a lesion was observed, its severity seemed to progress in relationship to the time-after-exposure. At lower doses, different lesions appeared distinctly in the following chronological order: metaplasia, adenomatous lesions, adenoma, cancer. At higher doses, this order was less evident, and all these types of lesion were found in the same lung. Mortality was concomitant with the appearance of tumors, at low doses. Death occurred before the tumors appeared if the doses were high, and the mortality rate increased as the periods of inhalation were lengthened.

Stable cerium hydroxide was an efficient cofactor, inducing cancers 2 or 3 months earlier. Uranium ore dust, on the other hand, did not influence the tumorigenesis.

The biological responses observed were in keeping with total exposure, expressed as cumulative WLM. The different equilibrium ratios of radon and radon decay products had no particular effect.

An experiment with tobacco smoke as a cofactor is now in progress. Thus far, 12 months after the beginning of exposure, the time of the first appearance of cancers does not seem to be shortened. However, precancerous lesions have been observed (PARK et al., 1970; STUART et al., 1970; CHRETIEN et al., no date).

Conclusion

These experiments confirmed the relationship of inhaled radon and its decay products to lung cancer, and lung cancer was induced at rather low doses. The evidence that stable cerium hydroxide is an efficient cocarcinogenic factor suggests that other cocarcinogenic factors may exist. Future studies will require investigation of the dose-effect relationships at lower exposure levels and evaluation of other cocarcinogenic factors in the pathogenesis of radon-induced lesions. Since the mortality rate at low doses was always higher, compared to controls, and was without infectious lesions, whether the animals developed cancer or not, future studies should also investigate the effects of radon exposure, other than cancer.

Acknowledgements

We would like to thank: L. CRUAUD and Y. FRANCOIS, Ph. DUPORT, E. BLONDEAU for their technical assistance.

References

BAIR, W.J.: Inhalation of radionuclides and carcinogenesis. In:
Inhalation Carcinogenesis (M.G. Hanna, Jr., P. Nettesheim, J.R.
Gilbert, eds). AEC Symposium Series no. 18, pp. 77-101. Oak Ridge,
Tennessee: U.S. Atomic Energy Commission, Division of Technical
Inf. 1970.
BLONDEAU, E., DUPORT, P., FRANCOIS, Y., MADELAINE, G.: Ensemble
d'étude expérimentale du cancer pulmonaire chez le rat par irra-
diation. Comm. Energie At. (France), Rappt. STEPPA-B.P. No.
1-87640 RAZES, 1973.
CHAMEAUD, J., PERRAUD, R., LAFUMA, J.: Cancers du poumon expérimen-
taux provoques chez le rat par des inhalations de radon. C.R. Acad.
Sci. (Paris) 273, 2388-2389 (1971).
CHRETIEN, J., HIRSCH, A., THIEBLEMONT, M.: Pathologie respiratoire
du tabac - l'expérimentation animale dans le monde - Objectifs et
méthodologie. Paris: Masson et Cie 1973.
Federal Radiation Council: Radiation exposure of uranium miners.
Report of an Advisory Committee from the Division of Medical
Sciences, National Academy of Sciences - National Research Council -
National Academy of Engineering. Washington, D.C. 1968.
HOWARD, E.G.: The morphology of experimental lung tumors in beagle
dogs. In: Morphology of Experimental Respiratory Carcinogenesis
(P. Nettesheim, M.G. Hanna, Jr., J.W. Deatherage, Jr., eds). AEC
Symposium Series no. 21, pp. 147-160. Oak Ridge, Tennessee: U.S.
Atomic Energy Commission, Division of Technical Inf. 1970.
KUSCHNER, M., LASKIN, S.: Pulmonary epithelial tumors and tumor-like
proliferation in the rat. In: Morphology of Experimental Respiratory
Carcinogenesis (P. Nettesheim, M.G. Hanna, Jr., J.W. Deatherage, Jr.,
eds). AEC Symposium Series no. 21, pp. 209-225. Oak Ridge, Tennessee:
U.S. Atomic Energy Commission, Division of Technical Inf. 1970.
LE BOUFFANT, L.: Etude quantitative de l'épuration pulmonaire chez
le rat. Comparaison entre poussières inertes et poussières nocives.
In: Inhaled Particles and Vapours. Proceedings of an Int. Symp.
organized by the British Occupational Hygiene Society, Oxford March
29 - April 1, 1960. Ed. by C.N. Davies, pp. 369-383.
LORENZ, E.: Radioactivity and lung cancer: A critical review of lung
cancer in the miners of Schneeberg and Joachimsthal. J. nat. Cancer
Inst. 5, 1-15 (1944).
PARK, J.F., HOWARD, E.B., STUART, B.O., WEHNER, A.P., DILLEY, J.V.:
Cocarcinogenetic studies in pulmonary carcinogenesis. In: Morphology
of Experimental Respiratory Carcinogenesis (P. Nettesheim, M.G. Hanna,
Jr., J.W. Deatherage, Jr., eds). AEC Symposium Series no. 21, pp.
417-436. Oak Ridge, Tennessee: U.S. Atomic Energy Commission, Division
of Technical Inf. 1970.
PERRAUD, R., CHAMEAUD, J., LAFUMA, J., MASSE, R., CHRETIEN, J.: Cancer
broncho-pulmonaire expérimental du rat par inhalation de radon. Comparaison avec les aspects histologiques des cancers humains. J. franç.
Méd. Chir. thor. XXVI., 172, 25-41 (1972).
PERRAUD, R., CHAMEAUD, J., MASSE, R., LAFUMA, J.: Cancers pulmonaires
expérimentaux chez le rat après l'inhalation de radon associé à des
poussières non radioactives. C.R. Acad. Sci. (Paris) 270, 2594-2595
(1970).
SACCOMANNO, G.: Uranium miners' health. In: Radiation Standards for
Uranium Mining. Hearings before the Subcommittee on Research, De-
velopment, and Radiation of the Joint Committee on Atomic Energy,
Congress of the United States. Washington, D.C. March 17 and 18 1969.
SACCOMANNO, G., SAUNDERS, R.P., ARCHER, V.E., AUERBACH, O., BRENNAN,
L.: Metaplasia to neoplasia. In: Morphology of Experimental Respira-
tory Carcinogenesis (P. Nettesheim, M.G. Hanna, Jr., J.W. Deatherage,
Jr., eds). AEC Symposium Series no. 21, pp. 63-80. Oak Ridge, Tennes-
see: U.S. Atomic Energy Commission, Division of Technical Inf. 1970.

SEVC, J., PLACEK, V., JERABEK, J.: Lung cancer risk in relation (to) exposure in uranium mines. In: Proceedings of 4th Conference on radiation hygiene. CSSR 1971.

SHABAD, L.M., PYLEV, L.N.: Morphological lesions in rat lungs induced by polycyclic hydrocarbons. In: Morphology of Experimental Respiratory Carcinogenesis (P. Nettesheim, M.G. Hanna, Jr., J.W. Deatherage, Jr., eds). AEC Symposium Series no. 21, pp. 227-242. Oak Ridge, Tennessee: U.S. Atomic Energy Commission, Division of Technical Inf. 1970.

SNIHS, J.O.: The approach to radon problems in non-uranium mines in Sweden. National Institute of Radiation Protection. Stockholm 1973.

STUART, B.O., WILLARD, D.H., HOWARD, E.B.: Uranium mine contaminants in dogs and hamsters. In: Inhalation Carcinogenesis (M.G. Hanna, Jr., P. Nettesheim, J.R. Gilbert, eds). AEC Symposium Series no. 18, pp. 413-427. Oak Ridge, Tennessee: U.S. Atomic Energy Commission, Division of Technical Inf. 1970.

WAGONER, J.K., ARCHER, V.E., LUNDIN, F.E., HOLADAY, DA. A., LLOYD, J.W.: Radiation as the cause of lung cancer among uranium miners. New Engl. J. Med. 273, 181-188 (1965).

Studies of Pulmonary Carcinogenesis in Rodents Following Inhalation of Transuranic Compounds*

Charles L. Sanders and G. E. Dagle

Biology Department, Battelle, Pacific Northwest Laboratories, Richland, WA 99352, USA

ABSTRACT

The influence of radiation dose and its distribution on pulmonary carcinogenesis in rats was examined following inhalation of ^{238}Pu from crushed $^{238}PuO_2$ microspheres, $^{238}PuO_2$, $^{239}PuO_2$, and $^{244}CmO_2$. A more uneven dose-distribution (e.g., $^{238}PuO_2$ or $^{239}PuO_2$) favored squamous carcinoma induction at high doses, while adenocarcinoma induction was more frequent at lower doses or at all doses having a more even dose-distribution in the lung (e.g., $^{244}CmO_2$). Squamous metaplasia and adenomatosis preceded the development of squamous carcinoma and adenocarcinoma, respectively. Pulmonary hemangiosarcomas were found only after high doses of inhaled $^{239}PuO_2$. These results suggest an influence of dose and dose-distribution on the type and incidence of pulmonary tumors from inhaled alpha emitters.

A.   Introduction

Pulmonary-deposited, alpha-emitting radionuclides are potent carcinogens in the lung of experimental animals. Among these radionuclides, the transuranic oxides, $^{238}PuO_2$, $^{239}PuO_2$, and $^{244}CmO_2$, constitute a potential health hazard to individuals in the nuclear industry.

LISCO (1959) described the morphogenesis of pulmonary tumors in rats following inhalation of $^{239}PuO_2$. He found 3 types of tumors: adenocarcinoma, squamous carcinoma, and hemangioendothelioma. Studies by BULDAKOV and LYUBCHANSKII (1970) with inhaled ^{239}Pu citrate and ^{239}Pu pentacarbonate in rats, showed that the predominant lung tumors were adenocarcinomas at lower radiation doses to the lung and squamous carcinomas at higher radiation doses; they also showed several pulmonary hemangiosarcomas at higher doses.

This paper describes the development of lung tumors in rats following pulmonary deposition of transuranic compounds. These compounds delivered a wide range of radiation doses to the lung with different spatial-temporal dose-distribution patterns. It was shown that both the tumor type and incidence were influenced by the amount of radionuclide deposited and by its distribution in the lung.

---

*This paper is based on research performed under United States Atomic Energy Commission Contract AT(45-1)-1830.

B. Methods

Wistar, SPF, female rats, about 70 days of age, were exposed in groups of 70 rats each to 4 to 5 dose levels of $^{238}PuO_2$, $^{239}PuO_2$, or $^{244}CmO_2$. The ^{244}curium oxide was a mixture of $^{244}CmO_2$ and $^{244}Cm_2O_3$ but is designated as $^{244}CmO_2$ since the ratio of Cm/O is not known. The studies with inhaled ^{238}Pu, derived from crushed $^{238}PuO_2$ microspheres in rats, have been previously published (SANDERS, 1973). Exposures were by nose-only inhalation for a period of 30 minutes. The $^{238}PuO_2$ and $^{239}PuO_2$ aerosols exhibited count median diameters that ranged from 0.1 μm to 0.3 μm, whereas the count median diameters of the ^{238}Pu or $^{244}CmO_2$ aerosols were 0.02 μm to 0.04 μm. Both ^{238}Pu and $^{244}CmO_2$ exhibited greater *in vivo* solubility than did PuO_2, as tested by ultra-filtration through Visking tubing; the ultrafilterability of PuO_2 was <0.5%, $^{244}CmO_2$ 2 to 3% and ^{238}Pu 70%. Two additional groups of rats were given either an intratracheal instillation of 29 nCi $^{239}PuO_2$ in saline or saline alone.

The experimental design and initial deposition levels in the lung are shown in Table 1. About half the lung of each of 5 rats per group at 1 day after exposure and the lungs of all rats which were autopsied when moribund or dead were fixed in 10% neutral buffered formalin, embedded in paraffin, and sections stained with eosin and hematoxylin, some after processing for autoradiographic examination. The remaining half of lung tissue was analyzed for transuranic contents by scintillation counting. The data with inhaled $^{238}PuO_2$, $^{239}PuO_2$, or $^{244}CmO_2$ represents an interim report of a lifespan study, emphasizing pathological alterations occurring in the lung for periods of up to 2 years post-exposure.

C. Results and Discussion

I. Lung Clearance

Inhaled $^{238}PuO_2$ or $^{239}PuO_2$ particles were cleared from the lung in a similar manner, with about 50% clearance of the initial alveolar deposition (1-day lung burden) in 30 to 50 days and a 225-day biological half-life for either isotope in the lung thereafter (Fig. 1). Only 10 to 15% of initial alveolar-deposited ^{238}Pu or $^{244}CmO_2$ remained in the lung at 50 days after inhalation with a 75 to 150 day biological half-life in the lung thereafter (Fig. 1). PuO_2 particles were cleared mostly within alveolar macrophages (SANDERS and ADEE, 1970; SANDERS, 1969), while $^{244}CmO_2$ or ^{238}Pu, because of their greater solubility, were cleared from the alveoli mostly into the blood (SANDERS, 1973).

II. Pulmonary Distribution

At 1 day after inhalation, both inhaled $^{238}PuO_2$ and $^{239}PuO_2$ particles were seen dispersed throughout the lung parenchyma, with a large range in the number of alpha tracks per star, indicative of a range of sizes of PuO_2 particles. These particles were usually seen within macrophages or alveolar septae. The more soluble transuranics, $^{244}CmO_2$ or ^{238}Pu, were initially distributed in the lung as single tracks or as loose aggregates of tracks mostly associated with the alveolar septae; stars, indicative of particles, were rare on auto-

Table 1. Incidence of pulmonary tumors in the rat following inhalation of transuranic compounds

Transuranic	Number dead rats[c]	Time after exposure, days[d]	Amount transuranic in lung, nanocuries[e]	Incidence of pulmonary tumors, %[f]			
				Adenocarcinoma	Squamous carcinoma	Hemangiosarcoma	Total
None[a]	146	600-980	0	0.7	0	0	0.7
$239PuO_2$	27	655	0.15 ± 0.07	0	0	0	0
$238PuO_2$	23	571	0.16 ± 0.04	0	0	0	0
$239PuO_2$	27	624	0.20 ± 0.05	0	0	0	0
$239PuO_2$	34	619	4.4 ± 1.6	2.9	0	0	2.9
$238PuO_2$	31	565	11 ± 3.6	9.7	0	0	9.7
$239PuO_2$[b]	19	730	29 ± 7.0	21.1	10.5	0	31.6
$239PuO_2$	29	620	56 ± 13	24.1	17.2	6.9	48.3
$239PuO_2$	31	608	180 ± 54	9.7	22.6	6.5	38.7
$238PuO_2$	32	544	690 ± 160	3.1	21.9	0	25.0
$238Pu$	30	930	1.6 ± 1.3	6.6	0	0	6.6
$238Pu$	30	930	5.9 ± 3.2	20.0	0	0	20.0
$238Pu$	32	790	69 ± 44	21.9	3.1	0	25.0
$244CmO_2$	4	393	0.22 ± 0.08	0	0	0	0
$244CmO_2$	5	389	2.8 ± 0.42	0	0	0	0
$244CmO_2$	4	387	15 ± 4.1	25.0	0	0	25.0
$244CmO_2$	34	421	790 ± 240	8.8	0	0	8.8

a) Includes 26 rats given an intratracheal instillation of saline.
b) Given by intratracheal instillation.
c) Treated groups consist of about 60 animals; 115 unexposed controls still alive.
d) Time of last recorded spontaneous death.
e) Mean ± standard deviation (number of samples = 5), at 1 day after exposure.
f) Percentage of dead rats.

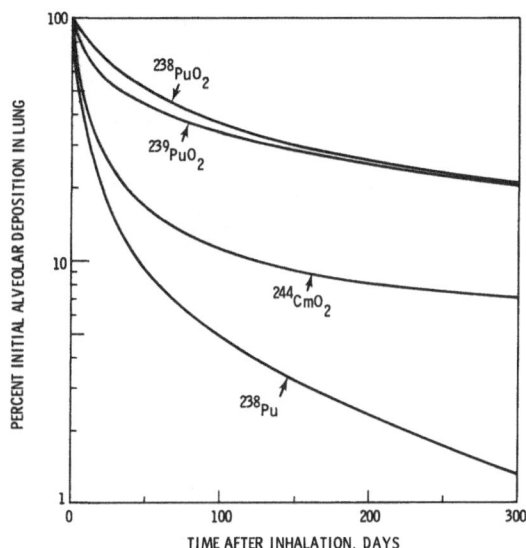

Fig. 1. Alveolar retention of inhaled transuranic compounds

radiograms (Fig. 2). The little remaining $^{244}CmO_2$ or ^{238}Pu activity seen on autoradiograms at 1 to 10 months after exposure was evenly spread over the parenchyma as single tracks or as loose aggregates within macrophages or associated with hemosiderin-like pigment in peribronchiolar, perivascular, or subpleural regions of the lung. At 1 to 10 months after exposure, many of the $^{238}PuO_2$ or $^{239}PuO_2$ particles had found their way from macrophages into the alveolar septae, concentrating in subpleural regions of the lung (Fig. 3), as well as in some peribronchiolar and perivascular regions of the lung. The pulmonary lymph nodes contained 2 - 4% of initially deposited $^{238}PuO_2$ or $^{239}PuO_2$, but little of $^{244}CmO_2$ or ^{238}Pu.

The major part of the total radiation dose was delivered to the lung in a shorter period of time from $^{244}CmO_2$ or ^{238}Pu than from $^{238}PuO_2$ or $^{239}PuO_2$ particles. However, $^{238}PuO_2$ or $^{239}PuO_2$ particles were seen concentrated in subpleural regions of the lung, causing higher radiation doses to this region of the lung from $^{238}PuO_2$ or $^{239}PuO_2$ particles than were seen following $^{244}CmO_2$ or ^{238}Pu dosages. Thus, the amount of radiation dose per µCi of transuranic deposited in the lung was significantly less but more evenly distributed in the lung for inhaled $^{244}CmO_2$ or ^{238}Pu than for $^{238}PuO_2$ or $^{239}PuO_2$ particles.

III. Development of Pulmonary Tumors

Plutonium dioxide particles concentrated in subpleural regions of the lung in the highest dose groups, produced a severe radiation pneumonitis with marked thickening and consolidation of the alveolar septae by connective tissue (Fig. 3). Plutonium particles became entrapped within fibrotic subpleural areas within a few months after inhalation. Within 3 months after inhalation, isolated islands of metaplastic squamous cells were found proliferating within these fibrotic areas, usually where the PuO_2 particle concentration was the greatest (Fig. 3). Squamous cells then began to proliferate and move towards the zones of lower PuO_2 concentration in the more central parts of the lung lobes, showing evidence more of carcinoma *in situ*, a histologic interim

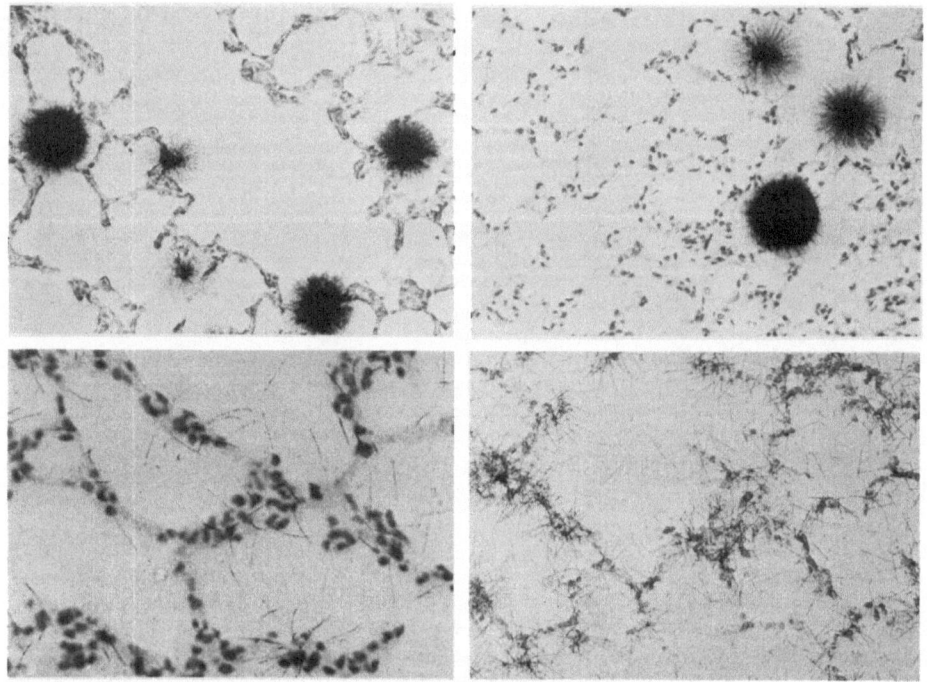

Fig. 2. Autoradiograms of lung at 1 day after inhalation of trans-uranic compounds. Upper left: $^{238}PuO_2$, 2 week exposure. X 176. Upper right: $^{239}PuO_2$, 2 week exposure. X 176. Lower left: ^{238}Pu, 3 day ex-posure. X 420. Lower right: $^{244}CmO_2$, 3 day exposure. X 176

stage between squamous metaplasia and squamous carcinoma. Squamous carcinomas exhibited varying degrees of differentiation. Those squamous carcinomas with abundant keratin tended to take up a large part of the lobe in which they originated, whereas less-differentiated tumors with little or no keratin formation, tended to spread to all lobes of the lung. These latter squamous carcinomas were seen growing into the pleu-ral cavity and in the pulmonary lymphatics. The development of squamous carcinoma from subpleural concentrations of PuO_2 particles was similar to that seen in the rat following "hot spots" of PuO_2 particle concen-tration after intrapulmonary injection of $^{239}PuO_2$ (SANDERS and PARK, 1972).

Rats exposed to high levels of ^{238}Pu or $^{244}CmO_2$, or to the lower dose levels of PuO_2, did not exhibit marked subpleural fibrosis or squamous metaplasia. Rats exposed to the highest amount of $^{244}CmO_2$ exhibited a generalized radiation pneumonitis with moderate thickening of the alveolar septae and an accumulation of protein and fluids in the al-veolar air spaces; rats living longer than 6 months after inhalation of $^{244}CmO_2$ exhibited only minimal-to-moderate alveolar septal thicken-ing due to radiation pneumonitis.

In contrast to squamous metaplasia, alveolar adenomatous metaplasia or adenomatosis was seen in all but control groups and the lower de-position level groups of rats exposed to all transuranics (Fig. 4). Areas of adenomatosis were more likely to be found in subpleural regions of PuO_2 particle concentration, although the association was

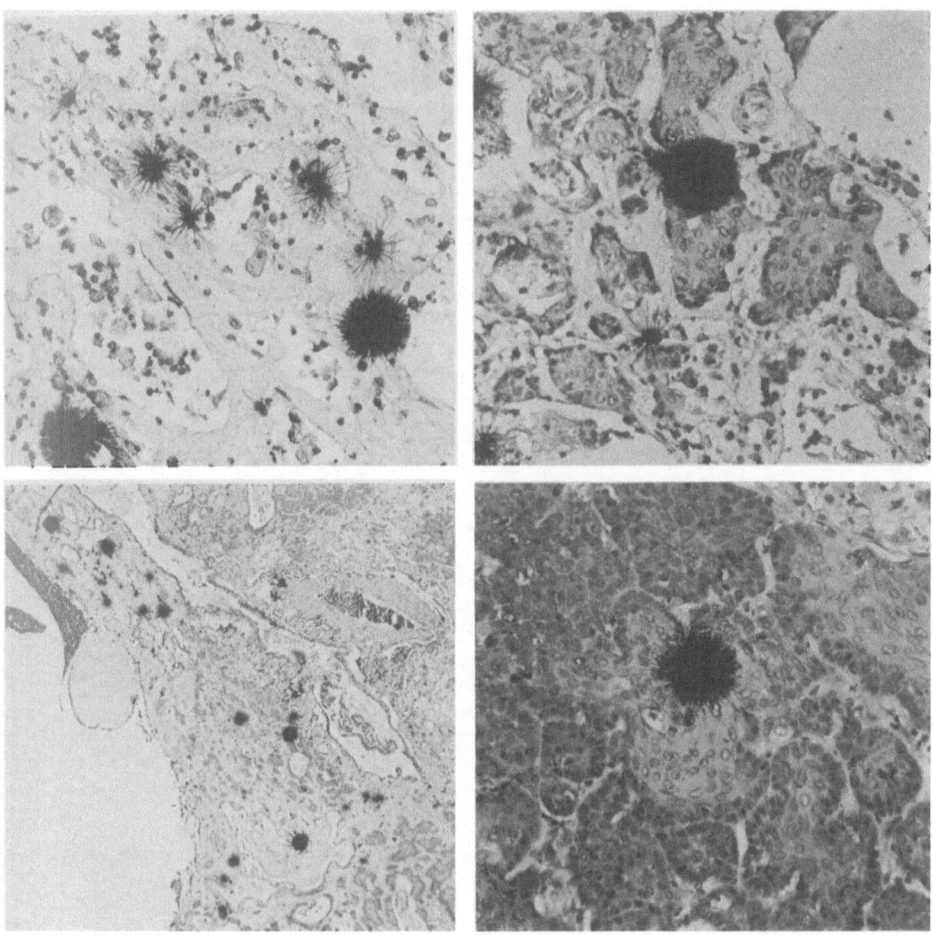

Fig. 3. Autoradiograms of lung at 6 to 8 months after inhalation of $^{238}PuO_2$. 2 week exposure of autoradiograms. Upper left: Subpleural PuO_2 concentration and severe radiation pneumonitis. X 176. Upper right: Squamous metaplasia in subpleural area of high PuO_2 concentration. X 176. Lower left: Early squamous carcinoma developing from subpleural area of PuO_2 concentration. X 43. Lower right: Squamous carcinoma surrounding a PuO_2 particle. X 176

much less apparent than it was with squamous metaplasia formation. Pulmonary adenocarcinomas varied from small, well-circumscribed, papillary well-differentiated tumors to undifferentiated tumors that had spread throughout the lung, in the pleural cavity, and in pulmonary lymph nodes (Fig. 4).

Four hemangiosarcomas were seen in rats which had inhaled $^{239}PuO_2$, and none in any of the other groups. These tumors were characterized by irregular islands of sarcomatous tumor cells, forming small-to-large cavities filled with red blood cells (Fig. 4).

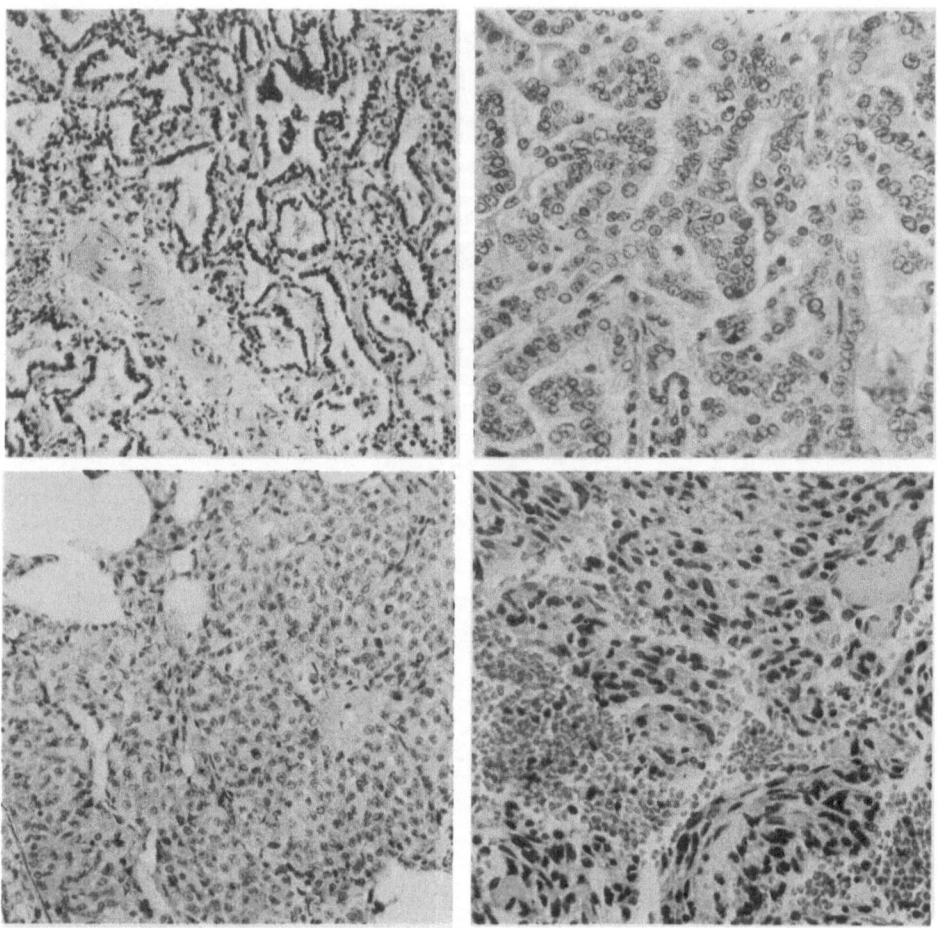

Fig. 4. Adenomatosis, adenocarcinoma and hemangiosarcoma in the lung
after inhalation of ^{239}PuO$_2$. Upper left: Adenomatosis at 293 days
after inhalation. X 176. Upper right: Papillary adenocarcinoma at
567 days after inhalation. X 448. Lower left: Undifferentiated adenocarcinoma at 619 days after inhalation. X 176. Lower right: Hemangiosarcoma at 560 days after inhalation. X 448

IV. Lung Tumors and Dose and Dose Distribution

There was a fairly clear temporal relationship between the development
of squamous metaplasia and the subsequent appearance of squamous carcinoma, and the development of adenomatosis and the subsequent appearance of adenocarcinoma. Thus, both squamous metaplasia and adenomatosis appeared to be preneoplastic stages in developing squamous
carcinoma or adenocarcinoma, respectively, since their incidence preceded and paralleled the incidences of frank carcinomas.

Squamous metaplasia and squamous carcinoma were seen only in rats with
the highest levels of ^{238}PuO$_2$ or ^{239}PuO$_2$ deposition with the exception
of 1 squamous carcinoma in a rat which had inhaled ^{238}Pu (Table 1).
The more uneven dose distribution of ^{238}PuO$_2$ or ^{239}PuO$_2$ particles with

physiological concentration of particles in the subpleural lymphatics, greatly favored the induction of squamous carcinoma at high initial lung depositions, while adenocarcinoma induction was greatly favored by a more even dose distribution, as was seen with inhaled ^{238}Pu or ^{244}CmO$_2$. For either ^{238}PuO$_2$ or ^{239}PuO$_2$, more squamous carcinomas were seen at radiation doses to lung of approximately greater than about 1,000 rads, corresponding to an initial alveolar deposition greater than 50 nCi ^{238}PuO$_2$ of ^{239}PuO$_2$, with adenocarcinomas predominating at lower doses of ^{238}PuO$_2$ or ^{239}PuO$_2$. Hemangiosarcomas were seen only at the 2 highest dose levels of ^{239}PuO$_2$. These interim results with inhaled ^{238}PuO$_2$ or ^{239}PuO$_2$ are somewhat similar to observations made by BULDAKOV and LYUBCHANSKII (1970) on rats following inhalation of ^{239}Pu citrate or ^{239}Pu pentacarbonate. Both total dose delivered to lung and its distribution in the lung influence the induction of adenocarcinoma, squamous carcinoma, and hemangiosarcoma in the lung of rats following inhalation of transuranic compounds, with adeno-carcinomas occurring more frequently following inhalation of "soluble" or more monomeric transuranic compounds, and squamous carcinomas and hemangiosarcomas occurring more frequently following inhalation of "insoluble" particulate or more polymeric transuranic compounds.

References

BULDAKOV, L.A., LYUBCHANSKII, E.R.: Experimental basis for maximum allowable load (MAL) of Pu-239 in the human organism, and maximum allowable concentration (MAC) of Pu-239 in air at work locations. Original source unknown. ANL-TRANS-864 (1970).

LISCO, H.: Autoradiographic and histologic studies in radiation carcinogenesis of the lung. Lab. Invest. 8, 162-170 (1959).

SANDERS, C.L.: The distribution of inhaled plutonium-239 dioxide particles within pulmonary macrophages. Arch. Environ. Hlth 18, 904-912 (1969).

SANDERS, C.L.: Carcinogenicity of inhaled plutonium-238 in the rat. Radiation Research 56, 540-553 (1973).

SANDERS, C.L., ADEE, R.R.: Ultrastructural localization of inhaled ^{239}PuO$_2$ particles in alveolar epithelium and macrophages. Health Physics 18, 293-295 (1970).

SANDERS, C.L., PARK, J.F.: Pulmonary distribution of alpha dose from ^{239}PuO$_2$ and induction of neoplasia in rats and dogs, p. 489-498. In: International Symposium on Inhaled Particles III, Vol. 1 (W.H. Walton, ed.). Oxford: Pergamon Press 1971.

Lung Irradiation with Static Plutonium Microspheres*

Ernest C. Anderson, Laurence M. Holland, James R. Prine, and
C. R. Richmond

Los Alamos Scientific Laboratory, University of California, Los Alamos, NM 87544, USA

ABSTRACT

Hamsters are exposed to selected lung burdens of plutonium contained
in 10 μm diameter inert microspheres of ZrO_2 ceramic. Injected into
the jugular vein, the microspheres lodge quantitatively in the lung
capillaries and remain immobile for the life of the hamster. Distribution through the lung is essentially random but shows a systematic
variation through a factor of about 2 from lobe to lobe.

The specific activity of the microspheres is varied from 0.01 to 100
pCi per sphere, spanning the range of respirable particles of $^{238}PuO_2$
and $^{239}PuO_2$. The number of spheres per animal varies from 2,000 to
1,000,000 and the lung burden from 0.1 to 1000 nCi. The fraction of
lung irradiated ranges from 0.01 to 0.98, and the calculated median
dose rate to the tissue exposed is from 0.5 to 700 krad per year. The
spheres are completely inert and provoke no foreign-body reactions.
In contrast to most methods of exposure by inhalation or insufflation,
the radiation is delivered essentially 100% to the lung. Because of
the immobility and uniformity of the microspheres, the distribution
of energy deposition can be calculated with precision on a microscale.

The most surprising result has been the minimal biological damage
even after exposure times in excess of 2 years. Not only are gross
effects (such as pneumonitis, hyperplasia, fibrosis, and tumors) insignificant, but little or no deterioration of parenchymal micro-
structure has been observed.

A. Introduction

The question of whether concentrated deposition of radiation dose in
a limited volume is more or less damaging than diffuse delivery of
the same quantity of energy has troubled health physicists for many
years. It has recently assumed new prominence with the potential risk
of exposure of large populations to PuO_2 aerosols from prospective
nuclear power generation with breeder reactors. The problem is complex, and theoretical calculations based on microdosimetry and assumed single-cell response are of little help since this response is subject to all the factors of biological regulation, control, repair, and

*This work is being performed under the auspices of the U.S. Atomic
Energy Commission.

other cooperative reactions characteristic of tissue. The primary
appeal must be to experimental data at this stage, until the limiting
mechanisms and interactions are identified. However, because of the
peculiar requirements of health protection, specifically the application of the data to human exposures of long duration and the desire
to limit the probability of damage to extremely low values, extrapolation of experimental results cannot be avoided. Extrapolation must be
made from animal to man, from short to long times of exposure and induction, and from measurable to indetectable probabilities. Such extra-
polations will be convincing in proportion to their basis on mechanistic
detail. Therefore, it is important that experiments correspond as
closely as possible to the actual situation to which they will be
applied and that, at the same time, enough independently controlled
variables be available to test various hypotheses and to identify the
controlling factors.

The hot particle studies in hamsters at the Los Alamos Scientific
Laboratory (LASL) are simulation experiments to the extent that the
target organ (the lung) and the radioactive sources replicate the
exposure to inhalation of PuO_2 aerosols to some extent. However, to
facilitate the analysis of the factors operating, certain unreal con-
straints have been introduced. A primary objective is determination
of the minimal conditions of exposure leading to tumor induction,
especially in terms of number and distribution of irradiation foci
and of volume and distribution of tissue at risk. Thus, animals are
exposed by jugular injection to a precise number of uniform microspheres which are retained quantitatively and permanently in the
capillary bed of the lung. The exposure is thereby limited strictly
to the lung itself, no other organ receiving a significant radiation
dose, and the dosimetric parameters can be varied in a controlled
manner.

B. Materials and Methods

Because of the limited space available here, experimental methods
will be presented only in outline. For details of procedures and
numerical confirmations, the reader is referred to our annual reports
(RICHMOND and VOELZ, 1972, 1973; RICHMOND and SULLIVAN, 1974).

The experimental animal chosen was the Syrian golden hamster. The
choice was primarily on the basis of the popularity of this animal
in many types of cancer experiments, both chemical- and radiation-
induced, that provide a large body of experimental data for comparison and interpretation of results, as well as its freedom from primary
lung disease. The route of exposure is unusual in that large (10 μm)
microspheres are injected into the jugular vein (HOLLAND et al., 1971)
and are trapped in the capillary bed of the lung. Since the range of
the alpha particle in the lung permits the traversal of several alveoli, the location of the source on the blood side of the membrane
is not physically important. The immobility results in significant
differences from inhaled aerosols; the local radiation fields are
higher in intensity and more circumscribed in volume than for mobile
particles of the same activity. However, by varying particle number
and specific activity, the dose distribution can be manipulated to
study the effects of this parameter.

The microspheres used are an inert, insoluble, high-fired ceramic of
ZrO_2 to which PuO_2 has been added at concentrations chosen to simulate

the radioactivity of respirable particles. They were prepared by generating, with a vibrating jet, uniform droplets of a ZrO_2/PuO_2 sol which were then gelled by dehydration and fired at 1000°C (FUL-WYLER et al., 1973). Extensive studies were made of the physical properties of the spheres, including diameter, mass, density, and radioactivity. Their uniformity is indicated by the coefficients of variation within a given batch for volume (better than 4%) and for plutonium activity (about 2.6%). The emergent alpha spectra showed the plutonium to be somewhat depleted toward the center of the micro-spheres by 20% to 40%, relative to the outer portions. Since the spheres are not large compared with the alpha range, energy degradation is not serious, the average energy loss being only about 1 MeV.

The range of plutonium activity covered in the microspheres is 0.01 to 59 pCi/sphere in 12 levels in an approximately geometric series. These activities correspond to pure PuO_2 particles in the diameter range of 0.06 to 0.9 μm for $^{238}PuO_2$ and 0.4 to 5.6 μm for $^{239}PuO_2$, thus spanning the range of respirable sizes. The actual chemical concentration of PuO_2 in ZrO_2 ranged from 0.04% to 1.1% by weight.

To facilitate measurement of the injected and retained dose, a low-level tag of ^{57}Co has been added to all batches of spheres. The only significant radiations from this nuclide are the gamma rays (122 and 136 keV). At a specific activity of 60 gammas/hr/sphere and a 3% absorption in the hamster, the calculated whole-body radiation dose is about 1.3 mR/yr or 1% of natural background, which is completely negligible in this experiment.

The first experiments were begun in early 1971, using 60 hamsters in each exposure group and 2000 spheres/animal at 8 exposure levels. Microsphere activity ranged from 0.07 to 59 pCi and total lung burden from 0.14 to 119 nCi. About 1% of the total lung volume was within the radiation fields, and the fields were far enough apart that there was no overlap. The median alpha dose to the population of cells at risk was calculated to range from 0.8 to 650 krad/yr, while the "average dose" from the deposition of total energy in 1 g of lung ranged from 13 to 12,000 rad/yr.

The possible tumor incidence from "hot particles" has been calculated by DEAN and LANGHAM (1969) and by GEESAMAN (1968) on the assumption that the rat skin tumor response curve observed by ALBERT et al. (1967) could be applied to the individual cells of the lung. Such models, when used with the distribution of dose over the cell population at risk in this experiment, predict tumor incidence per group ranging from 2 at the lowest activity group to a maximum of 60 in the middle group and then declining to 0 for the highest group. The total number of tumors predicted for the 480 hamsters is 162. As we shall show, this prediction is not confirmed by these experiments.

Additional experiments using larger numbers of microspheres have since been initiated. By the spring of 1974, a total of 1,900 hamsters had been exposed to 160,000,000 microspheres in various combinations of sphere activity and number to produce lung burdens in the range of 0.1 to 1,000 nCi, with particular emphasis on the 10 to 100 nCi range. LITTLE et al. (1973) have shown a very high tumor incidence in hamsters whose lungs were instilled with ^{210}Po solutions in this range of activity. (We have recently begun experiments duplicating LITTLE's polonium studies with our hamsters, but no results are yet available.)

Other experiments are in progress using microspheres loaded with ^{147}Pm to provide exposures to the entire lung with low LET radiation from the

225-keV beta rays. In addition, 115 rats have been exposed by the intravenous injection of 6000 plutonium-loaded microspheres per animal (4 pCi/sphere) to give lung burdens of 25 nCi and to provide evidence from another species.

C. Results

I. Distribution of Microspheres in the Lung

Measurements of distribution were made on hamsters which had received approximately 20,000 spheres of 4.3 pCi activity 4 weeks before sacrifice. Gamma counting of the specimens afforded a quick method of sphere counting, using the ^{57}Co tag. The lungs were inflated with formalin and fixed for 24 hr before analysis. The distribution of spheres between the divisions of the lungs is summarized in Table 1. The variability is not unexpected in view of the differences in blood supply. The range of concentrations (through a factor of 2) should not affect the interpretation of results, since the actual sphere content of a given lobe can be determined by gamma counting.

Table 1. Distribution of microspheres in hamster lung

Entity	Wet Weight (mg)	Spheres (number)	Concentration (spheres/mg)
Both lungs	2,844	23,600	8.3
Left lung	975	11,200	11.6
Right lung			
Diaphragmatic lobe	790	5,200	6.6
Cardiac lobe	408	2,300	5.6
Intermediate lobe	366	1,800	4.8
Right apical lobe	305	3,000	9.7

Following the above experiment, the left lung was minced by successive subdivision in halves. All pieces were measured at each level of division; an average and a coefficient of variation (CV) were calculated, and the results are given in Table 2. The constancy of the average concentration indicates the reliability of the measurements, and the CV indicates the degree of nonuniformity which increases with increasing subdivision but which appears to level out at about 30% to 40%.

To carry the study to the ultimate level, another lung was cut into 23 μm thick sections, which were scored visually for number of spheres. An examination of 16 sections showed 267 spheres. The CV among sections was 36%, of which 24% was expected from random statistics, leaving 26% for intrinsic variability. This is in good agreement with the larger dissection.

As a final test of the small-scale randomness of the distribution, the distances r between nearest-neighbor spheres in each section were measured with an optical micrometer. For a random distribution, the probability P(r) that the nearest-neighbor to a given sphere lies at

Table 2. Distribution of spheres within the left lung

Number of pieces	Average concentration (spheres/mg)	Coefficient of variation (%)
1	11.6	–
2	11.4	4
4	11.4	11
8	11.8	15
16	11.6	18
32	13.1	31
64	11.8	39

a distance r in a section of thickness δ with bulk sphere concentration C is given as (UNDERWOOD, 1970):

$$P(r) = 2\pi\delta Cr \exp(-\pi\delta Cr^2) \tag{Eq. 1}$$

From this equation we can calculate Δ_2, the mean value of r, to be

$$\Delta_2 = \Gamma(1.50)/\sqrt{\pi\delta C} = 1/2\sqrt{\delta C} \tag{Eq. 2}$$

(where Γ signifies the gamma function), and the variance (mean square deviation) of r with respect to Δ_2 is:

$$\mathrm{Var} = \frac{1 - \Gamma^2(1.5)}{\pi\delta C} = \frac{1 - \pi/4}{\pi\delta C} \tag{Eq. 3}$$

The distances observed between nearest-neighbors in 3 dimensions are, of course, different from those in a section. The mean in 3 dimensions, Δ_3, is given by:

$$\Delta_3 = \Gamma(1.33)/\sqrt[3]{4/3\ \pi C} \tag{Eq. 4}$$

The results of measurements of 114 nearest-neighbor distances in the 23 µm sections are shown in Fig. 1 as a histogram compared with the smooth curve given by Eq. 1. While there is a possible suggestion of structure, the general agreement is good. Statistically, the peak at 0 to 0.1 mm has an excess area above prediction of 2.5 times its standard deviation (SD), and the excess area between 1.4 and 1.8 mm is 2.2 times the SD. It is, of course, possible that geometric structure in the capillary bed could produce real effects of this sort. The variance of the data is 0.177 compared with 0.152 calculated from Eq. 3. It is concluded that at this level the distribution of spheres within the left lung is essentially random and that there is no large degree of clumping or association.

The measured Δ_2 was 768 µm in the sections. A contraction to 61% of original volume was measured for a similar left lung from fixation through paraffin embedding. The measured concentration of 11.6 spheres/mg in the fixed lung, therefore, corresponds to 19.2 spheres/mm³ in the sections. From this a Δ_2 of 750 µm is calculated using Eq. 2 – in excellent agreement with the 768 µm observed. The measured linear shrinkage from fresh lung to paraffin-embedded was to 0.72 of original dimensions; therefore, Δ_2 in fresh lung is 1,067 µm. Using the ratio of Δ_3/Δ_2 given by Eq. 4, the mean 3-dimensional nearest-neighbor distance in fresh lung is calculated to be 244 µm for 24,000 spheres and 559 µm for 2,000 spheres.

II. Retention and Excretion

Several methods have been used to determine retention of the microspheres in the animals. The most sensitive for short time scales is

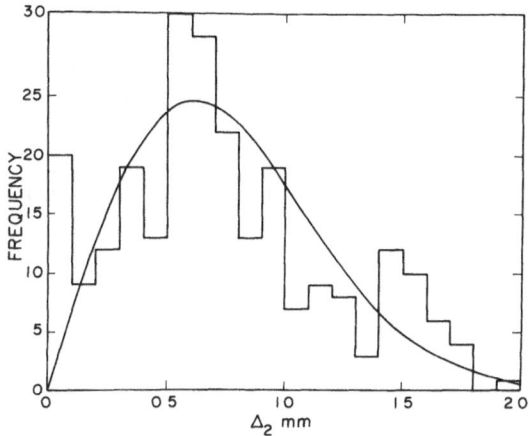

Fig. 1. Observed (histogram) and expected (smooth curve) frequency distribution of nearest-neighbor distances in lung section

the direct measurement of plutonium in the excreta. Results indicate an average rate of 0.032% ± 0.006% per day for the first 3 days and 0.000% ± 0.005% per day during the remainder of the first week (Table 3). These measurements were made with microspheres of Level 6, the highest specific activity. Total excretion over the first week measured 0.096%, corresponding to a half-time of 7,000 days.

Table 3. Excretion of plutonium-238 (% of injected dose/day ± S.E.)[a]

Day	Urine	Feces	Total
1	0.055 ± 0.013	0.003 ± 0.001	0.058 ± 0.013
2	0.011 ± 0.008	0.011 ± 0.006	0.022 ± 0.010
3	0.003 ± 0.004	0.013 ± 0.003	0.016 ± 0.005
4	-0.001 ± 0.001	-0.004 ± 0.004	-0.005 ± 0.004
5-7	+0.000 ± 0.002	+0.002 ± 0.002	+0.002 ± 0.003

[a]Average for 8 animals with 10,000 spheres each. S.E. = standard error of the mean calculated from the scatter of 3 determinations about their own mean. Negative excretion on day 4 results from random variations in counting statistics.

A summary of whole-body retention measurements is given in Fig. 2 (all curves are based on *in vivo* measurements of the 120 keV gamma ray from a ^{57}Co tag of the microspheres). The upper curve is for a group of animals (initially 8) that received intravenous injection of 2,000 microspheres of 60 pCi ^{238}Pu/sphere. Data extend to 500 days, at which time only 3 animals survive. The results give a biological half-time of the order of 7,000 days, corresponding to an excretion rate of 0.01% per day after the initial drop of 5% (which may be due to leaching of ^{57}Co from the surface of the spheres, since direct measurement of plutonium in the excreta did not indicate so large an initial loss).

The middle curve is a similar experiment in which 6 animals were injected with 300,000 spheres of 0.4 pCi ^{239}Pu/sphere. The slope corresponds to about 0.02% per day, or a half-time of some 3,500 days. The initial drop is not well documented, and there is a possibility of a

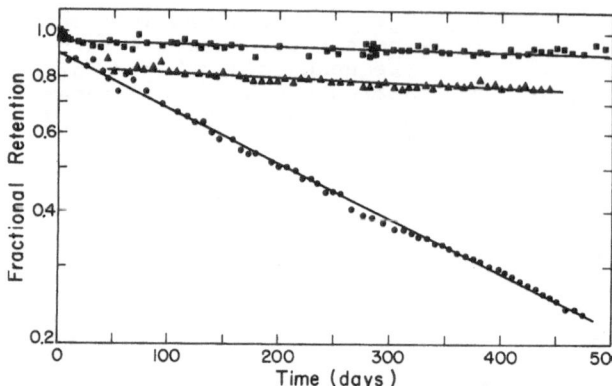

Fig. 2. The retention of microspheres as a function of time: (-■-) intravenous, 2,000 microspheres; (-▲-) intravenous, 300,000 microspheres; and (-●-) intratracheal, 500,000 microspheres

calibration shift during the first month. It is also possible that, due to the much larger number of spheres injected, some 20% may really have escaped the lung. The constant excretion rates observed in these experiments indicate that the lungs are sustaining no damage which could cause increased loss of microspheres. The bottom curve is for intratracheal instillation of 500,000 spheres tagged with ^{57}Co but without any plutonium. Initially, 24 animals were used; 6 remain (some were sacrificed). The half-time of the curve is 244 days, with no evidence of change with time.

Examination of lung sections shows that the intratracheal spheres which were driven into the lung by pulsed saline-jet injection are found in the alveolar spaces, often in association with macrophages. Therefore, the observed clearance time is apparently that associated with the deep lung and is in agreement with the range of half-times reported for plutonium and uranium oxides in rats (135 to 289 days), as summarized by the Task Group on Lung Dynamics (1966).

The data on retention of the intravenous spheres show that 90% to 95% of the initially retained dose is still in the body after almost 500 days, and measurements of body organs show no significant activity anywhere other than in the lung. Because of the measured rapid clearance from the alveoli, it would thus seem that the intravenous spheres must remain within the capillary bed of the lung. However, significant numbers appear to be outside the capillary bed in histological sections and associated with macrophages. The former criterion is not always rigorous because the extremely thin alveolar-capillary wall could be difficult to detect, but the latter suggests an alveolar location. If this is true, one must explain the failure to clear the lung as observed with the intratracheal spheres. Since the latter contained no plutonium, it may be that an alpha activity high enough to cause capillary wall breakage is also high enough to destroy macrophages attempting to transport spheres to the ciliary escalator. Movement of the spheres that have escaped the capillary bed could be limited to the dimensions of a small number of alveoli.

Another possibility of sphere movement which cannot be directly disproved is slow migration through the capillary bed. The retention data indicate that the spheres never escape into the postcapillary veinules; therefore, this movement would be limited by the diameter of the capillary network units, estimated by WEIBEL (1963) as 300 to 500 μm. A drift over distances of a few hundred microns at velocities of the order of 1 μm/day, therefore, is not inconsistent with the retention data. Since the mean range of an alpha particle in the lung of density 0.2 is 200 μm, the cumulation of dose to most of the cells at risk would be limited to a period of several months, and the number of such cells would be increased by a small factor.

The principal effect of both motion within a few alveoli and movement through the capillary bed would be to eliminate the extremely high end of the cell dose distribution function, which is of little biological significance in that the comparatively few cells involved are certainly subjected to extreme overkill and sterilization. The majority of the cells at risk lie in the outer portions of the alpha range and would not be markedly affected by sphere migration of this sort.

III. Survival

The fraction of animals surviving as a function of time is useful as an indicator of the health of the population and as a nonspecific signal of possible radiation damage. The hamsters used in our experiments generally show a mean survival time (MST) of about 700 days, indicating an unusual longevity. Typical curves for cumulative deaths as a function of time after injection (at age 100 days) are given in Fig. 3 for the original experimental groups receiving 2,000 spheres each with lung burdens of 0.1 to 120 nCi. The numbers at the beginning of each curve identify the plutonium level in the spheres. The line labeled "C" is for a control group receiving no spheres, and the line labeled "O" is for a group receiving nonradioactive spheres. Only the 4 extremes of the exposed groups are drawn for comparison. There seems to be no significant correlation of MST, nor of pattern of deaths with the activity of the particles. The shortest survival time is shown by Level 5, while the highest dose level (curve 6) is indistinguishable from the controls. The longest survivals are shown by Levels 2 and 3. The remaining dose levels fall within the range of those plotted. The data suggest that MST values vary by some ± 100 days under the conditions of our experiments; this large span is due, in part, to the small group sizes (60 animals). In many cases, MST curves are obtained which appear to be bimodal, with a high death rate at around 200 days which later declines. No specific pathology has been associated with these early deaths.

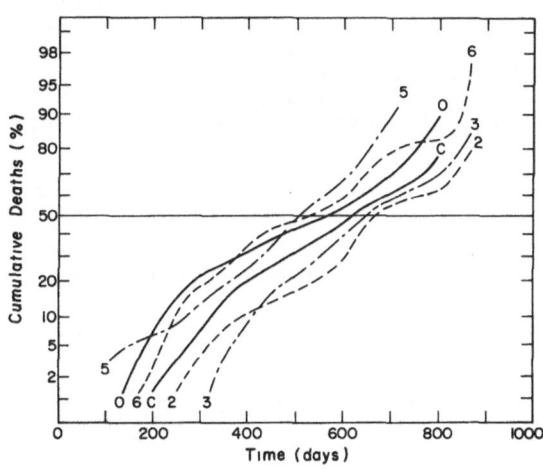

Fig. 3. Survival curves for hamsters receiving 2,000 microspheres intravenously. Time is in days postinjection (age = 100 days at injection). The number of each curve identifies specific activity level: (O) nonradioactive spheres and (C) control group, no spheres

IV. Pathological Results

The response elicited by the presence of the microspheres in the lung and the relationship of that response to carcinogenesis are the end points of primary interest in this research. The most striking feature of the results so far is the unobtrusive nature and limited extent of the observed tissue reactions.

The negative results of the survival time studies were reported above. Blood studies, including white cell counts, absolute lymphocyte counts, serum protein, and serum alkaline phosphatase, have been equally negative. Many studies in which radioactive materials have been administered by inhalation have resulted in early and prolonged lymphopenia. In these cases, there has usually been an accumulation of radioactive material in the regional lymph nodes as well as in the lung proper. In our studies, no activity has been found outside the lung parenchyma, and the lymphopoietic organs have not been irradiated. Since 50% of the radiation energy is absorbed by the circulating blood, the dose rate to that tissue is estimated to range from 1 to 900 rad/yr in the 2,000 sphere exposures. However, the hematopoietic system is not irradiated, and if any circulating blood elements are damaged, they appear to be adequately replaced from the unaffected stem-cell populations.

Turning to the lung itself, at the histological level the microspheres are found trapped in the interalveolar septa in both peripheral and central locations as well as in the other portions of the capillary bed. Because of the extreme thinness of the alveolar-capillary tissue layer, it is not always possible to demonstrate the continuity of the enclosure of the microsphere, but this can usually be inferred from the local morphology. Spheres have also been observed near respiratory bronchioles so that some portion of the bronchiolar epithelium is well within range of the alpha particles.

The microspheres themselves are chemically inert and do not appear to evoke any foreign body reactions as long as they remain within the capillaries. When microspheres of any radioactivity level are found extruded into an alveolar space, as they occasionally are, there is an associated, mild foreign body response with hemosidrin-bearing macrophage accumulation and occasional granuloma formation. The higher activity microspheres seem to be associated with macrophages containing more hemosidrin pigment. In the early experiments, macrophage accumulations were seen after about 30 days of exposure to Level 6 microspheres (59 pCi/sphere), as shown in Fig. 4. There seemed to be a progression of response with time, and by 4 months postinjection, occasional microgranulomas were seen, usually clearly associated with a microsphere. In Level 5 spheres (13 pCi/sphere), a similar response was observed at a later time.

Fig. 4. Mononuclear macrophage accumulation around a sphere of 59 pCi activity after 2 month exposure

Fig. 5. Alveolar epithelization near a sphere of 0.9 pCi activity after 7 month exposure

Fig. 6. Autoradiograph showing the radiation field and minimal tissue damage around a 4 pCi sphere after 15 month exposure

Fig. 7. Fibrosis and edema in a region of excessive sphere concentration resulting from nonuniform local deposition following injection of 1,000,000 spheres of activity 0.07 pCi (14 month exposure)

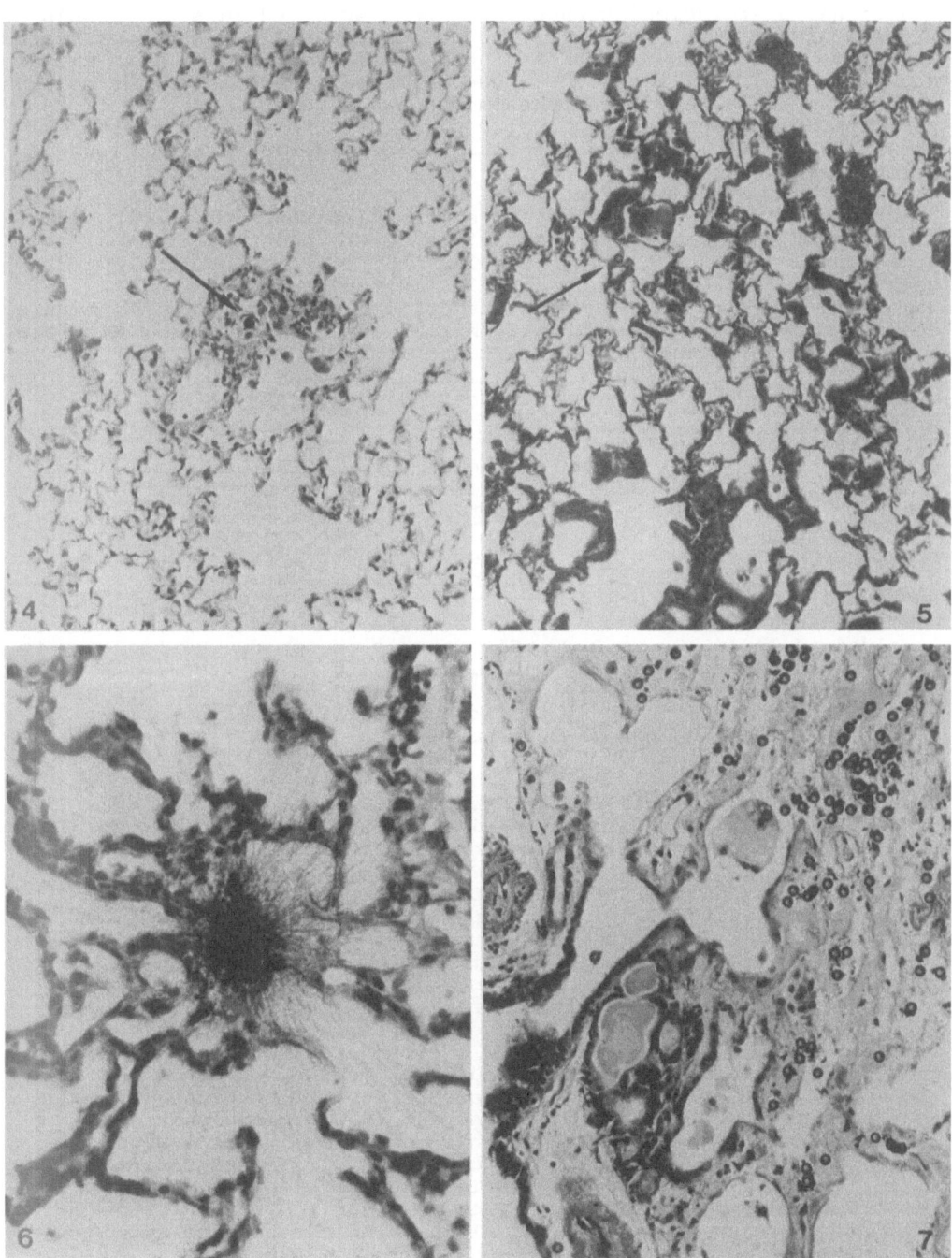

Legends see opposite page

Near the end of the normal life span (15 to 20 months postexposure), additional histological changes have been observed in some animals exposed at the 3 highest levels to relatively small numbers of spheres (2,000 to 6,000). An extension of bronchiolar epithelium into alveolar ducts has occurred, and alveoli become lined with cuboidal or columnar epithelial cells. A similar phenomenon has been noted with animals exposed to 60,000 spheres of 0.9 pCi per sphere for only 6 months, as shown in Fig. 5. These changes could be considered as precursors of peripheral adenomas.

In the experiments with comparatively small numbers of spheres (a few percent of the lung irradiated) of lower specific activity, no gross involvement of the lung results, but close inspection does reveal evidence of dead and dying cells in the midst of seemingly undamaged parenchyma that retains its delicate architecture. Even here one can note that a superficially normal alveolar wall near a sphere, on closer examination, may prove to be ischemic and acellular. An example of the minimal effects following prolonged exposure to a high radiation field is shown in the radioautograph in Fig. 6.

With the highest numbers of spheres (100,000 to 1,000,000), preliminary observations do show more extensive damage, similar to a radiation pneumonitis (Fig. 7). Sphere deposition is often nonuniform, and some regions of the lung show 1,000+ spheres in a low power field of a 6 μm tissue section, while other similar areas contain only 10 spheres/field. Those areas with large numbers of spheres reveal epithelization of alveoli, greatly thickened alveolar walls, and incipient fibrosis. The capillaries are devoid of red cells and are often surrounded by edematous connective tissue. While the specific activity of the spheres involved is low (0.02 to 0.07 pCi), the large number and tendency to cluster cause moderately high local radiation doses (tens of krad/yr) to extend over comparatively large volumes of tissue. Mechanical impairment of the blood supply to these areas by the large numbers of occluding spheres cannot be overlooked as a contributing factor to the fibrotic reaction.

Thus far, only 3 animals (out of some 1,900 total exposed) have died of neoplastic disease originating in the lung. Of these, 2 were from the original experimental group (and from the same dose level of 0.4 pCi/sphere, 2,000 spheres/animal). The other lung tumor was from a later group (59 pCi per sphere, 6,000 spheres/animal). Of the 2 pulmonary tumors in the original group, 1 was a hemangiosarcoma found 9.5 months after injection. This tumor replaced almost entirely the left lung and severely compressed the adjacent normal lung tissue. There was no evidence of metastases to the rest of the lung or to any other organ. The other tumor from this group was an undifferentiated sarcoma found after 1 year exposure. In this case, there were multiple nodules in both lungs. No microspheres were found within the tumor tissue in either case, but they were observed in the adjacent normal lung. A mucinous adenocarcinoma of the lung was found in a hamster after 2 years of exposure to 6,000 microspheres of the highest specific activity level. This tumor involved 1 lobe of the right lung and was locally invasive. Microspheres were observed in adjacent normal lung, showing little if any biological response. Several adrenal carcinomas have been seen during the course of the experiments. This is not an unusual tumor in the hamster and does not appear to be associated with the microsphere exposures.

D. Discussion

Our results confirm the observations of LITTLE et al. (1970, 1973) that locally concentrated alpha irradiation is less damaging in the hamster lung than the same amount of energy delivered over larger volumes. In their work, ^{210}Po was adsorbed onto ferric oxide particles to produce localization. Probably 10^8 to 10^9 particles were involved for 3 mg ferric oxide, compared with the 10^3 to 10^6 spheres used in the present experiments. Thus, our exposures are several orders of magnitude more extreme in terms of both limited number and high specific activity of the foci.

A number of other significant differences exist between the 2 experiments, including polonium vs plutonium, mobile vs fixed particles, and exposure of other organs by the polonium, but it seems probable that the degree of localization is the principal variable. The inefficiency resulting from localization is already evident in the polonium results and becomes extremely marked with the microspheres. Several factors no doubt contribute to the inefficiency of "hot particle" irradiations, including overkill in the extremely high fields close to the spheres, the ability of the tissue to control and repair such localized damage, the lack of synergistic involvement of other organs and other insults, and the probable importance of cooperative multi-cell interactions, which could result in a strong nonlinearity of response with respect to number of cells at risk.

Our results are in definite contradiction to all simplistic models (GEESAMAN, 1968; DEAN and LANGHAM, 1969; PEREZ and COLEMAN, 1969) that assume tumor induction can be calculated solely on the basis of cellular radiation exposure. The indication is that much more complicated mechanisms are involved and that the volume of tissue irradiated is an important factor. Of the experimental exposures, only the earliest ones have been completed in the sense that the animals have lived out their normal life spans. These involved comparatively small numbers of spheres irradiating only a few percent of the total lung mass. However, 1,142 hamsters were exposed to a total of some 5,700,000 spheres in these experiments, and only 2 lung tumors were observed, which already sets a very low limit on the probability of tumor induction per particle. The additional experiments begun through 1973 will raise the totals to 1,900 animals and 160,000,000 spheres and will greatly increase the fraction of lung irradiated.

Acknowledgements

We are indebted to S.G. CARPENTER, G.A. DRAKE, J.E. LONDON, J.S. WILSON, and R.H. WOOD for indispensable technical assistance. J.D. PERRINGS produced the microspheres, and P.N. DEAN has made basic contributions in experimental design and theoretical analysis. This work was performed under the auspices of the U.S. Atomic Energy Commission. The LASL animal colony is accredited by the American Association for Accreditation of Laboratory Animal Care.

442

References

ALBERT, R.E., BURNS, F.J., HEIMBACH, R.D.: Radiation skin tumorigenesis in the rat. Radiation Res. 30, 590-599 (1967).
DEAN, P.N., LANGHAM, W.H.: Tumorigenicity of small highly radioactive particles. Health Phys. 16, 79-84 (1969).
FULWYLER, M.J., PERRINGS, J.D., CRAM, L.S.: Production of uniform
microspheres. Rev. Sci. Instr. 44, 204-206 (1973).
GEESAMAN, D.P.: An analysis of the carcinogenic risk from an insoluble alpha-emitting aerosol deposited in deep respiratory tissue.
University of California Radiation Laboratory, report UCRL-50387
and Addendum (1968).
HOLLAND, L.M., DRAKE, G.A., LONDON, J.E., WILSON, J.S.: Intravenous
injection with a pulsed dental cleaning device. Laboratory Animal
Sci. 21, 913-915 (1971).
LITTLE, J.B., GROSSMAN, B.N., O'TOOLE, W.F.: Respiratory carcinogenesis in hamsters induced by Po-210 alpha radiation and benzo(a)-
pyrene. In: Morphology of Experimental Respiratory Carcinogenesis
(P. Nettesheim, M.G. Hanna, Jr., J.W. Deatherage, Jr., eds), pp.
383-394. AEC Symposium Series no. 21. Oak Ridge, Tennessee: U.S.
Atomic Energy Commission, Division of Technical Inf. 1970.
LITTLE, J.B., GROSSMAN, B.N., O'TOOLE, W.F.: Factors influencing
the induction of lung cancer in hamsters by intratracheal administration of Po-210. In: Radionuclide Carcinogenesis (C.L. Sanders, R.H.
Busch, J.E. Ballou, D.D. Mahlum, eds), pp. 119-137. USAEC Division
of Technical Information, Oak Ridge (1973).
PEREZ, L.J., Jr., COLEMAN, J.R.: Considerations of a tumor probabili-
ty function and micro-dosimetry for the deep lung. In: Report to
Space Nuclear Systems Division, USAEC report NUS-596, Part II (1969).
RICHMOND, C.R., VOELZ, G.L.: Annual report of the biological and
medical research group of the LASL Health Division, January through
December 1971. Los Alamos Scientific Laboratory report LA-4923-PR
(1972). (Available from the National Technical Information Service,
U.S. Department of Commerce, 5285 Port Royal Road, Springfield, Va.
22151).
RICHMOND, C.R., VOELZ, G.L.: Annual report of the biological and
medical research group of the LASL Health Division, January through
December 1972. Los Alamos Scientific Laboratory report LA-5227-PR
(1973). (Available from the National Technical Information Service,
U.S. Department of Commerce, 5285 Port Royal Road, Springfield, Va.
22151).
RICHMOND, C.R., SULLIVAN, E.M.: Annual report of the biomedical and
environmental research program of the LASL Health Division, January
through December 1973. Los Alamos Scientific Laboratory report LA-
5633-PR (1974). (Available from the National Technical Information
Service, U.S. Department of Commerce, 5285 Port Royal Road, Springfield, Va. 22151).
Task Group on Lung Dynamics: Deposition and retention models for
internal dosimetry of the human respiratory tract. Health Phys. 12,
173-207 (1966).
UNDERWOOD, E.E.: Quantitative Sterology, p. 84. Reading, Mass.:
Addison-Wesley Pub. Co. 1970.
WEIBEL, E.R.: Morphometry of the Human Lung, p. 86. Berlin-Göttingen-
Heidelberg: Springer 1963.

Respiratory Carcinogenesis in Rats after Inhalation of Radioactive Aerosols of Actinides and Lanthanides in Various Physicochemical Forms

Jaques LaFuma, J. C. Nénot, M. Morin, R. Masse, H. Metivier, D. Nobile, and W. Skupinski

Centre d'Etudes Nucleaires, Commissariat à l'Energie Atomique, Association Euratom, Fontenay-aux-Roses, France

ABSTRACT

To study the role of the distribution of local tissue irradiation on the toxicity of alpha emitters, groups of 50 to 165 rats were exposed to aerosols of $^{244}Cm(NO_3)_3$, $^{241}Am(NO_3)_3$, $^{238}Pu(NO_3)_4$, $^{235}Pu(NO_3)_4$, $^{239}PuO_2$, and $^{241}AmO_2$ and observed for effects. Curium-244 was most evenly distributed in the lung and most effective in reduction of survival time followed in descending order by $^{238}Pu(NO_3)_4$, $^{241}Am(NO_3)_3$, $^{241}AmO_2$, $^{239}Pu(NO_3)_4$, and $^{239}PuO_2$, which was more heterogeneously distributed in the lung as particulate. The toxicity had 2 results: shortening of life span and cancer induction (about 50% bronchogenic carcinoma and 40% bronchiolo-alveolar carcinomas). There appeared to be no correlation between survival time and cancer induction or localization of the element in the lung and the starting point of the tumors. This histologic type of cancer was independent of the nature of the element. Toxicity and cancer induction appeared to depend on the homogenicity of radiation dose with the more evenly distributed dose being most effective.

Introduction

Metabolic studies after inhalation of actinides and lanthanides by rats in various physicochemical forms have shown great differences in deposition, distribution of local activity, translocation pathways, and rate of clearance (BAIR, 1970; SANDERS, 1972; NENOT et al., 1972; MORIN et al., 1972). 5 years ago we began to study the role of the distribution of local radioactivity on the toxicity of the inhaled elements.

Methods

Table 1 summarizes the experimental design. Table 2 shows the values for lung clearance halftimes of the different compounds deposited in the lung during inhalation exposure (NENOT et al., 1971). For each compound there were 2 clearance fractions (F_1 and F_2), each with their own clearance halftimes expressed in days. Physicochemical parameters were selected to obtain lung clearance halftimes between 4 and 120 days. In order to have very short residence times in the lung, chronic treatment with calcium trisodium diethylenetriamineacetate (DTPA) was used (3 injections per week = 50 mg^2 per kg weight). Amer-

Table 1. α elements and activities deposited in alveoli

	nCi/g	Number of rats
^{244}Cm(NO$_3$)$_3$	20– 3500	140
^{241}Am(NO$_3$)$_3$	120– 2300	120
^{238}Pu(NO$_3$)$_4$	200– 1000	55
^{239}Pu(NO$_3$)$_4$	16– 2000	60
^{241}AmO$_2$	30–23000	150
^{239}PuO$_2$	80– 3300	165

Table 2. Lung clearance

	F_1	T 1/2 (days)	F_2	T 1/2 (days)
^{244}Cm(NO$_3$)$_3$	0.99	8	0.01	250
^{241}Am(NO$_3$)$_3$	0.99	12.5	0.01	250
^{238}Pu(NO$_3$)$_4$	0.99	15	0.01	250
^{239}Pu(NO$_3$)$_4$	0.98	60	0.02	250
^{241}AmO$_2$	0.99	12.5	0.01	250
^{239}PuO$_2$	0.96	120	0.04	500

With chronical DTPA treatments

^{244}Cm	0.998	4	0.002	250
^{241}Am	0.998	6	0.002	250

F - fraction

Legend to Table 2. Particle sizes were respectively for ^{239}PuO$_2$ and ^{241}AmO$_2$ 2.06 μm (σ 1.28) and 2.12 μm (σ 1.68) CMAD. For liquid aerosols 95% of the droplet sizes were smaller than 5 μm in the generator. The droplets dissolved more or less in the alveolar fluid, leading to variable and unknown size emitters.

icium-241 oxide and ^{241}Am(NO$_3$)$_3$ have the same lung clearance halftimes but not the same initial deposition.

Autoradiographic studies have shown that the local distribution of dose was quite different for the different compounds. Plutonium-239 nitrate and ^{239}PuO$_2$ are in particulate forms (Fig. 1). Plutonium-238 nitrate and americium compounds have 2 different distributions: 1 part is particulate and the other part widely dispersed in the lung. Curium-244 nitrate is only widely dispersed in the lung (Figs 2 and 3).

3 days after exposure the rats were counted with an external counter to determine their lung burdens. Some of the rats were killed and their lungs analyzed for radionuclides to calibrate external counting (LAFUMA, 1962).

The rats were sacrificed when moribund. All of the organs were fixed in Bouin-Hollande solution and counted with an x-ray detector to measure their radionuclide content. The whole respiratory system was embedded in paraffin and serial sections of 20 μm were prepared and observed for macroscopic lesions. Sections of gross lesions were prepared and examined microscopically. When a tumor was seen during autopsy, a sample was taken for electron microscopy.

For each rat, we determined the initial and the final lung burdens. Using these 2 values and the lung clearance halftime, we computed a total α activity per gram lung. For each animal we have the total α activity and the survival time; and for each group of animals with the same total α activity, we have a survival curve and a median value between dose and survival time. For each element and for each physicochemical compound we have a relationship between total α activ-

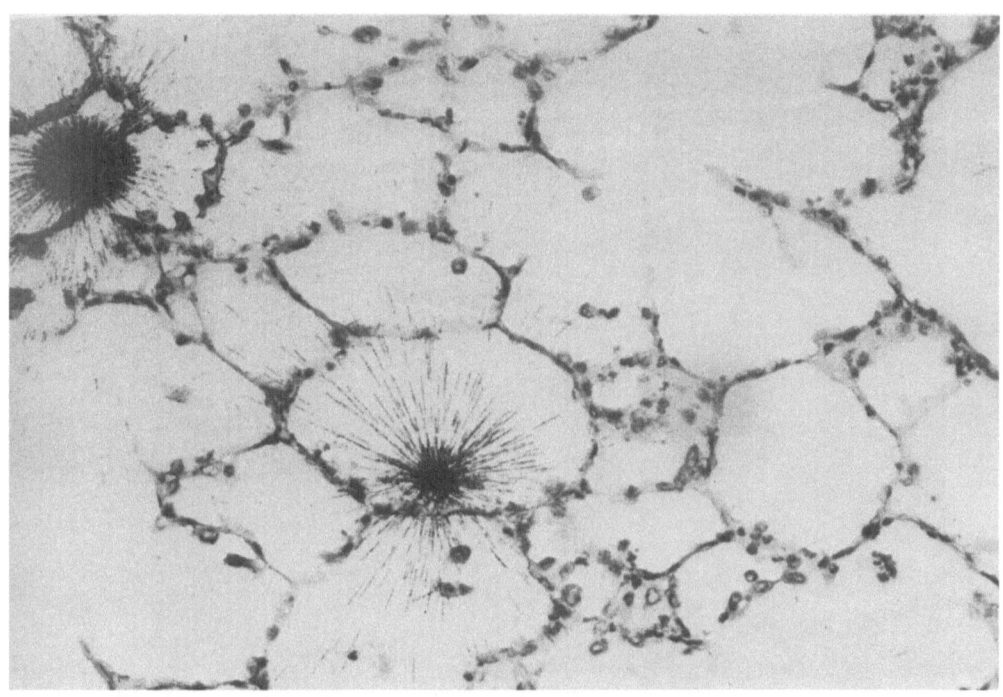

Fig. 1. Baboon 200 days after inhalation. $^{239}PuO_2$ particles. Note alveolar areas free of any particle. Paraffin section, HE (x 188)

ity and survival. Fig. 4 shows this relationship for 4 compounds. One can see that for the same α total activity, the life span increases with the heterogenicity of the local distribution of dose. The most toxic element is the Curium-244 nitrate, which is the most widely dispersed element. For this reason we have made direct calculation of radiation dose only for Curium-244 nitrate.

For these elements we have a relative heterogenicity factor based on the curve of survival time with Curium-244: the heterogenicity factor is the ratio of the total α activity of the elements and of the Curium-244 which are sufficient to kill rats after 1 year. Table 3 shows the heterogenicity factor. For each compounds there is a value (R), which is the product of activity times energy, divided by the heterogenicity factor.

Fig. 5 shows the relationship between the doses expressed in "rads equivalent curium" and the reduction in the life span of rats. The reduction is calculated in percentage of the normal life span of the control animals.

We have observed many lung carcinomas in the rat lungs. Figs 6 to 8 resume the data for 4 compounds: $^{239}PuO_2$, $^{239}Pu(NO_3)_4$, $^{238}Pu(NO_3)_4$, $^{241}Am(NO_3)_3$. All of the rats in these 4 groups were Sprague-Dawley S.P.F. rats. There is one point per animal and each rat is characterized by the following data: dose, survival time, and lesion. "2 carcinomas" means that 2 different histological types of lung carcinomas were observed in the same animal. For the same total dose the cancers appear in the animal with the greatest survival time.

446

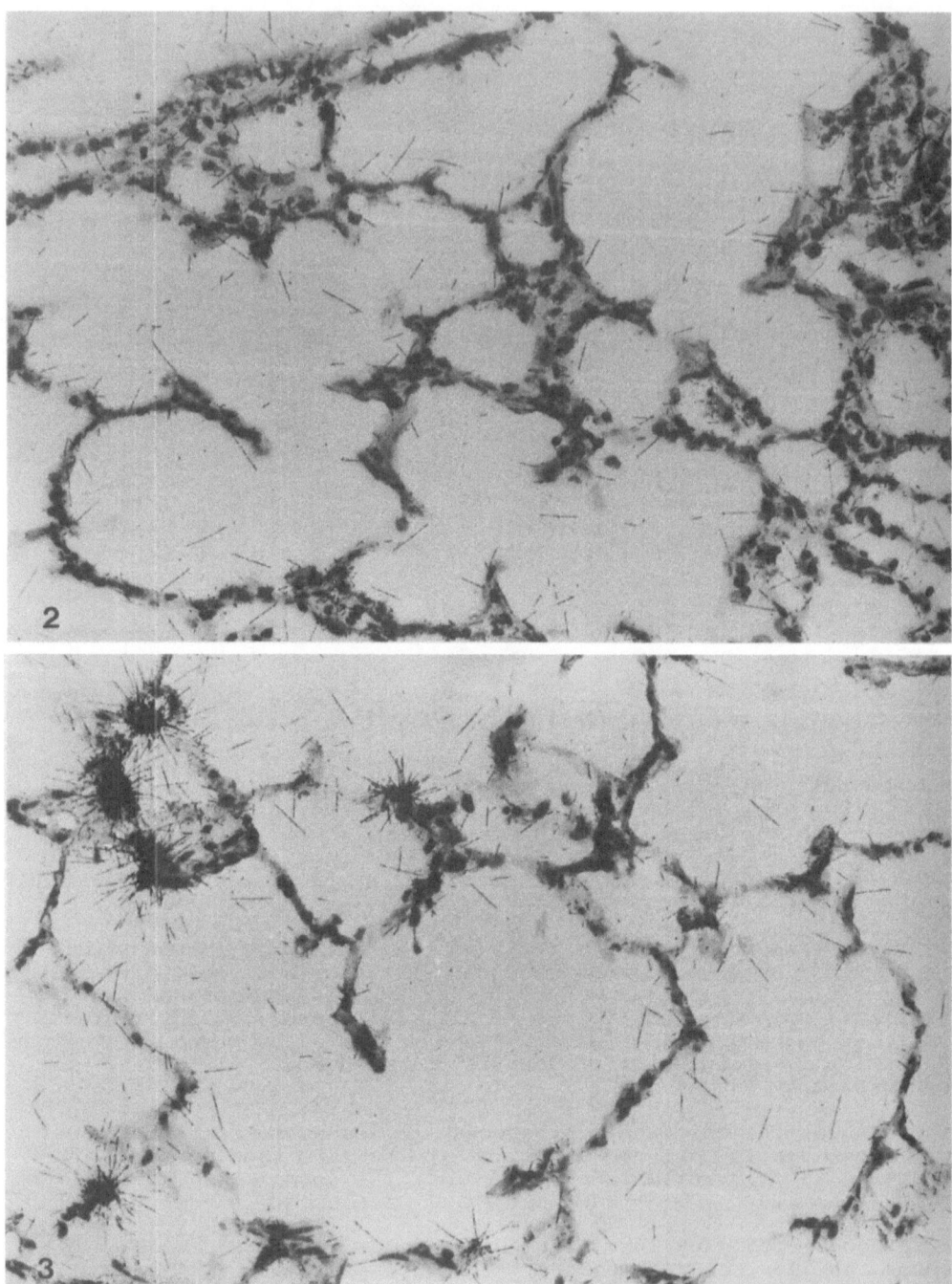

Fig. 2. Rat 20 days after inhalation. ^{244}Cm nitrate. Note lack of particle like emitters. Paraffin section, HE (x 188)
Fig. 3. Rat 60 days after inhalation. ^{241}Am nitrate. Note formation of aggregates among isolate α tracks. Paraffin section, HE (x 188)

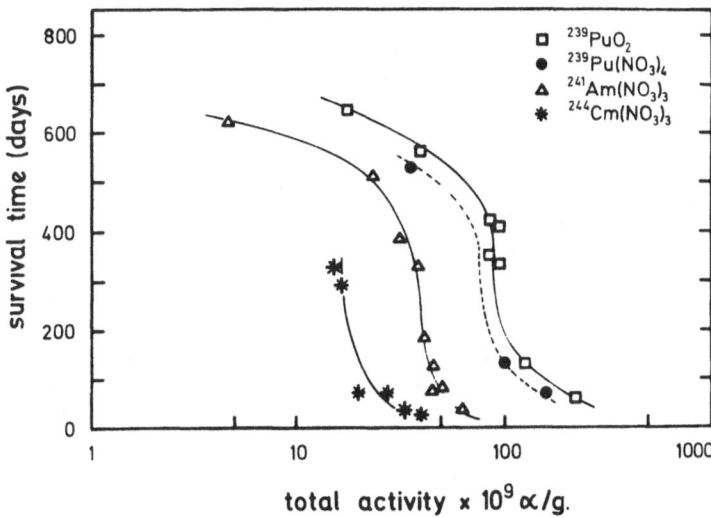

Fig. 4. Relationship between total α activity per gram of rat lung and survival of rats

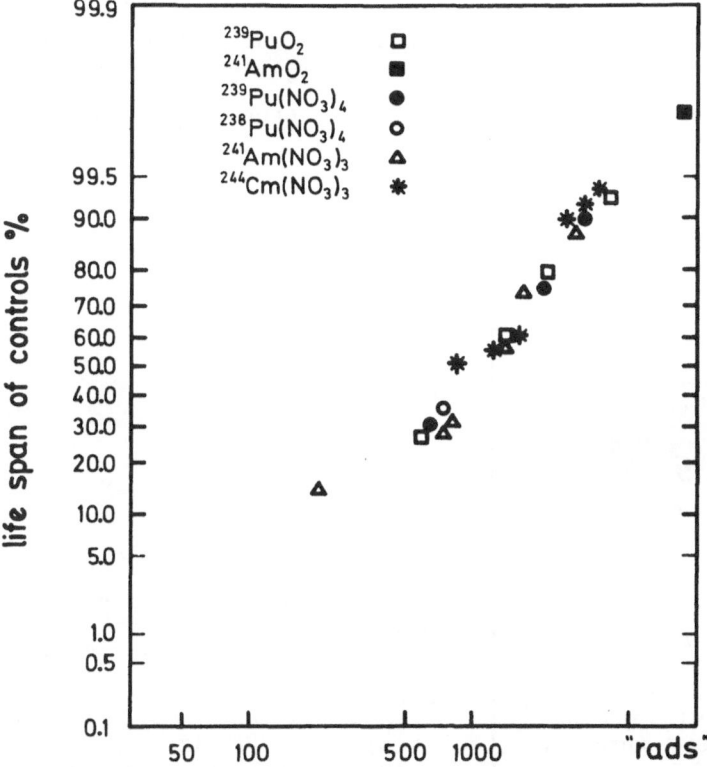

Fig. 5. Relationship between dose expressed in "rads equivalent curium" and reduction in the life span of rats

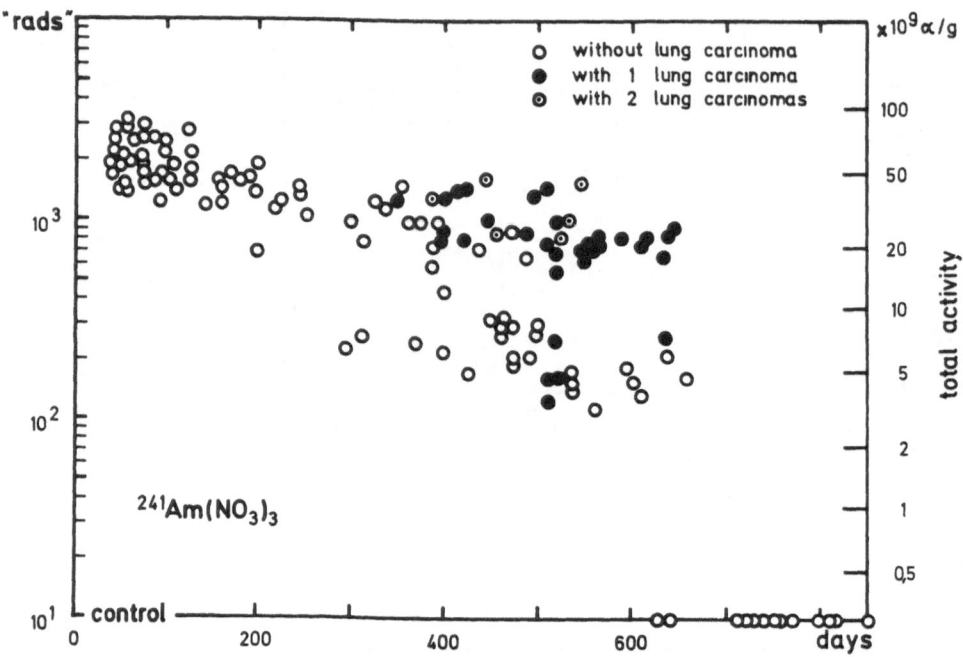

Fig. 6. Relationship between dose ("rads equivalent curium", α activity per gram rat lung), survival (days), and tumor induction in Sprague-Dawley S.P.F. rats after inhalation of $^{239}PuO_2$. Each point represents 1 rat. 2 lung carcinomas means 2 different histological types of tumor in the same animal

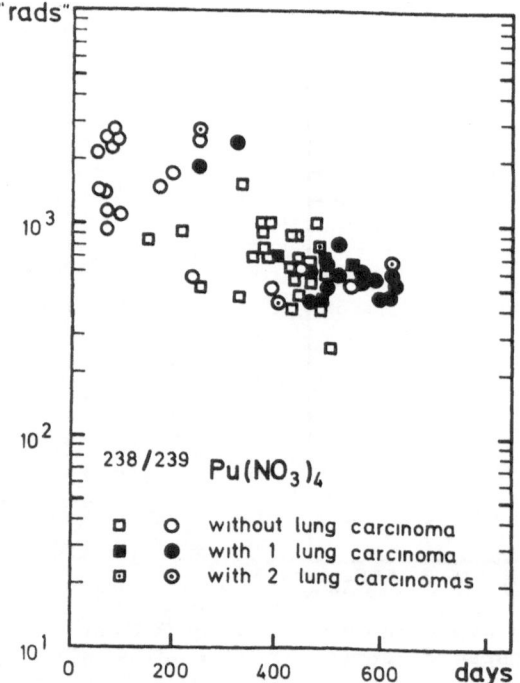

Fig. 7. Relationship between dose ("rads equivalent curium", activity per gram rat lung), survival (days), and tumor induction in Sprague-Dawley S.P.F. rats after inhalation of ^{238}Pu $(NO_3)_4$ or $^{239}Pu(NO_3)_4$. Each point represents 1 rat. 2 lung carcinomas means 2 different histological types of tumor in the same animal

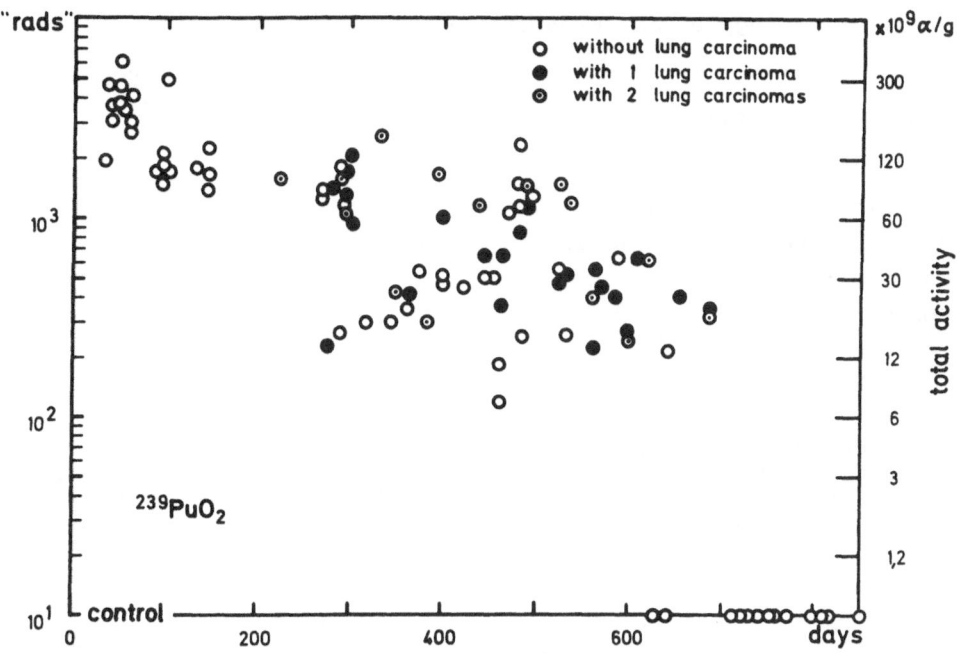

Fig. 8. Relationship between dose ("rads equivalent curium", α activity per gram rat lung), survival (days), and tumor induction in Sprague-Dawley S.P.F. rats after inhalation of ^{241}Am(NO$_3$)$_3$. Each point represents 1 rat. 2 lung carcinomas means 2 different histological types of tumor in the same animal

Table 3. Heterogeneity factors based on total α activity which reduced life span of a factor 2. ^{244}Cm the most homogenous dispersed element is the reference value

	H.F.	R
^{244}Cm(NO$_3$)$_3$	1	93
^{241}Am(NO$_3$)$_3$	3	38
^{238}Pu(NO$_3$)$_4$	2	44
^{239}Pu(NO$_3$)$_4$	5	16
^{241}AmO$_2$	3	29
^{239}PuO$_2$	5.5	15

H.F. = heterogeneity factors
R   = rads/10^{9}α/g

More than 190 lung tumors have been observed, Table 4 shows the percentage of histological types observed. The classification used is based on electronmicroscopic examinations, and is not based on morphology of tumors but on histogenesis of cells.

Table 4. Histology of observed lung tumors

		Percentages
Bronchogenic carcinomas		56.7
squamous-cell	51.9	
bronchogenic adeno-carcinomas	3.7	
anaplastic (great cells)	1.0	
Bronchiolo alveolar carcinomas		39.6
Alveolar carcinomas		1.0
Sarcomas		2.6
reticulo-sarcomas	1.6	
hemangio-sarcomas	1.0	

For each compound we determined the ratio between squamous cell carcinoma and bronchiolo-alveolar carcinomas (Figs 9 and 10). This ratio changes with survival time. Table 5 summarizes the data. Since survival time depends on the dose, it is not possible to say if the differences observed are related to survival time or to dose.

Table 5. Histological types of lung tumors

Survival time days		<300	300-400	400-500	500-600	<600	Σ
$^{239}PuO_2$	S	14	7	7	9	6	43
	B	6	9	8	12	9	44
$^{239}Pu(NO_3)_4$	S	2		3	4	1	10
	B	1	1	1	8	5	16
$^{238}Pu(NO_3)_4$	S			1	1		2
	B			4			4
$^{241}Am(NO_3)_3$	S		2	8	9		19
	B		2	4	11		17

S = squamous cell carcinoma
B = bronchiolo-alveolar carcinoma

The location of the cancers was mostly peripheral in the lung. With the smallest tumors (<10,000 cells), the location of the tumors did not depend on the compound inhaled. At death, the size of the cancer varied from one animal to another. The range of volumes was from 0.2 mm^3 to 10 cm^3. The cancers had no extra thoracic metastasis but were often very invasive.

Rarely was the lung carcinoma the cause of death. The cause of death was unknown and seemed to vary with the different compounds: fibrosis for ^{239}Pu and ^{238}Pu, interstitial pneumonitis for ^{241}Am, immunological deficiency with ^{244}Cm. We do not know if the same mechanism induced the death and the tumors.

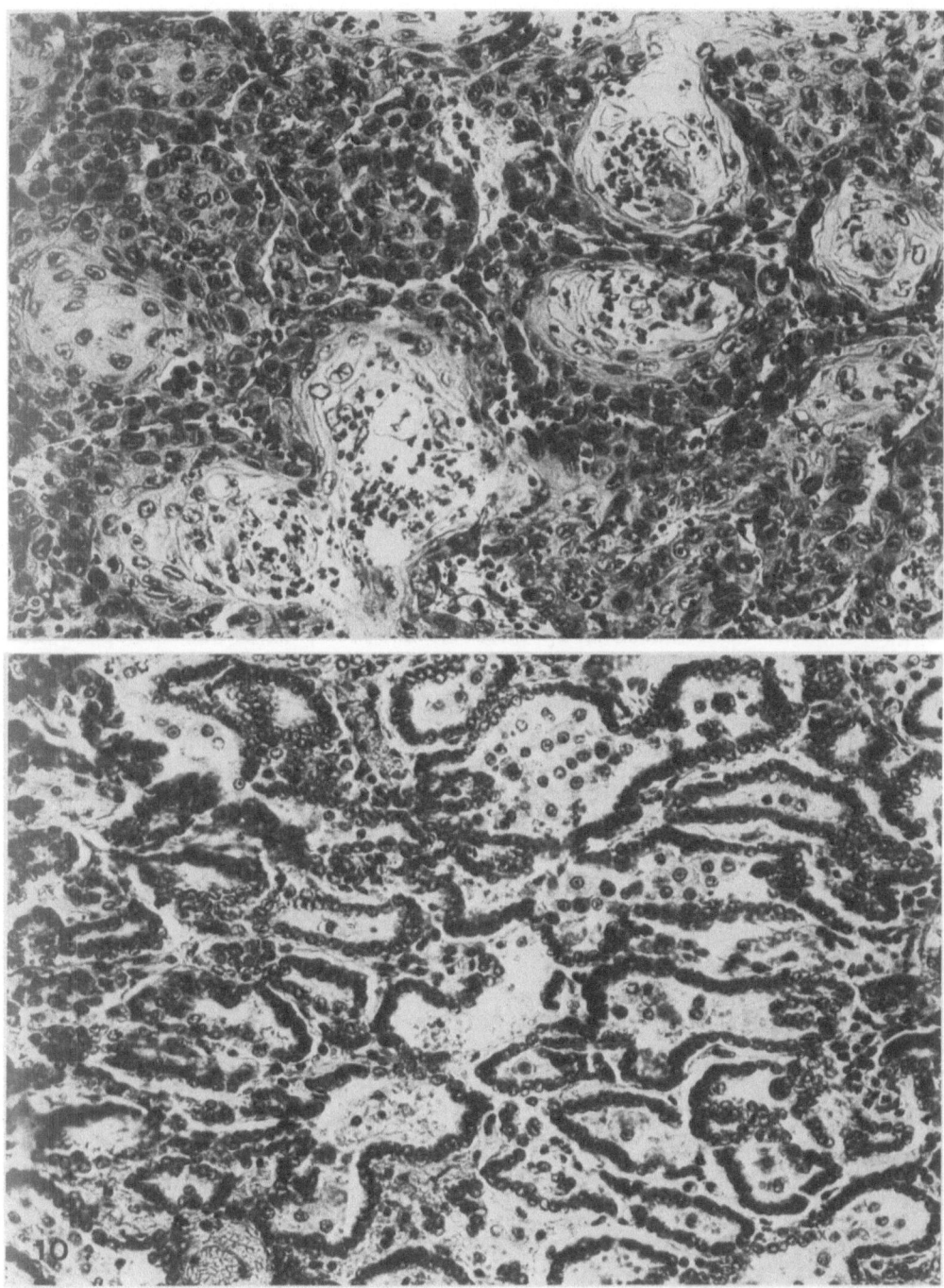

Fig. 9.   Squamous cell carcinoma. Rat. Paraffin section, HE (x 188)

Fig. 10. Bronchiolo-alveolar carcinoma. Rat. Paraffin section, HE
(x 188)

452

Discussion

Experiments with β emitters are now in progress. Rats have been exposed to aerosols of cerium-144 chloride, cerium-144 nitrate, cerium oxide, and yttrium-90 chloride. A few cancers have been observed with cerium, but results have shown that induction of the tumors may be related to the amount of stable carrier. We have observed no relationship between dose and effect (HAHN et al., 1973a, 1973b).

Monkeys have been exposed to ^{239}PuO$_2$ aerosols, and although adenomatous focal growth was observed with a very short latency period in 4 occasions, they seem to be due to a vitamin A deficiency combined with α irradiation (METIVIER, 1972, in press). Preliminary results have clearly demonstrated that baboons are more sensitive than beagle dogs to inhaled ^{239}PuO$_2$, succombing earlier to the same dose levels. We do not know whether a similar difference exists for sensitivity to tumor induction.

Conclusion

These results suggest that the toxicity of inhaled α emitters depends on the homogenicity of local distribution of dose. The toxic action has 2 results: shortening of life span and cancer induction. There appears to be no relationship between survival time and the presence of a cancer. The size of the tumors did not depend on the survival time. There was no correlation between the localization of the element in the lung and the starting point of the tumors. The histological types of the cancer were independent of the nature of the element inhaled. With Curium-244, we have observed only a small number of cancers because the animals were exposed just 15 months ago. Thus far, it seems that for lung cancer induction, this element, widely dispersed in the lung, is more effective than those elements in particulate form.

References

BAIR, W.J.: Plutonium inhalation studies. BNWL-1221 (1970).
HAHN, F.F., SNIPES, M.P., HOBBS, C.H.: Pulmonary hemangiosarcomas in beagle dogs that inhaled ^{90}Sr fused-clay. Radiat. Res. 55, 3, 534 (1973a).
HAHN, F.F., BENJAMIN, S.A., BOECKER, B.B., CHIFFELLE, T.L., HOBBS, C.H., JONES, R.K., MCCLELLAN, R.O., PICKRELL, J.A., REDMAN, H.C.: Primary pulmonary neoplasms in beagle dogs exposed to aerosols of ^{144}Ce in fused-clay particles. J. nat. Cancer Inst. 50, 3, 675 (1973b).
LAFUMA, J.: Mesure précise de la radioactivité de l'animal vivant. J. Rad. et d'Elec. 43, 67, 109 (1962).
METIVIER, H., NOLIBE, D., MASSE, R., LAFUMA, J.: Cancers provoqués chez le singe babouins (papio-papio) par inhalation de PuO$_2$. C.R. Acad. Sci. 275, D, 25, 3069 (1972).
METIVIER, H., NOLIBE, D., MASSE, R., LAFUMA, J.: Excretion and acute toxicity of inhaled ^{239}PuO$_2$ in baboons. Health Phys., in press.
MORIN, M., NENOT, J.C., LAFUMA, J.: Metabolic and therapeutic study following administration to rats of ^{238}Pu nitrate - a comparison with ^{239}Pu. Health Phys. 23, 473 (1972).

NENOT, J.C., MASSE, R., MORIN, M., LAFUMA, J.: An experimental comparative study of the behaviour of ^{237}Np, ^{238}Pu, ^{239}Pu, ^{241}Am, and ^{242}Cm in bone. Health Phys. <u>22</u>, 657 (1972).

NENOT, J.C., MORIN, M., LAFUMA, J.: Etude métabolique et thérapeutique des contaminations respiratoires par certains actinides en solutions. Health Phys. <u>20</u>, 167 (1971).

SANDERS, C.L.: Deposition patterns and the toxicity of transuranium elements in lung. Health Phys. <u>22</u>, 609 (1972).

Pulmonary Carcinogenesis and Chronic Beta Irradiation of Lung

Robert K. Jones, Fletcher F. Hahn, C. H. Hobbs, S. A. Benjamin,
B. B. Boecker, R. O. McClellan, and D. O. Slauson

Inhalation Toxicology Research Institute, Lovelace Foundation for Medical Education and Research,
Albuquerque, NM 87108, USA

ABSTRACT

Light water nuclear power reactor fuel cycles at various stages contain substantial quantities of β-emitting radionuclides. Thus, in
the event of an accident, there is potential for inhalation exposure
of man to various types and forms of β-emitting radionuclides. In
order to study the biological effects of such potential exposures,
a series of life span studies have been initiated in which beagle
dogs have been exposed to inhalation to achieve graded lung burdens
of a relatively insoluble fused clay form of β-emitting radionuclides.
The specific radionuclides, ^{90}Y, ^{91}Y, ^{144}Ce, or ^{90}Sr, were selected
on the basis of physical half-life to produce a variety of radiation-
dose patterns to the lung. Early effects have been the development
of radiation pneumonitis and progressive pulmonary fibrosis. In
general, dogs which receive high- and rapidly-declining dose-rate
exposure from ^{90}Y or ^{91}Y die earlier and at lower cumulative doses
than dogs exposed to ^{144}Ce or ^{90}Sr. By contrast, the incidence of
later-occurring malignant lung tumors and the degree of inflammatory
response is greater in dogs which received protracted low dose-rate
exposure associated with ^{144}Ce and ^{90}Sr. Of particular note is the
nature of the lung tumors thus far observed. These have been of endothelial origin - hemangiosarcomas rather than the epithelial carcinomas that are seen in uranium miners or dogs exposed to $^{239}PuO_2$.
This association between β-radiation exposure and vascular neoplasms
will be discussed further.

A.   Introduction

Human epidemiological and animal dose-response studies have revealed
that chronic or intermittent radiation exposure of the lung may result in a variety of later-occurring sequelae, including pulmonary
fibrosis and the development of malignant neoplasms. This apparent
association between pulmonary radiation exposure and lung cancer was
first documented in 1879 when lung cancer was initially diagnosed in
Joachimsthal and Schneeberg miners (HARTING and HESSE, 1879). Additional evidence was added in 1933 when lung cancer was also reported
in fluorospor miners of Newfoundland (DEVILLER and WINDISH, 1964).
Finally, the more recent experience with uranium miners of the Colorado plateau (LUDIN et al., 1969; ARCHER and WAGONER, 1973) has further substantiated the apparent relationship between chronic inhalation of radon and radon daughters and the development of malignant
pulmonary neoplasms. Unresolved is the question of the degree to
which other inhaled substances, such as cigarette smoke or fossil

fuel combustion products, interact with damage produced by ionizing radiation in a synergistic manner to produce lung cancer.

Further evidence for the pulmonary carcinogenicity of ionizing radiation is available from laboratory studies in which several animal species have received both beta and alpha pulmonary radiation exposure through the use of tracheobronchial implants (LASKIN et al., 1964; WARREN and GATES, 1968) or intratracheal instillation of radionuclides (CEMBER, 1966). Interpretation of the results of these studies, largely performed in small animals, is complicated by the trauma associated with the surgical manipulation and unnatural pulmonary deposition patterns and thus atypically nonuniform radiation dose-distribution associated with both techniques. Relatively few studies have been done in which radionuclides have been deposited in the respiratory tract by inhalation and, other than the early work of LISCO and FINKEL (1949), most have involved the use of alpha-emitting radionuclides. The most important of these latter studies is the work reported by PARK et al. (1972), in which beagle dogs were exposed by inhalation to $^{239}PuO_2$. The results conclusively indicated that inhaled alpha-emitters are extremely carcinogenic, resulting in a high incidence of pulmonary epithelial neoplasms, primarily of the bronchiolo-alveolar type.

With the increased use of light water reactors for the production of electrical power, there exists an increased potential for occupational exposure to beta-gamma-emitting fission products associated with the uranium fuel cycle. Accidental inhalation exposure might occur as a result of a reactor accident or in fuel-reprocessing operations. The lack of available information on the response of the lung to chronic radiation from beta-gamma-emitting radionuclides prompted the initiation of a program with 2 purposes: 1. to define the biological hazards associated with human accidental inhalation exposure to relatively insoluble beta-gamma-emitting radionuclides, and 2. to establish the relationship between radiation-dose pattern and the incidence and nature of late-occurring pulmonary sequelae. In order to provide information which might be most meaningfully extrapolated, the beagle dog was chosen as the primary experimental subject. Its selection not only permitted intensive clinical evaluation on a continuous basis, but also provided an animal having a life span long enough to observe neoplastic changes occurring after a latent period on the order of 10 years. The following report summarizes the current status of 4 major studies in which beagle dogs were exposed by inhalation to fused clay aerosols contaminated with either ^{90}Y, ^{91}Y, ^{144}Ce, or ^{90}Sr. The major emphasis will relate to the distribution and nature of pulmonary neoplasms observed to date.

B. Materials and Methods

The basic experimental approach for these studies has been previously described (MCCLELLAN et al., 1970). Equal numbers of male and female beagle dogs raised in this colony were exposed by inhalation to achieve graded initial lung burdens of one of the beta-gamma radionuclides ^{90}Y, ^{91}Y, ^{144}Ce, and ^{90}Sr. The aerosol was prepared by cation exchange into montmorillonite clay with subsequent high temperature fusion, to form relatively insoluble clay-particle aerosols containing 1 of the 4 radionuclides. Each dog received a single nose-only inhalation exposure when approximately 13 months old and then was maintained for observation over its life span. The radiolabeled fused-clay aerosols were polydisperse, with activity median aerodynamic diameters ranging from 0.8 to 2.7 µm with geometric standard deviations of 1.4 to 2.7.

The experimental design utilized a randomized block design schematically illustrated in Fig. 1. Alternate blocks of male or female dogs were periodically introduced until each study contained 12 complete blocks. This resulted in differences in total current observation period from animals in the first block to the last block of up to 3.8 years. Each block contained 1 control dog exposed to unlabeled fused clay and a number of dogs exposed to radiolabeled fused-clay aerosols to achieve the desired lung burdens. In each study, the highest projected initial lung burden was predicted to result in significant radiation pneumonitis, fibrosis, and death of the animals within approximately 1 year of inhalation exposure. By contrast, the lowest initial lung burden was anticipated to result in little detectable difference in life span from the controls and in 1 instance, [144]Ce fused clay, to represent the canine equivalent of current maximal permissible lung burdens for man. This figure also illustrates that inhalation exposure results in a continuum of initial lung burdens rather than distinct graded-dose levels.

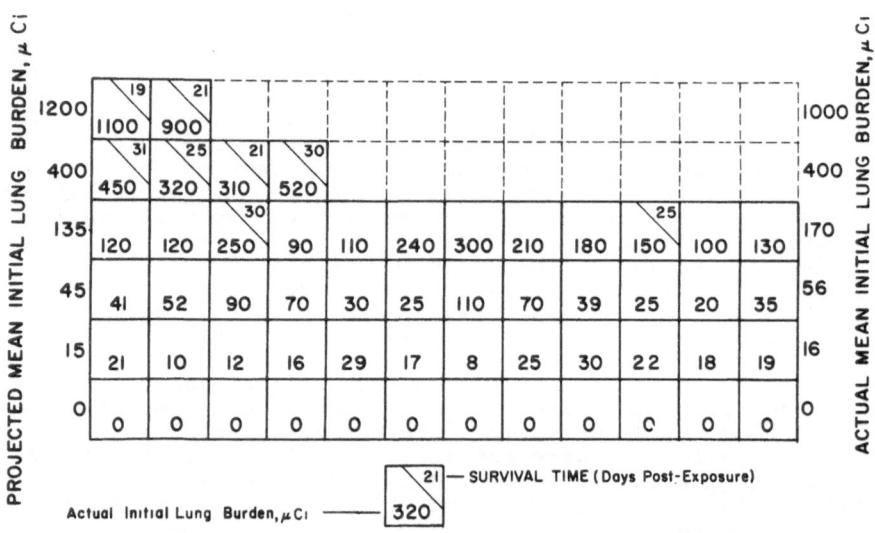

Fig. 1. Experimental design for dose response studies on the effects of inhaled radionuclides in beagle dogs

The effective half-life in lung and the activity levels containing a complete complement of 12 dogs for each of the studies are shown in Table 1. The total number of graded levels differs from study to study but the [144]Ce in fused clay represents the greatest range in initial lung burdens, and thus in cumulative doses. Also shown is the elapsed period of observation for animals contained in the last block introduced into each study. Although this ranges from 947 to 1156 days, many animals in each experiment have been under observation for considerably longer periods of time.

After inhalation exposure, each dog received periodic whole-body counts or lung scans to ascertain the initial lung burden and thus

Table 1. Representative parameters for the 4 dose-response studies
with dogs exposed to beta-emitting radionuclide aerosols

Radionuclide and form	Effective half-life in lung in days	Activity levels containing 12 dogs (μCi/kg body weight)	Minimum observation period since introduction of last block
^{90}Y in fused clay	2.6	0, 100, 200, 300, 400, 600, 800	1156
^{91}Y in fused clay	50	0, 12, 25, 50, 75, 100, 125, 150	980
^{144}Ce in fused clay	180	0, .0009, .045, 0.23, 1.2, 6, 12.5, 25, 50	1024
^{90}Sr in fused clay	370	0, 5, 10, 20, 40, 60, 80	947

to assist in determining the cumulative radiation dose to lung with
time. Further, the health status of each dog was assessed on a regular basis by physical examination, radiographic surveys, clinical
chemistry, and hematologic evaluation, and in some instances, by the
measurement of pulmonary function profiles. Each dog was continuously
observed until death occurred spontaneously or the animal was euthanized in a moribund condition. Following death, animals were given a
detailed post-mortem examination that included observation of all
organ systems. Tissue sections of all major organs and all lesions
were made for histologic evaluation. Formalin-fixed tissues were
routinely processed, sectioned, and stained with hematoxylin and
eosin, and selected sections were stained with elastic masson, periodic acid shift, and Alcein blue. Autoradiographs were made from lung
and tracheobronchial lymph node sections and, where appropriate, radio-
analyzed along with other major tissues for the radionuclide content.

C. Results

I. Radiation Dose Patterns

The 4 radionuclides selected for study were chosen not only because
of their abundance in the inventory of operational reactors, but because they provided distinct radiation dose-patterns to lung, typical
of a variety of radionuclides to which humans might be accidentallly
exposed by inhalation. Since fused clay particles are relatively insoluble, having a biological half-time in lung on the order of 300 to
400 days, the radiation-dose pattern observed in each instance was
largely due to the physical half-life of the radionuclides. Fig. 2
shows the change of radiation-dose rate to lung with time for the 4
radionuclides under investigation. Each is normalized to 100 rads per
day initial dose rate. Thus, animals exposed to ^{90}Y clay received
their total radiation dose over a relatively short time, as compared
with those exposed to ^{90}Sr clay where the radiation dose rate remained substantial over the first 1,000 days post-inhalation exposure.
Dogs exposed to ^{144}Ce and ^{91}Y clay received their radiation dose to

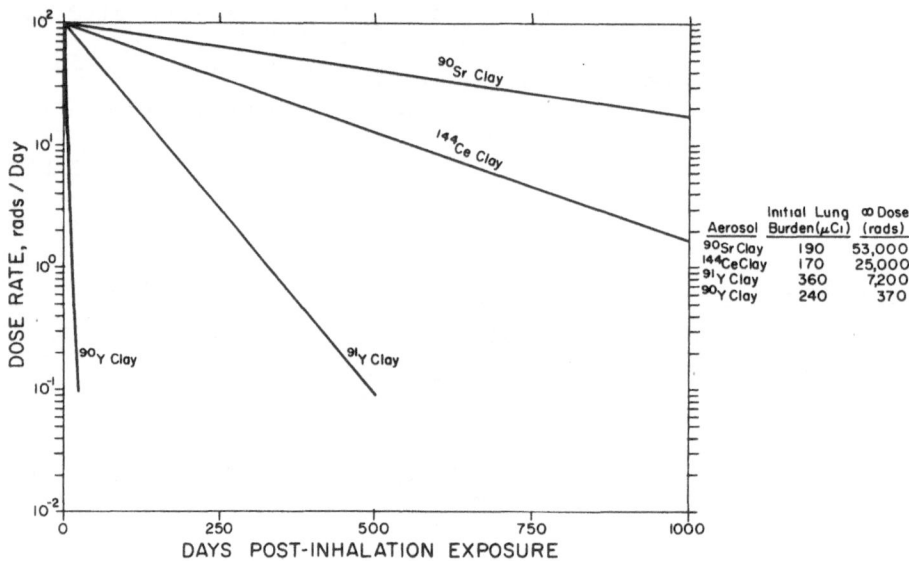

Aerosol	Initial Lung Burden(μCi)	∞ Dose (rads)
^{90}Sr Clay	190	53,000
^{144}Ce Clay	170	25,000
^{91}Y Clay	360	7,200
^{90}Y Clay	240	370

Fig. 2. Absorbed beta radiation dose-rate-to-lung of beagle dogs exposed by inhalation to various radioactive aerosols (^{90}Sr in fused clay, ^{144}Ce in fused clay; ^{91}Y in fused clay, and ^{90}Y in fused clay). Initial dose rate normalized to 100 rads/day. Lung weight assumed to be 110 gm

lung over intermediate time periods between the 2 aforementioned cases. Also shown are the initial lung burdens in microcuries required to achieve an initial radiation dose rate of 100 rads and the infinite cumulative radiation dose that would result for each animal, were it to live a normal life span. The selection of graded levels of these radionuclides not only provides the opportunity to study the relationship between total radiation dose and pulmonary carcinogenesis, but also to investigate the relative carcinogenicity of brief relatively high-dose rate beta irradiation versus protracted low-dose rate pulmonary exposure.

II. Death Distribution and Nature of Radiation-Induced Disease

All dogs which died or were euthanized in all 4 studies within 500 days after inhalation exposure had a varying mix of severe radiation pneumonitis and pulmonary fibrosis. In general, dogs exposed to ^{90}Y and ^{91}Y had a shorter survival time than those which received ^{144}Ce or ^{90}Sr. Further, in part due to the longer survival times, dogs exposed to ^{144}Ce and ^{90}Sr had a more substantial development of pulmonary fibrosis than did those which were exposed to the shorter-lived radionuclides and which died at earlier times.

A total of 25 dogs, 22 with primary pulmonary neoplasms, have died at times beyond 500 days, ranging from 644 to 1318 days after inhalation exposure. The incidence and nature of primary pulmonary neoplasms are shown in Table 2. All 4 dogs in the ^{90}Y and ^{91}Y study died as a result of extensive pulmonary fibrosis and none was found to have a primary malignant pulmonary neoplasm. A small localized benign pulmonary adenoma was observed as an incidental finding in 1 dog from

Table 2. Pulmonary neoplasms observed to date in dogs surviving beyond 500 days

Radionuclide	Number of dogs dead at from 644 to 1318 days post-inhalation exposure	Dogs with one or more primary pulmonary neoplasms listed by type			
		Pulmonary adenoma	Bronchiolo-alveolar carcinoma	Hemangio-sarcoma	Fibro-sarcoma
^{90}Y in fused clay	1	1[a]	0	0	0
^{91}Y in fused clay	3	0	0	0	0
^{144}Ce in fused clay	7	0	1	7	1
^{90}Sr in fused clay	14	0	1	14	0

[a]Incidental finding at necropsy.

the ^{90}Y study. By contrast, aggressive, widely-disseminated primary pulmonary hemangiosarcomas contributed to the death of all 7 dogs in the ^{144}Ce studies and the 14 dogs in the ^{90}Sr studies. A second form of malignant pulmonary neoplasm was observed concurrently in 2 dogs in the ^{144}Ce group. In 1 case, the second tumor was a bronchiolo-alveolar carcinoma, and in the other a fibrosarcoma. Similarly, a concurrent bronchiolo-alveolar carcinoma was found in 1 dog in the ^{90}Sr group.

III. Clinical and Pathologic Findings

Other than the development of a progressive absolute lymphopenia and the occasional appearance of slight anemia, no clinical abnormalities were apparent prior to the clinical diagnosis of a primary lung tumor. In most instances, the diagnosis was established on the basis of radiographic examination, the development of hemoptysis, or clinical abnormalities referable to distant metastasis. Once a diagnosis was established, the subsequent survival time was less than 3 months.

At necropsy, the hemangiosarcomas were characterized by irregular purple nodular pulmonary infiltrates, measuring from a few millimeters in diameter up to large variegated blood-filled sacs measuring up to 10 centimeters in greatest dimension. Many of the smaller nodules collapsed upon sectioning and contained partially-organized thrombi. Although the initially-observed hemangiosarcomas in the ^{144}Ce fused-clay group appeared to have a predilection for the anterior lobes, this was not borne out in dogs with hemangiosarcomas in the ^{90}Sr study where the lobar distribution appeared to be more random. Distant metastases were observed in all but 1 dog, and the most frequent sites of involvement were tracheobronchial lymph nodes, brain, kidney, adrenal, and heart. The histologic appearance, although varied, was similar in lung and distant metastasis, and consisted of blood-filled capillary to cavernous sinoids lined by plump pleomorphic angioblasts occasionally undergoing mitosis (Fig. 3). In some areas, the sinusoids contained partially-organized thrombi, and hemosiderin-laden macrophages were present both within the infiltrate and at their periphery. Collections of tumor cells were frequently present around bronchioles, bronchi, and in blood vessels. In many areas, neoplastic cells were accompanied by a fine-to-coarse trabecullar fibrous stroma but, other than in the central portion of large necrotic masses, dense pulmonary fibrosis was not a characteristic feature.

The bronchiolo-alveolar carcinomas observed in 2 dogs had a distinctly different gross appearance at necropsy. The lobe involved was more
uniformly consolidated, having a greyish-yellow gelatinous appearance
on cut section. Distant metastases were not evident grossly; however,
metastatic foci were found in tracheobronchial lymph nodes. The histologic characteristics are illustrated in Fig. 4. The cells, medium-
sized, round, or cuboidal, occurred in clumps or ribbons and had
distinct cytoplasmic borders. Individual cells had a moderate amount
of eosinophilic cytoplasm and an intermediate-sized round or oval
nucleus with sparse chromotin and occasionally a prominent nucleus.
The distinct characteristic of the cells was their growth along alveolar walls and the tendency to fill alveoli with little alteration
of alveolar architecture. Neoplastic cells were frequently found in
peribronchial lymphatics in lobes adjacent to the primary tumor. As
was the case for the hemangiosarcomas, extensive pulmonary fibrosis
was not a major associated feature.

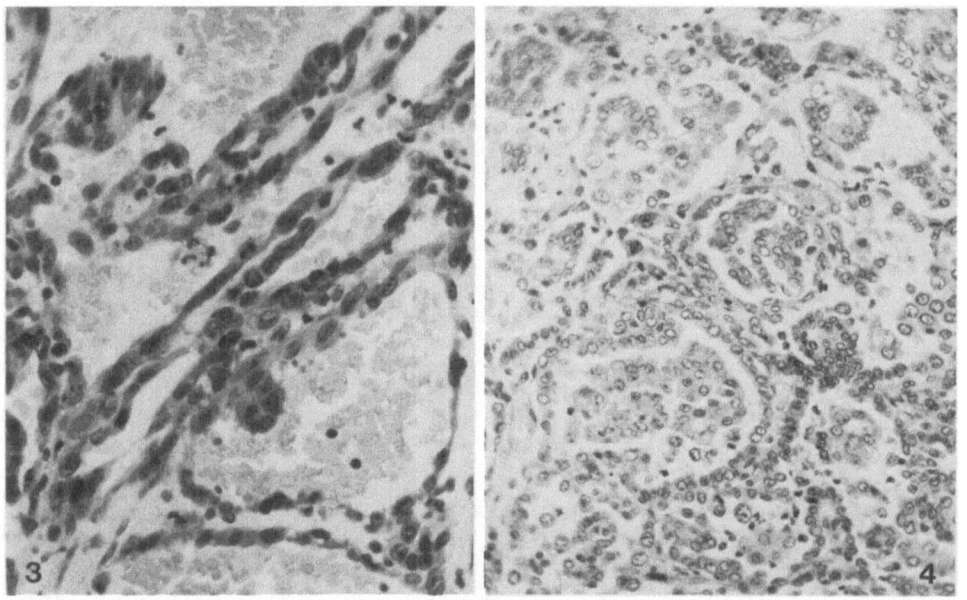

Fig. 3. Photomicrograph of a pulmonary hemangiosarcoma showing
cavernous sinusoids with lining of plump angioblasts. HE (x 266)

Fig. 4. Photomicrograph of a bronchiolo-alveolar carcinoma showing
lining of the alveolar wall with cuboidal cells and sloughing of
these cells into the alveoli. HE (x 203)

The fibrosarcoma observed in 1 dog exposed to ^{144}Ce in fused clay
had gross and histologic features quite different from areas of hemangiosarcomas seen in the same dog. The right cardiac lobe and a portion of the right apical lobe were replaced by a large 10 x 7 x 6
centimeter fibrotic yellow mass, showing areas of central necrosis.
The right diaphragmatic and left apical cardiac lobes contained
similar small yellowish nodules. Distant metastases were found in
the myocardium, wall of the ileum, kidney, and brain. The histologic

detail varied greatly from nodule to nodule. In some areas, it was characterized by broad swirling masses of mature connective tissue with interspersed well-differentiated fibroblasts. Plump anaplastic cells containing frequent mitotic figures were generally seen at the periphery of such masses (Fig. 5). More aggressive foci contained greater numbers of anaplastic cells, more frequent mitotic figures, and considerably less collagen. It is interesting to note that, although the fibrosarcoma and hemangiosarcoma were interspersed within the lung, distant metastases were entirely distinct, with no intermixture of histologic types observed.

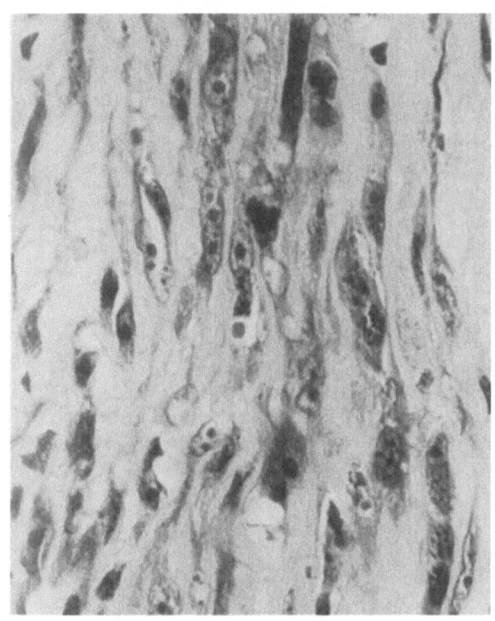

Fig. 5. Photomicrograph of a fibrosarcoma of the lung showing plump anaplastic fibroblasts. HE (x 490)

IV. Dose-Response Relationships

Fig. 6 shows the cumulative radiation dose in rads and death distribution of the 7 dogs which developed malignant pulmonary neoplasms in the ^{144}Ce in fused-clay study. To date, the lowest radiation dose that has resulted in the development of a hemangiosarcoma is 29,000 rads. Currently, 4 dogs are surviving with cumulative radiation doses in excess of this value, and 1 has radiographic evidence of a pulmonary neoplasm. Exclusive of controls, 81 additional dogs are currently under study with ranges of doses and current observation periods as indicated in Fig. 6. Fig. 7 shows similar data for tumor-bearing dogs in the ^{90}Sr in fused-clay study. The lowest radiation dose to result in the development of a pulmonary angiosarcoma was 34,000 rads. Exclusive of controls, 26 additional animals are currently under study with cumulative radiation doses falling between the highest and lowest levels indicated in the figure.

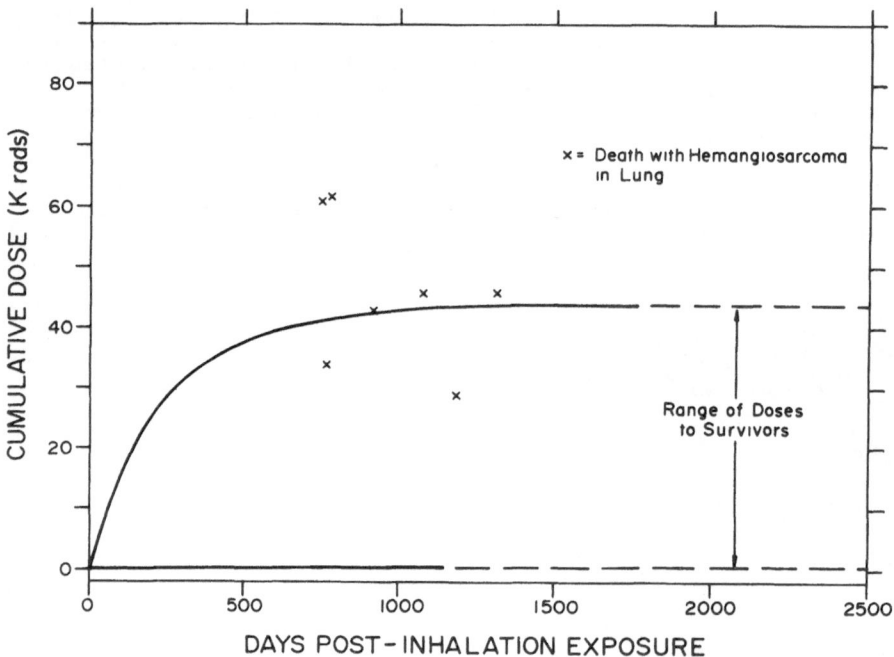

Fig. 6. Cumulative beta radiation dose to lung following inhalation of ^{144}Ce in fused clay in beagle dogs dying with pulmonary hemangiosarcomas. Solid lines represent dose to highest and lowest surviving animals to date. Dashed lines project the dose to 2,500 days

D. Discussion

Although malignant pulmonary neoplasms have been observed to date only in dogs exposed by inhalation to ^{144}Ce and ^{90}Sr fused clay, the observation period is inadequate to firmly establish the relative carcinogenicity associated with the 4 distinct radiation dose patterns produced by ^{144}Ce, ^{90}Sr, ^{91}Y, and ^{90}Y fused clay. Primary lung neoplasms have thus far been observed only in dogs receiving cumulative radiation doses in excess of 29,000 rads and surviving beyond 644 days after inhalation exposure. Because of the higher initial radiation dose rates associated with lung burdens required to produce a similar cumulative radiation dose in dogs exposed to ^{90}Y and ^{91}Y, the dogs in these 2 studies did not survive long enough to be at risk for the development of primary lung tumors. In fact, a cumulative radiation dose of 29,000 rads resulted in death at approximately 70 and 250 days after inhalation exposure, respectively, in dogs exposed to ^{90}Y and ^{91}Y in fused clay.

The current status of the surviving dog with the highest cumulative radiation dose in each of the 4 studies is illustrated in Fig. 8. The continuous line represents the observation period to date and the dashed line represents the projected cumulative dose to 2,500 days. This represents the maximum range of radiation doses that encompasses all of the surviving dogs in each study. To illustrate the overlap in cumulative doses, the infinite cumulative dose for the lowest dog

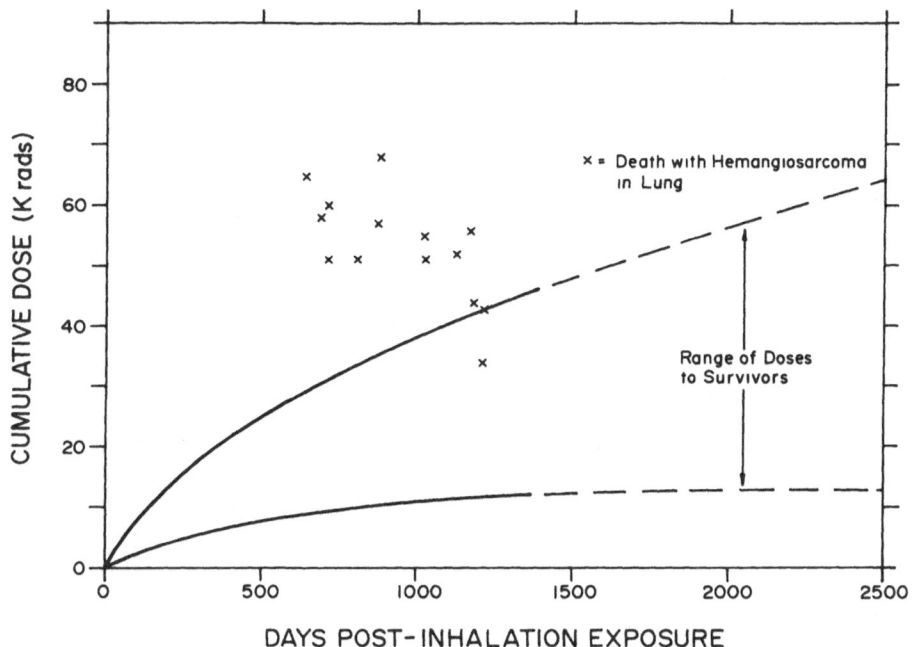

Fig. 7. Cumulative beta radiation dose to lung following inhalation of ^{90}Sr in fused clay in beagle dogs dying with pulmonary hemangiosarcomas. Solid lines represent dose to highest and lowest surviving animals to date. Dashed lines project the dose to 2,500 days

in each study is 900, 1900, 2.7, and 7200 rads for ^{90}Y, ^{91}Y, ^{144}Ce, and ^{90}Sr, respectively. Thus, more protracted observation periods will permit a comparison of biological response in dogs receiving similar cumulative radiation doses delivered in 4 distinct radiation-dose patterns. Thus far, however, it would appear that protracted low-dose rate beta irradiation does result in adequately long-term survival and accumulation of sufficient beta-irradiation to the lung to produce primary pulmonary neoplasms. It would then follow that accidental exposure of relatively insoluble forms of long-lived radionuclides may be considerably more hazardous with respect to pulmonary cancer than inhalation of a similar µCi amount of shorter-lived isotopes.

Although HAHN et al. (1973) have previously reported on the first 5 cases of primary pulmonary hemangiosarcoma in dogs inhaling ^{144}Ce in fused clay, the uniformity of subsequent results from the ^{144}Ce and ^{90}Sr fused-clay studies is quite startling and relatively unique to this form of radiation exposure. At least 1 other study has been performed in which dogs have been exposed by inhalation to a relatively insoluble form of ^{144}Ce (STUART et al., 1964). Although no neoplasms were observed in this study, the observation period of 480 days was in all probability too short for the development of such lung tumors. Hemangiosarcomas have also been extremely rare in other species following inhalation exposure to radionuclides. LISCO (1959) observed 1 hemangiosarcoma in a rat exposed to ^{239}PuO$_2$ fumes, and CEMBER (1964) described 1 case in a rat which had been exposed to ^{144}CeCl$_3$ and received greater than 25,000 rads to the lung.

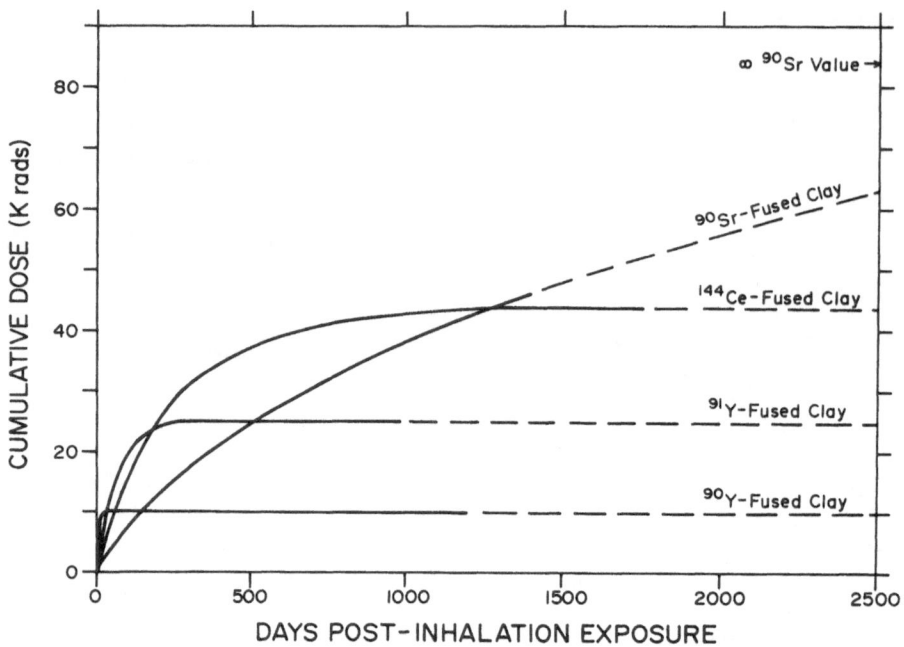

Fig. 8. Cumulative beta radiation doses as of 6/1/74 to the surviving dog with the highest cumulative dose to lung in each study (^{90}Sr in fused clay, ^{144}Ce in fused clay, ^{91}Y in fused clay, ^{90}Y in fused clay). Dashed line represents dose projected beyond current observation period

The significance of the observed incidence of hemangiosarcoma in dogs exposed by inhalation to ^{144}Ce or ^{90}Sr in fused clay is underscored by the fact that primary pulmonary hemangiosarcoma has not previously been reported as a spontaneous tumor in canine species, although such neoplasms are not uncommon in other locations. To date, 7 of 11 dogs with initial lung burdens of ^{144}Ce in fused clay ranging from 27 to 46 µCi/kg, and which lived for at least 790 days, have died with primary pulmonary hemangiosarcomas. 1 of the 4 surviving dogs has radiographic evidence of a pulmonary neoplasm. Similarly, 14 of 17 dogs with initial lung burdens of ^{90}Sr in fused clay ranging from 15 to 30 µCi/kg and which survived beyond 693 days after inhalation exposure, have died with primary pulmonary hemangiosarcomas. The 3 remaining dogs currently show no evidence of pulmonary neoplasms.

It is interesting to note the substantial difference in the type of lung neoplasms observed at Battelle-Northwest Laboratory in dogs with chronic alpha irradiation of lung from inhaled ^{239}PuO$_2$, to those resulting from chronic beta radiation exposure (Table 3). Of 35 dogs exposed by inhalation to ^{239}PuO$_2$, 24 have thus far shown primary lung neoplasms (BAIR, personal communication, 1974). All of the animals were found to have peripheral bronchiolo-alveolar carcinomas and 10 animals had, in addition, concurrent epithelial or mesenchymal tumors. Although all animals exposed to β-emitting radionucludes which developed malignant lung tumors were found to have hemangiosarcomas, only 2 hemangiosarcomas were found in the 24 tumor-bearing dogs following in-

Table 3. Nature of primary malignant pulmonary neoplasms in dogs exposed by inhalation alpha- or beta-emitting radionuclides

Radionuclide and form	Radiation type	Bronchiolo-alveolar carcinoma	Hemangio-sarcoma	Other mesenchymal neoplasms	Other epithelial neoplasms	Mean survial time in all tumor bearing dogs in days
^{144}Ce fused clay	Beta	1	7	1	0	971
^{90}Sr fused clay	Beta	1	14	0	0	943
^{239}PuO$_2$	Alpha	24	2	3	7	2230

halation of alpha-emitting radionuclides. The peripheral tumors were generally associated with significant pulmonary fibrosis, epithelial hyperplasia, and metaplasia, findings which were considerably less striking in the beta-emitter studies. This may relate in part to the longer latent period between inhalation-exposure and the development of lung tumors in dogs which inhaled ^{239}PuO$_2$. The mean survival time for tumor-bearing dogs in the ^{239}PuO$_2$ study was 2230 days, whereas the mean survival time thus far in dogs with hemangiosarcomas is 971 days for the ^{144}Ce, and 943 for the ^{90}Sr groups. If pulmonary fibrosis and associated metaplastic changes are a prerequisite for the development of epithelial neoplasms, and progressive pulmonary fibrosis occurs as a result of chronic beta irradiation of the lung, then with increasing time, dogs exposed to relatively insoluble beta-emitting radionuclides may well develop a spectrum of lung tumors similar to those observed in dogs which inhaled ^{239}PuO$_2$. Results of earlier studies conducted in our institute, in which dogs were exposed to more soluble forms of beta-emitting radionuclides, would suggest that pulmonary fibrosis is not an essential prerequisite for the development of such primary lung tumors. 3 primary pulmonary neoplasms have been observed to date in these studies (Table 4). All 3 were epithelial in origin, 2 were malignant and all were observed at survial times beyond 1632 days. In these dogs, only 1 showed very impressive interstitial fibrosis of a generalized nature, and in none was dense pulmonary fibrosis associated with the tumors. It is important to note the low cumulative radiation dose-to-lung of these 3 dogs at time of death. The occurrence of lung neoplasms at doses on the order of 3000 to 4000 rads would suggest that a considerable number of primary lung tumors may be expected in surviving dogs, currently under observation in all 4 studies involving more insoluble forms of beta-emitting radionuclides. It should be recognized, however, that due to the more soluble aerosol form the cumulative doses delivered to the lungs of these 3 dogs, were delivered at a relatively high dose rate and over a relatively short period of time. It remains to be seen whether later-occurring neoplasms will develop in dogs which received cumulative doses of several thousand rads delivered over longer periods of time and, if so, whether they will be of endothelial or epithelial origin.

Regardless of the future results of these studies, it is apparent that significant differences in the nature of primary lung cancer have been observed between dogs exposed by inhalation to beta- versus alpha-emitting radionuclides, and one can only speculate as to the pathogenic nature of these observed differences. 1 possibility, already alluded to, relates to differences in the destructive nature of these 2 forms of radiation. High LET alpha-irradiation may result in greater

Table 4. Pulmonary neoplasms observed in other dogs exposed by inhalation to β-emitting radionuclides

Radionuclide and form	Nature of pulmonary neoplasm	Survival time (days)	Cumulative dose to lung to time of death (rads)
$^{91}YCl_3$	Bronchiolo-alveolar carcinoma	2109	3300
$^{144}CeCl_3$	Pulmonary adenoma	1632	6200
$^{144}CeCl_3$	Adenocarcinoma	2773	3900

localized nonreparable cell injury with subsequent cellular death and initiation of reparative processes, including connective tissue proliferation, epithelial hyperplasia, and metaplasia, all of which may be prerequisites for the subsequent development of epithelial neoplasms. By contrast, lower LET and more diffuse beta-irradiation may result in more reparative cell damage, less cell death, and thus less reparative fibrosis and epithelial response. Also, because endothelial cells have a relatively slow turnover time, they may accumulate considerable nonlethal cytogenetic damage which, following ultimate cell division, may result in the development of endothelial neoplasms. However, until we better understand the normal function and kinetics of cells comprising the lung and the relative sensitivity of such cells to localized radiation dose, the explanation for these observed differences must remain only speculative.

E. Acknowledgements

The generous assistance of the staff of the Inhalation Toxicology Research Institute, Lovelace Foundation for Medical Education and Research, in the conduct of this study is gratefully acknowledged. These studies could not have been performed without the input of a number of individuals with diverse skills. This research was performed under AEC Contract No. AT(29-2)-1013 between the U.S. Atomic Energy Commission and the Lovelace Foundation for Medical Education and Research in animal facilities fully accredited by the American Association for Accreditation of Laboratory Animal Care.

References

ARCHER, V.E., WAGONER, J.K.: Lunc cancer among uranium miners in the United States. Health Phys. 25, 351-371 (1973).
BAIR, W.J.: Personal communication, 1974.
CEMBER, H.: Radiogenic lung cancer. Prog. exp. Tumor Res. 4, 251-303 (1964).
CEMBER, H.: Progress in radiogenic lung cancer. In: Lung Tumors in Animals (L. Siveri, ed.), pp. 321-330. Italy: University of Perugia 1966.
DEVILLER, A.J., WINDISH, J.P.: Lung cancer in a florospar mining community. I. Radiation, dust, mortality experience. Brit. J. Med. 21, 94-109 (1964).

HAHN, F.F., BENJAMIN, S.A., BOECKER, B.B., CHIFFELLE, T.L., HOBBS, C.H., JONES, R.K., MCCLELLAN, R.O., REDMAN, H.C.: Primary pulmonary neoplasms in beagle dogs exposed to aerosols of ^{144}Ce in fused clay particles. J. nat. Cancer Res. 50, 675-698 (1973).

HARTING, F.H., HESSE, W.: Der Lungenkrebs, die Bergkrankheit in den Schneeberger Gruben. Vierteljahrsschr. gerichtl. Med. Offenth Gesundkertswesen, (N.F.), 30 (1879), 296-309, 102-129, 313-337.

LASKIN, S., KUSCHNER, M., ALLSHULER, B., NELSON, N.: Tissue reactions and dose relationships in rats following intrapulmonary beta radiation. Health Phys. 10, 1229-1233 (1964).

LISCO, H., FINKEL, M.P.: Observations on lung pathology following inhalation of radioactive cerium. Federation Proc. 8, 360-361 (1949).

LISCO, H.: Autoradiographic studies in radiation carcinogenesis of the lung. Lab. Invest. 8, 1-21 (1959).

LUDIN, F.E., Jr., LLOYD, J.W., SMITH, E.M., ARCHER, V.E., HOLADAY, D.A.: Mortality of uranium miners in relation to radiation exposure, hard rock mining and cigarette smoking - 1950 through September 1967. Health Phys. 16, 571-578 (1969).

MCCLELLAN, R.O., BARNES, J.E., BOECKER, B.B., CHIFFELLE, T.L., HOBBS, C.H., JONES, R.K., MAUDERLY, J.L., PICKRELL, J.A., REDMAN, H.C.: Toxicity of beta-emitting radionuclides inhaled in fused clay particles - an experimental approach. In: Morphology of Experimental Respiratory Carcinogenesis (P. Nettesheim, M.G. Hanna, Jr., J.W. Deatherage, Jr., eds), pp. 395-415. AEC Symposium Series no. 21. Springfield, Va.: U.S. Department of Commerce 1970.

PARK, J.F., BAIR, W.J., BUSCH, R.H.: Progress in beagle dog studies with transuranium elements at Battelle-Northwest. Health Phys. 22, 803-810 (1972).

STUART, B.O., CASEY, H.W., BAIR, W.J.: Acute and chronic effects of inhaled ^{144}CeO$_2$ in dogs. Health Phys. 10, 1203-1209 (1964).

WARREN, S., GATES, O.: Cancers induced in different species by continuous gamma-radiation. Arch. Environ. Hlth 17, 697-704 (1968).

Histologic Observations on the Pathogenesis of Lung Cancer in Hamsters Following Administration of Polonium-210*

Hermann Lisco, Ann R. Kennedy, and John B. Little

Department of Anatomy, Harvard Medical School, and Department of Physiology, Harvard School of Public Health, Boston, MA 02115, USA

ABSTRACT

A serial sacrifice experiment was carried out to study the site of origin and the stages in development of lung cancer in hamsters induced by polonium-210 (^{210}Po). 1 or 2 animals were sacrificed weekly during and after a course of 7 intratracheal instillations of 0.1 µCi of ^{210}Po in saline. This exposure produced a transient radiation pneumonitis of moderate severity during, and for several weeks after, the instillation period. Subsequent pathological changes included hyperplasia of bronchiolar epithelium, and focal proliferation of epithelial cells in peribronchiolar and more remote alveoli, termed epithelialization of alveoli. Hyperplastic bronchiolar epithelium frequently showed numerous Clara cells which exhibited pleomorphism of cells and nuclei, multinucleated cells, and striking changes in staining characteristics of secretory granules. Epithelialization of alveoli showed steady progression from well-circumscribed small foci to larger confluent lesions which were composed of various cell types and resembled tumors. Malignant tumors occurred in many animals surviving more than 24 weeks after the last instillation of ^{210}Po.

Introduction

In earlier experiments we have shown that polonium-210 (^{210}Po), an alpha particle emitting radionuclide, is a potent lung carcinogen in Syrian golden hamsters (LITTLE et al., 1970, 1973, 1974). Tumor incidence and induction time were related to dose over a range of 300 to 5000 rads to the whole lung. Most of the tumors arose in the periphery of the lung, and have been classified as combined epidermoid and adenocarcinomas (LITTLE et al., 1970, 1974). The present experiments were designed to study the site of origin and sequential stages in the development of benign and malignant changes in the lungs of hamsters under conditions of exposure comparable to those of earlier experiments. 1 or 2 animals were sacrificed weekly during and after a course of 7 intratracheal instillations of 0.1 µCi of ^{210}Po in saline. The lungs were examined with 1 µm sections from glycol methacrylate embedded tissue which allowed high resolution in the identification of cell types. A preliminary survey of lungs from animals sacrificed up to 25 weeks after the last instillation of ^{210}Po has been made and is presented here.

*Supported by Grants DT-37B from the American Cancer Society, and ES-00002 from the National Institutes of Health.

Materials and Methods

Male Syrian golden hamsters, 100 to 125 g, obtained from Dennen Animal Industries in Gloucester, Massachusetts, were given 7 weekly intra-tracheal instillations of 0.1 µCi ^{210}Po in 0.2 ml saline as described by LITTLE et al. (1970, 1974). 1 or 2 animals were sacrificed 7 days after each instillation, and then weekly following the instillation period for 60 weeks. The present histopathologic observations include animals only up to 25 weeks after the last instillation of ^{210}Po.

Animals were sacrificed by sodium brevital overdose and exsanguination from a renal artery. After puncturing the diaphragm near the apex of the heart, the trachea and collapsed lungs were removed en bloc, wrap-ped in saline-soaked gauze, and evacuated at -740 mm Hg for 10 minutes. The trachea was cannulated with PE 190 polyethylene tubing, and lungs filled at a pressure of 30 cm water with glutaraldehyde fixative (3% glutaraldehyde in TC-199, 1x, Grand Island Biological Company) at pH 7.2. The trachea was occluded and lungs suspended in a glutaraldehyde-filled beaker for 1 hour at room temperature. The lungs were then cut with a scalpel into pieces no larger than 12 x 6 x 2 mm. Tissue sam-ples were cut from the trachea, from each lobe of the lungs in a plane including a longitudinal section of the major bronchus, and from areas suspected of pathology. At least 6 samples were thus taken from each lung. The tissue samples were dehydrated, infiltrated in a desiccator jar evacuated to -740 mm Hg for 1 hour, and embedded in glycol metha-crylate. 1-micron sections were cut on a Sorvall JB-4 microtome (Ivan Sorvall, Norwalk, Connecticut) and stained with hematoxylin-phloxine and PAS-hematoxylin.

Results

4 major types of lesions were seen: 1. acute and subacute inflammation (radiation pneumonitis) which was transient; 2. hyperplasia of bron-chiolar epithelium, particularly of the Clara cells, often associated with focal proliferative lesions involving alveoli (epithelialization of alveoli); 3. extensive multiple areas of epithelialization of al-veoli consisting of a variety of cell types and simulating tumors; and 4. invasive malignant tumors. These lesions were observed in this general sequence, but with a certain amount of overlap.

During the period of administration of ^{210}Po, and for a few weeks thereafter, the sequence of events was as follows. Definite evidence of injury was first observed after the second instillation, whereas only minor irregularities were noted after the first. The changes con-sisted of dilatation of alveolar capillaries, some swelling of alveolar septa, and accumulation of pale pink staining fluid in the alveoli. A few inflammatory cells were scattered about, but the process consisted chiefly of interstitial and alveolar edema. There also appeared to be some loss of alveolar lining cells and of great alveolar cells, and some of the nuclei of septal and great alveolar cells were hyperchromat-ic and irregular. All of these changes were focal in character and other parts of the lung did not differ from controls.

Following further instillations of ^{210}Po, edema became more copious and more inflammatory cells were seen. There were polymorphonuclear leukocytes as well as many mononuclear cells (Fig. 1). Small hemorrhages were noted occasionally and the lesions tended to involve larger areas

of lung tissue. Radiation pneumonitis was especially pronounced after
the fifth, sixth, and seventh instillations. In some specimens, the
exudate consisted chiefly of large mononuclear cells, macrophages,
and cellular debris mixed with a few leukocytes as shown in Fig. 2.
Great alveolar cells, which were diminished in number at earlier intervals, appeared to be more numerous than usual at later intervals and
during the resolution of the pneumonic lesions. They tended to accumulate in small clusters (Fig. 3).

With the exception of a few animals, none of those examined 5 weeks
or more after the last instillation of ^{210}Po showed evidence of radiation pneumonitis or residual earmarks of an earlier pneumonic process,
except for thinning of alveolar septa and focal areas of emphysema.
There was no fibrosis, although a few animals showed an occasional
small subpleural scar.

Nothing unusual was seen in the epithelium of bronchi and bronchioles
during the instillation period except for an increase in the number of
dead or dying cells. It is noteworthy that there was no evidence at
any time of squamous metaplasia of bronchial or bronchiolar epithelium.
5 of the 7 animals sacrificed between 18 and 25 weeks after the last
instillation, however, showed very striking hyperplasia of Clara cells
in large and small bronchioles (Figs 4 through 7). In some instances,
Clara cells were also noted in alveolar regions where they are not
usually seen. Not only were these cells much more numerous than usual,
but they also were considerably larger than normal and variable in
size. They contained large pale nuclei with excessive margination of
chromatin, and many cells showed 2 and sometimes 3 nuclei (Fig. 6).
Some of these cells showed giant nuclei with prominent multiple nucleoli. There also was a change in the nature of the secretion of these
cells as shown by the PAS stain. Clara cell granules ordinarily stain
light pink with this stain, but in the hyperplastic cells these granules stained bright red (Fig. 7). In the extreme case, many bronchioles and terminal airways showed hyperplasia of Clara cells, but in
most of the animals Clara cell hyperplasia was moderate and involved
relatively few bronchioles.

Epithelialization or bronchiolization of alveoli refers to a well-
known condition in which various types of epithelial cells, including
ciliated cells, are found illegitimately to line the surface of alveoli. We have observed this condition in almost all of those animals
sacrificed from 4 to 25 weeks after the last instillation of polonium,
although it was seen as early as 7 days after the second instillation.
Foci of alveolar epithelialization were usually seen in connection
with or adjacent to bronchioles or terminal bronchioles, as shown in
Fig. 8. There were several instances, however, where scattered, isolated foci of epithelial cells were found in the periphery of the lung,
near the pleura, and seemingly not connected with airways, as shown
in Figs 9 and 10. A point worth mentioning in connection with the type
of lesion shown in Figs 9 and 10 is that it occurred in areas of otherwise normal lung tissue.

The number and size of areas of alveolar epithelialization increased
with time after the administration of polonium. This condition was the
predominating pathologic lesion in all animals in the post-instillation
period of the experiment. Increasingly, these lesions exhibited very
active proliferation and migration of cells from one alveolus to another,
and not infrequently the alveolar septa, which serve as a scaffold for
the growth of these cells, were lined by 2 or more layers of cells. An
example of a very actively proliferating, rather aggressive and tumor-
like lesion of this type is shown in Figs 11 and 12. This animal was

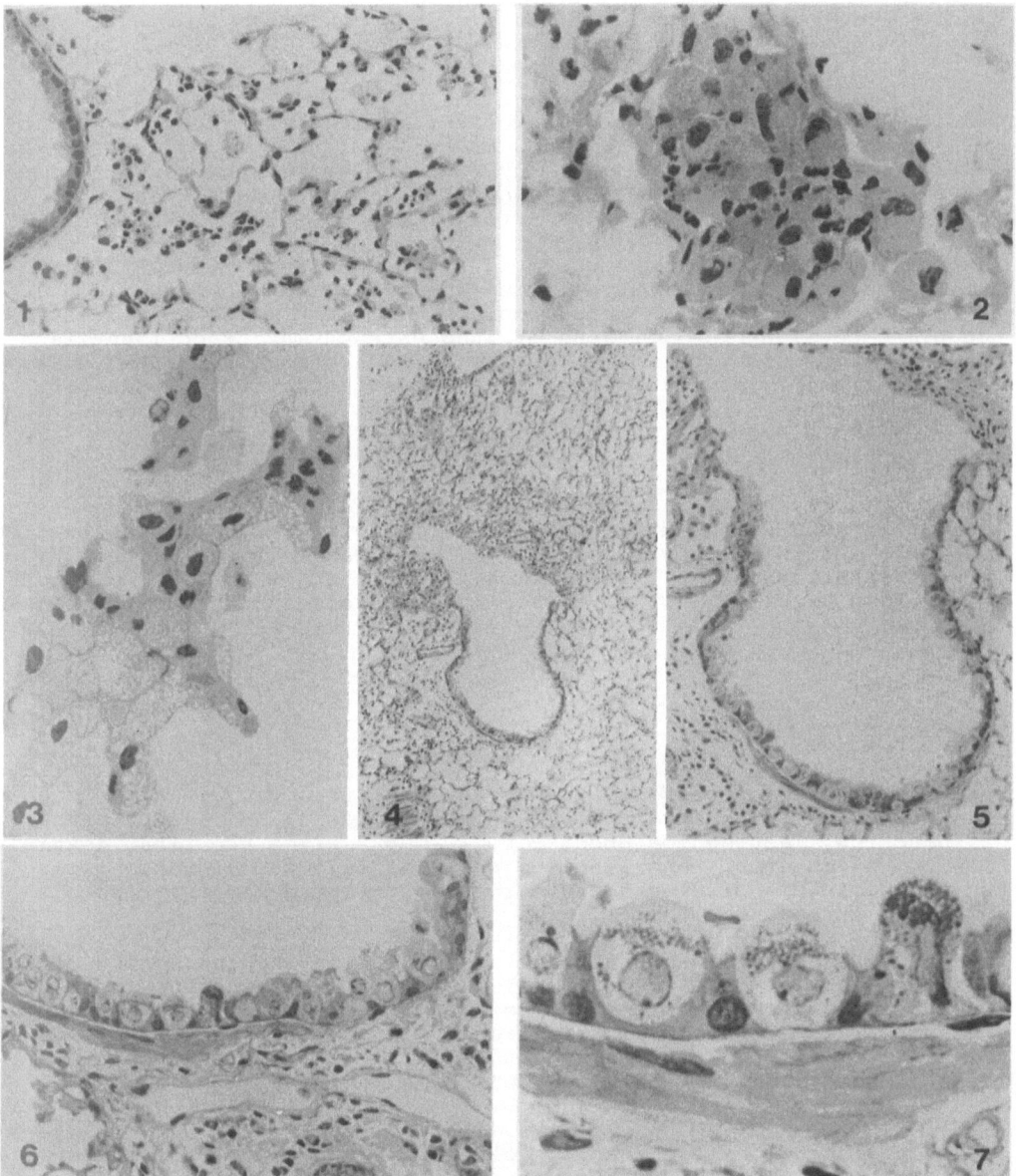

Fig. 1.   Mild radiation pneumonitis showing alveolar exudate with cell debris, leukocytes, and many macrophages. 7 days after fourth ^{210}Po instillation. Hematoxylin-phloxine. (x 84)

Fig. 2.   Alveolar exudate consisting chiefly of large mononuclear cells, macrophages and cellular debris mixed with a few leukocytes. 7 days after fifth ^{210}Po instillation. Hematoxylin-phloxine. (x 338)

Fig. 3.   Accumulation of enlarged great alveolar cells containing increased number of cytosomes. Hematoxylin-phloxine. (x 338)

Fig. 4.   Chronic mild interstitial pneumonitis associated with hyperplasia of Clara cells of dilated terminal bronchiole. 18 weeks after instillation period. Hematoxylin-phloxine. (x 34)

Fig. 5.   Same bronchiole as in Fig. 4 showing numerous Clara cells. Hematoxylin-phloxine. (x 83)

Fig. 6.   Same bronchiole as in Fig. 5 at higher magnification. Note irregular size and shape of Clara cells, several of which contain 2 nuclei. PAS-hematoxylin. (x 169)

Fig. 7.   Higher power view of bronchiolar epithelium shown in Fig. 6. Note atypical Clara cells with numerous PAS positive granules. PAS-hematoxylin. (x 658)

sacrificed 10 weeks after the last instillation of ^{210}Po. The lesion was situated adjacent to a dilated bronchiole and composed of somewhat polymorphous epithelial cells, many of which showed numerous PAS positive cytoplasmic granules secreting abundant mucous-like material into the intervening and adjacent alveolar spaces.

As mentioned earlier, there was a steady progression from well-circumscribed small foci of alveolar epithelialization to larger confluent aggregates of epithelial cells completely filling alveolar spaces and occupying considerable portions of lung parenchyma. Exact identification and classification of the epithelial cells involved in alveolar epithelialization in this series of animals has not been completed. Suffice it to say that we have seen columnar, cuboidal, ciliated, squamous and Clara cells; usually more than 1 cell type was found in any given lesion.

Categorical classification of these very cellular and often aggressive lesions is difficult and problematical, and will require more detailed study and analysis. Provisionally, of the 30 animals sacrificed up to 25 weeks after the last instillation, 7 are thought to have malignant lung tumors (Fig. 13), primarily of combined epidermoid-adenocarcinoma type.

Discussion

The carcinogenic process in the hamster lung following multiple instillations of ^{210}Po may be divided into 2 phases: an initial phase of induction, lasting for about 9 to 10 weeks after the first instillation of the material, and a second phase of cell proliferation which began immediately afterward and effectively lasted for the rest of the life of the animal.

The induction period was characterized by the waxing and waning of radiation-induced inflammatory lesions, e.g., radiation pneumonitis. These changes were transient and left no discernable gross lesions in the lung. The geographic distribution of inflammatory changes could be correlated with the distribution of polonium as determined by autoradiographs and described in the following paper (KENNEDY and LITTLE, 1974).

The second phase, namely that of cell proliferation, was characterized by the gradual emergence of permanent anatomical changes in the lungs. These involved the bronchioles and alveolar tissues. To our knowledge, hyperplasia of Clara cells as seen in our animals has not been described previously. These cells were shown in the autoradiographic studies of KENNEDY and LITTLE (1974) to have received a high dose of alpha radiation as compared to other cells in the bronchiolar epithelium. It is likely that the very active proliferation of Clara cells and the appearance of many atypical cells among them, which was seen at late intervals after the instillations of polonium, was the result of this exposure. The role that these atypical cells may have played in subsequent proliferative processes in the alveoli has not been determined, although such cells could clearly be identified in the complex cellular aggregates characterizing advanced stages of alveolar epithelialization.

Epithelialization of alveoli represents a proliferative response to injury on the part of bronchiolar or alveolar duct epithelium. There

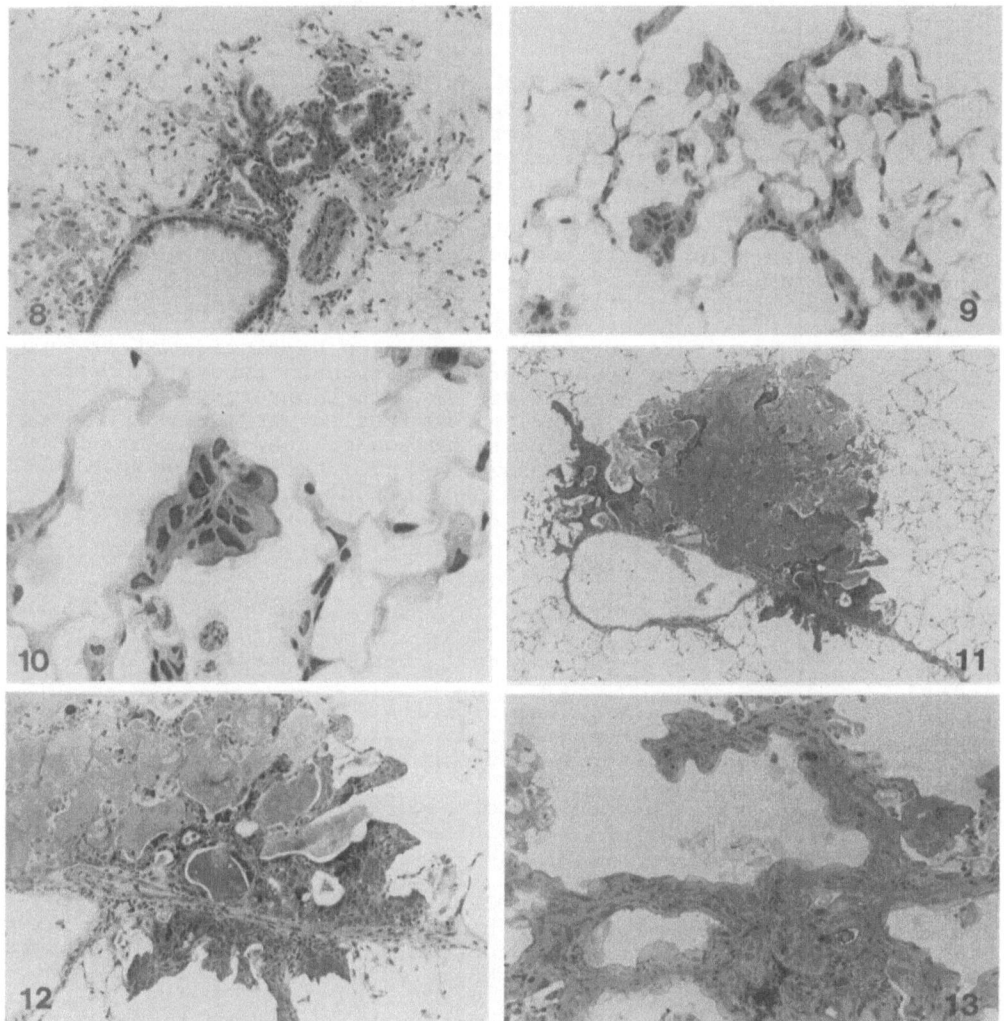

Fig. 8.   Small focus of alveolar epithelialization adjacent to bronchiole. 7 days after fifth ^{210}Po instillation. Hematoxylin-phloxine. (x 84)

Fig. 9.   Scattered foci of epithelial cells lining alveolar septa in periphery of lung. 2 weeks after instillation period. Hematoxylin-phloxine. (x 169)

Fig. 10.   Higher magnification of Fig. 9. Note well-developed cilia on many cells. (x 338)

Fig. 11.   Peribronchiolar, actively proliferating lesion of lung. Note accumulation of PAS positive material spreading into adjacent lung tissue. 10 weeks after ^{210}Po instillation period. PAS-hematoxylin. (x 34)

Fig. 12.   Higher power view of Fig. 11. (x 84)

Fig. 13.   Carcinoma of lung showing distortion of pulmonary parenchyma and many tumor cells containing PAS positive granules. 20 weeks after instillation period. PAS-hematoxylin. (x 84)

is evidence that in some instances alveolar epithelialization is due to extension and migration of bronchiolar epithelium into adjacent alveoli (NETTESHEIM and SZAKAL, 1972), but the possibility has not been excluded that under certain conditions, epithelialization may occur through a process of special differentiation of autochthonous

alveolar epithelium. The condition has been observed in human lungs
and in experimental animals as a result of a variety of insults including noxious gases, chemical irritants, carcinogens (including
radiation) and prolonged respiratory infections. The exact pathogenesis of the condition is not clear.

Alveolar epithelialization was the predominating feature in practical-
ly all of the animals sacrificed between 4 and 25 weeks after the
last ^{210}Po instillation. Different types of epithelial cells were
found in these lesions - ciliated, squamous, and Clara cells among
them. The exact development of alveolar epithelialization, under
the conditions of this experiment, remains to be elucidated in future
studies. There is little doubt that the malignant tumors which were
seen in this and earlier experiments in this laboratory, arose from
preexisting areas of alveolar epithelialization. It is likely that,
as in other types of carcinogenesis, malignant lung tumors emerge
as a result of a stepwise progression of qualitative changes (FOULDS,
1969) - in this case, the progression from the ectopic epithelial
cells in the alveolar tissue to frank carcinomas.

References

FOULDS, L.: Neoplastic development. London-New York: Academic Press
    1969.
KENNEDY, A.R., LITTLE, J.B.: Cellular localization of intratracheally
    administered ^{210}Po in the hamster lung using autoradiography of
    thin sections from plastic embedded tissue. In: These Proceedings.
LITTLE, J.B., GROSSMAN, B.N., O'TOOLE, W.F.: Respiratory carcino-
    genesis in hamsters induced by polonium-210 alpha radiation and
    benzo(a)pyrene. In: Morphology of Experimental Respiratory Carcino-
    genesis (P.Nettesheim, M.G. Hanna, Jr., J.W. Deatherage, Jr., eds).
    AEC Symposium Series 21, 383-392 (1970).
LITTLE, J.B., GROSSMAN, B.N., O'TOOLE, W.F.: Factors influencing
    the induction of lung cancer in hamsters by intratracheal administra-
    tion of polonium-210. In: Radionuclide Carcinogenesis (C.L. Sanders,
    R.H. Busch, J.E. Ballou, D.D. Mahlum, eds). AEC Symposium Series
    29, 119-137 (1973).
LITTLE, J.B., O'TOOLE, W.F.: Respiratory tract tumors in hamsters
    induced by benzo(a)pyrene and polonium-210 alpha radiation. Cancer
    Res., in press.
NETTESHEIM, P., SZAKAL, A.K.: Morphogenesis of alveolar bronchioliza-
    tion. Lab. Invest. 26, 210-219 (1972).

Cellular Localization of Intratracheally Administered ^{210}PO in the Hamster Lung Using Autoradiography of Thin Sections from Plastic Embedded Tissue*

Ann R. Kennedy and John B. Little

Department of Physiology, Harvard School of Public Health, Boston, MA 02115, USA

ABSTRACT

The cellular localization of polonium-210 (^{210}Po), given intratracheally either alone in saline or adsorbed onto ferric oxide carrier particles, has been studied using autoradiography of 1 μm sections from glycol methacrylate embedded tissue. Within the first week after instillation, ^{210}Po administered in saline was localized in the alveolar region primarily in type 1 epithelial - endothelial cells and macrophages, and to a lesser extent in great alveolar cells. In the larger airways, ^{210}Po was localized primarily in ciliated and Clara cells. Following administration adsorbed onto ferric oxide carrier particles, ^{210}Po was found primarily in alveolar macrophages surrounding respiratory bronchioles and alveolar ducts.

^{210}Po localization in relation to the pathologic changes reported in the previous paper (LISCO et al., these Proceedings) is presented here. At later times, significant numbers of alpha tracks were found in the lesions, but they were almost entirely absent in areas of the lung which appeared to be normal.

Introduction

We have previously shown polonium-210 (^{210}Po), an alpha emitter, to be a potent lung carcinogen in Syrian golden hamsters when given alone in saline or adsorbed onto ferric oxide carrier particles as a series of 7 or 15 weekly intratracheal instillations (LITTLE et al., 1970, 1973, 1974). We have been studying the transport and localization of ^{210}Po in the lung: the regional distribution by freeze-dry, frozen section autoradiography to avoid translocation of the carcinogen (KENNEDY and LITTLE, 1974a), and the distribution by cell type within a region by plastic (glycol methacrylate) section autoradiography.

The results of the freeze-dry study for regional localization will not be presented here, but may be summarized as follows: following intratracheal administration, ^{210}Po-saline was diffusely distributed throughout the peripheral lung, while the distribution of ^{210}Po ferric oxide was nonhomogeneous, with "hot spots" massively irradiating respiratory bronchiole and alveolar duct regions only. In either case, the major dose of radiation was to the peripheral lung, the site where

*Supported by Contract CP-33273 from the National Cancer Institute and NIH Grant ES-00002.

tumors develop. Most of the ^{210}Po given in saline solution was deposited in the alveolar region, with clearance being primarily via the airways and blood stream. The airway clearance had 2 components: 1. an early phase of extracellular ^{210}Po clearance that took place within the first 8 hrs after an intratracheal instillation and 2. a later phase of clearance from the alveolar region involving the movement of macrophages that had engulfed ^{210}Po. These macrophages migrate to the mucous ciliary escalator, which carries them out of the lung. This late phase reached a peak at 2 to 5 days after a single intratracheal instillation. The statistical methods used to determine the above results will be described elsewhere.

After intratracheal instillation, most of the ^{210}Po ferric oxide was deposited on the ciliated epithelium of the large airways, although some reached the respiratory bronchiole and alveolar duct regions where it settled into the proximal alveoli (KENNEDY and LITTLE, 1974b). Most of the ^{210}Po ferric oxide deposited on the mucous ciliary escalator was rapidly cleared from the lung (within the first day), whereas ^{210}Po ferric oxide reaching the respiratory bronchiole and alveolar duct regions was trapped in the cup-shaped alveolar structures where it was phagocytized by macrophages. These alveolar macrophages may remain *in situ* for a long period of time, or migrate to the terminal bronchiole where they are carried upward on the mucous ciliary escalator.

In the present report, the results of the cellular localization study utilizing thin plastic sections will be presented. We will try to correlate the localization of ^{210}Po and the resultant distribution of radiation dose with the early pathologic changes that were described by LISCO et al. (these Proceedings).

Materials and Methods

Male Syrian golden hamsters, 100 to 125 g (Dennen Animal Industries, Gloucester, Massachusetts), were given single or multiple intratracheal instillations of 0.1 µCi ^{210}Po in 0.2 ml saline or of 0.1 µCi ^{210}Po bound to 3 mg ferric oxide particles suspended in 0.2 ml saline as described by LITTLE et al. (1970, 1974). The sacrifice schedule for the animals following a single instillation of ^{210}Po-saline or ^{210}Po ferric oxide was as follows (2 animals per time): immediately following the instillation, and hourly for the first 6 hrs, at 12 hrs; daily for the first week; and at 1, 2, 4, and 8 months. For multiple instillations, animals were sacrificed at 7 days after each instillation, then weekly thereafter until 34 weeks, and then monthly up to 60 weeks after the instillation period.

Animals were sacrificed and tissues prepared as described by LISCO et al. (these Proceedings). Sections were cut at 1 µm on a Sorvall JB-4 microtome (Ivan Sorvall, Norwalk, Connecticut), stained with PAS, dipped into undiluted Kodak NTB-3 autoradiographic emulsion, exposed at 4°C for 6 months to 2 years (depending on the length of time elapsed since ^{210}Po instillation), developed, and stained with hematoxylin.

Results

<u>Loss of radioactivity in plastic sections: comparison of freeze-dried</u>
<u>and plastic section autoradiographs.</u> The plastic section technique
utilizes many tissue processing fluids that could remove the ^{210}Po
from the lungs or translocate the carcinogen and result in a false
redistribution of activity. The very different exposure times required
for freeze-dried and plastic section lung autoradiographs (0.5 to
30 days vs 6 to 24 months) prepared from animals sacrificed at the
same time after ^{210}Po-saline instillation indicates that a substantial
fraction of the ^{210}Po was lost in the processing fluids used in the
preparation of plastic sections. To obtain a rough estimate of the
amount of ^{210}Po washed out by the plastic section technique, the total
number of alpha tracks in the same histologic structures was counted
in both freeze-dried and plastic sections and corrected for exposure
time, radioactive decay, and tissue section thickness (freeze-dried
sections were 4 μm). When sacrifices were made soon after instillation (0 to 2 hrs), 99% of the radioactivity was lost in plastic sections compared to freeze-dried sections. The amount of ^{210}Po lost
progressively decreased with time, but still remained at 86% 1 month
after instillation.

This loss of ^{210}Po from the tissue during processing raised the question
as to whether the results of a plastic section localization study would
be meaningful. To determine whether there had been a selective loss of
^{210}Po by a particular histologic region in the lung, total alpha tracks
were counted in 100 epithelial cells for each major region (trachea,
bronchi, bronchioles, and alveoli), and the ratios of counts made on
plastic and freeze-dried sections compared. It was found that the ratios
derived from the 2 methods of processing were comparable for the times
studied, up to 1 week after ^{210}Po instillation. At later times, most
of the activity was localized in the alveolar region for both freeze-
dried and plastic sections. Thus, our results give no indication that
there is a selective loss of ^{210}Po from particular tissues or cell
populations in the lungs due to the liquid processing procedure.

^{210}Po-saline: All of the alpha tracks were counted in sections from
the major regions of each lung at each time period. The tracks were
furthermore identified as originating in specific cell types in the
trachea, bronchi, bronchioles, alveoli, and the blood and lymph. The
percent of tracks in a given cell type (tracks in a cell type per
total tracks counted) was determined in each section for each time.
The percent of cell types in each slide was not determined. Since,
at the light microscope level, type 1 epithelial cells are very
difficult to distinguish from endothelial cells in the alveolar
region, these 2 cell types were counted together (Fig. 2 below).

During the first week after a single ^{210}Po instillation and during
the period of multiple instillations, alpha tracks were found in all
regions of the lung. Beyond 1 week, after either single or multiple
instillations, alpha tracks were found only in the alveolar region
and occasionally in the bronchioles. Only rarely were tracks ever
seen in the trachea; these were present in the connective tissue
and ciliated epithelial cells. In the bronchi, the muscle and connective tissue contained variable amounts of activity. Within the epithelium, goblet cells contained a negligible amount of ^{210}Po, and
basal cells only occasionally contained alpha tracks. Most of the
alpha tracks were found in ciliated and Clara-type cells, even though
relatively few of these Clara-type cells were present in the bronchial
epithelium. (It was not clear at the light microscope level whether

these were true Clara cells in the bronchi; electron microscopic
studies will be done in the future to establish their identity.)
In the bronchioles, the muscle and connective tissue contained variable amounts of activity. Within the epithelium, Clara cells consistently contained more activity than ciliated cells. In fact, Clara
cells contained a sizable fraction of the total tracks counted in
any section (Fig. 1). In the alveolar region, alpha tracks were found
primarily in type 1 epithelial-endothelial cells (Fig. 2) and in macrophages (Figs 3 and 4), although occasional tracks were found in great
alveolar cells (Fig. 5). Occasional tracks were also found in interstitial cells (Fig. 6), most of which were probably macrophages. The
few ^{210}Po aggregates or sunbursts (Fig. 3) usually occurred in macrophages. They appear to become disorganized, or no longer radiate from
a single point (Fig. 4), a few days after the ^{210}Po instillation.
A similar finding was reported by CASARETT and MORROW (1964).

The blood and blood vessel walls showed variable amounts of activity
as long as 4 months after a single instillation of ^{210}Po-saline. The
alpha tracks usually appeared to originate from red blood cells. The
lymph contained a negligible fraction of the ^{210}Po except in a few
animals, and in only 1 animal was activity found in the tracheobronchial lymph nodes.

In general, very few alpha tracks remained in the lungs for more than
a few weeks after multiple instillations of ^{210}Po-saline. Those remaining were usually in type 1 epithelial-endothelial cells, macrophages, or in the blood. In addition, however, residual alpha tracks
were also associated with foci of atypical great alveolar cells (Fig.
7), areas of hyperplastic Clara cells (Fig. 8), areas of "epithelialization of alveoli" (NETTESHEIM and SZAKAL, 1972; LISCO et al., 1974),
and with hyperplastic foci of epithelial cells in which they occurred
in large numbers (Fig. 9). As described in LISCO et al. (these Proceedings), these cellular changes all appear to be associated with the
development of malignant tumors in ^{210}Po treated animals. Alpha tracks
were also scattered apparently at random throughout the tumors which
developed (Fig. 10). Interestingly, lungs in which these pathologic
lesions were observed were remarkably free of alpha tracks in areas
that appeared histologically normal. There were also lungs in which
no alpha activity was found, but when present it was highly correlated with the lesions.

In a preliminary experiment designed to study the proliferation rates
of cells in normal hamsters as compared to ^{210}Po treated hamsters,
tritiated thymidine was injected ip to normal control animals and to
animals which had received 7 weekly ^{210}Po instillations 60 weeks previously; the animals were sacrificed 2 hrs to 4 weeks after injection,
autoradiographs prepared, and labeled nuclei scored as a measure of
proliferative activity. The cellular proliferation rates in the alveolar
region of the ^{210}Po-treated animals (Fig. 11) were markedly greater
than in comparable controls, both in pathologic areas and in foci of
normal appearing cells. We plan to initiate a serial sacrifice experiment after ^{210}Po instillations using the tritiated thymidine method
to determine the increase in proliferation rates of specific cell
types with time.

^{210}Po ferric oxide: All alpha tracks in slides from animals sacrificed
at 1 hr and 2 days after ^{210}Po ferric oxide instillation were counted.
For the rest of the times studied, only "ionic" ^{210}Po alpha tracks
not associated with visible ferric oxide particles were counted. The
same cell types were scored as for ^{210}Po-saline animals, and the percent of tracks per cell type was determined.

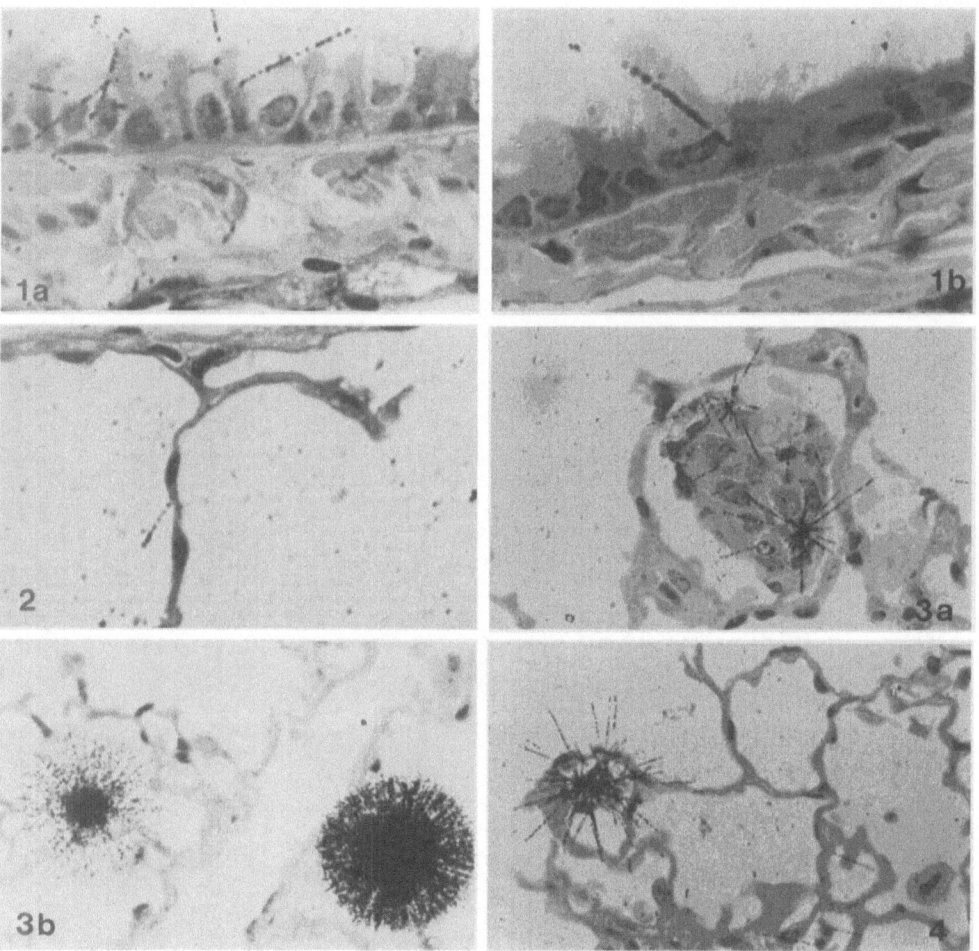

Fig. 1 a and b. Alpha tracks in Clara cells in bronchiolar epithelium.
(a) ^{210}Po-saline, 7 days after fourth instillation. PAS-hematoxylin.
(x 675). (b) High power view of alpha track originating in Clara cell.
PAS-hematoxylin. (x 845)

Fig. 2. Alpha track originating from type 1 epithelial-endothelial
cell in alveolar region. ^{210}Po-saline, 12 hours after instillation.
PAS-hematoxylin. (x 675)

Fig. 3. (a) Clump of macrophages from which alpha tracks originate.
^{210}Po-saline, 2 days after instillation. PAS-hematoxylin. (x 338).
(b) Alpha track "sunbursts" (^{210}Po aggregates). ^{210}Po-saline,
after instillation. PAS-hematoxylin. (x 338)

Fig. 4. Alpha track sunburst (in macrophage) becoming "disorganized
Note that tracks are not radiating from a single point. ^{210}Po-saline,
3 days after instillation. PAS-hematoxylin. (x 338)

480

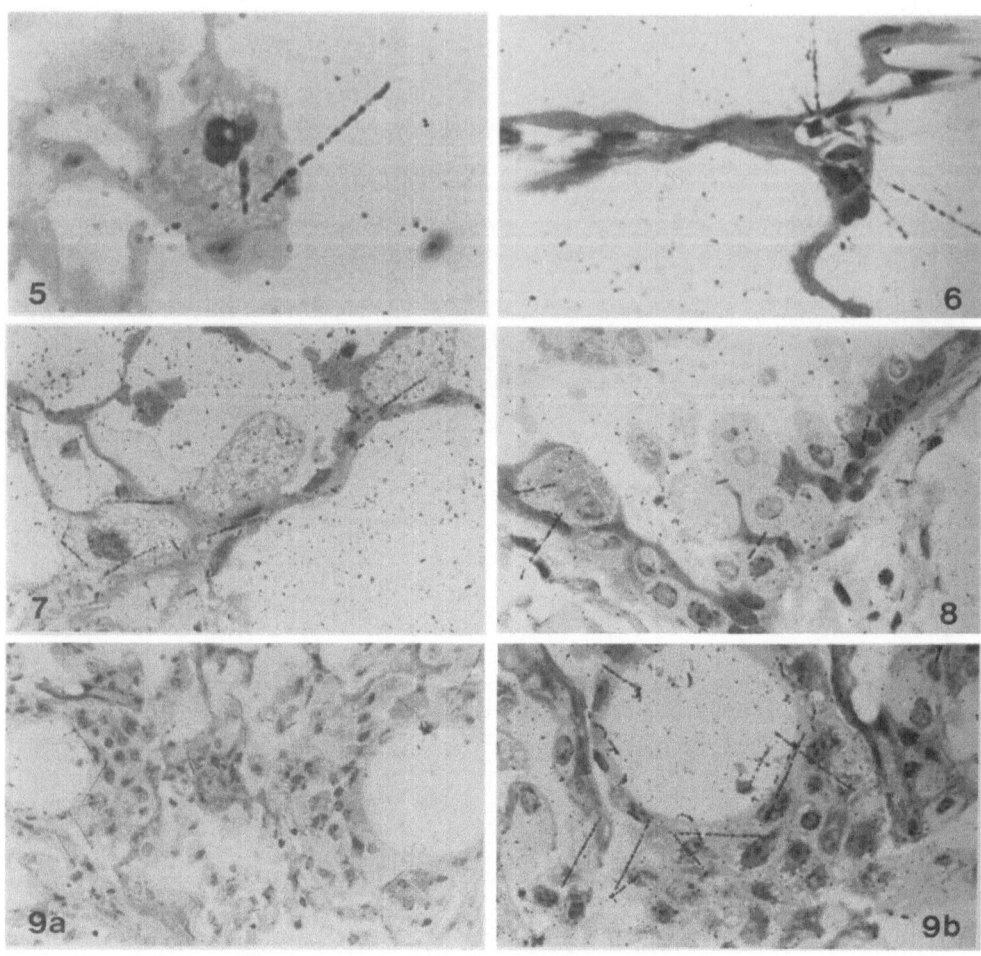

Fig. 5. High power view of great alveolar cell with 2 alpha tracks.
^{210}Po-saline, 7 days after instillation. PAS-hematoxylin. (x 845)

Fig. 6. Interstitial cell, probably a macrophage, with alpha tracks.
^{210}Po-saline, 12 hours after instillation. PAS-hematoxylin. (x 675)

Fig. 7. Focus of atypical great alveolar cells with alpha tracks.
^{210}Po-saline, 7 weeks post instillation period. PAS-hematoxylin.
(x 338)

Fig. 8. Atypical Clara cells in bronchiole with alpha tracks. ^{210}Po-saline, 18 weeks post instillation period. PAS-hematoxylin. (x 338)

Fig. 9 a and b. Alpha tracks originating from hyperplastic focus of
epithelial cells in alveolar region. (a) ^{210}Po-saline, 12 weeks post
instillation period. PAS-hematoxylin. (x 169). (b) Higher power view
of hyperplastic epithelial cell focus shown in 9a. PAS-hematoxylin.
(x 338)

From the analysis of the ^{210}Po ferric oxide slides, it was obvious that most of the activity at any time studied was in macrophages in respiratory bronchiole and alveolar duct regions. Actually, ^{210}Po ferric oxide is also initially deposited on the mucous sheet in the larger airways (KENNEDY and LITTLE, 1974b), but the processing fluids necessary for the preparation of plastic sections washed out all of this superficial material in the larger airways. Of the ^{210}Po ferric oxide remaining in the lungs processed for plastic sections at 1 hr after instillation, 75% was in macrophages. The total amount in macrophages increased to 94% by 2 days after a single instillation. Almost all of the remaining 25% of the activity at 1 hr was found lining the respiratory bronchiole and alveolar duct areas as patches of ^{210}Po ferric oxide (Fig. 12) not yet phagocytized by any cell. The first few alveoli of the respiratory bronchioles and alveolar ducts seemed to collect the ferric oxide: first as patches of ^{210}Po ferric oxide (Fig. 12), then later as clumps of macrophages filled with ^{210}Po ferric oxide (Figs 13 and 14). Patches of ^{210}Po ferric oxide were not seen in the peripheral alveolar areas of the lung, but occasional tracks were seen in these areas as "ionic" ^{210}Po (that is ^{210}Po either not bound to ferric oxide or bound to submicroscopic particles of ferric oxide). The distribution of alpha tracks not attached to ferric oxide particles was very much like that of ^{210}Po-saline. The effect of giving several instillations of ^{210}Po ferric oxide to animals was to increase the number of single tracks in the lung parenchyma with each successive instillation. With time, more and more ionic ^{210}Po (single alpha tracks) appeared in the same cell types as in the ^{210}Po-saline animals.

Discussion

The results of the thin plastic section localization study indicate that following administration in saline solution, ^{210}Po is distributed throughout the peripheral lung, while ^{210}Po ferric oxide is localized primarily in aggregates surrounding respiratory bronchioles and alveolar ducts. This difference in distribution of activity leads to a homogeneous diffuse radiation dose to the entire bronchiolar-alveolar region of the lung following ^{210}Po-saline administration, whereas ^{210}Po ferric oxide results in a concentration of activity in discrete areas of the lung, leading to the distribution of radiation dose in "hot spots". Much consideration has been given to "hot spots" vs diffuse radiation as being the more effective for the induction of cancer. Previous experiments done in our laboratory (LITTLE et al., 1973) indicated that diffuse radiation (^{210}Po-saline) was at least as effective as hot spot (^{210}Po ferric oxide) radiation. The work presented here suggests that ^{210}Po-saline may be more effective owing to the distribution of radiation dose among cell types. Macrophages, shown to be relatively radioresistant (GILMAN and TROWELL, 1965; JORDAN, 1967; KORNFELD and GREENMAN, 1966), receive the bulk of the radiation dose from ^{210}Po ferric oxide. In the serial sacrifice tumor induction study (LISCO et al., 1974), there was no histologic evidence that macrophages had malignant potential. Thus, with ^{210}Po ferric oxide, much of the radiation energy is deposited in cells not involved in the development of tumors. With ^{210}Po-saline, on the other hand, all cell types in the peripheral lung share in the radiation exposure, among them, the cell or cells of origin of the tumors.

Although it is very difficult to identify the exact cell of origin of the tumors, distinct morphologic changes do occur in specific cell

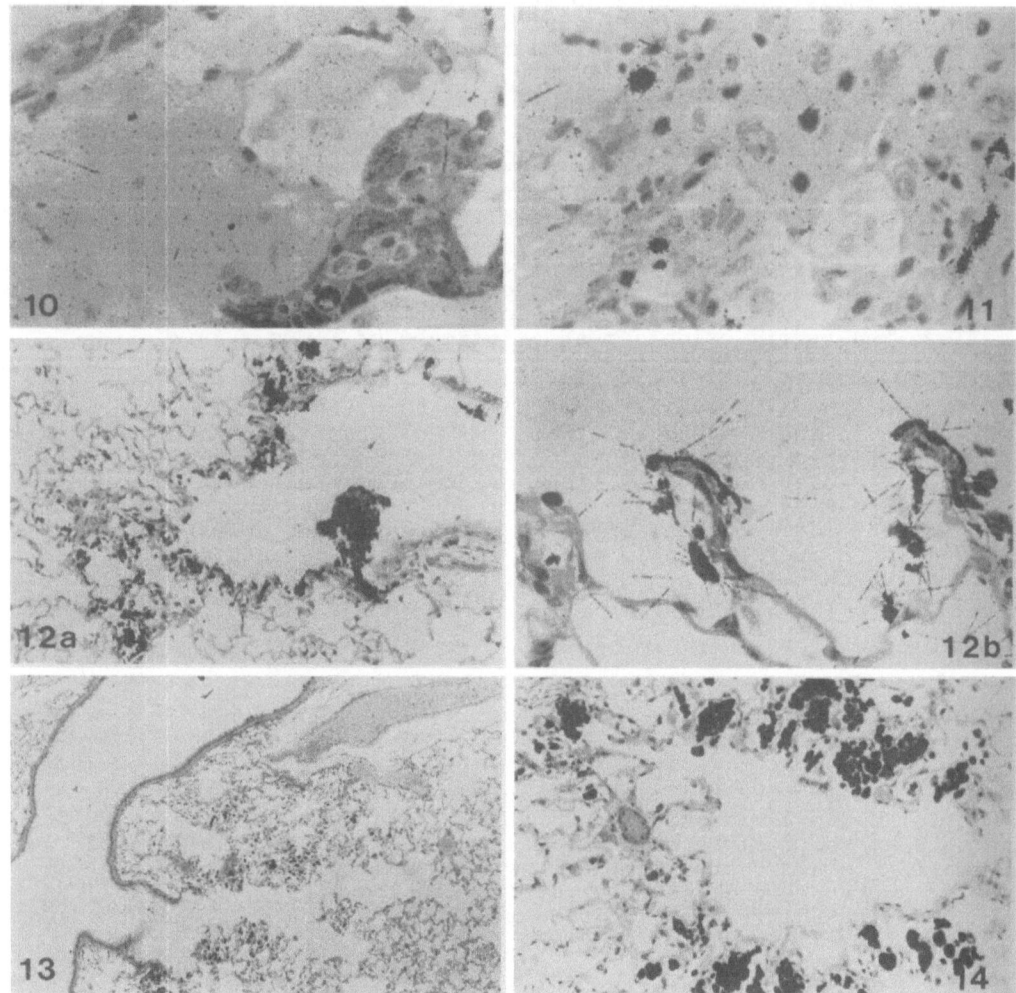

Fig. 10. Alpha tracks originating from tumor area described in LISCO et al. (these Proceedings). (Figs 11 and 12). ^{210}Po-saline, 10 weeks post instillation period. Alpha tracks can be seen originating from the epithelial cells (right center) and within the PAS positive material (center left). PAS-hematoxylin. (x 338)

Fig. 11. Proliferating lesion in alveolar region of ^{210}Po-saline tumor bearing animal showing that cells have taken up tritiated thymidine (grains) in areas where ^{210}Po alpha tracks are present. Note tuft of cells resembling bronchiolar epithelium (top center). ^{210}Po-saline, 60 weeks post instillation period. Animal sacrificed 2 hrs after ^{3}H-T (ip) injection. PAS-hematoxylin. (x 338)

Fig. 12 a and b. Alveolar duct region immediately after an instillation of ^{210}Po ferric oxide. (a) Ferric oxide film on surface of alveoli, and clump of macrophages containing ^{210}Po ferric oxide between alveolar duct and terminal bronchiole. PAS-hematoxylin. (x 84). (b) Higher power view of alveolar duct region. PAS-hematoxylin. (x 338)

types after instillation of ^{210}Po (LISCO et al., 1974). In the pathologic study of animals receiving ^{210}Po-saline, for example, the great
alveolar cell showed the most obvious changes. It responded to the
radiation fairly early (within 7 days after the second instillation)
with hypertrophy, hyperplasia, and an increased number of lipid-filled
cytoplasmic inclusions. Whether this response of the great alveolar
cell is really due to ^{210}Po is a matter of speculation: a similar
response of the great alveolar cell has been reported in response to
noncarcinogenic irritants (SHORTER, 1970; YUEN and SHERWIN, 1971).
Interestingly, the great alveolar cell did not particularly localize
^{210}Po when compared to other alveolar cells.

On the other hand, alpha tracks were notably concentrated in the Clara
cells in the bronchioles; these Clara cells showed a striking proliferative response to the treatment (LISCO et al., 1974). Although the
response was not an immediate one, the Clara cell appears to play a
later role in the development of premalignant changes and frank tumors.
As Clara cell hyperplasia is not known to be a response to irritation,
it is most likely due specifically to the radiation.

The 2 cell types in the lung which contained the most activity after
^{210}Po-saline instillation, macrophages and type 1 epithelial-endothelial cells, did not appear to undergo morphologic change. Macrophages take up most of the ^{210}Po ferric oxide and a large portion of
the ^{210}Po-saline, but do not appear to show morphological evidence
of radiation damage. The type 1 epithelial-endothelial cells also remained relatively unchanged during the course of ^{210}Po instillations.
Even though they appeared to be grossly intact, their permeability
must have been changed to result in the edema found in the pathological
analysis of the slides (LISCO et al., 1974). Future work will include
electron microscope autoradiographic studies to determine whether it
is the type 1 epithelial cell or the endothelial cell in the alveolar
region which take up the major fraction of the ^{210}Po. There is some
evidence that type 1 epithelial cells are phagocytic and take up
^{239}Pu (SANDERS and ADEE, 1970).

Whether a cell actually localizes ^{210}Po may not be the important factor in carcinogenesis. A cell can receive alpha radiation from ^{210}Po
localized in another cell type. Secondary irradiation may be more carcinogenic to either cell than if the alpha particle deposits its full
5.3 Mev in 1 cell. BARENDSON (1962) maintains that a direct nuclear
hit from an alpha particle should kill a cell: the energy that is
deposited is all that is necessary to stop cell division. An alpha
particle grazing the nucleus may sublethally damage a cell without
interfering with mitosis: these are the cells which most likely give
rise to neoplastic growth (BEVAN and HAQUE, 1968).

In conclusion, the plastic section ^{210}Po localization study has
demonstrated that most of the activity is deposited and retained in

Fig. 13. Low power view of lung 7 days after the third instillation
of ^{210}Po ferric oxide. Note that ^{210}Po ferric oxide extends only a
short distance into the respiratory bronchiole and alveolar duct regions and is absent in the rest of the lung parenchyma. PAS-hematoxylin.
(x 34)

Fig. 14. Alveolar duct region seen in cross section. Note presence of
macrophages containing ferric oxide in the alveolar duct region. ^{210}Po
ferric oxide, 7 days after instillation. (Not an autoradiograph.)
PAS-hematoxylin. (x 84)

cells in the peripheral lung, the site where the pathologic lesions occurred (LISCO et al., 1974). In the bronchioles, alpha tracks were found primarily associated with Clara cells, and it is noteworthy that LISCO et al. (1974) observed marked morphological changes in these Clara cells. Another interesting finding was that alpha activity was clearly associated with the cells that showed early pathologic changes, as well as with hyperplastic foci of epithelial cells and other later pathologic lesions.

References

BARENDSON, G.W.: Dose survival curves of human cells in tissue culture irradiated with alpha-, beta-, 20 kv, X- and 200 kv irradiation. Nature 193, 1153-1155 (1962).
BEVAN, J.S., HAQUE, A.K.M.M.: Some speculations on the carcinogenic effect of inhaled alpha active material. Phys. Med. Biol. 13, 105-112 (1968).
CASARETT, L.J., MORROW, P.E.: Distribution and excretion of polonium-210. XI. Autoradiographic studies after intratracheal administration in the rabbit. Rad. Res. Suppl. 5, 175-186 (1964).
GILMAN, R., TROWELL, O.R.: The effect of radiation on the activity of reticuloendothelial cells in organ cultures of lymph node and thymus. Intern. J. Radiation Biol. 9, 313-322 (1965).
JORDAN, S.W.: Ultrastructure studies of spleen after whole body irradiation of mice. Exp. Mol. Pathol. 6, 156-171 (1967).
KENNEDY, A.R., LITTLE, J.B.: Autoradiography using dry-mounted, freeze-dried sections for localization of carcinogens in the lung. J. Histochem. Cytochem. 22, 361-367 (1974a).
KENNEDY, A.R., LITTLE, J.B.: The transport and localization of benzo-(a)pyrene-hematite and ^{210}Po-hematite in the hamster lung following intratracheal instillation. Cancer Res. 34, 1344-1352 (1974b).
KORNFELD, L., GREENMAN, U.: Effects of total body X-irradiation on peritoneal cells of mice. Rad. Res. 29, 433-444 (1966).
LITTLE, J.B., GROSSMAN, B.N., O'TOOLE, W.F.: Respiratory carcinogenesis in hamsters induced by polonium-210 alpha radiation and benzo(a)pyrene. In: Morphology of Experimental Respiratory Carcinogenesis (P. Nettesheim, M.G. Hanna, Jr., J.W. Deatherage, eds). AEC Symposium Series 21, 383-392 (1970).
LITTLE, J.B., GROSSMAN, B.N., O'TOOLE, W.F.: Factors influencing the induction of lung cancer in hamsters by intratracheal administration of polonium-210. In: Radionuclide Carcinogenesis (C.L. Sanders, R.H. Busch, J.E. Ballou, D.D. Mahlum, eds). AEC Symposium Series 29, 119-137 (1973).
LITTLE, J.B., O'TOOLE, W.F.: Respiratory tract tumors in hamsters induced by benzo(a)pyrene and polonium-210 alpha radiation. Cancer Res., in press.
LISCO, H., KENNEDY, A.R., LITTLE, J.B.: Histologic observations on the pathogenesis of lung cancer in hamsters following administration of polonium-210. These Proceedings 1974.
NETTESHEIM, P., SZAKAL, A.K.: Morphogenesis of alveolar bronchiolization. Lab. Invest. 26, 210-219 (1972).
SANDERS, L.L., ADEE, R.R.: Ultrastructural localization of inhaled ^{239}PuO$_2$ particles in alveolar epithelium and macrophages. Health Phys. 18, 293-294 (1970).
SHORTER, R.G.: Cell kinetics of respiratory tissues, both normal and stimulated. In: Morphology of experimental Respiratory Carcinogenesis (P. Nettesheim, M.G. Hanna, Jr., J.W. Deatherage, Jr., eds). AEC Symposium Series 21, 45-57 (1970).
YUEN, T.G.H., SHERWIN, R.P.: Hyperplasia of type 2 pneumocytes and nitrogen dioxide (10 ppm) exposure. A quantitation based on election micrographs. Arch. Environ. Hlth 22, 178-188 (1971).

Experimental Respiratory Carcinogenesis: Interaction between Alpha Radiation and Benzo (a) pyrene in the Hamster*

Robert B. McGandy, Ann R. Kennedy, Margaret Terzaghi, and John B. Little

Department of Physiology, Harvard School of Public Health, Boston, MA 02115, USA

ABSTRACT

We have previously shown that a high incidence of lung cancer can be induced in hamsters by multiple intratracheal instillations of either benzo(a)pyrene (BaP) or polonium-210 (^{210}Po). The present experiments have used low doses of these 2 carcinogens, singly and together, in simultaneous and sequential designs. In terms of unequivocal lung tumors, 15 weekly instillations of ^{210}Po (total 0.05 μCi) and BaP (total 4.5 mg) given simultaneously on the same carrier particles induced twice the prevalence of lung tumors expected from the additive effect of either carcinogen alone. In a separate experiment, a single instillation of 0.04 μCi ^{210}Po led to only 1 tumor in 139 animals (0.7%) in contrast to 23 tumors among 135 animals (17%) when it was followed 18 weeks later by 7 weekly instillations of BaP (total 2.1 mg). These results suggest synergistic action between alpha radiation and BaP in the induction of lung cancer.

Introduction

Ionizing radiation is known to be a potent initiator of cancer in most tissues of most species tested, and alpha radiation from inspired radon daughter products has been shown to be a cause of the very high mortality rate from lung cancer in the Colorado Plateau uranium miners (WAGONER et al., 1965). Interestingly, however, a significant excess of lung cancer deaths has been found only among those miners who were also cigarette smokers (LUNDIN et al., 1971). Alpha radiation has also been implicated as a cofactor in the increased lung cancer mortality found among the West Cumberland ferric oxide miners in England (BOYD et al., 1970). The naturally occurring alpha-emitting radioisotope polonium-210 (^{210}Po) is present in cigarette smoke and has been shown to accumulate in areas of the bronchial epithelium of cigarette smokers (LITTLE et al., 1965). Recently, MARTELL (1974) has shown that lead-210 (the parent isotope of ^{210}Po) is present in tobacco smoke in the form of very high specific activity "hot" particles, which may penetrate the bronchial epithelium and lead to the accumulation of high local concentrations of ^{210}Po. The alpha particle from ^{210}Po has an energy and path length (37 μm) similar to those of the radon daughters.

*Supported by Contract CP-33273 from the National Cancer Institute and Grants DT-37B from the American Cancer Society and ES-00002 from the National Institute of Environmental Health Sciences.

Although the radiation dose from ^{210}Po in the epithelium of smokers appears to be too small to explain by itself the observed lung cancer incidence in smokers, the alpha radiation could well be acting as an important cocarcinogen with known chemical components of cigarette smoke. That this may occur is actually suggested by the epidemiologic evidence of a synergistic effect between alpha radiation and cigarette smoke in the Colorado Plateau miners.

The fact that human populations are continuously exposed to these carcinogens emphasizes the importance of studying the interactions between alpha radiation and chemical carcinogens in the pathogenesis of experimental lung cancer. During the past 3 years we have developed a model system with which we can consistently produce a high incidence of respiratory cancers in hamsters with either ^{210}Po or BaP along (LITTLE et al., 1970, 1973, 1974). This system involves multiple intratracheal instillations of the carcinogen adsorbed onto ferric oxide particles in the manner originally described by SAFFIOTTI and coworkers (SAFFIOTTI et al., 1968).

The present series of experiments has used low levels of these 2 carcinogens, singly and together, in a design aimed at investigating synergistic effects.

Materials and Methods

Male golden Syrian hamsters (Dennen Animal Industries, Gloucester, Massachusetts) were utilized. This species is not only resistant to acute and chronic inflammatory lung diseases but has an essentially zero incidence of spontaneous respiratory tumors (LITTLE et al., 1970; SAFFIOTTI et al., 1968). The animals were caged individually in a controlled-environment animal room.

Ferric oxide particles (98% with a diameter less than 0.75 μm) were used as carrier particles. Previous studies (LITTLE et al., 1970, 1973) have shown that these particles do not have a carcinogenic or cocarcinogenic effect in themselves. The adsorption of ^{210}Po and BaP to these carrier particles and the instillation procedure have been previously published (LITTLE et al., 1970).

Each animal was sacrificed when moribund. The formalin-inflated lungs were embedded in paraffin after fixation and routine 5 μm sections of lungs and trachea were prepared. Sections were interpreted and graded as to presence or absence of unequivocal lung tumors. Since these experiments are still in progress, final lung tumor prevalence, as well as the incidence of premalignant and borderline lesions, and tumors of other locations will be reported subsequently.

Table 1 summarizes the design of this series of studies in which low levels of the 2 carcinogens were administered either singly, simultaneously, or sequentially. The treatment periods began when the animals were approximately 12 weeks of age. Animals dying during the treatment periods were excluded from the calculation of prevalence rates.

Table 1. Treatment groups

Group	Treatment	Approximate radiation dose[a]
	Simultaneous series	
1	210Po ferric oxide (0.0025 μCi x 15 weeks)	60 rads
2	210Po ferric oxide (0.0005 μCi x 15 weeks)	12 rads
3	BaP ferric oxide (0.3 mg x 15 weeks)	
4	(1) and (3) - simultaneously (on same ferric oxide particles)	
5	(2) and (3) - simultaneously (on same ferric oxide particles)	
	Sequential series	
6	210Po ferric oxide (0.04 μCi, single instillation)	60 rads
7	210Po-saline (0.04 μCi, single instillation)	25 rads
8	(6) and, 18 weeks later, BaP ferric oxide (0.3 mg x 7 wks)	
9	(7) and, 18 weeks later, BaP ferric oxide (0.3 mg x 7 wks)	

[a]Approximate dose to whole lung based on preliminary radiochemical analyses.

Results and Discussion

As shown in Table 2 for the simultaneous series, the prevalence of unequivocal malignant lung tumors in groups 1 and 2 (210Po ferric oxide alone) was 12 and 11% respectively. There was thus no difference in tumor rate related to dose of 210Po at these low exposure levels. Moreover, the sequence of appearance of lung tumors was almost identical in these 2 groups; only the data for group 1 are plotted in Fig. 1. In group 3 (BaP ferric oxide alone), the net tumor yield was 8%, the first tumor appearing on the 72nd week and the second not until the 87th week (Fig. 1). Simultaneous exposure to both carcinogens (groups 4 and 5) led to a similar percentage and time sequence of tumors among group 5 hamsters as in groups 1 and 2. On the other hand, the net prevalence of lung tumors in group 4 was 34%, about twice the rate expected from the simple additive effect of 210Po and BaP alone (groups 1 and 3).

Table 2 also presents the prevalence of tumors among the 4 groups in the sequential series. There was only 1 tumor (arising at 73 weeks) among 139 animals in groups 6 and 7 (210Po alone). Yet, in groups 8

Table 2. Prevalence of malignant lung tumors

	Group	Number of animals at risk	Number of animals with lung tumors	Percent with tumors
Simultaneous series	1	82	10	12.2
	2	83	9	10.8
	3	66	5	7.6
	4	73	25	34.2
	5	74	8	10.8
Sequential series	6	65	0	0.0
	7	74	1	1.4
	8	72	13	18.0
	9	63	10	15.9

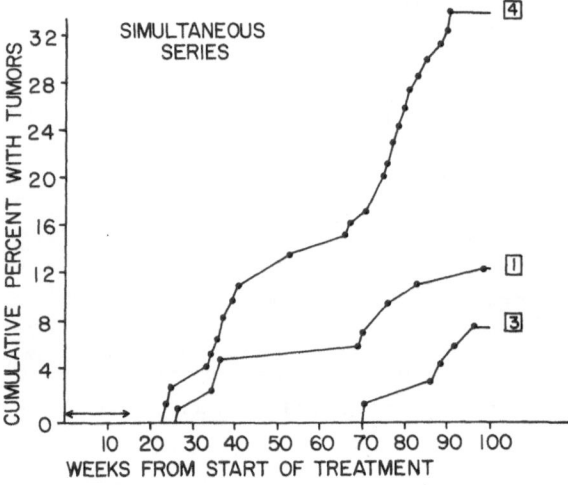

Fig. 1. Simultaneous series. Cumulative percentage of tumors vs time after the beginning of intratracheal instillation in groups 1, 3, and 4. Treatments ended on the 15th week

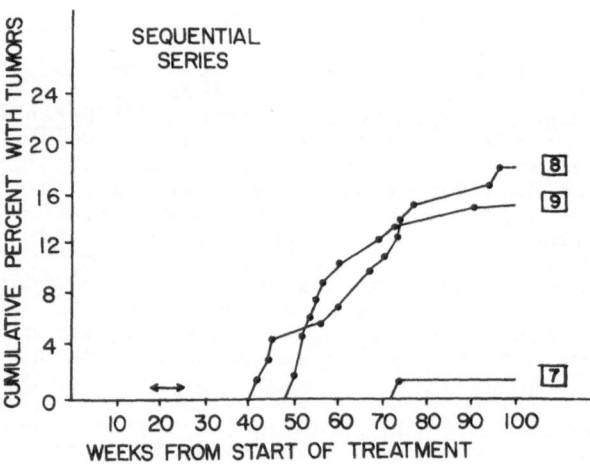

Fig. 2 Sequential series. Cumulative percentage of tumors vs time after a single intratracheal instillation of 0.04 µCi ^{210}Po. BaP was also instilled in groups 8 and 9 from the 18th to 25th week (7 weekly instillations of 0.3 mg BaP each on 3 mg ferric oxide particles). No tumors were found in group 6

and 9 (^{210}Po followed by BaP ferric oxide) tumors were found in 18 and
16% respectively. The time course of appearance of these lung tumors
is shown in Fig. 2. The yield of tumors was much higher than expected
from a single instillation of ^{210}Po alone (essentially zero) plus a
total dose of BaP only half as great (2.1 mg) as that administered
to group 3 hamsters in the previous series (4.5 mg).

All the tumors in these experiments were of the combined adenocarcino-
ma-epidermoid carcinoma type; all arose in peripheral lung fields and
were, for the most part, multicentric in location. Details of the
histopathology of these tumors have been already reported (LITTLE and
O'TOOLE, 1974). Several representative examples are shown in Figs 3
through 5.

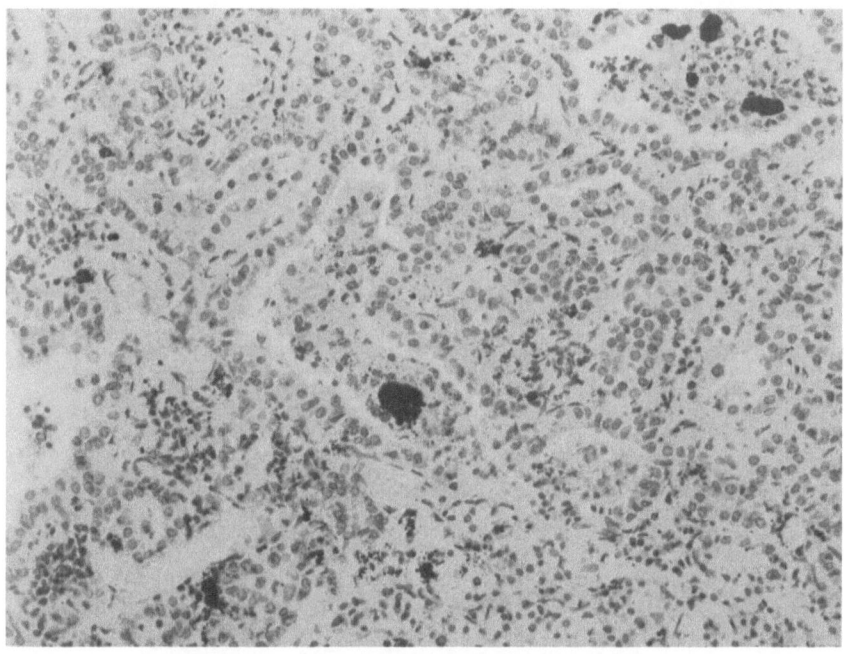

Fig. 3. Peripheral lung tumor from group 4 showing glandular pattern.
Note ferric oxide particles. PAS-hematoxylin. (x 135)

We interpret these data to be consistent with a synergistic effect
between ^{210}Po and BaP following both simultaneous (group 4) and sequential (groups 9 and 10) administration. It is not clear why this
synergistic effect in the simultaneous series appeared to be associated only with the higher radiation exposure group.

The induced tumors were all peripheral, combined lesions typical of
those associated with ^{210}Po alone. These lesions have also constituted
a major proportion of the lung tumors found after BaP administration.
Higher doses of BaP, however, also led to epidermoid carcinoma of the
trachea and major bronchi (LITTLE and O'TOOLE, 1974). Such major airway carcinomas were not found in the present series. The findings that
all of the tumors in the combined treatment groups were in the peri-

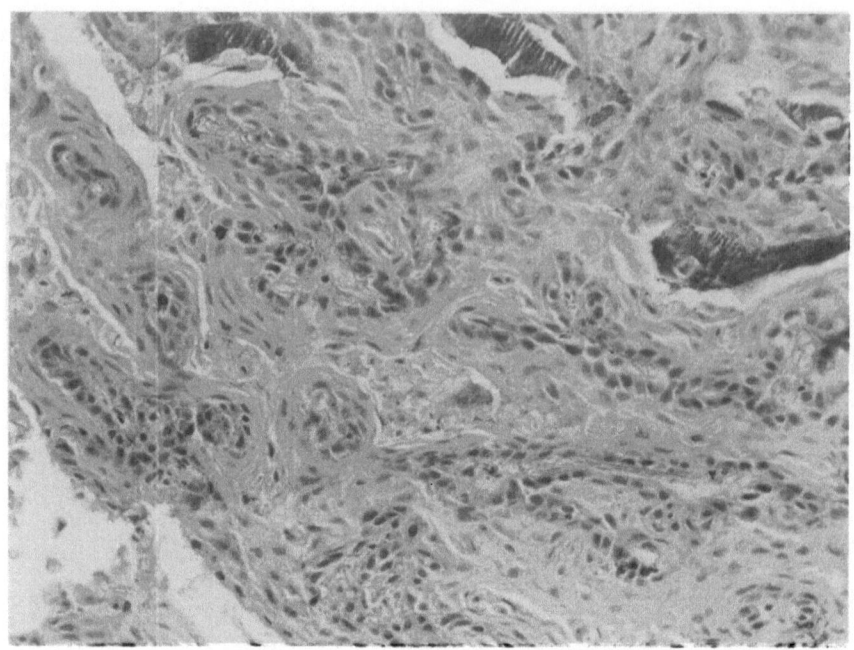

Fig. 4. Peripheral lung tumor from group 4 showing area of epidermoid differentiation. PAS-hematoxylin. (x 150)

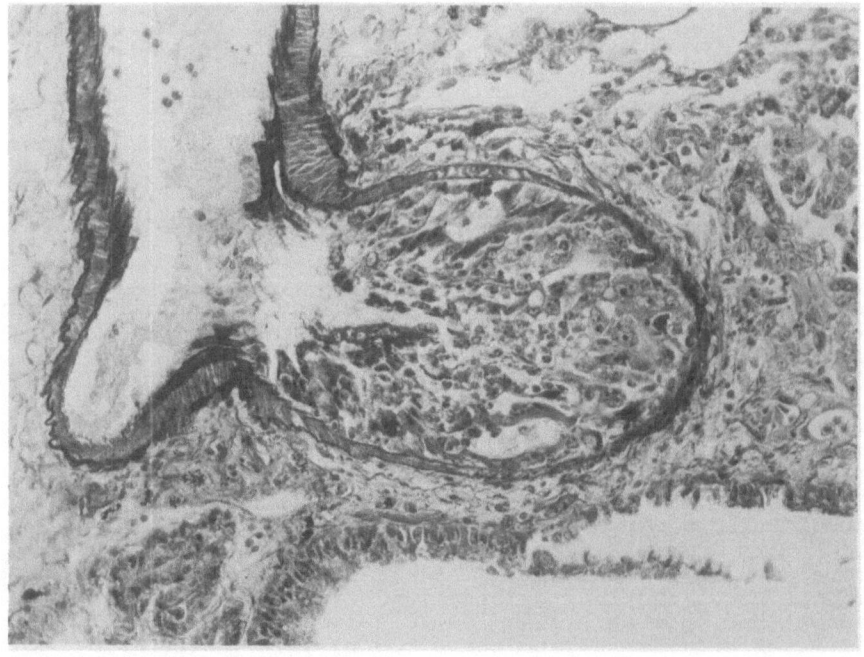

Fig. 5. Area of vascular invasion in poorly differentiated adeno-carcinomatous tumor. Verhoeff-VanGieson. (x 135)

pheral lung is consistent with the results of our localization studies (KENNEDY and LITTLE, 1974a, 1974b). Both central and peripheral airways receive exposure from BaP, whereas the radiation dose from ^{210}Po is largely confined to the bronchiolar-alveolar region - the area of origin of the pathological changes reported here.

References

BOYD, J.T., DOLL, R., FAULDS, J.S., LEIPER, J.: Cancer of the lung in iron ore (hematite) miners. Brit. J. Ind. Med. 27, 97-105 (1970).

KENNEDY, A.R., LITTLE, J.B.: The transport and localization of benzo (a)pyrene-hematite and ^{210}Po-hematite in the hamster lung following intratracheal instillation. Cancer Res. 34, 1344-1352 (1974a).

KENNEDY, A.R., LITTLE, J.B.: Cellular localization of intratracheally administered ^{210}Po in the hamster lung using autoradiography of thin sections from plastic embedded tissue. These Proceedings . 1974b.

LITTLE, J.B., GROSSMAN, B.N., MCGANDY, R.B., O'TOOLE, W.F.: Influence of genetic strain on the induction of lung cancer in hamsters by alpha radiation. Europ. J. Cancer 9, 825-828 (1974).

LITTLE, J.B., GROSSMAN, B.N., O'TOOLE, W.F.: Respiratory carcinogenesis in hamsters induced by polonium-210 alpha radiation and benzo(a)pyrene. In: Morphology of Experimental Respiratory Carcinogenesis (P. Nettesheim, M.G. Hanna, Jr., J.W. Deatherage, Jr., eds). AEC Symposium Series 21, 383-392 (1970).

LITTLE, J.B., GROSSMAN, B.N., O'TOOLE, W.F.: Factors influencing the induction of lung cancer in hamsters by intratracheal administration of polonium-210. In: Radionuclide Carcinogenesis (C.L. Sanders, R.H. Busch, J.E. Ballou, D.D. Mahlum, eds). AEC Symposium Series 29, 119-137 (1973).

LITTLE, J.B., O'TOOLE, W.F.: Respiratory tract tumors in hamsters induced by benzo(a)pyrene and polonium-210 alpha radiation. Cancer Res., in press.

LITTLE, J.B., RADFORD, E.P., Jr., MCCOMBS, H.L., HUNT, V.R.: Distribution of polonium-210 in pulmonary tissues of cigarette smokers. New England J. Med. 273, 1343-1351 (1965).

LUNDIN, F.E., Jr., WAGONER, J.K., ARCHER, V.E.: Radon daughter exposure and respiratory cancer quantitative and temporal aspects. NIOSH-NIEHS Joint Monograph No. 1, June 1971.

MARTELL, E.A.: Radioactivity of tobacco trichomes and insoluble cigarette smoke particles. Nature 249, 215-217 (1974).

SAFFIOTTI, U., CEFIS, F., KOLB, L.H.: A method for the experimental induction of bronchogenic carcinoma. Cancer Res. 28, 104-124 (1968).

WAGONER, J.K., ARCHER, V.E., LUNDIN, F.E., HOLADAY, D.A., LLOYD, J.W.: Radiation as the cause of lung cancer among uranium miners. New England J. Med. 273, 181-188 (1965).

Session V   *In vitro* Bioassays of Respiratory Carcinogens

Chairman: Michael B. Sporn

Lung Cancer Branch, National Cancer Institute, Bethesda, MD 20014, USA

Review and Introductory Remarks: The Role of Organ Culture and Cell Culture Methods in Studies of Respiratory Carcinogenesis and Anti-Carcinogenesis

Michael B. Sporn

Lung Cancer Branch, National Cancer Institute, Bethesda, MD 20014, USA

The ultimate goal of experimental respiratory carcinogenesis studies is the prevention of lung cancer in man. There would appear to be two general approaches to achieve this goal. The first would be to further our understanding of the process of respiratory carcinogenesis, which entails the identification of respiratory carcinogens and co-carcinogens, as well as elucidation of their cellular and molecular mechanism of action. If this approach is pursued vigorously, we hopefully can lessen the degree of human exposure to carcinogens and co-carcinogens, and thus reduce incidence of disease. However, given the fact that it appears unlikely that man will ever eliminate all of the respiratory carcinogens in his environment, a second approach, namely the development of new means of anti-carcinogenesis, is also required if we are to achieve our goal. By anti-carcinogenesis, I mean the inhibition of development of cancer, even though the organism has been exposed to a significant dose of carcinogen sufficient to cause cancer if no further measures are taken.

There are two general types of anti-carcinogenic agents that one may consider. The first type would prevent the activation of a carcinogen to a true proximate carcinogen, or inhibit the binding of such a proximate carcinogen to a critical cellular receptor, such as DNA or a regulatory protein. To be effective, such anti-carcinogenic agents would have to be administered *during* the period of exposure to carcinogen. I would like to call such agents "anti-initiation agents". A second type of anti-carcinogenic agent would not affect the immediate metabolism of a carcinogen, but rather would modify the development of neoplasia *after* biologically significant initiation of cancer had occurred, that is *after* a significant dose of carcinogen had bound either to DNA, a regulatory protein, or whatever other critical cellular receptors are involved in the initiation of cancer. This second type of anti-carcinogenic agent would *not* have to be given during the period of exposure to carcinogen and would be effective if given during the latent period for development of cancer; I would like to call such agents "anti-promotion agents".

I would now like to turn to the immediate problem of our current session, namely: How can organ and cell culture methods further the development of studies in respiratory carcinogenesis and anti-carcinogenesis? I will not attempt a comprehensive review of *in vitro* methodology or results, but will rather attempt to point out some highlights. In particular, I would like to discuss some of the strengths, as well as the weaknesses, of *in vitro* methods, as compared to more classical *in vivo* studies.

The most obvious strength of the *in vitro* approach is the ability to evaluate directly and rapidly the effect of either a prospective carcinogenic or anti-carcinogenic agent on a target tissue. Although

the end points with *in vitro* methods are certainly much more controversial than the end points in whole animal studies (in which one can
measure incidence and properties of tumors), the saving of time and
the ability to investigate large numbers of variables that may modify
the response of the system now make the use of *in vitro* methods a necessary supplement to *in vivo* studies of respiratory carcinogenesis or
anti-carcinogenesis. Indeed, there are questions of mechanisms that
can *only* be answered with *in vitro* experiments.

Since almost the entire session will deal with organ culture experiments, I will say little about the important topic of cell culture
methods in carcinogenesis studies; moreover, this topic has recently
been very well reviewed by experts this area (CASTO and DiPAOLO, 1973;
HEIDELBERGER, 1973). Suffice it to say that cell culture methods,
which employ *homogeneous* cell populations, lend themselves uniquely to
answering questions about mechnisms of transformation, as will presented in the first paper in the session, which deals with the synergism
between radiation and a chemical carcinogen.

In contrast to the *homogeneous* cell populations used in cell culture
experiments, in organ culture we have the simplest *heterogeneous* cellular
system that maintains the normal physiological structure of the tissue,
so that the cells of that tissue can interact with one another in their
presumably normal physiological manner. Since a great deal of carcinogenesis research deals not with "the cancer cell" but rather with the
cancerous behavior of a heterogeneous population of cells, we have in
organ culture the simplest experimental tool to study these heterogeneous cell populations. Since cellular differentiation is maintained
in organ culture, the activation and further metabolism of carcinogens
may be meaningfully studied in appropiate target tissues. Thus, the
biochemical and cellular responses leading to carcinogenesis can be
identified in an isolated experimental system.

Further, organ culture methodology offers a unique opportunity to
identify new anti-carcinogenic agents, both anti-initiating agents
and anti-promoting agents, and to study their mechanism of action.
In particular, there is unique potential in organ culture to study
the repair, healing, or arrest of a lesion induced by a carcinogen,
and this will be discussed in more detail later in the session.

A final strength of the organ culture approach is the ability to study
directly the effects of carcinogens on human target tissues. This
method thus presents a unique opportunity to correlate results obtained on the same tissues, treated in analogous fashion, from both
man and the experimental animal.

So much for the strengths of the organ culture method. It is not without its weaknesses, which we will now discuss briefly. Perhaps the
most fundamental weakness is the lack of sharp or quantitative end
points to measure the effects of a carcinogen or anti-carcinogen on
a target tissue. Morphological end points may be very subjective and
difficult to relate to experiments in whole animals. Well-defined,
sophisticated, and meaningful biochemical end points do not exist.
A second weakness in organ culture methodology in the past has been
the relatively limited capacity to maintain tissue *in vitro* for long
periods of time in a viable state. Thus, it has not been possible to
allow full development of a tumor *in vitro*; it has only been possible
to study the early cellular changes associated with initiation. However, as we shall hear, important methodological advances are being
made in this area. A final major problem in respiratory carcinogenesis
studies using the organ culture method has been the inability to dem-

onstrate the progression of preneoplastic explants to true neoplastic tumors, when the explants have been transplanted back into appropriate host animals. This problem is not limited to studies on respiratory tissue; for example, ROLLER and HEIDELBERGER (1967), working with prostate treated with carcinogenic polycyclic hydrocarbons in organ culture, were able to induce massive hyperplasia, anaplasia, abnormal mitoses, and invasion of pleomorphic epithelial cells through the basement membrane. However, when pieces of prostate from these cultures were implanted into over 8oo syngeneic animals, no tumors developed. It was suggested that failure to produce tumors under these circumstances may have been the result of inoculation of too few preneoplastic or neoplastic cells. Therefore, in other experiments, HEIDELBERGER and IYPE (1967) established cell cultures from the prostate explants that had been treated *in vitro* with the carcinogens. When 1 to 2 million cells from these cultures were inoculated into recipients, both carcinomas and sarcomas did indeed develop. More recent work by DAO and SINHA (1972), using mammary gland explants treated *in vitro* with 7,12-dimethylbenz(a)anthracene, suggests that direct transplantation of organ cultures into host animals can in fact lead to development of carcinoma. This entire problem has, of course, not yet been clarified with respect to respiratory tissue, and I look forward to the new data that will be presented in our session.

Whatever the limitations of organ culture methods may be, there is no question that they have already made important contributions to our understanding of respiratory carcinogenesis. Organ culture studies have by now shown that purified hydrocarbons, as well as cigarette smoke condensate, can directly cause preneoplastic lesions of tracheo-bronchial epithelium of both man and experimental animals (CROCKER et al., 1965; CROCKER and SANDERS, 1970; LASNITZKI, 1956, 1958; PALEKAR et al., 1968). Organ cultures studies have also shown that respiratory epithelium itself has enzymatic mechanisms to activate carcinogenic polynuclear hydrocarbons and to bind them to cellular DNA (KAUFMAN et al., 1973). A more complete explanation of the relationship of the preneoplastic phenomena that have been observed in organ culture to the ultimate development of cancer is obviously critically needed at present. Equally needed, if we are to achieve our goal of prevention of lung cancer, are some new approaches to the study of anti-carcinogenesis *in vitro*. As we turn now to review some of the latest research in the organ culture and cell culture field, it should be apparent that this field is now in a very productive state, that important new findings on the causation of lung cancer are being made, and that we may cautiously hope that this field will play an increasingly important role in our attempts to develop effective means for prevention of lung cancer.

References

CASTO, B.C., DiPAOLO, J.A.: Virus, chemicals, and cancer. Prog. Med. Virol. 16, 1-47 (1973).
CROCKER, T.T., NIELSEN, B.I., LASNITZKI, I.: Carcinogenic hydrocarbons. Effects on suckling rat trachea in organ culture. Arch. Environ. Health 10, 240-250 (1965).
CROCKER, T.T., SANDERS, L.L.: Influence of vitamin A and 3,7-dimethyl-2,6-octadienal (citral) on the effect of benzo(a)pyrene on hamster trachea in organ culture. Cancer Res. 30, 1312-1318 (1970).
DAO, T.L., SINHA, D.: Mammary adenocarcinoma induced in organ culture by 7,12-dimethylbenz(a)anthracene. J. nat. Cancer Inst. 49, 591-593 (1972).

HEIDELBERGER, C.: Chemical oncogenesis in culture. Advanc. Cancer
    Res. 18, 317-366 (1973).
HEIDELBERGER, C., IYPE, P.T.: Malignant transformation *in vitro* by
    carcinogenic hydrocarbons. Science 155, 214-217 (1967).
KAUFMAN, D.G., GENTA, V.M., HARRIS, C.C., SMITH, J.M., SPORN, M.B.,
    SAFFIOTTI, U.: Binding of ^{3}H-labeled benzo(a)pyrene to DNA in
    hamster tracheal epithelial cells. Cancer Res. 33, 2837-2841 (1973).
LASNITZKI, I.: Effect of 3,4-benzpyrene on human foetal lung grown
    in vitro. Brit. J. Cancer 10, 510-516 (1956).
LASNITZKI, I.: Observations on effects of condensates from cigarette
    smoke on human foetal lung *in vitro* . Brit. J. Cancer 12, 547-554
    (1958).
PALEKAR, L., KUSCHNER, M., LASKIN, S.: Effect of 3-methylcholanthrene
    on rat trachea in organ culture. Cancer Res. 28, 2098-2104 (1968).
ROLLER, M.R., HEIDELBERGER, C.: Attempts to produce carcinogenesis
    in organ cultures of mouse prostate with polycyclic hydrocarbons.
    Int. J. Cancer 2, 509-520 (1967).

Interactions between Radiation and Benzo(a)pyrene in an *in vitro* Model for Malignant Transformation*

Margaret Terzaghi and John B. Little

Department of Physiology, Harvard School of Public Health, Boston, MA 02115, USA

ABSTRACT

Malignant transformation, confirmed by reinjection of transformed cells into syngeneic mice, has been induced by both BaP and X-irra-- diation in a C3H mouse embryo cell line (1oT-1/2). A synergistic ef- fect was found when both agents were given sequentially; maximum synergism occurred when 15 to 2o hours elapsed between treatments. Both survival and transformation frequency per surviving cell were enhanced by maintaining cells in conditions of growth inhibition for 4 hours after radiation, suggesting that repair processes may be involved in the transformation process. Such an *in vitro* transformation system, particularly involving plateau phase cultures, appears to be valuable adjunct to the study of interactions between chemical carci- nogens and radiation that may occur in critical cell populations in the lung.

A. Introduction

Experiments reported elsewhere in this symposium (McGANDY et al.), indicate possible synergistic interaction between alpha radiation and benzo(a)pyrene (BaP) in the induction of experimental lung cancer. The work presented in this paper represents preliminary data obtained in the course of developing an *in vitro* system which may be of predic- tive value in projected experiments on the interaction of respiratory carcinogens *in vivo*. An *in vitro* transformation system allows investi- gation of the dynamics of the interaction in greater detail.

Our general approach has been to study the effects of growth phase (exponential, serum-deficient, or contact inhibited plateau) and re- pair state of cultures on sensitivity to transformation by X-radiation and BaP, and to correlate transformation with the lethal effects of these agents. In the initial experiments, the agents were given indi- vidually to cells in the exponential phase of growth. Transformation frequencies, survival rates, and the effects on growth kinetics, as ascertained by growth curves, are described. Exponentially growing cultures were then exposed to radiation and BaP given in sequence, with varying time intervals between treatments. In order to progress to a system which more closely approximates the cell proliferation kinetics observed in tissues *in vivo* (ZINNINGER and LITTLE, 1973),

*Supported by Contract CP-33273 from the National Cancer Institute, and NIH Grant ES-ooo2.

preliminary experiments have been carried out with plateau phase cultures in which cells are not proliferating exponentially at the time of exposure to these carcinogenic agents.

B. Material and Methods

The cell line used in these experiments was C3H/1oT-1/2 clone 8, kindly provided by C. REZNIKOFF and C. HEIDELBERGER (McArdle Laboratory for Cancer Research, University of Wisconsin). These cells are a line of C3H mouse embryo cells which are highly sensitive to postconfluence inhibition, and are readily adapted to transformation studies. The establishment and characterization of this cell line was reported by REZNIKOFF and HEIDELBERGER (1973). Adaptation of this system to transformation was similarly described by REZNIKOFF et al. (1973). Experiments presented in this paper were all done with cells in passages 8 to 28.

Stock and experimental cultures were maintained in Eagle's Basal Medium supplemented with 1o% heat inactivated fetal calf serum in accordance with the protocol outlined by REZNIKOFF et al. (1973). BaP was obtained from Eastman Organic Chemical Co. A stock solution was made up in DMSO (Sigma Chemical Co.) for each experiment, and diluted with fresh medium just before addition to the cell culture. The final concentration of DMSO in the culture medium never exceeded o.4%. DMSO was added to all control plates in an amount which was commensurate with that in the plates containing BaP. The cells were irradiated at 37°C at a dose rate of 83.5 rads/min.

For the standard transformation assay, experiments were designed such that all experimental and control plates had $1o^3$ viable cells per 1oo mm petri dish. The treatment protocol was initiated 24 hours after plating the cells. Cells were exposed to BaP for 24 or 48 hours. BaP treatment was terminated by removal of the old media followed by replacement with fresh medium. Control plates with added DMSO were given fresh medium at the same time as BaP-containing plates. In all experiments, the medium was changed twice a week until the cells reached confluency, and once a week from confluency until termination of the experiment at 6 weeks. Upon termination, plates were washed with o.85% saline, fixed in Bouin's solution, washed with ethanol, and stained with trypan blue. Plating efficiencies (PE) were determined for each experimental group where appropriate. Standard plating efficiency plates (those seeded at low density and treated at the same time as experimental plates) were terminated at 1o to 15 days, stained as described above, and colony counts were done. Plating efficiency was defined as the percentage of cells plated that form colonies of more than 5o cells.

For plateau phase experiments, the cells were grown until confluent and a stable plateau phase of growth was reached. The medium was changed 24 hours before treatment. The cells were irradiated while confluent, then trypsinized and subcultured at various times after irradiation to assay for the surviving fraction and transformation frequency.

The procedure for scoring experimental plates was the same as outlined by REZNIKOFF, BERTRAM et al. (1973). Morphologically-altered foci on the plates were divided into three classes, types I, II, and III. Type I foci exhibited a slightly denser growth than normal cells, but were not scored as transformed. Types II and III formed piled-up foci with varying degrees of disorganization and alterations in nu-clear-cytoplasmic ratios. Types II and III may be of solid or "corded" morphology. REZINIKOFF, BERTRAM et al. (1973) reported that the degree of tumorigenicity in X-irradiated syngeneic mice correlated with the morphological classification of foci.

C. Results

I. Transformation: Single Doses of Radiation and BaP

X-rays and BaP both induced morphologically-altered foci on plates allowed to grow beyond confluency. The types of foci observed in both cases appeared to fall into classes that are analogous to those des-cribed by REZNIKOFF, BERTRAM et al. ·(1973). No transformed foci were found on untreated control plates in any of the experiments included in this report. Experiments were performed in order to establish that the morphological transformation we observed represented malignant transformation, defined as the ability of the cells to produce upon reinjection into mice. Morphologically-distinct foci were picked using the cylinder isolation technique, and the clones were dispersed and grown in glass culture bottles. Areas from treated and control plates which appeared normal were also picked and treated in a manner similar to that for the morphologically-altered foci. Recipient syngeneic mice were irradiated with 35o rads 24 hours prior to inoculation with the test-cell cultures. Cell suspensions were injected subcutaneously in the interscapular region in a total volume of o.3 ml of complete medi-um. Results to date are summarized in Table 1.

Table 1. Inoculation of C3H1OT-1/2 clone 8 normal and radiation-transformed cells into syngeneic mice

Treatment	(Morphology) Classification	* Cells injected mouse	Tumor incidence (* tumors/ * mice)
None	(control) Normal	$2-5 \times 10^6$	0/4
600 rads	III	$2-4 \times 10^6$	3/4
600 rads	II	$2-4 \times 10^6$	2/4
600 rads	I	$2-4 \times 10^6$	0/4
600 rads	I	10^7	0/4
600 rads	Normal	$2-4 \times 10^6$	0/4
600 rads	Normal	10^7	0/4

In order to ascertain whether the carcinogenic effect of radiation was related to the presence of dead or dying cells, viable 1OT-1/2 cells were either plated on irradiated feeder layers of 1OT-1/2 cells or incubated with conditioned medium therefrom. No evidence of trans-formation was seen in either experimental group. These results do not support the hypothesis recently put forward by KLEIN (1974).

Further characterization of one radiation-transformed foci (F-5) was carried out. Growth properties in medium with 10%, 5%, and 0% fetal calf serum were compared to normal cells and methylcholanthrene-transformed clone 15 (kindly provided by REZNIKOFF and HEIDELBERGER). Results are summarized in Table 2.

Table 2. Growth properties of control and transformed C3H1OT-1/2 clones

Cell doubling time	Rad. Tr. clone (F-5)	MCA Tr-Clone 15	Control (1OT-1/2 clone 8)
FCS - 0%	24 hours	26 hours	36 hours
5%	23 hours	26 hours	16 hours
10%	23 hours	25.5 hours	15.6 hours
	F-5	MCA	Control
	Saturation density (cells cm^2)		
FCS - 0%	2.8×10^4	1.1×10^4	0.5×10^4
5%	14.0×10^4	3.5×10^4	1.8×10^4
10%	18.0×10^4	7.1×10^4	2.5×10^4

II. Toxicity: BaP and Radiation

C3H/1OT-1/2 cells were found to have a characteristic mammalian cell survival curve in response to X-radiation (Fig. 1). There is a shoulder in the lower dose range, the magnitude of which is reflected in an extrapolation number of ($\tilde{n}$) = 2.7. The D_0 (inverse of the slope on the linear portion of the survival curve) is 185 rads.

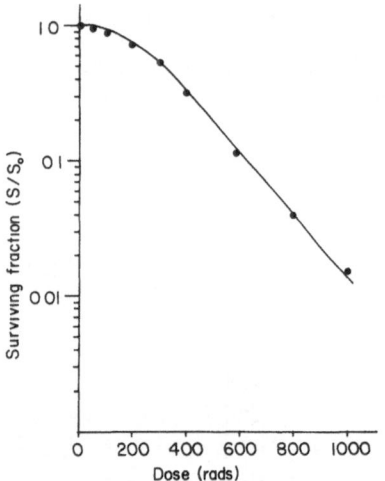

Fig. 1. Cell survival following radiation

The toxicity of BaP was measured over a dose range of 1 to 6 µg/ml of medium. Survival (expressed as the plating efficiency with BaP/plating efficiency with DMSO only) dropped from 46% with 1 µg/ml to 16% with 16 µg/ml. The decrease in survival within this dose range was linear when plotted as a semilogarithmic function.

Growth curves following treatment with BaP (2.5 µg/ml for 24 or 48 hours) or radiation, are shown in Fig. 2. Cells were plated at an initial density of 5×10^4 per 6o mm petri dish. Treatment was initiated 24 hours after plating the cells.

III.   Transformation Dose-Response: Single Doses of BaP or Radiation

The dose-response relationship for transformation with radiation is
shown in Fig. 3. Doses used ranged from 0 to 800 rads. Below 200 rads,
the response is linear on a semilog plot. At doses greater than 200
rads, the efficiency of radiation for the induction of transformation
reaches a plateau which is maintained at least up to doses of 800 rads.

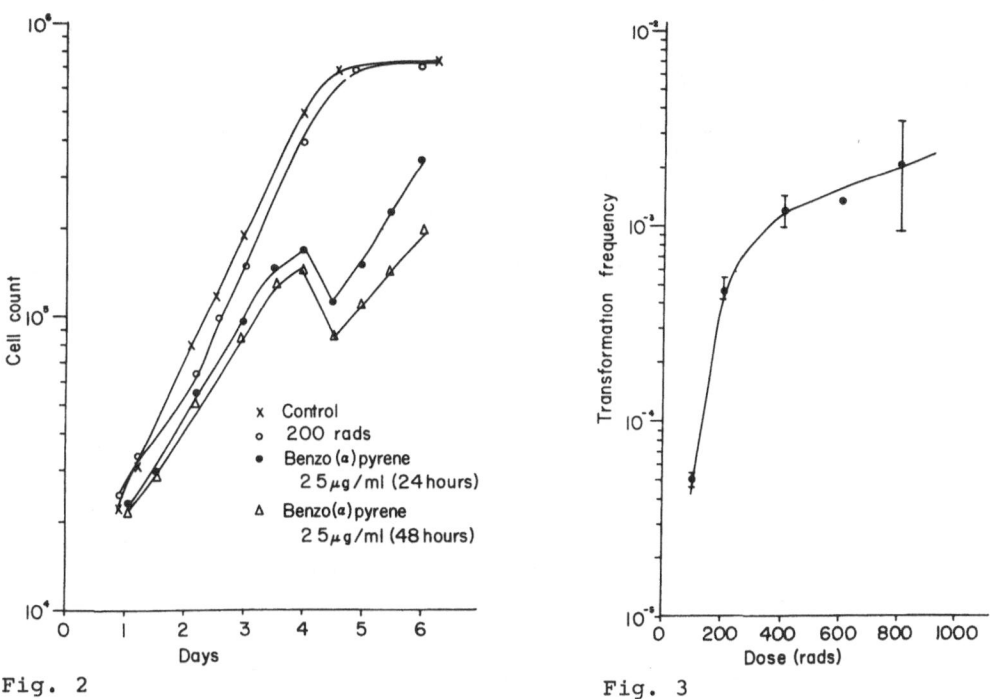

Fig. 2   Fig. 3

Fig. 2. Growth curves. Cells treated with 200 rads of radiation,
2.5 µg BaP/ml for 24 hours, or 2.5 µg BaP/ml for 48 hours. Cell count
per 60 mm petri dish vs. time

Fig. 3. Transformation induction by radiation. Transformants per
viable cell vs. dose (rads)

Less extensive data has been collected with respect to dose-related
transformation and BaP. BaP has been extensively studied in other
systems (e.g., HUBERMAN and SACHS, 1966); our primary purpose was to
establish a baseline for radiation - BaP interaction studies. A dose
of 2.5 or 3 µg BaP per ml of medium was found to produce a reproducible
transformation frequency of 2.5 to 4 per 10^3 viable cells.

IV.   BaP - Radiation Interaction

Preliminary experiments have been performed to investigate interaction
between BaP and X-rays in exponentially growing cells. The magnitude
of the interaction observed is expressed as the Transformation Enhancement Ratio (TER).

$$TER = \frac{(BaP - Rad)_{together}}{(BaP)_{alone} + (Rad)_{alone}}.$$

If one plots TER against the time interval elapsing between treatment with either agent, two different patterns of interaction emerge. There was an increase in the TER as the time between treatments was increased up to 15 to 20 hours; at this point, there was maximum synergistic effect. If BaP was given prior to radiation, there was a gradual decline in synergism from this maximum as the time between treatments was increased. If radiation preceded BaP, there was a rapid drop in synergism with increasing time intervals between treatments. The result of an experiment in which these patterns of interaction were particularly striking are shown in Fig. 4. This general response pattern was observed in four similar experiments.

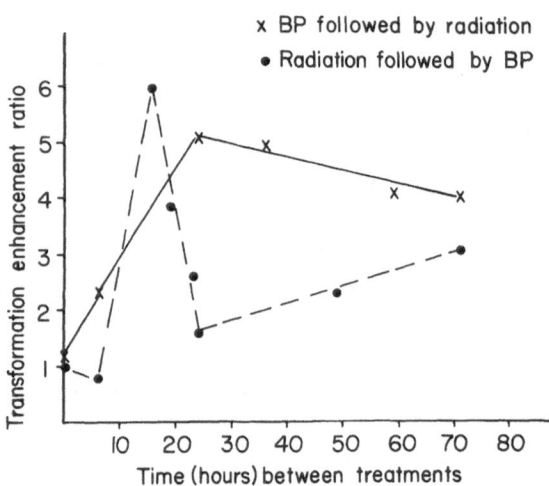

Fig. 4. Transformation enhancement with combined BaP-radiation treatments. Magnitude of enhancement above that induced by radiation alone plus BaP alone vs. time between the two treatments

The data presented in Fig. 4 is based on transformation frequencies in which cells at risk to transformation were computed by use of the product of the individual toxicities of the two treatments involved. Technically speaking, this is accurate only when the two treatments are given simultaneously. In future experiments involving multiple treatments, a more precise measurement of cells at risk in each experimental group will be used.

V. Plateau Experiments: Radiation

The effect on transformation frequency of holding cells in confluent or plateau phase growth for 1 to 3 days after exposure to various types of carcinogens has been studied by other groups (BOREK and SACHS, 1966; TODARO and GREEN, 1966; KAKANUGA, 1972). As indicated in experiments reported by LITTLE (1969, 1973), there are significant variations in survival when cells are held in plateau phase growth for various time intervals up to 10 hours after irradiation. This effect most likely represents a significant pattern of underlying molecular repair processes. Experiments were thus performed in order to assess whether such survival-related repair occurs in 1OT-1/2

cells held in plateau phase after irradiation, and whether it correlates with changes in transformation frequency. Simultaneous survival
experiments (1200 rads) and transformation experiments (200 rads) were
carried out as outlined above (Materials and Methods). The results are
summarized in Fig. 5. Both survival and transformants per surviving
cell were enhanced when cultures were maintained in plateau growth
for 3 to 4 hours after irradiation.

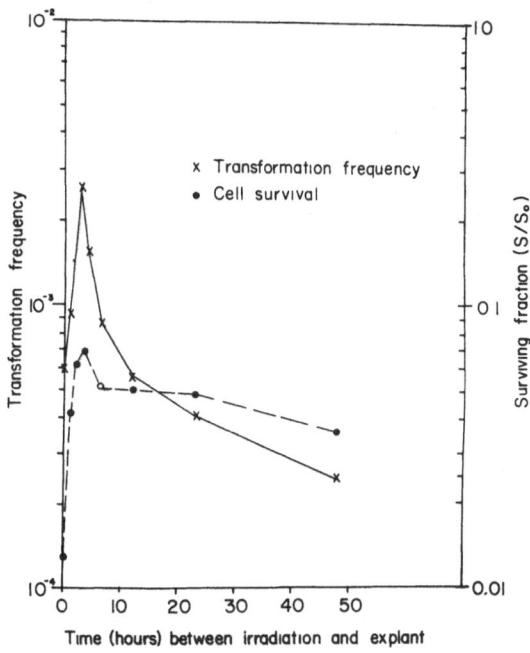

Fig. 5. Plateau phase cultures: Survival and transformation (transformants per
viable cell) vs. time after
irradiation and before explant at low cell concen-
trations

VI.   Serum Deprivation: BaP

Parallel with the above experiments, we have attempted to determine
whether the ability of BaP to induce transformation in plateau phase
cultures could be altered in a way which is analogous to that seen
with radiation. Clearly, one has the problem of defining the point
in time at which exposure of the cultures to BaP has occurred. BaP
cannot be given in a short, well-defined pulse. For purposes of definition, the time of addition of BaP is considered to be time zero.
In this set of experiments, the cells were allowed to reach a plateau
phase of growth by placing the cells in medium with no fetal calf
serum. The cells were allowed to resume proliferation by the addition
of complete medium at various times after treatment with BaP. Data
obtained to date are summarized in Table 3.

D.   Discussion

Radiation transformation *in vitro* was initially reported by BOREK and
SACHS (1966), and later by BOREK and HALL (1973). The transformation
frequency observed by these authors in hamster embryo cells irradiated
with 250 rads was 7 to 8 x 10^{-3} transformants per cell. In our labo-

504

Table 3

Time of release from block[a]	TER[b]
Control[c]	1
0 hours	1.9
24 hours	2
48 hours	1.6
72 hours	1.6

[a]Cells blocked by 24 hours incubation in serum-free medium. Block reversed by adding medium containing 10% fetal calf serum. BaP added at 0 hour.

[b]$TER = \dfrac{\text{Transformation in cultures blocked by 24 hours in serum-free medium}}{\text{Transformation in exponentially dividing cultures}}$

[c]Controls were exponentially dividing cultures in medium with 10% fetal calf serum

ratory, using mouse 10T-1/2 cells, 6×10^{-4} transformants per cell were observed following a dose of 250 rads. The explanation for this difference is not immediately apparent. Possibly, the response is highly sensitive to specific parameters which characterize any given cell system. Differences in protocol with respect to such factors as media and growth state may influence the magnitude of the transformation frequency observed.

Important parallels between BOREK's results and ours become apparent if one considers relative changes in the survival curves and dose-response transformation frequency data obtained in the two laboratories. Using hamster embryo cells, BOREK and HALL (1973) observed a radiation survival curve with a D_q (the dose at which the linear portion of the survival curve extrapolates to 100% survival) of 250 rads. The transformation frequency, observed in the same cell system, reaches a plateau between 150 and 300 rads. In our laboratory, 10T-1/2 cells were found to have a survival curve (Fig. 1) with $D_q = 200$ rads. The point of inflection seen in the transformation frequency curve (Fig.3), which represents the beginning of the plateau, occurs at approximately 200 rads. The above observations suggest that, although the absolute quantitative results obtained in the two laboratories are not comparable, more fundamental aspects of radiation transformation, such as the involvement of repair processes associated with cell survival, are common to both cell systems. Further work with doses greater than 800 rads is planned in our laboratory; BOREK and HALL (1973) have observed a sharp decline in transformation at higher doses, an observation which may be of critical importance when planning *in vivo* experiments with radiation or radiation in conjunction with other carcinogens.

Data on BaP-induced transformation reported by other laboratories are variable. DIPAOLO et al. (1971) report 1.33×10^{-3} transformants per cell in a hamster embryo cell system with 2.5 µg BaP per ml of medium. Later, DIPAOLO et al. (1972) using a Balb/3T3 cell line, reported approximately 3×10^{-2} transformants per cell with the same dose of BaP. Clearly, the quantitative response to BaP varies among cell systems, and the transformation frequency observed in our laboratory (3×10^{-3} with 3 µg/BaP for 24 hours) is presumably reflective of the cell line and specific protocol used.

DIPAOLO et al. (1971) have also investigated the interaction between BaP and radiation. They found no transformation with radiation, and no interaction when radiation followed exposure of the cells to BaP. Synergism was found to be maximal when radiation (250 rads) was followed 48 hours later by 2.5 µg BaP/ml of medium. The results obtained by DIPAOLO and our laboratory thus differ; the reasons for these differences are not clear at present. Possibly, the fact that 10T-1/2 cells can be transformed by exposure to radiation alters the dynamics of the interaction. As is shown in the growth curves (Fig. 2), BaP and radiation affect the cell proliferation kinetics of 10T-1/2 cells in characteristic ways which might be quite different from other cell systems. Further investigation of the effects of radiation and BaP on cell proliferation and repair may shed more light on the mechanisms involved in their interactions.

To date, much of the work done with *in vitro* transformation has involved exponentially growing cells. The exponential *in vitro* model lacks any real resemblance to the proliferation kinetics of most critical cell populations *in vivo*. Plateau phase cultures, as described by ZINNINGER and LITTLE (1973), exhibit a number of properties characteristic of cell populations *in vivo*, such as a significant population of nonproliferating but viable cells which are able to initiate DNA synthesis of transformation in this system. Radiation transformation in plateau cultures has been investigated by BOREK and SACHS (1966). In similar experiments, chemical transformation with methylcholanthrene has been reported by KAKANUGA (1972), and viral transformation by TODARO and GREEN (1966). One observation made, and reported separately, by the above authors is the decline in transformation as the time interval between treatment (in plateau phase), and subculture at low concentration to assay for transformation frequency, is extended beyond 24 hours. This result has been interpreted as indicating the need for cell proliferation after the initiating event to "fix" the transformed state. None of these workers, however, reported data for subculture between 0 and 24 hours after treatment.

Data reported by LITTLE (1969, 1973) indicate that important repair processes occur during the first few hours after treatment and before subculture of plateau phase cells, as reflected by a marked enhancement in surviving fraction following radiation. Given that there is enhancement of repair activity during this time interval, it seemed appropriate to study transformation during the time period up to 24 hours after radiation in greater detail. As is shown in the results presented, there is a high degree of correlation between the repair interval which allows the maximum enhancement of survival. These data open up the question of whether either initiation or expression of the transformed state is at least in part dependent upon the occurrence of certain DNA repair processes such as those necessary for cell survival.

Clearly, there is a need to further investigate the interaction between cell proliferation kinetics, molecular repair processes, and oncogenic agents. Plateau phase cultures are perhaps the best cell culture model for studying these effects. These factors will be considered in our future work on the interactions between chemical carcinogens and radiation *in vitro*, as they may apply to cell populations in the lung.

506

References

BOREK, C., HALL, E.J.: Transformation of mammalian cells *in vitro* by low doses of X-rays. Nature 243, 45o–453 (1973).

BOREK, C., SACHS, L.: *In vitro* cell transformation by X-irradiation. Nature 21o, 276–278 (1966).

DIPAOLO, J.A., DONOVAN, P.J., NELSON, R.L.: X-irradiation enhancement of transformation by benzo(a)pyrene in hamster embryo cells. Proc. nat. Acad. Sci. (Wash.) 68, 1734–1737 (1971).

DIPAOLO, J.A., TAKANO, K., POPESCU, N.C.: Quantitation of chemically induced neoplastic transformation of BALB/3T3 cloned cell lines. Cancer Res. 32, 2686–2695 (1972).

HUBERMAN, E., SACHS, L.: Cell susceptibility to transformation and cytotoxicity by the carcinogenic hydrocarbon benzo(a)pyrene. Proc. nat. Acad. Sci (Wash.) 56, 1123–1129 (1966).

KAKANUGA, T.: In: Nakahara, W., Takayuma, S., Sugimura, T., Odashima, S. (eds.), Topics in Chemical Carcinogenesis, pp. 32–34. Japan: Univ. of Tokyo Press 1972.

KLEIN, J.C.: Evidence against a direct carcinogenic effect of X-rays *in vitro*. J.N.C.I. 52, 1111–1116 (1974).

LITTLE, J.B.: Repair of sub-lethal and potentially lethal radiation damage in plateau phase cultures of human cells. Nature (London) 224, 8o4–8o6 (1969).

LITTLE, J.B.: Factors influencing the repair of potentially lethal radiation damage in growth-inhibited human cells. Radiation Res. 56, 32o–333 (1973).

REZNIKOFF, C.A., BERTRAM, J.S., BRANKOW, D.W., HEIDELBERGER, C.: Quantitative and qualitative studies of chemical transformation of cloned C3H mouse embryo cells sensitive to postconfluence inhibition of cell division. Cancer Res. 33, 3239–3249 (1973).

REZNIKOFF, C.A., BRANKOW, D.W., HEIDELBERGER, C.: Establishment and characterization of a cloned line of C3H mouse embryo cells sensitive to postconfluence inhibition of division. Cancer Res. 33, 3231–3238 (1973).

TODARO, G.J., GREEN, H.: Cell growth and the initiation of transformation by SV4o. Proc. nat. Acad. Sci. (Wash.) 55, 3o2–3o8 (1966).

ZINNINGER, G.G., LITTLE, J.B.: Proliferation kinetics of density-inhibited cultures of human cells, a complex *in vitro* cell system. Cancer Res. 33, 2343–2348 (1973).

Dose Dependence of Carcinogen-Induced Changes in Tracheal Epithelium in Organ Culture

Bernard P. Lane and Sandra L. Miller

Department of Pathology, State University of New York at Stony Brook, Stony Brook, NY 11790, USA

ABSTRACT

The effect of varying concentration of a chemical carcinogen on the histology and cytology of tracheal epithelium exposed to the agent was studied in order to determine a maximally effective concentration and duration of exposure for tumorigenesis. Organ cultures consisting of segments of rat tracheas sectioned transversely into rings were incubated in McCoy's 5A medium (modified) with 10% calf serum to which benzo(a)pyrene (BaP) had been added in concentrations of 0.1, 0.5, 1.0, 1.5, 2.0, 3.0 or 4.0 μg/ml. Replicate cultures from these carcinogen-exposed groups and from control groups exposed to medium alone or medium containing Tween 60, the vehicle for the BaP, were sampled at regular intervals.

At the two lowest dose levels, 0.1 and 0.5 μg/ml, squamous hyperplasia developed after 3 months but no cellular atypias or histologic changes of disorderly growth appeared. At 1.0, 1.5, and 2.0 μg/ml the hyperplasia was followed by cellular atypias and nodular intraepithelial growth. The changes did not meet histopathologic criteria for neoplasia but did suggest mutagenic effect of the agent. The time of appearance of the sequential stages was roughly proportional to the dose. At the two highest concentrations, 3.0 and 4.0 μg/ml, there was early and extensive cell death without hyperplasia of disordered growth.

The results indicate that, under these conditions of continuous exposure of tracheal epithelium in organ culture, concentrations of 0.1 and 0.5 μg/ml of BaP are below the effective level for mutagenicity or malignant transformation while concentrations of 3.0 and 4.0 μg/ml are too cytotoxic to permit long term studies. The intervening range of concentrations do induce sequential changes but there is no evolution to histologic malignancy.

Since high rates of cell turnover were observed at all concentrations of carcinogen and the life span of the cultures, when compared to the controls, was shortened in proportion to the level of carcinogen, cytotoxicity may interfere with emergence of a transformed population at any level of continuous exposure. Substitution of protocols which involve discontinuous exposure or incorporate techniques for dissociating cytotoxicity and carcinogenicity, cell cloning or establishment of new criteria for malignant change may be required for exploitation of this organ culture carcinogenesis model.

Introduction

Organ cultures serving as assay systems for chemical carcinogens can
be expected to exhibit the cytotoxic as well as the carcinogenic effects of these agents. Protocols for exposure of organ cultures to
carcinogens, known or suspected, must therefore take into account both
types of effect. We continuously exposed cultures composed of rat tracheal epithelium and associated connective tissues to a known *in vivo*
carcinogen, benzo(a)pyrene, independently varying concentration of the
chemical and duration of the application. Dose- and time-dependence
of the effects were observed, and there was an overall shortening of
the life of the culture which was also a function of the concentration
of carcinogen.

Materials and Methods

Female Sprague-Dawley rats weighing 150 ± 20 g were anesthetized with
an intraperitoneal injection of sodium pentabarbital and the treacheas
excised sterilely. Mechanical transverse sectioning yielded 14 uniform
rings from each trachea. Several hundred rings were prepared at one
time, randomized, and immersed in groups of 3 or 4 in 35 mm disposable
Petri dishes containing McCoy's 5a (modified) medium with 10% calf
serum and buffered with sodium bicarbonate. The cultures were incubated for 5 days at $37^\circ C$ in an atmosphere of 5% CO_2 in air, and those
exhibiting epithelial confluence over the surface were transferred to
the same medium to which benzo(a)pyrene stabilized in solution by
Tween 60 had been added. Concentrations of 0.0, 0.1, 0.5, 1.0, 1.5,
2.0, 3.0, and 4.0 µg of carcinogen per milliliter of culture medium
were employed.

Of over 450 rings treated, 300 were used in experiments in which the
effects of exposure to 1.0, 1.5, or 2.0 µg/ml of the agent was studied.
These cultures were examined weekly by phase microscopy, and after
periods ranging from 4 days to 3 months, were sacrificed in groups
of 3 or more rings to be sectioned and studied by light and electron
microscopy. The cultures exposed to lower doses were also monitored
vitally by phase microscopy and were sacrified monthly in groups of
3 while those subjected to higher doses were sampled at twice weekly
intervals.

Prior to fixation the rings were transferred to a medium containing
5 µCi of tritiated thymidine. After 3o min the medium was replaced
by an aliquot containing non-radioactive thymidine at a tenfold higher
concentration so that the labelled base not incorporated into the DNA
but bound to the tissue, would be diluted.

After fixation in 3% glutaraldehyde buffered with sodium cacodylate
to pH 7.3, all specimens were embedded in plastic and sectioned
through their equators so that the complete circumference of inner
and outer epithelial surfaces could be examined. Alternate sections
were prepared as autoradiograms by coating with Kodak NTB2 emulsion,
exposing for an appropriate period, developing, fixing, and staining
with a thionine dye. Selected areas of representative blocks were
sectioned for transmission electron microscopy.

Results

Cultures grown for periods of 2 weeks to 5 months in a medium free of carcinogen exhibited flattened epithelium with persistent pseudo-stratification and motile cilia. In specimens maintained for more than 2 weeks in culture, only an occasional cell was radioactively labelled.

Cultures exposed to 0.1 or 0.5 µg/ml of benzo(a)pyrene demonstrated focal fatty or vacuolar degenerative changes after a few days of exposure. Approximately 4% of epithelial cell nuclei was labelled with radioactive thymidine by the end of the first week and this degree of apparent cell replication was sustained over the period of exposure. The epithelium became hyperplastic after 2 months but never included significant numbers of atypical cells. These cultures degenerated and died after 4 months of exposure to benzo(a)pyrene, at least a month sooner than the controls.

Cultures exposed to 1.0, 1.5, or 2.0 µg/ml showed early severe fatty or vacuolar change (Fig. 1) and then became hyperplastic (Fig. 2). Over 10% of nuclei contained radioactive thymidine (Fig. 3). Atypical nodular hyperplasia (Fig. 4) appeared by 5 weeks of culture in a medium containing 2 µg/ml of the carcinogen but this stage took 3 or 4 weeks longer to develop at the lower concentration. Nuclear and cell surface features seen in preneoplastic and neoplastic lesions induced *in vivo* with benzo(a)pyrene were present at this and later points (Fig. 5). All cultures ultimately degenerated with spotty dropout of basal cells and keratinizing, desquamating superficial cells (Fig. 6) and died after 3 months of continuous exposure.

Cultures incubated in a medium containing either 3 or 4 µg/ml were not distinguishable from one another. All specimens from early showed coincident cellular atypia, focal hyperplasia, and focal cell death and all cultures were dead by the end of 6 weeks.

Discussion

Organ cultures can offer a tissue-specific test system for identifying carcinogens or a model system for studying the process of carcinogenesis. They are less expensive and are more easily monitored and controlled than whole animal assays; cell populations similar to those in tissues at risk in the intact animal are retained, a feature not shared by cell cultures. The use of organ cultures, however, not only requires development of techniques of long term culture (LANE and MILLER, 1973), but also of protocols for exposure to carcinogens and methods of assessing malignant transformation.

Studies of effects of carcinogens on cell cultures have demonstrated a concomitant cytotoxicity which must be considered in divising protocols (DIPAOLO et al., 1971). This problem was not apparent in short-term studies of the effects of carcinogens on organ cultures (DIRKSEN and CROCKER, 1968; PALEKAR et al., 1968), but we found in the present investigation that continuous exposure to any level of carcinogen causes cell death, increases the rate of cell replication, and eventuates in the death of treated cultures sooner than untreated cultures. This early death may reflect the same fundamental biologic property observed in the limited life spans of primary cell lines (HAYFLICK,

1965). The continuous cell death due to the toxic chemical, in provoking a high mitotic rate, could propel the epithelial cell population through its preprogrammed finite number of cell generations in a much shorter time than would be observed for the same number of generations in an unstimulated population. Concentrations of benzo(a)pyrene over 2 µg/ml resulted in death of the culture in 6 weeks or less, rendering this concentration or equivalent concentrations of other agents unsuitable for continuous exposure protocols. Since there is evidence from cell culture studies that these concentrations exceed the metabolic capacity of the cell to activate the carcinogen (DUNCAN and BROOKES, 1970), our data suggests that cytotoxicity may be at least in part independent of activation, and this provides an additional reason for selecting lower concentrations.

We also identified a lower limit of concentration at which there is no evidence of atypia suggestive of carcinogenic effect. Therefore, while avoiding the pitfall of cytotoxicity, concentrations of benzo-(a)pyrene below 1.0 µg/ml used without additional factors do not appear to be appropriate for use in a carcinogenesis model, and equivalent concentrations of other agents being screened as potential carcinogens would probably not exhibit their tumorigenic effects under these conditions of exposure.

At concentrations from 1.0 to 2.0 µg/ml, the range between the lethal and non-tumorigenic levels, described above, cytologic abnormalities, distorted histologic patterns and ultrastructural features seen in neoplastic and preneoplastic lesions (TARIN, 1967; HARRIS et al., 1971; HARRIS et al., 1973), were produced. The times of appearance of the various stages depended upon the dosage level, with the changes appearing earlier in specimens treated with higher concentrations of carcinogen. However, in no specimen did transformation to histopathologically recognizable malignancy appear. One possible explanation for the lack of development of overtly malignant cell populations may relate to cytotoxicity. The carcinogen was continuously present in the culture in the protocol used and, while transformed cells may be more resistant than normal cells, such resistance is, of course, not absolute. The agent may kill enough transformed cells under these conditions to suppress the emergence of a malignant population.

Our studies have identified an effective concentration for continuous exposure to carcinogenic agents and quantitated cytotoxic effects at these levels, at dosages below the carcinogenic level, and at still

---

Fig. 1. In a culture specimen incubated for a week in medium containing 2 µg/ml of benzo(a)pyrene, the basal cells are finely vacuolated and surface cells are coarsely vacuolated. The desquamated or partially detached cells are frequently present but are not seen in all specimens. x 200

Fig. 2. After 3 weeks of continuous exposure to 2 µg/ml of benzo(a)-pyrene, there is a hyperplastic stratified squamous metaplasia. Degenerative changes at this stage are less pronounced. x 80

Fig. 3. An autoradiograph of specimen exposed for one week to 2.0 µg/ml of benzo(a)pyrene reveals that over 10% of the epithelial cells have incorporated tritiated thymidine during a 3o minute pulse shortly before fixation of the tissue. The labelled cells are uniformly distributed over the surface of the culture. x 80

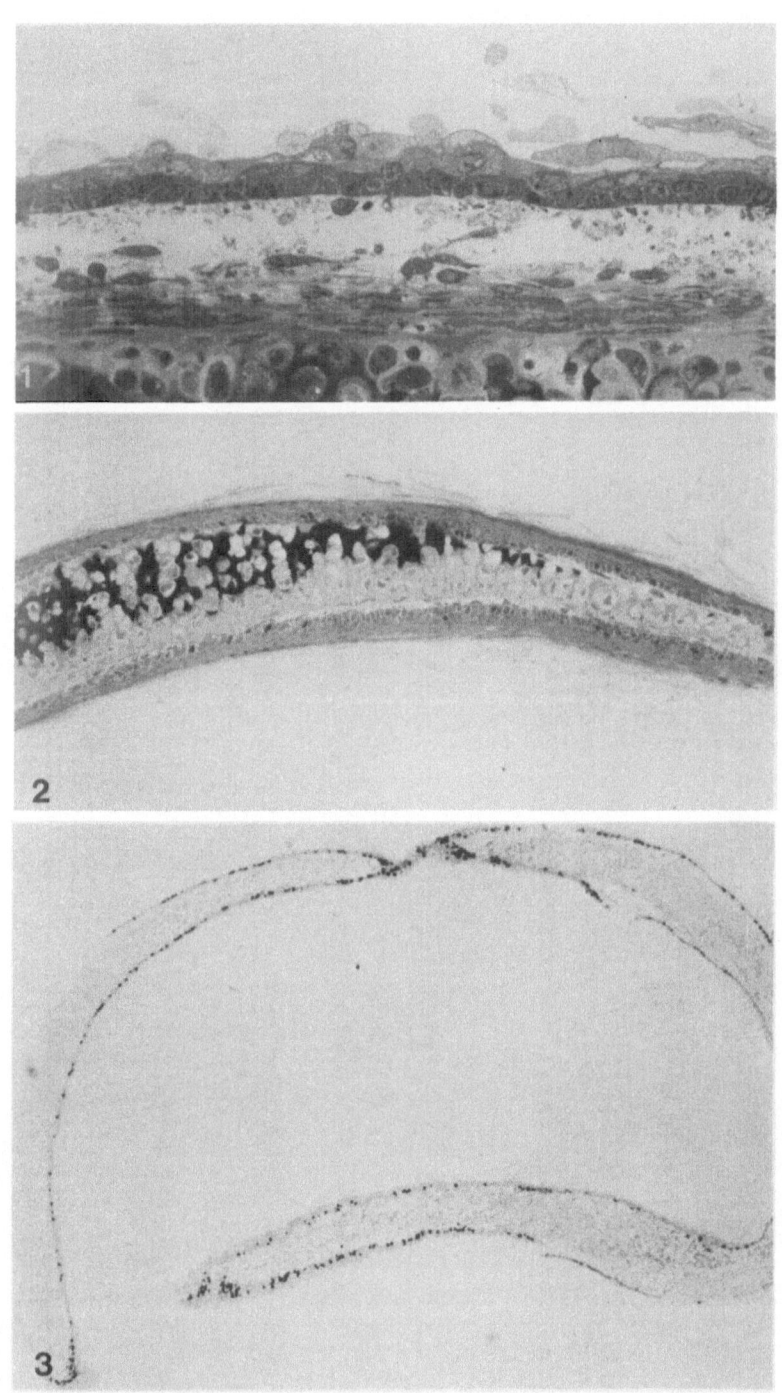

Legends see opposite page

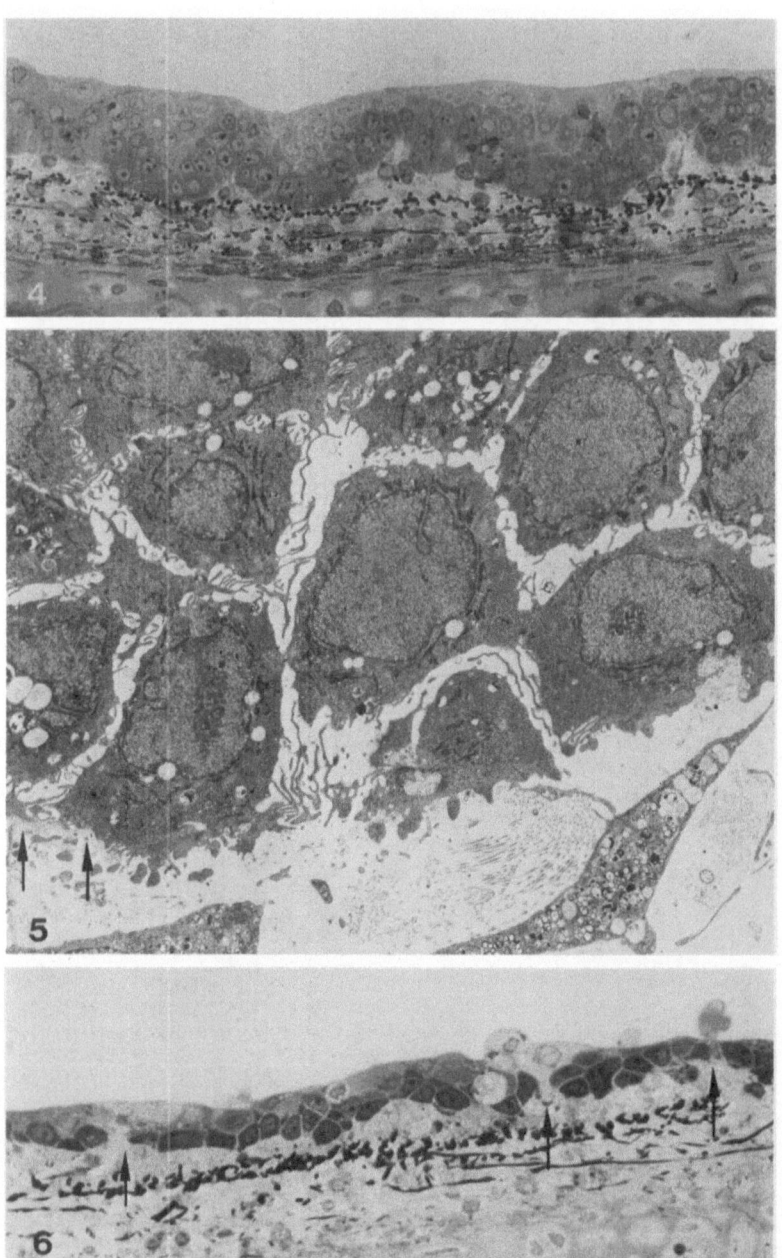

Legends see opposite page

higher concentrations. They suggest that more elaborate protocols
utilizing discontinuous exposure, addition of cofactors, or more sensitive criteria for malignant transformation than classical diagnostic
histopathologic alterations, may be required to realize the potential
of organ cultures as carcinogenesis models or screening systems.

References

DI PAOLO, J.A., DONOVAN, P.T., NELSON, R.L.: Transformation of hamster
    cells in vitro by polycyclic hydrocarbons without cytotoxicity.
    Proc. nat. Acad. Sci. (Wash.) 68, 2958-2961 (1971).
DIRKSEN, E.R., CROCKER, T.T.: Ultrastructural alterations produced
    by polycyclic aromatic hydrocarbons on rat tracheal epithelium in
    organ culture. Cancer Res. 28, 906-923 (1968).
DUNCAN, M., BROOKES, P.: The relation of metabolism to macromolecular
    binding of the carcinogen benzo(a)pyrene, by mouse embryo cells in
    culture. Int. J. Cancer 6, 496-505 (1970).
HARRIS, C.C., KAUFMAN, D.G., SPORN, M.B., SMITH, J.M., JACKSON, F.,
    SAFFIOTTI, U.: Ultrastructural effects of N-methyl-N-nitrosourea
    on the tracheobronchial epithelium of the Syrian Golden Hamster.
    Int. J. Cancer 12, 259-269 (1973).
HARRIS, C.C., SPORN, M.B., KAUFMAN, D.G., SMITH, J.M., BAKER, M.S.,
    SAFFIOTTI, U.: Acute ultrastructural effects of benzo(a)pyrene
    and ferric oxide in the hamster tracheobronchial epithelium. Cancer
    Res. 31, 1977-1989 (1971).
HAYFLICH, L.: The limited in vitro lifetime of human diploid cell
    strains. Exp. Cell. Res. 37, 614-636 (1965).
LANE, B.P., MILLER, S.: Benzo(a)pyrene-induced changes in tracheal
    epithelium in organ culture. Fed. Proc. 32, 825 (1973).
PALEKAR, L., KUSCHNER, M., LASKIN, S.: Cancer Res. 28, 2098-2104
    (1968).
TARIN, D.: Sequential electron microscopical study of experimental
    mouse skin carcinogenesis. Int. J. Cancer 2, 195-211 (1967).

Fig. 4. Several weeks after the appearance of hyperplasia, the regular
linear array of basal cells is focally or diffusely replaced by nodular aggregates or, in other cases not illustrated, by more irregular
spike-line downward growth. Basal-type cells are heaped up in 3 to 5
layers. These cells have a high nucleocytoplasmic ratio, irregularly
spaped nuclei and clear mucleoplasm with active large nucleoli. x 200

Fig. 5. The basal cells in the hyperplastic epithelium exhibit loss
of basal lamina (arrow) with small cytoplasmic projections extending
into lamina propria. Cells are separated by wide interspaces and have
relatively large numbers of fingerlike surface projections and relatively few desmosomes. These changes, together with high nuclear-
cytoplasmic ratio and irregular nuclear outlines, have been described
in premalignant and early malignant lesions in vivo. Fine fatty vacuo-
lization is frequently present and may be evidence of sustained cytotoxicity but few obviously necrotic cells are encountered. x 2800

Fig. 6. By 8 weeks of continuous exposure to 2 µg/ml of benzo(a)pyrene,
hyperplasia is no longer a prominent feature and most areas of epithelium consist of 2 cell layers. The basal cell layer in many areas
is discontinuous (arrows) and superficial cells are frequently vacuolated. x 200

Topical Application of Polycyclic Hydrocarbons to Differentiated Respiratory Epithelium in Long-Term Organ Cultures

Brooke T. Mossman and John E. Craighead

Department of Pathology, Medical Alumni Building, University of Vermont, College of Medicine, Burlington, VT 05401, USA

ABSTRACT

Polycyclic hydrocarbons are insoluble in the nutrient medium used to support cells and tissues *in vitro*. These substances must be incorporated into organic solvents which in turn are mixed with the culture medium. This approach raises questions regarding the exposure of individual cells since the carcinogen may separate out or adhere to the walls of the culture vessel.

Recently, we undertook studies to assess the carcinogenic properties of selected hydrocarbons using the differentiated respiratory mucosa of the hamster trachea maintained in organ culture. Borosilicate glass fibers (diameter 3×10^{-2} mm) were flushed with solutions of radiolabeled hydrocarbons in acetone and applied (after evaporation of the acetone) to the epithelial surface of the organ culture. This permitted us to vary the concentration of the carcinogen and allowed a systematic evaluation of epithelial changes at a defined site over a range of time periods. Presumably, the connective tissue elements subjacent to the mucosa were not exposed to the carcinogen.

In our studies, cultures are maintained in a viable, differentiated state for two or more months as confirmed by histologic study and radioautography. Epithelial cells exhibit cytologic alterations and changes in ^{3}H-thymidine uptake at sites of fiber application after brief periods of exposure. Proliferation of the affected mucosa and loss of orientation of epithelial cells is noted. Possible neoplastic transformation of affected cells is currently being tested by implantation of cultures subcutaneously into syngeneic animals.

A. Introduction

Chemical carcinogens are toxic for cells in monolayer culture at high concentrations, but cause a variety of cytologic alterations at lower concentrations (DIAMOND, 1969; DIPAOLO et al., 1971). The introduction of water-insoluble polycyclic hydrocarbons into cell cultures poses technical problems since these compunds must be incorporated into organic solvents which in turn are mixed with the medium. As a result, quantitative effects are difficult to assess since the carcinogen might separate out or adhere to the walls of the culture dish in an unpredictable fashion.

---

*This work was supported by contract PHSCP33360 from the National Cancer Institute.

Organ cultures of respiratory tract mucosa provide a system for assessing the carcinogenic effects of polycyclic hydrocarbons on differentiated epithelial cells over prolonged periods of time. In our studies, radiolabeled 3-Methylcholanthrene (MCA) was applied to fibers
of glass which were then layered onto the epithelial surface of hamster tracheal organ cultures. This permitted us to vary the concentration of carcinogen and allowed a systematic evaluation of epithelial changes at a defined site in the mucosa.

The present report describes our methods and preliminarily documents
the cytologic alterations which develop in the respiratory epithelium
exposed to MCA.

B. Materials and Methods

I. Organ Culture Preparation

Organ cultures were prepared from the tracheas of adult hamsters of
the 87.20 strain (TELACO, Bar Harbor, Me.) by previously described
methods (MOSSMAN and CRAIGHEAD, in press). In brief, approximately
1.0×1.0 mm^3 segments were incubated in groups of 4 in 35 mm plastic
Petri dishes containing 0.5 ml of Eagle's Minimum Essential Medium
(Earle's base) with added Gentamicin (50 µg/ml) and chicken serum
(2% final concentration). Explants were maintained in a 95% air -
5% CO_2 water-saturated environment at 35°C and the medium changed
twice weekly. Preliminary experiments showed that the respiratory
epithelium of the explants maitained a normal pseudostratified appearance in this medium for long as 20 weeks *in vitro*.

II. Preparation and Use of MCA-Glass Fibers

Fibers of borosilicate glass (approximate diameter 3.0×10^{-2} mm,
length 2.3 mm) were washed in acetone, placed in glass Petri dishes
and sterilized. Three-methylcholanthrene -6^{14}C (New England Nuclear,
Boston, Mass., ca. 98% purity, S.A., 5.47 mc/mM) was dissolved in
acetone (Fisher Certified, 99% purity) to make a final concentration
of 2.5×10^3 µg/ml. Serial 10-fold dilutions of this stock solution
were prepared and assayed by scintillation spectrophotometry using
the least squares fit of the logs to analyze data. Aliquots (0.5 ml)
of the diluted MCA solution were introduced into the dishes containing
fibers and the acetone evaporated at 25°C. Individual fibers were then
removed from the dishes with fine forceps and applied to the epithelial surface of explants. During the course of these experiments,
fibers were assayed for ^{14}C activity after their removal from the
cultures and the MCA dosage calculated.

III. Histological Techniques

At weekly intervals 0.5 µc thymidine-^{3}H was added to each of several
culture dishes. Eighteen hours later the thymidine-^{3}H containing medium was removed and the tissue washed twice with balanced salt solution. Explants were fixed in culture dishes using 4% glutaraldehyde
in 0.1 M sodium cacodylate buffer. The fibers were then removed, and
the area of the explant which had been exposed directly to the carcinogen excised.

After 18 hours the tissues were post-fixed in 1% osmium tetroxide, dehydrated, and embedded in Epon by standard methods. Sections (ca. 1 µ thickness) were prepared with an ultramicrotome and stained with toluidine blue.

Radioautography was done by the method of KAUFMAN et al. (1972). Ultrathin sections were stained with uranyl acetate and lead citrate and examined with a Phillips 300 electron microscope.

C. Results

I. Properties of MCA-Glass Fibers

Radioactive MCA was deposited on glass fibers as the volatile component of the acetone-MCA solution evaporated. Although the quantity of MCA which accumulated on individual fibers varied somewhat, the relative amount was roughly proportional to the concentration of the polycyclic hydrocarbon in the stock solution. In preliminary studies it was found that approximately 10% of the MCA on the fibers was lost into the culture medium after two weeks of incubation *in vitro*. By washing the fibers in distilled water, it was possible to remove this labile component of the MCA before exposing cultures to the fiber (Fig. 1).

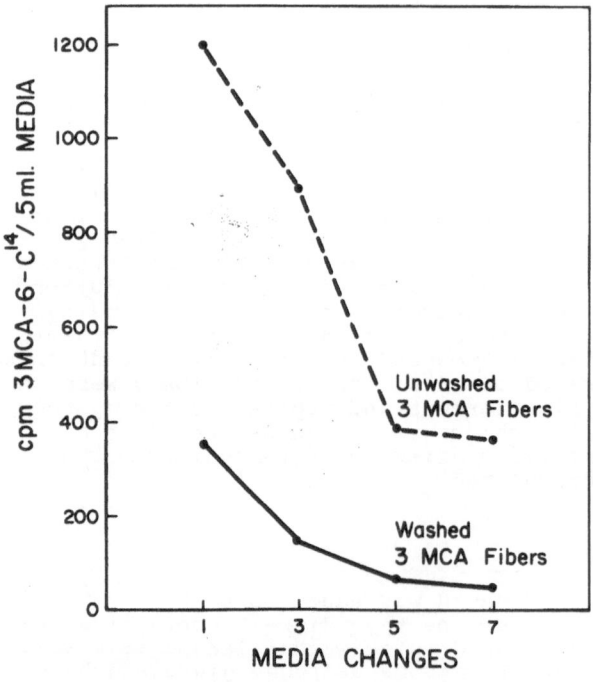

Control media values 22.6 ± 2.3 s.d.

Fig. 1. Release of radiolabeled MCA into culture medium from unwashed and washed glass fibers. Rinsing of the filaments in distilled water prior to their application to explants removed excess amounts of the hydrocarbon

II. Morphologic Observations

Thus far, detailed morphological studies have been carried out on tracheal explants exposed to MCA-treated fibers for periods of as long as 4 weeks. In these experiments it was assumed that the effect of the carcinogen was confined largely to the cells of the respiratory mucosa in immediate proximity to the fiber. Since the changes appeared to be dosage-dependent, and varied in extent from one explant to another, only a brief summary of our findings is recorded here.

Cells of the organ culture epithelium promptly proliferated adjacent to, and over, the surface of the glass fiber (Fig. 2). This apparently was a non-specific response to the foreign glass filament since it was observed in cultures exposed to fibers which had not been treated with MCA. As might be expected, portions of the outgrowth of cells were torn from the mucosal surface of the explants when fibers were physically removed after glutaraldehyde fixation.

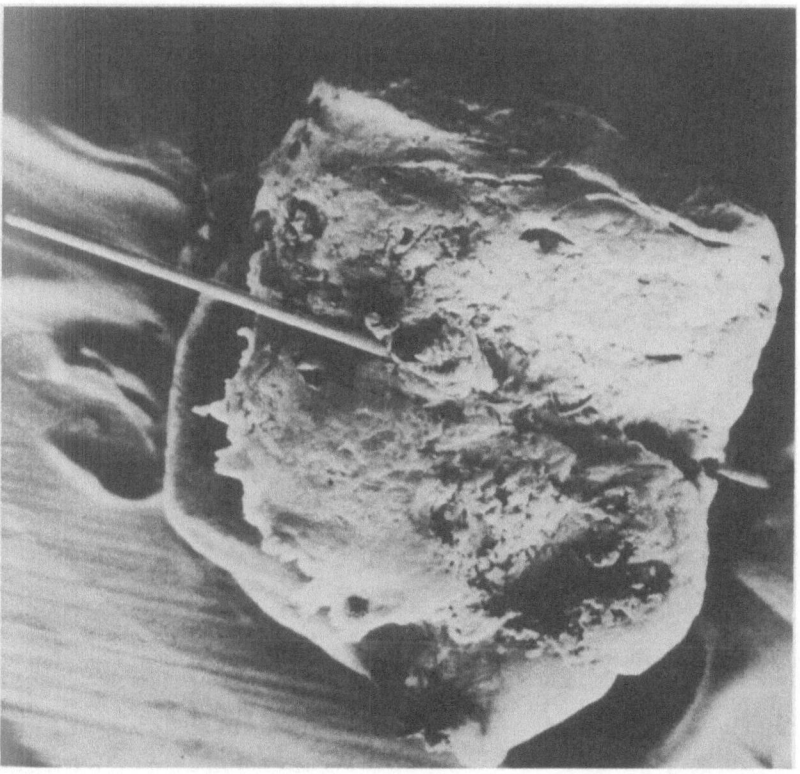

Fig. 2. Scanning electron photomicrograph of explant 2 weeks after application of carcinogen fiber. After critical point freeze-drying, the tissue was coated with gold-paladium in a vacuum evaporator and viewed with a Cambridge Stereoscan (x 120)

The morphologic features of the excrescence of cells which formed adjacent to the glass fibers are illustrated in Fig. 3. As can be seen, the epithelial elements of the MCA-exposed mucosa exhibited

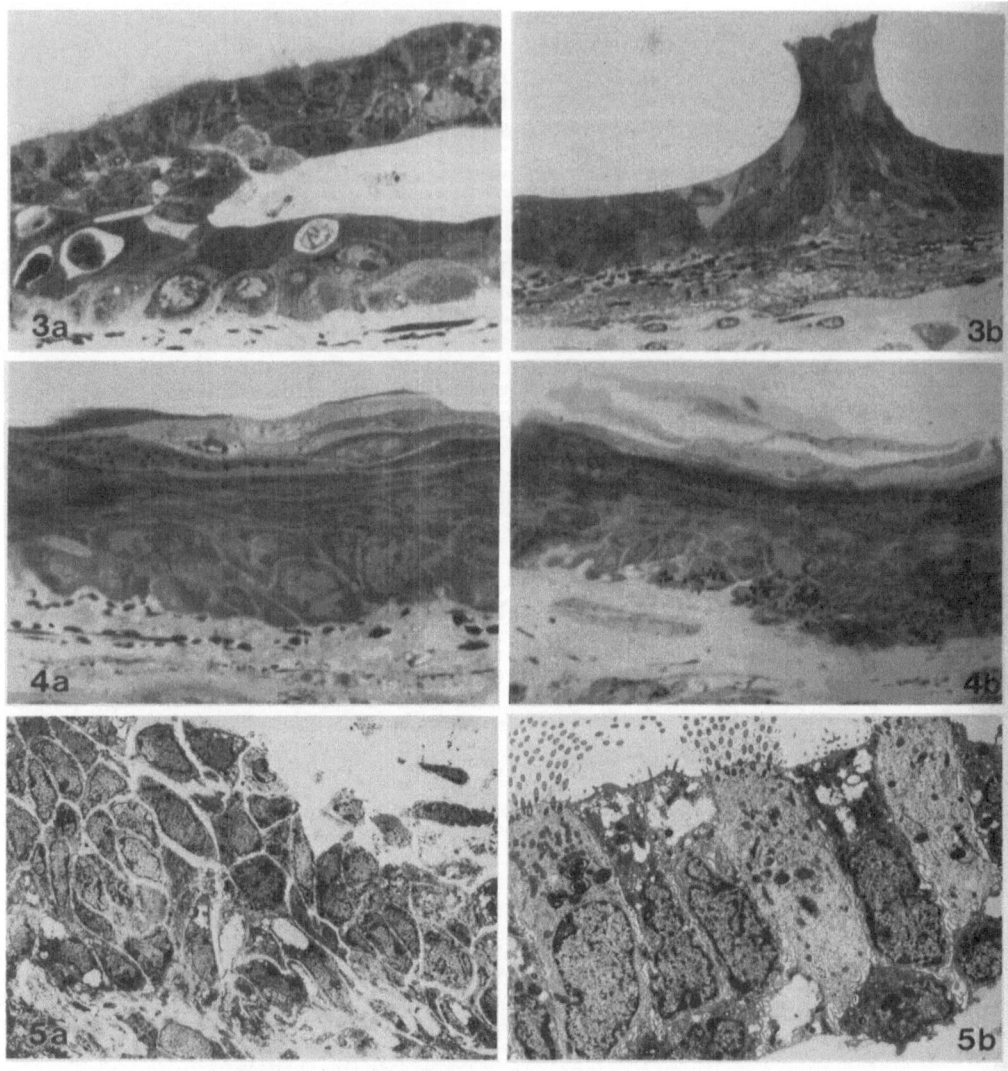

Fig. 3 a and b. Outgrowths of cells adjacent to fiber site. (a) Fiber
exposure - 3 weeks (3.4 μg MCA). (x 1200). (b) Fiber exposure - 2 weeks
(control). (x 1350). Note the irregular proliferation of atypical polygonal cells from the basal layer in the MCA exposed tissue

Fig. 4 (a) Squamous metaplasia at fiber site. Fiber exposure - 2 weeks
(6.5 x 10⁻² μg MCA). (b) Autoradiogram of corresponding lesion exhibiting intensive labeling of basalar cell layer

Fig. 5 (a) Proliferation of affected tracheal mucosal cells adjacent
to fiber site. Note the irregular arrangement of cells having polygonal configurations. Fiber exposure - 4 weeks (2.7 x 10⁻³ μg MCA).
(x 1580). (b) Normal tracheal mucosa after 5 weeks *in vitro*. Fiber
exposure - 4 weeks (control). (x 2730)

cytologic alterations which were not observed in control cultures. These changes were prominent in cultures exposed to fibers coated with approximately 1 x 10^{-3} µg of MCA. They were not found when smaller amounts of the hydrocarbon were employed.

Ciliated cells in MCA-treated cultures often appeared distended and exhibited supranuclear vacuoles. Frequently the ciliated mucosa was replaced by basal cells having a polygonal outline and cuboidal cells which lacked cilia. Occasional cultures showed prominent features of squamous metaplasia (Fig. 4).

The ultrastructural features of the carcinogen-exposed cells were complex (Fig. 5a). The nuclei exhibited increased numbers of nucleoli and an irregular configuration. Often they appeared enlarged. Cyto-plasmic organelles were prominent in these cells and lysosomes were increased in number. Nonetheless, basal bodies and cilia occasionally were observed on some distorted superficial cells. Alterations in the submucosa occasionally were prominent. Mesenchymal cells appeared to proliferate or accumulate subjacent to the fiber site. Occasionally these cells encroached on the mucosal basement membrane where they came in close proximity to the basal layer of the epithelium. Epi-thelial cells of explants which had not been exposed to MCA exhibited the features of the normal tracheal mucosa. Mucin-secreting cells occasionally showed supranuclear vacuoles (Fig. 5b).

D. Discussion

Experimental attempts to induce bronchogenic carcinomas in laboratory animals with polycyclic hydrocarbons have yielded variable and unpre-dictable results. Moreover, relatively large amounts of the carcinogen must be instilled into the tracheobronchial tree over extended periods of time using foreign substances as carriers. Clearly, animals provide an unsatisfactory means for assaying the properties of new or suspected carcinogens, and are an unreliable system for testing possible prophy-lactic or chemotherapeutic agents.

Monolayer cell cultures have been employed extensively to assess the carcinogenic potential of hydrocarbons and to explore the mechanism of neoplastic transformation. These systems are imperfect for studies of this type because the cells usually are modified by growth *in vitro* and often exhibit features of neoplastic tissues. Inasmuch as water-insoluble organic substances must be introduced into the liquid medium of the cell culture, it is difficult to quantitate dosages and reliably define the duration of exposure.

The methods described in this report were developed to overcome many of these practical and theoretical considerations. By annealing hydro-carbons onto the surface of glass fibers which are then applied to the mucosa of organ cultures, it is possible to expose localized areas of the differentiated respiratory epithelium to known quantities of car-cinogen. Our techniques allow the investigator to carry out studies with replicate cultures and thus to define systematically the sequen-tial morphologic changes which accompany transformation. Since organ cultures of the type described can be transplanted into syngeneic animals, it is feasible to determine the neoplastic potentials of carcinogen-treated cells in a reproducible fashion.

It was of interest to observe in our morphologic studies the growth of epithelial cells over the surfaces of the glass fibers. These changes undoubtedly illustrate a mechanism whereby the respiratory mucosa responds to the presence of foreign materials. At this juncture, one can only speculate as to the role of this process in neoplasia in the intact animal. However, it seems likely that a reactive change of this type would enhance the exposure of epithelial cells to carcinogens when these substances are deposited on inhaled inorganic particulate matter.

The morphologic alterations observed in our carcinogen-exposed organ cultures are similar to those described in the respiratory mucosa of animals administered polycyclic hydrocarbons by the intratracheal route (STENBACK, 1974; HENRY et al., 1974). Thus far in our experiments, explants of tissue treated with MCA have failed to exhibit neoplastic epithelial growth after transplantation into syngeneic hamsters.

Acknowledgements

BRENDA LEY and JUDITH KESSLER provided valuable technical assistance. Dr. ARNOLD BRODY prepared the scanning electron micrographs.

References

DIAMOND, L.: The interaction of chemical carcinogens and cells *in vitro*. In: Progress in Experimental Tumor Research (ed. S. Karger), Vol. II. pp. 364-383. Basel-New York: F. Holmburger 1969.

DIPAOLO, J.A., NELSON, R.L., DONOVAN, P.J.: Morphological, oncogenic, and karyological characteristics of Syrian hamster embryo cells transformed *in vitro* by carcinogenic polycyclic hydrocarbons. Cancer Res. 31, 1118-1127 (1971).

HENRY, M.C., PORT, C.D., KAUFMAN, D.G.: Role of particles in respiratory carcinogenesis bioassay (these proceedings).

KAUFMAN, D.G., BAKER, M.S., HARRIS, C.C., SMITH, J.M., BOREN, H., SPORN, M.B., SAFFIOTTI, U.: Coordinated biochemical and morphologic examination of hamster tracheal epithelium. J. nat. Cancer Inst. 49, 783-792 (1972).

STENBACK, F.: Experimental lung carcinogenesis in hamsters: effect of carrier dust (these proceedings).

The Bioassay of Carcinogenesis: Effects on the Epithelial Cell Complement of Rat Tracheae Maintained *in vitro*

David W. Lindsay, J. R. Jones, W. J. Higgins, and P. W. Brown

Carreras Rothmans Ltd., Research Division, Basildon, Essex, England

ABSTRACT

The effects on the epithelium of suckling rat tracheae in organ cultures of three polycyclic hydrocarbons, 7,12-dimethylben(a)anthracene
and benzo(a)pyrene which are carcinogenic and pyrene which is not
carcinogenic, of diethylnitrosamine and of cigarette smoke condensates
prepared from two types of cigarettes were studied. The changes found
in the epithelial cell complement were analyzed by differential cell
counts which revealed the relative numbers of undifferentiated, normally differentiated and abnormally differentiated cells present. It
was found that the same general pattern of change, involving a reduction in the proportion of differentiated cells at low concentrations
of test material and an increasing proportion of abnormally differentiated cells at higher concentrations was found with all the carcinogens and the cigarette smoke condensates but not with the noncarcinogen. Some evidence suggesting that this constant pattern of change
was induced in a different manner by different materials was found.
The total cell number per unit length of epithelium was also recorded
and it was found that all of the active materials caused an increase
in total cell number except in the case of 7,12-dimethylben(a)anthra-
cene which was markedly toxic and reduced cell number at relatively
low concentrations. Differences in the magnitude of effect on the
level of differentiation in the epithelium between the two cigarette
smoke condensates were found and were similar in extent to differences
which have been found in skin painting experiments. It is suggested
that the method has potential appplication as a predictive bioassay
for carcinogenic materials.

A. Introduction

A number of reports, using both *in vitro* and *in vivo* techniques, have
described the changes induced in respiratory epithelia by carcinogenic
compunds (LASNITZKI, 1951, 1955, 1958, 1973; CROCKER and SANDERS,
197o; PALEKAR et al., 1968). Changes in the appearance of such epithelia are clearly the result of changes in the number and distribution of different cell types within the epithelial cell complement,
and it is likely that some indication of the mode of action of chemical carcinogens could be given by an analysis of changes in the epithelial cell population. In addition, since such an analysis would be
amenable to quantitative expression, information permitting a comparison of the effectiveness of different compunds, and hence a form
of assay of potential carcinogenicity, might be obtained.

This report describes an attempt to make an analysis of this type. The effects of a number of compounds with carcinogenic activity as compared with noncarcinogens and cigarette smoke condensate, an undefined material of possible carcinogenic significance obtained from cigarettes which had been tested tumorigenicity in skin-painting procedures, were examined in tracheal epithelia by means of differential cell counts. The investigation was carried out *in vitro* using rat tracheae maintained in organ culture, to exploit the greater reproducibility and precision of dosage obtainable with such techniques with a view to developing a bioassay technique for carcinogenic activity.

B. Materials and Methods

I. Animal Tissue

Tracheae for culture were obtained from 4-to-5-day-old Wistar rats.

II. Test Materials

7,12 dimethylbenz(a)anthracene (DMBA) and benzo(a)pyrene (BaP) were obtained from Koch-Light Laboratories Limited, pyrene from Hopkin and Williams Limited, and diethylnitrosamine (DENA) from Eastman Organic Chemicals. Smoke condensate was prepared from each of two plain cigarettes, manufactured for the Tobacco Research Council from the lamina (L) and stem (S) of a composite blend of flue-cured tobacco. (The cigarettes had the following characteristics: length 7o mm, circumference 25.3 mm, average weight 1.12 g (L) and 1.19 g (S).) This tobacco was similar to that used in the major cigarette brands smoked in the United Kingdom at the time of manufacture. Cigarettes were smoked on a Mason rotary smoking machine to the standard parameters of one 35 ml puff of 2 second duration per minute continuing to a 23 mm butt length, and a nonvolatile whole smoke condensate collected in an impaction trap.

In all cases, analytical grade acetone was used as solvent.

III. Organ Culture

Tracheae were cultured by a modification of Trowell's method (TROWELL, 1959) in which tissue was supported on a stainless steel mesh raft covered by lens tissue that dipped into the culture medium. The medium consisted of medium 199 65%, calf serum 25%, and chick embryo extract 10%, plus penicillin and streptomycin at concentrations of 100 units/ml and 50 µ/ml respectively. Test materials in acetone solution were mixed with calf serum, and aliquots of this mixtures were added to the medium as part of the total serum complement. The final acetone concentration in the medium was in all cases 0.2%.

Cultures were exposed to an atmosphere of 5% carbon dioxide in oxygen and incubated at 36.5°C. The atmosphere was changed daily and the medium replaced every other day.

Explants were cultured for 7 days in the presence of test material plus 0.2% acetone, 0.2% acetone, or culture medium only and then for a further 4-day period in culture medium without test material or acetone. The final 4 day-period was included as an attempt to exclude any changes resulting simply from the actual presence of test material.

Each dose level of test material and each control was represented by 8 explants.

At the end of the culture period explants were removed from the lens tissue, rinsed free of culture medium, fixed in Bouin's fluid, and embedded in paraffin wax. Serial transverse sections, 5 µm thick, were cut from the entire length of each explant and stained with haematoxylin and eosin.

IV. Assessment

Differential cell counts were performed on cultured material by examining fixed lengths of epithelium and assigning the constituent cells to three groups similar to those described by CROCKER et al. (1965). Undifferentiated cells, corresponding closely to the basal cells of CROCKER et al. (1965) were small cells, with round nuclei, adjacent to the basement membrane or belonging to groups of such cells whose most distal members were in contact with the basement membrane. Normally differentiated cells (the differentiated epithelial cells of CROCKER et al., 1965) were cells that were elongate in a plane perpendicular to the basement membrane and containing elongate nuclei. Abnormally differentiated cells (the metaplastic or flattened epithelial cells of CROCKER et al., 1965), were irregular cells that frequently contained pleomorphic nuclei. Such cells tended to be elongate parallel to the basement membrane, to have an altered nuclear-cytoplasmatic ratio, and to be eosinophilic.

Counts were made on 6 randomly selected sections of each explant, with a randomly chosen length of epithelium and the length of epithelium diametrically opposite this being counted in each section. The length counted was 201 µm per observation, and with 8 explants per treatment, a total length of about 20 mm (which in control tissue contained 3.000 to 4.000 cells) was examined for each dose level of a treatment.

Results of such counts for each cell are here expressed as percentages of the total number scored together with the total cell number per 100 µm. Each point represents the mean value of 12 counts on each of 8 explants with 95% confidence limits added.

C. Results

I. Control Material

Differential cell counts on material exposed to culture medium or medium plus 0.2% acetone suggested that the presence of acetone had no marked effect on the parameters used.

Total cell number in control tissue varied from 17 to 28 cells per 100 µm, with one isolated observation of 43 cells per 100 µm. The percentage of undifferentiated cells commonly fell in the range of 32% to 33%, with occasional scores of 37% to 38%, while normally differentiated cells fell in the range 67% to 68% with a few scores of 58% to 60%. These values agree with published findings for rat tracheal epithelium (RHODIN and DALHAMN, 1956). In all but one case, abnormally differentiated cells accounted for less than 1% of the population.

The appearance of cultured epithelium (Fig. 1a) was closely similar
to that of the material used to initiate the organ cultures (Fig. 1b).

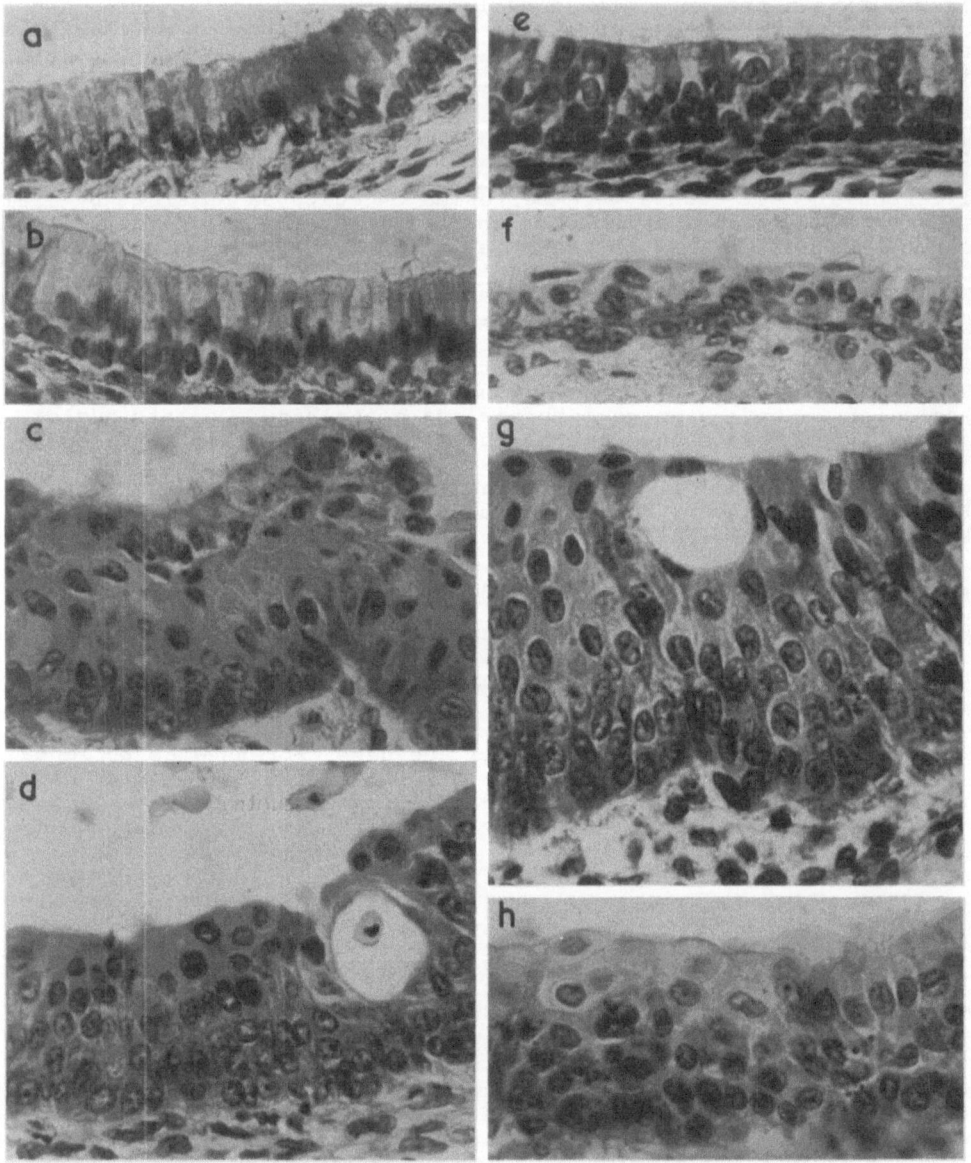

Fig. 1 a–h. Photomicrographs of transverse sections of cultured tracheae, stained with haematoxylin and eosin (x 540). (a) Control-exposed
to 0.2% acetone for first 7 days of 11-day culture period; (b) uncul-
tured trachea; (c–h) exposed to test material for first 7 days of
11-day culture period, as follows: (c) 5 μg/ml DMBA, (d) 20 μg/ml
BaP, (e) 100 μg/ml pyrene, (f) 1.000 μg/ml DENA, (g) 500 μg/ml condensate L, (h) 250 μg/ml condensate S

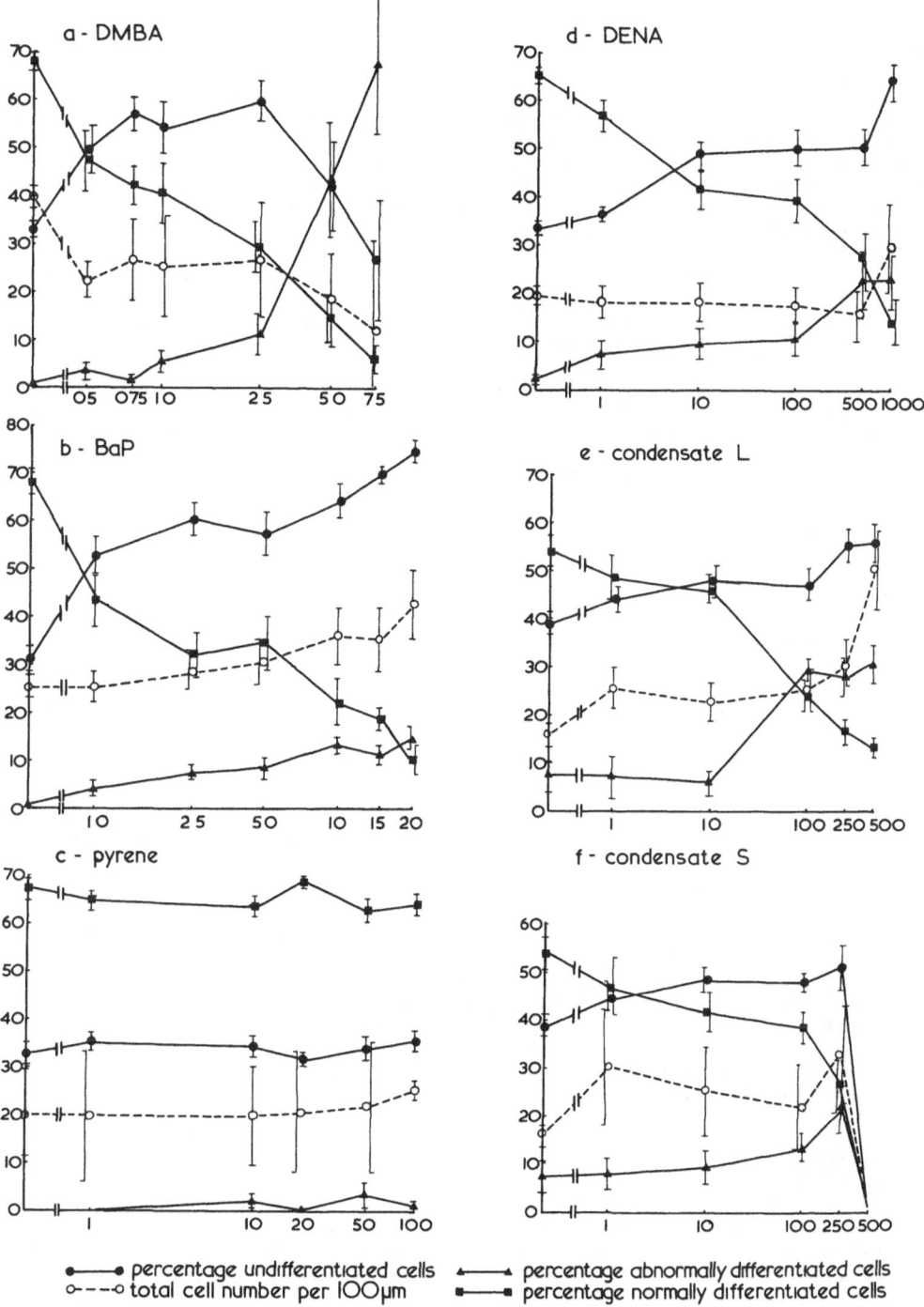

Fig. 2. Effect of test materials on the epithelial cell complement of trachease exposed to these test materials for the first 7 days of an 11-day culture period. *Ordinate* - Percentage of total epithelial cell complement represented by given cell type *or* total cell number per 100 μm. *Abscissa* - Concentration of test substance (μg/ml)

526

II. Effect of DMBA

The effect of a range of concentrations of DMBA is shown in Fig. 2a.
Three marked patterns of change with increasing concentrations were
noted. First, a progressive decrease in the proportion of normally
differentiated cells with increasing DMBA concentration was apparent.
Second, the proportion of undifferentiated cells increased with concentrations up to 0.75 µg/ml at which level the epithelium contained
more undifferentiated than differentiated cells, a balance that was
maintained at higher concentrations. Finally, at concentrations in
excess of 0.75 µg/ml, DMBA induced increasing proportions of abnormally differentiated cells in the epithelium. It may also be seen
that after an initial decrease with the addition of DMBA, total cell
number remained relatively constant with increasing concentrations
up to 2.5 µg/ml. At higher concentrations, total cell number decreased
as the toxic concentration of DMBA was approached.

It can be inferred from these results that low concentrations of DMBA
reduce the proportion of cells in the epithelium that differentiate.
At concentrations above 1.0 µg/ml, there was no change in the overall
proportion of differentiated cells until toxic levels were approached
but there was a progressive change of balance from normal to abnormal
differentiation within the differentiated population.

The appearance of epithelium exposed to 5 µg/ml DMBA is shown in
Fig. 1c.

III. Effect of BaP

The effect of increasing concentrations of BaP in the range 0 to
20.0 µg/ml, shown in Fig. 2b, was similar but not identical to the
changes induced by DMBA. Low concentration were associated with a
reversal of the proportions of differentiated and undifferentiated
cells, while an increase in BaP concentration led to a continued reduction in the proportion of normally differentiated cells and an
increase in the proportion of abnormally differentiated cells. This
was similar to the findings with DMBA, but differences exist. Whereas
after an initial change at low concentrations increasing levels of
DMBA did not have further effects on the proportion of undifferentiated
cells until toxicity became apparent, increasing BaP concentrations led
to further increases in the proportion of these cells. High concentrations of BaP led to an increase in total cell number in contrast to
the findings with DMBA. Finally, abnormally differentiated cells were
noted at the lowest BaP concentrations tested, whereas, with DMBA,
there was some indication concentration for their induction.

The appearance of epithelium treated with high BaP concentrations is
shown in Fig. 1d.

IV. Effect of Pyrene

Pyrene was chosen as an example of a noncarcinogenic polycyclic hydrocarbon rather than benzo(e)pyrene, the noncarcinogenic analog of BaP,
because difficulty was experienced in obtained samples of benzo(e)-
pyrene that were not contaminated with BaP.

Pyrene was tested over as wide a concentration range as solubility
permitted, namely from 0 to 100 µg/ml. It was immediately apparent
from the results of this treatment, shown in Fig. 2c, that no changes

of the magnitude induced by carcinogenic compounds took place. There was little alteration in the proportions of normally differentiated cells, while the highest level of abnormal cells observed was 3%. The only pronounced change noted was an increase in total cell number at high concentrations. This is in accord with the appearance of the epithelium which at the highest concentration tested differed from control material only in showing a moderate hyperplastic response (Fig. 1e).

V.   Effect of DENA

DENA was examined to give some indication of the effect of a carcinogen not related chemically to polycyclic hydrocarbons. It was found that over a wider concentration range (0 to 1,000 µg/ml), the response was similar to that found with DMBA and BaP. It can be seen from Fig. 2d that lower concentrations altered the relative proportions of normally differentiated and undifferentiated cells, so that the latter become predominant in the epithelium. At higher concentrations the proportion of normally differentiated cells decreased in conjunction with an increase in the proportion of abnormally differentiated cells. In common with BaP, high DENA concentrations induced a further increase in the proportion of undifferentiated cells associated with an increase in total cell number.

The appearance of epithelium treated with 1.000 µg/ml DENA is shown in Fig. 1f.

VI.   Effect of Cigarette Smoke Condensate

Both types of condensate (L and S) were tested in the range 0 to 500 µg/ml. The results for condensate L are shown in Fig. 2e and for condensate S in Fig. 2f.

The pattern found with other active materials was observed - namely a change from a predominance of undifferentiated cells in the epithelium at low concentrations and a replacement of normally differentiated cells by abnormally differentiated cells within the differentiated population at higher concentrations. At higher concentrations the proportion of undifferentiated cells and total cell number increased in parallel.

A number of particular points, concerning differences between the two condensates, can be drawn from these results. First, the change in relative proportions of differentiated and undifferentiated cells took place at lower concentrations with condensate S than with condensate L, whereas an increase in the proportion of abnormally differentiated cells occurred at lower concentrations of condensate L.

Further, at the concentrations tested, condensate L induced a higher proportion of abnormally differentiated cells. In addition, condensate S was markedly toxic at a concentration of 500 µg/ml while condensate L was not toxic at this level. It is thus apparent that although there is a close similarity in the response of the tissue to the two condensates, a number of differences in activity can be discerned.

The appearance of epithelium treated with 500 µg/ml of condensate L and 250 g/ml of condensate S is shown in Figs 1g and 1h respectively.

D. Discussion

The work reported here has demonstrated that the epithelium of cultured rat tracheae responds to a number of carcinogens and to cigarette smoke condensate in a manner that can be interpreted in terms of changes in the level and pattern of differentiation. The responses can be considered in terms of the percentage of differentiated cells present in the epithelium and in terms of the form of such differentiation as takes place. In addition, observed changes in the total number of cells in unit length of epithelium may permit some conclusions regarding overall changes in cell number and net proliferation rates associated with changes in the pattern of differentiation.

The three carcinogenic compounds and the two cigarette smoke condensates tested all gave closely similar results which were not reproduced by the noncarcinogen pyrene. The response illicited by the active materials appeared to have two phases. First, at low concentrations, the proportion of differentiated cells in the epithelium decreased and the proportion of undifferentiated cells increased. In most cases, the concentrations active in producing this change did not induce a large proportion of abnormally differentiated cells within the differentiated population. The type of change found could result from a selective loss of differentiated cells, from an increase in proliferation rate without a corresponding increase in differentiation rate, or from a decrease in differentiation rate. The present data do not yield decisive information on which, if any, of these mechanims are involved, but the data on total cell number permit some speculation. Thus, it was found with DMBA that the decreased proportion of differentiated cells was accompanied by a decrease in total cell number, suggesting a selective loss of differentiated cells. In contrast, over the corresponding part of the concentration range, cigarette smoke condensate induced an increase in total cell number in parallel with the increased proportion of undifferentiated cells, allowing the possibility that the observed change was a consequence of a change in net proliferation rate. Finally, BaP did not affect total cell number over the appropriate concentration range, implying that the change in pattern of differentiation was a consequence of a change in differentiation rate. Such suggestions emphasize the fact that there is no a-priori reason to assume that different compounds induce a given change by the same mechanisms, and it may be noted that other workers examining the effects of carcinogenic polycyclic hydrocarbons in organ culture, notably LASNITZKI (1956) and CROCKER et al. (1965), have observed differences in response to closely related compounds. CROCKER and NEILSEN (1967) suggested that the use of tissue in culture may emphasize differences that are less apparent *in vivo*.

At higher concentrations of active materials, a second form of change in the cell complement of the tracheal epithelium was apparent as a reduction in the proportion of normally differentiated cells and an increase in the proportion of abnormally differentiated cells. Curves showing the proportions of these cell types at different concentrations of active material tend to be mirror images of each other and this, together with the fact that such changes could occur without marked alteration in total cell number, suggests that the effect is the result of a change in the type of differentiation taking place rather than some form of selective cell loss. This need not be, however, the only mechanism whereby abnormally differentiated cells become predomonant at higher concentrations since the possibility exists that abnormal cells may be more resistant to the toxic effects of the active compounds. There is a parallel to this suggestion in the observation by DIAMOND (1965) that cells that have undergone a malignant transformation tend to have a greater resistance to the toxicity of the transforming agent than the parent cell type. Some response of this type may have taken place with DMBA as the curve for abnormally differentiated cells tended to mirror that for total cell number.

It has been noted that all of the active compounds tested affected both the extent and form of differentiation in the cultured epithelium. There is some indication, particularly with DMBA and the cigarette smoke condensates, that the quantitative and qualitative effects occurred in distinct parts of the concentration ranges. This raises the possibility that the two effects are, to some extent at least, independent of each other.

In some cases, a third form of response is discernable in the induction of a state resembling basal cell hyperplasia. From the present data, this could be identified from the observed increase in the proportion of undifferentiated cells accompanied by an increase in total cell number. The number of undifferentiated cells per unit length, support the use of these criteria (unpublished data). On this basis, the results indicate that a marked basal cell hyperplasia was induced by BaP, DENA, and the cigarette smoke condensates but not by DMBA. It should be noted that the increase in total cell number associated with high concentrations of pyrene was not accompanied by any marked change in the proportion of different cell types, suggesting that an increase in the net proliferation rate is not necessarily associated with a disruption of the pattern of differentiation.

The effects of carcinogens on ciliated columnar epithelia in organ culture have been described by a number of workers. In particular, LASNITZKI has examined the effect of polycyclic hydrocarbons on mouse prostate (LASNITZKI, 1951, 1955), human fetal lung (LASNITZKI, 1956), and of cigarette smoke condensate on human fetal lung (LASNITZKI, 1958), and mouse trachea (LASNITZKI, 1968). From this work, the general finding emerged that both polycyclic hydrocarbon carcinogens and cigarette smoke condensate induced basal cell hyperplasia and squamous metaplasia, the latter tending to occur at higher concentrations. These changes were accompanied by a loss of secretory cells. CROCKER and SANDERS (1970) reported similarly that in cultured hamster tracheae, BaP treatment led to the development of zones of pleimorphic undifferentiated cells and the appearance of abnormal dysplastic or squamous metaplastic lesions. ALTHOFF et al. (1971) studied the effect of DENA on hamster tracheae *in vivo* and found that the first changes involved an increased density of basal cells and a loss of ciliated cells followed by the appearance of several layers of variously differentiated cells. Thus, the present observations of reduced total differentiation and increased proportions of abnormally differentiated cells are supported by the existing literature.

LASNITZKI considered that the changes induced in culture have some preneoplastic significance (LASNITZKI, 1951, 1955, 1973), while CROCKER (1970) found that organ cultures treated with polycyclic hydrocarbon carcinogens histologically resembled cultures from the bronchial mucosa of human carcinoma patients. In addition, CROCKER and NEILSON (1967), suggesting that the squamous metaplastic changes induced in organ culture bear some relation to the carcinogenic properties of the experimental compounds have shown similarities between effects *in vivo* and *in vitro*. A relationship between squamous metaplasia and neoplasia *in vivo* has been discussed by a number of workers (BLACK and ACKERMAN, 1952; AUERBACH et al., 1957; SAFFIOTTI et al., 1967; CROCKER, 1970), and it has been suggested that squamous metaplasia

may represent one or more stages in a series of events leading ultimately to neoplasia (SAFFIOTTI et al., 1967). Further, it has been
demonstrated that tissues grown in organ culture and treated with
carcinogenic chemicals or cigarette smoke condensate induce tumours
after implantation in animals (LAWS and FLAKS, 1966; DAVIES et al.,
197o). It is thus possible that the changes in epithelial cell complement described in this report have some connection with the early
stages of neoplastic development.

The possible preneoplastic significance of the observed changes means
that the precise numerical nature of the data presented here may be
of value in the assessment of the potency of carcinogens and in the
screening of putative carcinogens. In this context, it is useful to
consider the effects of the two cigarette smoke condensates. From an
examination of the data, it might be considered that condensate S is
the less potent since, compared with condensate L, a lower proportion
of abnormal cells was produced at a higher concentration and the increase in total cell number was lower. These condensates have been
examined in mouse skin painting experiments, which have demonstrated
that condensate L had a tumorigenicity of 2.1 (1.3 to 3.4) times that
of condensate S (Tobacco Research Council, 1969). Thus, the extent of
the activity *in vitro* is paralleled by an effect *in vivo*, and it is of
interest to note that over the concentration range in which the two
condensates effect the greatest changes in the proportion of abnormally differentiated cells, the ratio of activity of condensate L to
condensate S approximates the ratio found in skin painting (e.g., at
a concentration of 100 µg/ml, the ratio of abnormally differentiated
cells was 28%:14% or 2:1). This provides a further parallel between
the production of abnormally differentiated cells *in vitro* and tumours
in vivo. Further work to determine those areas of the spectrum of
quantitative change that are most suitable for the comparison of activity of different materials is in progress.

Acknowledgments

The authors wish to thank the Board of Directors of Carreras-Rothmans
Limited for permission to publish this work. We are also grateful to
Dr. W.D. ROWLAND and his staff for computing the confidence limits of
the means.

References

ALTHOFF, J., WILSON, R., MOHR, U.: Diethylnitrosamine induced alter-
    ations in the tracheo-bronchial system of the Syrian Golden Hamster.
    J. nat. Cancer Inst. 46, 1o67-1o71 (1971).
AUERBACH, O., GERE, J.B., FORMAN, J.B., PETRICK, T.G., SMOLIN, H.J.,
    MUEHSAM, G.E., KASSOUNY, D.Y., STOUT, A.P.: Changes in the bron-
    chial epithelium in relation to smoking and cancer of the lung.
    New Engl. J. Med. 256 (3), 97-1o4 (1957).
BLACK, H., ACKERMAN, L.V.: Importance of epidermoid carcinoma in
    situ on the histogenesis of carcinoma of the lung. Ann. Surg. 136,
    45-55 (1952).
CROCKER, T.T.: Bronchial mucosa of Monkey and Man in organ culture
    application to the study of bronchial carcinogenesis. Amer. Rev.
    Resp. Dis. 1o1, 443-445 (197o).

CROCKER, T.T., NEILSEN, B.I.: Effect of carcinogenic hydrocarbons on suckling rat trachea in living animals and in organ culture in 'Lung Tumours in Animals' (ed. L. Severi), pp. 765-787. Perugia: University of Perugia 1967.

CROCKER, T.T., NEILSEN, B.I., LASNITZKI, I.: Carcinogenic hydrocarbons; effect on suckling rat trachea in organ culture. Arch. Environ Hlth. 1o, 24o-25o (1965).

CROCKER, T.T., SANDERS, L.L.: Influence of Vitamin A & 3, 7, Dimethyl-2,6-octadienal (Citral) on the effect of Benzo(a)pyrene on hamster trachea in organ culture. Cancer Res. 3o, 1312-1318 (197o).

DAVIES, R.F., MAJOR, I.R., ABERDEEN, E.R.: Pulmonary adenomata induced by carcinogen treatment in organ culture: Influence of increasing amounts of carcinogen. Brit. J. Cancer 24, 785-787 (197o).

DIAMOND, L.: The effect of carcinogenic hydrocarbons on rodent and primate cells in vitro. J. cell. comp. Physiol. 66, 183-198 (1965).

LAWS, J.O., FLAKS, A.: Pulmonary adenomata induced by carcinogen treatment in organ culture. Brit. J. Cancer 2o, 55o-554 (1966).

LASNITZKI, I.: Precancerous changes induced by 2o-methyl-cholanthrene in mouse prostates grown in vitro. Brit. J. Cancer 5, 345-352 (1951).

LASNITZKI, I.: The influence of hypervitaminosis on the effect of 2o-methylcholanthrene on mouse prostates gland grown in vitro. Brit. J. Cancer 9, 434-441 (1955).

LASNITZKI, I.: The effect of 3,4 Benzyprene on human foetal lung grown in vitro. Brit. J. Cancer 1o, 51o-516 (1956).

LASNITZKI, I.: Observations on the effects of condensates from cigarette smoke on human foetal lung in vitro. Brit. J. Cancer 12, 547-552 (1958).

LASNITZKI, I.: The effect of a hydrocarbon-enriched fraction from cigarette smoke on mouse tracheas grown in vitro. Brit. J. Cancer 22, 1o5-1o9 (1968).

LASNITZKI, I.: Seventh Paterson Symposium on Carcinogenesis in vitro. Brit. J. Cancer 27, 92-96 (1973).

PALEKAR, L., KUSCHNER, M., LASKIN, S.: The effect of 3-Methylcholanthrene on rat trachea in organ culture. Cancer Res. 38, 2o98-21o4 (1968).

RHODIN, J., DALHAMN, T.: Electron microscopy of the tracheal ciliated mucosa in rat. Z. Zellforsch. 44, 345-412 (1956).

SAFFIOTTI, U., MONTESANO, R., SELLAKUMAR, A.R., BORG, S.A.: Experimental cancer of the lung: Inhibition by Vitamin A of the induction of tracheobronchial squamous metaplasia and squamous cell tumors. Cancer 2o, 857-865 (1967).

Tobacco Research Council, London. Review of Activities, 1969.

TROWELL, O.A.: The culture of mature organs in a synthetic medium. Exp. Cell Res. 16, 118-147 (1959).

Effects of Cigarette Smoke Condensate (CSC) on Rat Fetal Lung in Organ Culture

Ivan Chouroulinkov and M. Michiels

Institute de Recherches Scientifiques sur le Cancer, Villejuif, France

A. Introduction

The first studies on the effect of chemical carcinogens on the lung in organ cultures were done by ILSE LASNITZKI (1956). She also used this method to study the effects of cigarette smoke condensate and a 3,4-benzopyrene-enriched fraction on the human fetal lung (LASNITZKI, 1958, 1968). The lung tissue treated with these agents showed a hyperplasia of the bronchiolar epithelium, indicating a qualitative difference between the various treatments. To our knowledge, there is no other report on the activity of smoke condensate nor whole tobacco smoke on the lung in organ culture.

SHABAD et al. (1971), after an extensive investigation of the transplacental blastomogenesis in organ cultures of embryonic lung tissue, concluded that "finally, organ cultures of lung tissue can be used to screen and test the oncogenic activity of some new or insufficiently studied chemicals".

Despite the technical difficulties indicated by SHABAD et al. (1971), we have undertaken a comprehensive study of fetal lung tissue of rats and mice in organ cultures which have been treated with various chemicals including the cigarette smoke condensate (CSC). This paper will describe some of the results obtained from this study.

B. Materials and Methods

A modified version of a technique used by TROWELL (1954) was used in this study.

Lungs from 15- and 16-day-old rat embryos, maintained in 199 liquid (Difco), were used. Before starting the cultures, the lungs were cut in 1-mm fragments. The culture medium 199 with 20% horse serum contained 100 units of penicillin and 50 µg/ml streptomycin. Each fragment was explanted on a 0.45-µm Millipore membrane in a Falcon organ tissue culture dish (ref. 3010). The dishes were incubated in Lwoff's box with 5% carbon dioxide at 37°C.

The condensates A, B, and C (CSC-A, -B, and -C), prepared by the "Service d'Exploitation Industrielle des Tabacs et Allumettes" (SEITA – The French Tobacco Monopoly), were added to the medium as acetone/methanol (v/v) solution in doses of 50, 100, and 150 µg/ml of medium. The solvent with or without condensate did not exceed 0,5% of the medium.

The medium with the solvent or with the CSC was changed every third day. After 16 days of culture, the explants were fixed in Bouin's solution, embedded in paraffin, and serial slides were stained with hematoxylin-eosin.

C. Results

I. Strain Susceptibility to the Toxic Effect of CSC-A in Organ Culture

For this experiment, 15-day-old embryonic lung from 3 different rat strains was used. Table 1 shows that the lung of the WAF rat strain is very sensitive to the treatment. In a complementary experiment with doses of 100 µg/ml, 1 explant out of 14 survived in a degenerative state. The same sensitivity was observed with lung fibroblasts from this strain. It was found that this sensitivity is related to the growing activity of explants. The control explants of WAF lung were very proliferative, and the corresponding fibroblasts show a high mitotic index in tissue culture.

Table 1. Number of surviving embryonal rat lung explants treated with CSC-A in organ culture

| Treatment | Rat strain[a] | | |
	WAG[b]	Hollande	WAF[c]
Solvent	30/37 (81%)	21/24 (87,5%	31/38 (82%)
CSC-A (150 µg/ml)	31/37 (84%)	23/31 (74%)	0/36 (0%)

[a]Rats obtained from the local breeding house.

[b]WAG: Wistar rats, conventional.

[c]WAF: Wistar rats, pathogen-free.

II. Activity of CSC-B and CSC-C on the 16-Day-Old Embryonic Lungs of WAG rats

In 448 explants from two consecutive experiments (224 explants each time), we did not observe any case of total degeneration. During these experiments, we lost only 7 explants due to technical problems.

After 16 days of organ culture, the control explants showed four histological types:

1. "Normal" explants showed an organoid structure with considerable development of the bronchiolar tree lined by columnar or cuboidal epithelium. The connective tissue was relatively well developed. Compared with the embryonic lung, these explants showed a normal differentiation with or without alveolar formation (Fig. 1).

2. "Bronchiolar"-type explants showing predominately bronchiolar structure with columnar or cuboidal epithelium (Fig. 2).

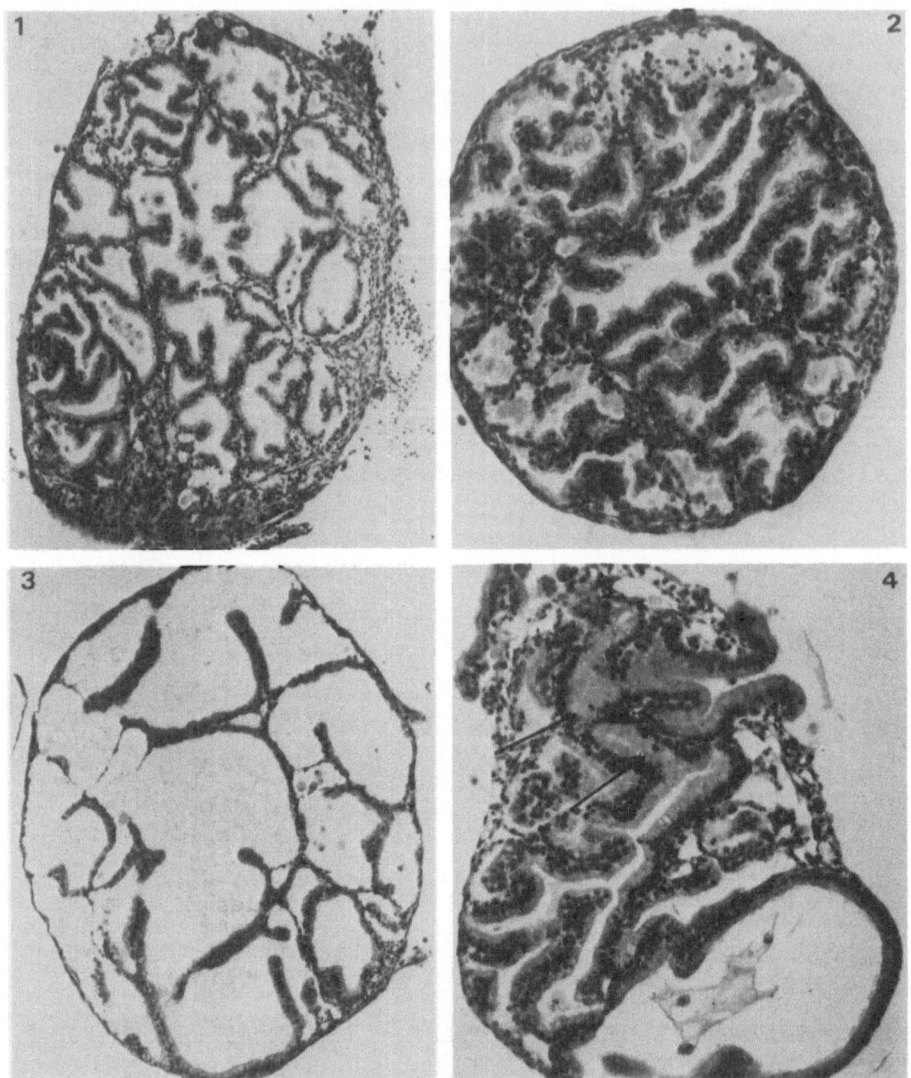

Fig. 1. Embryonic rat lung explant (control) after 16 days of organ culture: Normal type (x 120)

Fig. 2. Embryonic rat lung explant (control) after 16 days of organ culture: Bronchiolar type with predominance of bronchioli (x 200)

Fig. 3. Embryonic rat lung explant (control) after 16 days of organ culture: Polycystic type (x 120)

Fig. 4. Embryonic rat lung explant after 16 days treatment with CSC in organ culture: CSC-C (50 μg/ml). Degenerative type of explant with cyst and proliferative columnal epithelium. Presence of two mitotic figures (→) (x 200)

3. "Polycystic" explants, another aspect of degenerative change showing well-differentiated lung tissue where the lining epithelium is
columnar, cuboidal, or flat (alveolar). The connective tissue is almost nonexistent (Fig. 3).

4. "Degenerative" explants with partial necrosis, edematous connective
tissue, and quiescent bronchioli (Fig. 4).

Table 2. Distribution of the explants according to treatment and
morphological aspect

Treatment	Dose (μg/ml)	"Normal"	"Bron-chiolar"	"Poly-cystic"	"Degene-rative"	Total
Solvent		22	18	13	10	63
CSC-B	50	27	17	9	11	64
	100	27	14	3	19	63
	150	59	3	-	2	64
CSC-C	50	42	4	5	10	61
	100	33	14	4	13	64
	150	34	21	-	7	62

Table 2 presents the distribution of the explants according to the
histologic type. In the controls, the first two types are most frequent. The treatment increased the number of the "normals", which
indicates that the connective tissue remains in better condition when
treated with CSC. Apparently, the only similarity between the control
explants and the treated ones was the presence of epithelial and connective tissue. The organoid structure of the treated explants was
completely modified by: (a) a diffuse or local hyperplasia (*pseudostratified hyperplasia* - PSH), characterized by an epithelial proliferation, hyperchromatic nucleus, mitosis, and high secretory activity
(Figs 5 - 8); (b) *papillary* or *free outgrowth* (OG) (Figs 5 and 6), showing a proliferation of the bronchial epithelium as described by SHABAD
et al. (1971); and (c) a *basal hyperplasia* (BH), like metaplasia that
occurred generally near of the explant support (Millipore membrane)
(Figs 8 - 10). It should be mentioned that these changes were observed
less frequently in the other morphologic groups of the explants.

Table 3. Incidence of pseudostratified hyperplasia (PSH), basal hyperplasia (BH), and "outgrowth" (OG) in rat fetal lung treated with CSC
in organ culture

Treatment	Dose (μg/ml)	Total number of explants	PSH	BH	OG
Solvent		63	27 (42.9%)	1 (1.6%)	1 (1.6%)
CSC-B	50	64	42 (66.0%)	5 (8.0%)	12 (18.8%)
	100	63	55 (87.3%)	26 (41.3%)	32 (51.0%)
	150	64	62 (97.0%)	49 (76.6%)	50 (78.1%)
CSC-C	50	61	50 (82.0%)	28 (46.0%)	28 (46.0%)
	100	64	44 (68.8%)	40 (62.5%)	29 (45.3%)
	150	63	48 (76.2%)	39 (62.0%)	9 (14.3%)

Table 3 gives the frequency of the PSH, BH, and outgrowths. It is clear from these data that CSC-B stimulates the explant growth, which is dose-dependent. This is shown by the increase of the number of the "normal" explants (Table 2), and increase of the PSH, BH, and of the outgrowths.

The same stimulating effect is shown for CSC-C when compared to the controls; however, dose dependency of this effect is prevented by an increase of toxicity with the dose. The decrease of the incidence of the outgrowths is very significant; moreover, the explants treated with a dose of 100 µg/ml showed a significant reduction in size, which was even more evident at a dose of 150 µg/ml. Chronologically, the CSC-C originally manifested a toxic effect, inducing degeneration, and later a stimulation of the proliferation of the cells characterized by the presence of mitosis in spite of the small size of the explants.

Comparing the activity of the two condensates, it appears that: (a) the CSC-B is more stimulating and the CSC-C more toxic; (b) the CSC-C is twice as active as the CSC-B. The CSC-C at a dose of 50 µg/ml is as active as CSC-B at 100 µg/ml. The incidence of BH induced by CSC-C with dose of 100 µg/ml is similar to the BH induced by CSC-B at 150 µg/ml.

D. Discussion

The strain susceptibility of the lung to chemical carcinogens is well known in animals and especially in mice (CHOUROULINKOV et al., 1966). Our results show that this susceptibility persists in organ culture. The phenomenon is typical not only for the toxic effect but also for the various lesions described above (unpublished data). This raises the question of whether humans from different geographical areas have the same susceptibility to chemical carcinogens. LASNITZKI (1956) observed precancerous lesions in human fetal lung treated with CSC in organ culture. We treated more than 150 human fetal lung explants with CSC under the same conditions using the same doses as LASNITZKI. Only the age of the fetus was different. Our findings did not show the lesions described by LASNITZKI (1956). The epidemiological study showed that in England the incidence of lung cancer is higher than in France. At this time, we cannot speculate reagarding the results of our work.

Fig. 5. CSC-B (100 µg/ml). Pseudostratified hyperplasia of the bronchial epithelium and multiple outgrowths (x 120)

Fig. 6. CSC-B (150 µg/ml). Pseudostratified hyperplasia, outgrowths and secretory activity (x 120)

Fig. 7. CSC-C (100 µg/ml). Pseudostratifeid hyperplasia (upper right), basal hyperplasia (→), and mitotic figures (x 200)

Fig. 8. CSC-C (150 µg/ml). General pseudostratified and basal hyperplasia (→) (x 200)

Fig. 9. CSC-C (150 µg/ml). Basal hyperplasia, oblique section (x 200)

Fig. 10. CSC-C (50 µg/ml). Basal hyperplasia (metaplasia) similar to adenoma (x 300)

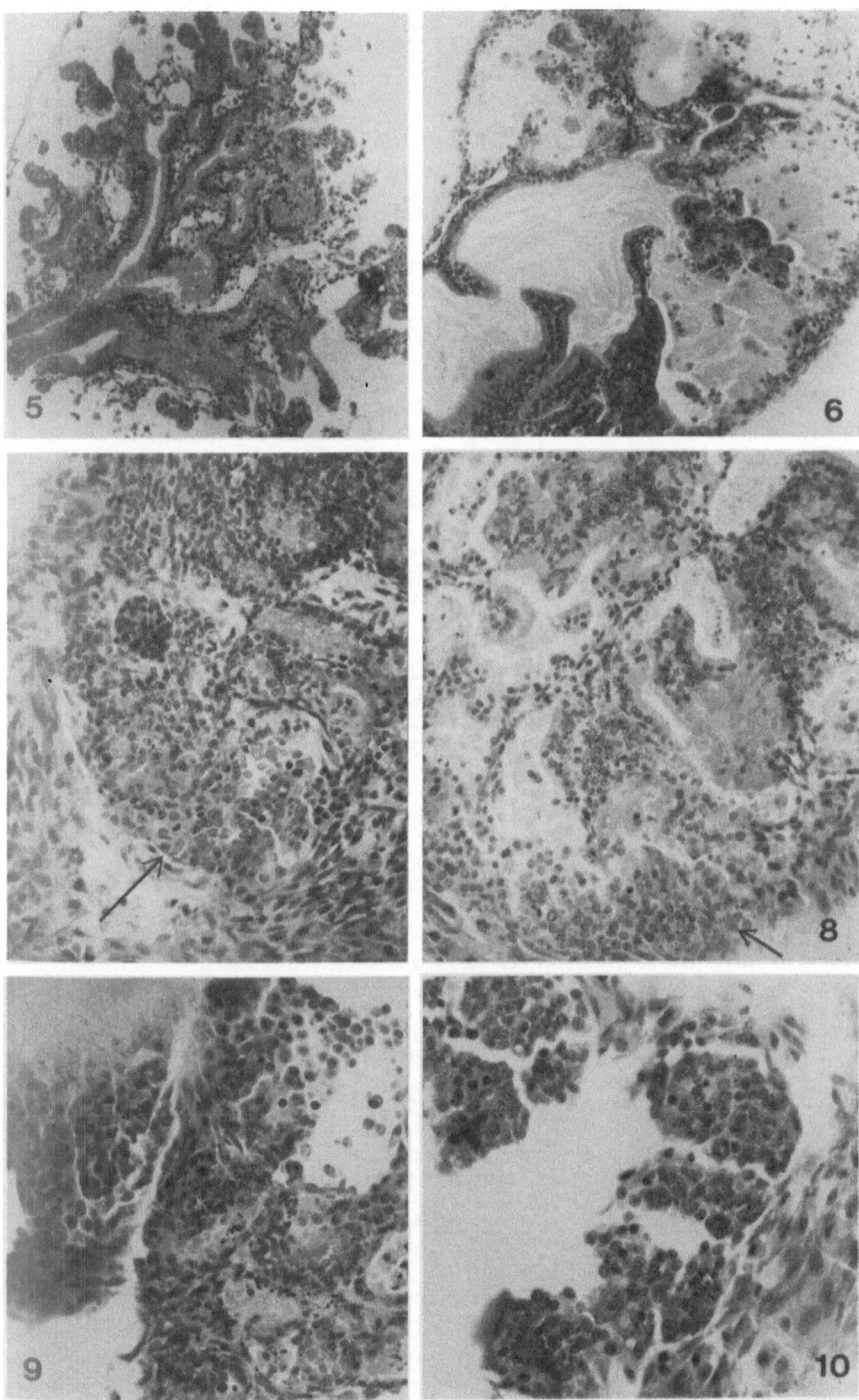

Legends see opposite page

To appreciate the activity of the chemical carcinogens on the human
lung in organ culture, LASNITZKI (1956) classified the lesions as a
basal cell hyperplasia with or without secretory activity and a squamous metaplasia of the bronchial epithelium. SHABAD et al. (1971)
employed the term "diffuse or focal hyperplasia". Using mouse lung,
they did not observe squamous metaplasia. Differentiating a pseudostratified hyperplasia (PSH), which is equivalent to the Lasnitzki
secretory basal hyperplasia and to Shabad's hyperplasia, we should
state that this proliferation is still within the normal limits. The
basal hyperplasia (BH), which is metaplastic but not yet squamous
metaplasia, is abnormal and may be present in a pretumorous lesion.
The same is valid for papillary outgrowths, which sometimes may resemble the papillary adenoma. These lesions could be graded from the
normal to the tumorous as follows: normal, pseudostratified hyperplasia, outgrowths, basal hyperplasia, squamous metaplasia, and, finally,
tumors.

The real value of these histological criteria could be appreciated if
there were a correlation between the effect of the activity of the
condensates on the lung in organ culture and the carcinogenicity *in
vivo*. In another unpublished work of these authors, after intrasplenic
grafting of the treated lung explants a long survival was observed
(several months) but tumor development never took place. Nevertheless,
with the skin test we found that CSC-C was about twice as carcinogenic
than CSC-B. This observation correlates well with the results obtained
in our lung organ culture study.

In conclusion, the dose response of rat fetal lung tissue in organ
culture using cigarette smoke condensate and the correlation with the
in vivo skin carcinogenic activity of this condensate allows us to
utilize the lung organ culture method for studing the effect of various cigarette smoke products.

References

CHOUROULINKOV, I., RIVIERE, M.R., ARNOLD, J., GUERIN, M.: Étude du
dévelopment d'adénomes pulmonaires chez des souris de souches
variées après traitement par l'uréthane associée aux rayons X.
C.R. Soc. Biol. (Paris) 16o, 234-237 (1966).
LASNITZKI, I.: The effect of 3.4-benzopyrene on human foetal lung
grown in vitro. Brit. J. Cancer 1o, 51o-516 (1956).
LASNITZKI, I.: Observations on the effects of condensates from cigarette smoke on human foetal lung in vitro. Brit. J. Cancer 12,
547-552 (1958).
LASNITZKI, I.: The effect of a hydrocarbon enriched fraction of
cigarette smoke condensate on human fetal lung grown in vitro.
Cancer Res. 28, 51o-516 (1968).
SHABAD, L.M., KOLESNICHENKO, T.S., SMETANIN, E.T.: Transplacental
blastomogenesis in organ cultures of embryonic lung tissue. J.
nat. Cancer Inst. 47, 987-1oo5 (1971).
TROWELL, O.A.: A modified technic for organ culture in vitro. Exp.
Cell Res. 6, 246-248 (1954).

Tracheal Grafts*

Richard A. Griesemer, J. Kendrick, and Paul Nettesheim

Biology Division, Carcinogenesis Program, Oak Ridge National Laboratory, Oak Ridge, TN 37830, USA

ABSTRACT

To learn when transplanted trachea becomes established and is suitable
for experimentation, a serial sacrifice study was performed on rats.
After transplant to a subcutaneous site, tracheal grafts survived by
diffusion until the fourth day when the blood supply was re-established. Further improvement occurred in the mucosal epithelium, so
that by the seventh day after transplanting, the graft was again lined
by tall columnar ciliated cells and scattered secretory cells. The
mucosal epithelium remained separated from the submucosal elastic
layer, however, until 14 days after transplanting, when the established
grafts resembled untransplanted tracheas histologically. When exposed
to 7,12-dimethyl(a)benzanthracene, the mucosa underwent squamous metaplasia that progressed to squamous carcinoma as early as 3 months after
treatment. A major advantage of the tracheal graft as a research tool
is that neoplasia can be induced in a respiratory tissue without interfering with respiration.

Introduction

Recently, we reported the development of techniques for grafting whole
tracheas in the subcutis of mice, rats, and hamsters, as well as the
successful production of carcinomas in tracheal grafts by polycyclic
hydrocarbons (KENDRICK et al., 1974). Since then, the techniques have
been further refined and extended to include guinea pigs.

To learn when a transplanted trachea becomes established and is suitable for experimentation, a serial sacrifice study was performed in
male rats. Secondary objectives were to evaluate two methods of transplanting the grafts, and to compare the structure of grafted tracheas
with normal ungrafted tracheas.

Another experiment was designed to learn the response of rat tracheal
grafts to 7,12-dimethyl(a)benzanthracene (DMBA) and to compare the
effects of DMBA on recently-transplanted, versus established, grafts.

*Research supported jointly by the National Cancer Institute and the
U.S. Atomic Energy Commission under contract with Union Carbide Corporation

Materials and Methods

Animals. Ten-week old isogenic rats of the Fischer 344 strain were bred and reared in an animal isolation facility. They were demonstrated to be free of the common infectious diseases of rats, including pneumonia.

Grafting Technique. The technique for transplanting entire tracheas from donor animals to the subcutis of recipient animals has been described (KENDRICK et al., 1974). To prevent curling and to facilitate the insertion of carcinogen pellets, two modifications of the grafting technique were employed. In the first method, the trachea was sutured at both ends to sterile polyethylene tubing and the trachea, together with the tubing, was inserted under the skin. In the second method, tracheas were stretched to their original length and sutured directly to the fascia overlying the dorsal cervical or lumbar muscles. 2 or 4 grafts (cervical and lumbar pairs on either side of the midline) were placed in the subcutis of each rat so that the grafts were at least 1.0 cm apart.

Normal Graft Establishment. To learn the sequence of events during establishment of tracheal grafts, a serial sacrifice study was conducted in male rats. 2 grafts attached to tubing, and 2 sutured in place, were collected at each time interval, days 0, 1, 2, 3, 4, 5, 6, 7, 10, 14, 21, and 28, after transplanting (a total of 48 grafts).

Histology. For histological evaluation, 2 transverse rings were fixed in 2.3% glutaraldehyde, embedded in epon, sectioned at 1μ, and stained with toluidine blue. The remainder of each graft was transected at 2 mm intervals, embedded on end in paraffin, sectioned at 6μ, and stained with hematoxylin and eosin, periodic acid-Schiff (PAS), or trichome stains and reagents.

Autoradiography. All animals used to characterize normal grafts were injected with 2 μC/g body weight tritiated thymidine 45 minutes before harvesting the tracheal tissue. Epon-embedded, 1μ thick sections of tracheal grafts were coated with Kodak NTB-2 emulsion, and exposed at 4°C for 4 weeks before developing. Host trachea and intestine served as tissue controls.

Colloidal Carbon. To demonstrate blood vessels in tracheal grafts, selected animals were injected intravenously under anesthesia with 2.5 ml of a colloidal carbon suspension (100 mg/ml). The grafts were fixed in a mixture of formaldehyde, alcohol, and acetic acid, cleared in cedarwood oil and methyl salicylate, and examined macroscopically and histologically.

Carcinogen Pellets. DMBA was obtained from Eastman Kodak Co. in the form of a powder. Beeswax was used as a vehicle for sustained release of carcinogen. To prepare pellets, DMBA was melted at 122°C, added to melted beeswax, mixed while hot with a vortex mixer and sonicator, and formed into pellets in a pellet maker. Control pellets contained only the beeswax vehicle.

The pellet maker (Fig. 1) consisted of two matching cylinders. One contained a well in which the carcinogen mixture was placed. When the matching half was apposed, the carcinogen mixture was forced from the well into holes where, following rapid chilling, cylindrical pellets were formed. The pellets were expelled from the pellet maker with a metal rod.

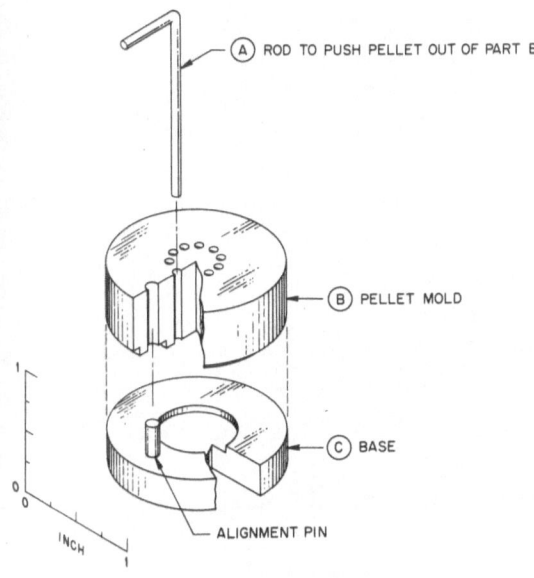

— (A) ROD TO PUSH PELLET OUT OF PART B

— (B) PELLET MOLD

— (C) BASE

— ALIGNMENT PIN

PELLETIZER

Fig. 1. Schematic diagram of a pellet maker used to make uniform carcinogen pellets

Beeswax pellets had a volume of 30 µl, weighed 24.5 mg, and contained 2.98 mg DMBA. Assays for carcinogen were performed by extraction in benzene and fluorometry. Spectral analysis revealed no interference from beeswax.

Exposure of tracheal grafts to carcinogens was performed by incising one end of a graft that had been established for 4 weeks, aspirating mucus when necessary, inserting the carcinogen pellet, and ligating the end of the graft. In one experiment, carcinogen pellets were inserted at the time of transplanting.

Effect of DMBA on Tracheal Grafts. 48 established tracheal grafts in male rats and 48 grafts in female rats were exposed to DMBA to learn the response of tracheal grafts to a relatively large dose (2.98 mg) and to determine the rate at which the carcinogen is released from beeswax pellets *in vivo*. Control beeswax pellets without carcinogen were implanted in 48 grafts in male rats. 8 treated grafts and 4 control grafts were harvested at each of the following time intervals: 4 days, 1 week, 2 weeks, 1 month, 2 months, 3 months, and 4 months. The remaining animals bearing 40 treated- and 20 control-grafts are still alive and under observation. At the time of harvest, the pelle s were removed for carcinogen assay and the grafts fixed and processed for histopathology.

DMBA and Non-established Grafts. In view of the partial degenerat and rapid regeneration in the first few days after grafting, one m predict the response to the carcinogen of newly-transplanted tracheal tissue would be different from that of a well-established graft. To test this hypothesis, beeswax pellets containing 2.98 mg DMBA were inserted in each of 10 tracheas at the time of grafting in male rats. 2 were harvested at 1 and 2 weeks and at 1, 2, and 3 months after grafting, to compare with those in the previous experiment.

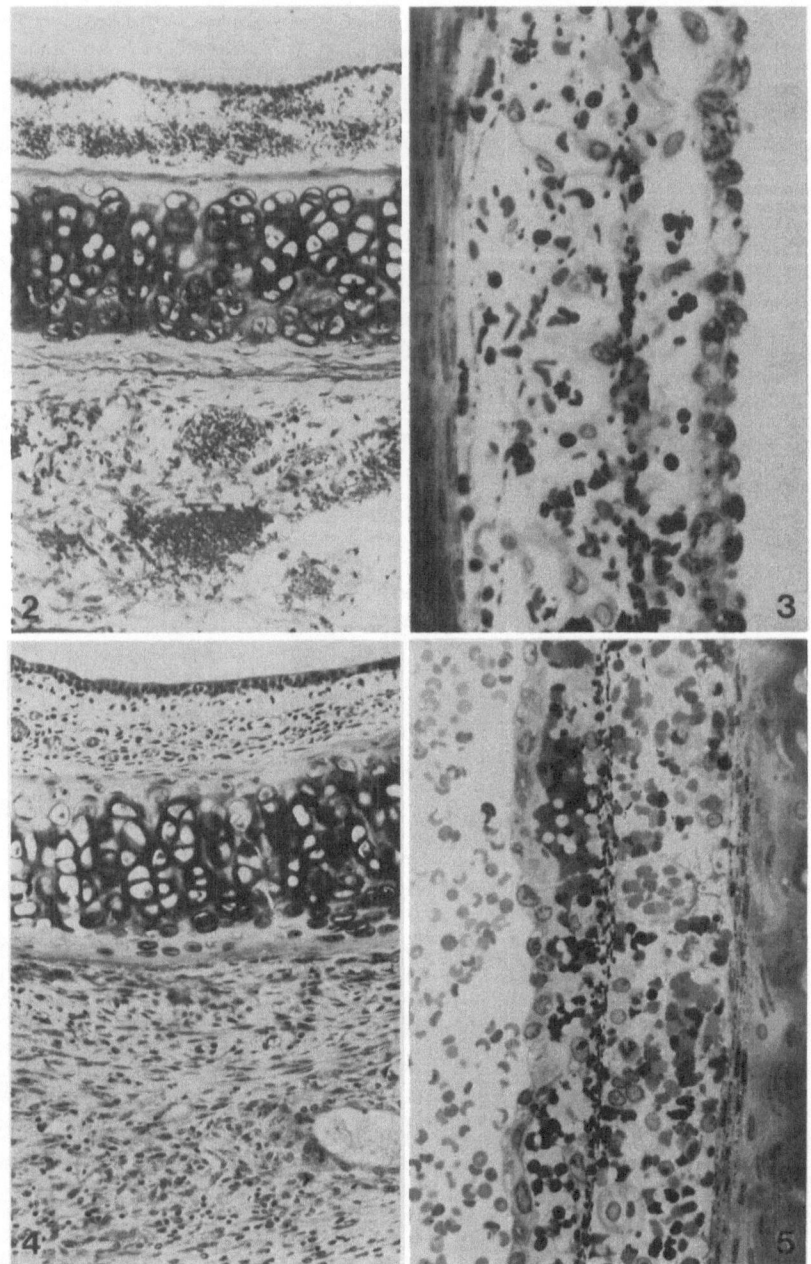

Fig. 2. Photomicrograph of a tracheal graft 3 days after transplanting. Severe circulatory changes with congestion and hemorrhage in the submucosa and adventitia and hemorrhage in the lumen

Fig. 3. Higher magnification of the mucosa in Fig. 2. One micron, epon-embedded, toluidine blue-stained section. The mucosal epithelium is vacuolated and degenerating. The epithelium is separated from the underlying elastica (narrow, middle layer of black fragments) by edema. Scattered erythrocytes appear black in this photomicrograph

Results

<u>Normal Graft Establishment.</u> All grafts were accepted without evidence
of histoincompatibility. There was no evidence of infection, and no
microorganisms could be cultured from the graft contents. In 4 of 12
rats with grafts sutured to fascia and 2 of 11 rats with grafts attached to tubing, hematomas about 1.0 cm diameter formed in the subcutis between the grafts, shortly after surgery. The hematomas persisted as hematocysts for several weeks but had no demonstrable effect
on the grafts themselves. It was not necessary to tie off the ends of
the grafts. A thin layer of fibrin and granulation tissue occluded
the ends of open grafts in 1 or 2 days and the luminal surface soon
became lined by epithelium.

1 day after transplanting, there were mild changes in the grafts.
The lumens were filled with proteinic fluid resembling serum and blood.
The mucosal epithelial cells were retracted into low columnar cells
with short cilia and no secretory activity, but the mucosa was intact.
The submucosa was slightly edematous and the submucosal capillaries
were distended with blood that was partially hemolyzed. The cartilage
appeared normal. The adventitia was moderately congested and edematous
and coated with a thin layer of fibrin.

On the second day after transplanting, a thick layer of fibrin covered
the graft and an advancing front of new capillaries penetrated the
outer layers. The mucosal epithelial layer contained scattered necrobiotic and karyorrhetic cells.

On the third day after transplanting, circulatory and retrogressive
changes were severe (Fig. 2). The lumen contained considerable blood.
The mucosal lining was intact but the lining epithelium was damaged
(Fig. 3), with scattered vacuolation, karyorrhexis and pycnosis. The
number of epithelial cells per transverse section was reduced to 55%
of that of nontransplanted tracheas. Tritiated thymidine reached the
mucosa, but only 0.03% of cells were labeled, compared with 0.26% of
host tracheal epithelial cells. The submucosa was congested and edematous with scattered, small hemorrhages. The adventitial layers were
severely congested and edematous, but without cellular inflammatory
infiltrates. Organization of the fibrin clot progressed with penetration of many capillary sprouts and early fibroplasia. Cartilage and
nerves appeared normal.

On the fourth day, a striking improvement in circulatory changes occurred (Figs 4 and 5), when the proliferating blood vessels in the
surrounding granulation tissue reached the graft and blood flow was
re-established. Vascularization of the entire graft was readily demonstrated by the colloidal carbon method (Figs 6 and 7). The mucosal
epithelium became taller with a burst of secretory and mitotic activity.
Labeled epithelial cells increased to 7.5%.

Further improvement occured in the mucosal epithelium during the next
several days, so that by the seventh day after transplanting the graft

<u>Fig. 4.</u> Four days after transplanting, the circulatory changes have
subsided and adventitial granulation tissue is prominent

<u>Fig. 5.</u> Higher magnification of Fig. 4, embedded in epon and stained
with toluidine blue. The mucosal epithelium is still separated from
the submucosal elastic layer by edema and hemorrhage, but correlative
studies indicate a burst of secretory and mitotic activity

544

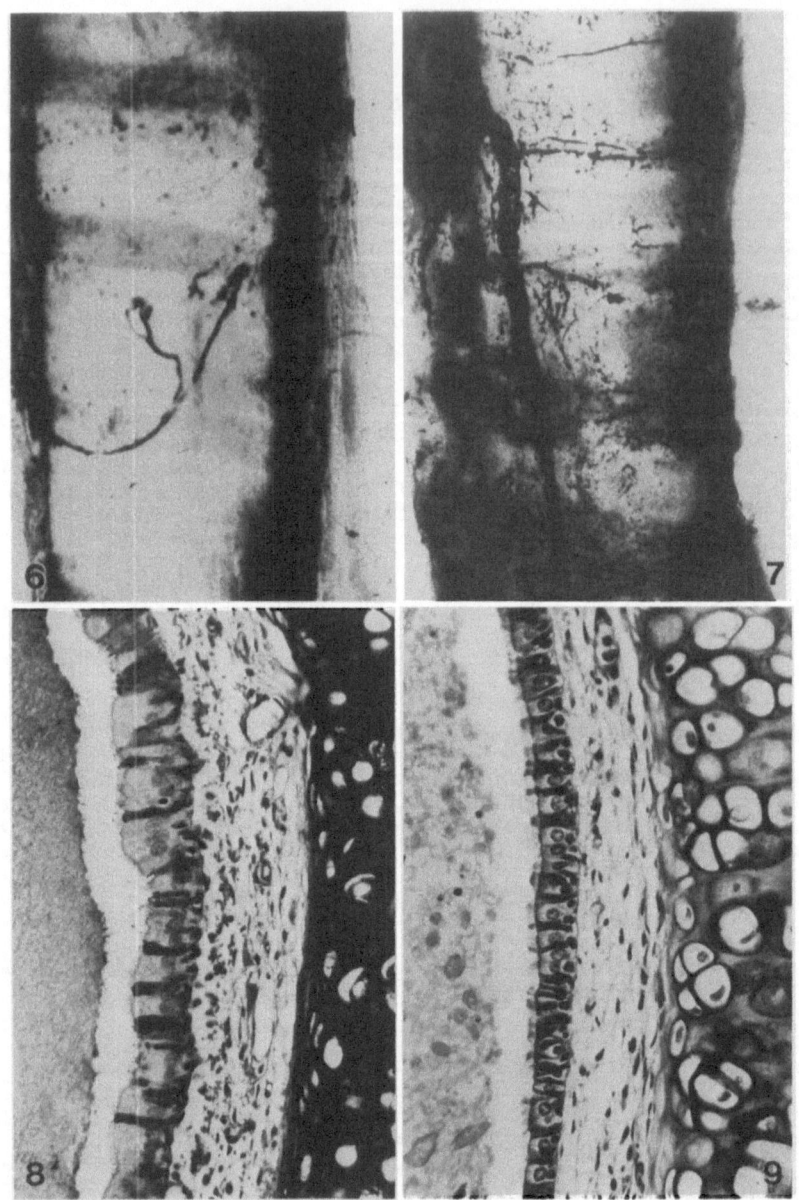

Fig. 6. Unstained, whole mount, cleared trachea from an animal which had been injected with colloidal carbon. 3 days after grafting, there is a single, large, brached vessel on the surface of the graft

Fig. 7. Colloidal carbon injection. Four days after grafting, vascular arborization on and in the graft is apparent. Compare with Fig. 6

Fig. 8. Tall columnar and secretory cells 7 days after grafting. Subepithelial edema is still present. PAS reaction

Fig. 9. An established graft, 2 months after grafting with partially-inspissated mucus in the lumen

was again lined by tall columnar ciliated cells and scattered secretory cells (Fig. 8). The number of labeled cells approached pre-transplant levels. The grafts were surrounded by organized collagenous granulation tissue. Transplanted thyroid tissue also remained viable.

The mucosal epithelium remained separated from the submucosal elastic layer, however, until 14 days after transplanting. Thereafter, the grafts resembled untransplanted tracheas (Fig. 9), except for the autonomic nerve trunks which had started to demyelinate on the fourth day after transplanting. The nerves along with their ganglia survived, but were completely unmyelinated from the tenth day through the remainder of the 28-day observation period.

Effect of DMBA on Tracheal Graft. The only change in grafts exposed to beeswax control pellets was a slight increase in secretory activity for several weeks. Tracheal grafts exposed to DMBA, however, developed metaplastic and neoplastic lesions. No appreciable differences were found in grafts from male or female rats.

On the fourth day after implantation, the mucosal epithelium was thickened by basal-cell hyperplasia, with elevation of ciliated cells. The submucosa was widened by edema and infiltration of heterophils. On the seventh day, the columnar epithelium was replaced by stratified, squamous, keratinizing epithelium (Fig. 10). The second week after treatment began, squamous metaplasia was more severe, and the carcinogen pellets were surrounded by keratin that filled the lumen.

2 months after the start of carcinogen treatment, proliferating epithelium extended outside the confines of the original graft into the surrounding connective tissue, where it formed keratinic cysts with dysplastic linings. 3 months after the start of treatment, the grafts had increased in size 3- to 4-fold over control grafts, due to continued disorderly epithelial growth and enlargement of keratinic cysts (Fig. 11).In addition, the proliferating squamous epithelium was no longer confined to the cysts, but penetrated the graft wall and invaded the subcutis. After 4 months' exposure to DMBA, the lesions were characteristic of invasive squamous carcinoma (Fig. 12), although no metastases were found at necropsy. The host tracheas appeared unchanged, grossly and microscopically.

When assayed for DMBA, pellets recovered from grafts 2 months after treatment contained 77% of the original dose and 53% remained after 3 months.

DMBA in Non-established Grafts. When DMBA beeswax pellets were inserted at the time of grafting, the resulting squamous metaplasia and early invasive squamous carcinoma were comparable in type and time of occurrence to those in the previous experiment with established grafts.

Discussion

The trachea with its several tissues survived for 3 days after implantation, presumably by diffusion, until a new blood supply was established. In parallel studies with organ cultures, we have learned that whole tracheas, ligated at each end, survive 4 (but not 5) days at 37°C in Hank's balanced salt solution without serum and can be successfully transplanted *in vivo*.

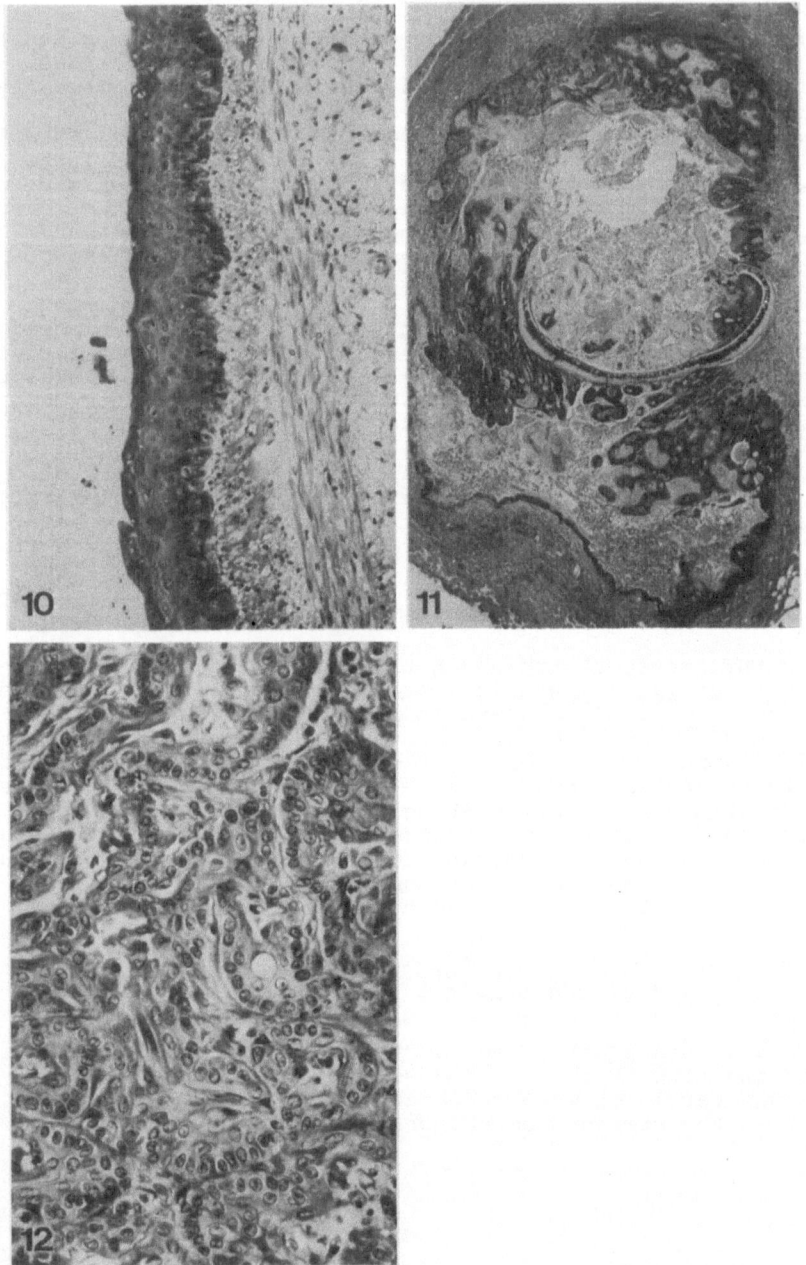

Fig. 10. One week after exposure to DMBA in beeswax, the entire tra-cheal graft mucosa has undergone squamous metaplasia

Fig. 11. Three months after exposure to DMBA, the original graft is largely replaced by proliferating dysplastic squamous epithelial cells. Note surviving cartilaginous ring in the center

Fig. 12. Well differentiated carcinoma, 4 months after exposure to DMBA

The production of pre-neoplastic and neoplastic lesions in the tracheal graft makes it a useful tool for studies on respiratory carcinogenesis, where a restricted target organ can be uniformly to carcinogens, and dose-response relationships can be established. In our experience, the tracheal graft lends itself to experimental manipulations, including multiple treatments, cytological sampling, and subtransplantation. Through the use of tracheal grafts, neoplasia can be produced in a respiratory tissue without interfering with respiration or exposing the gastrointestinal tract to carcinogens.

Reference

KENDRICK, J., NETTESHEIM, P., HAMMONS, A.S.: Tumor induction in tracheal grafts: a new experimental model for respiratory carcinogenesis studies. J. nat. Cancer Inst. $\underline{52}$, 1317-1325 (1974).

Studies of Ultrastructure, Cytochemistry, and Organ Culture of Human Bronchial Epithelium*

Benjamin F. Trump, Elizabeth M. McDowell, Lucy A. Barret, Arthur L. Frank, and Curtis C. Harris

Department of Pathology, University of Maryland, Baltimore, MD 21201, USA, and Lung Cancer Branch, Carcinogenesis Program, National Cancer Institute, Bethesda, MD 20014, USA

ABSTRACT

In these studies human bronchi removed at time of surgery of "immediate autopsy" from both cancer and non-cancer patients are studied by light and electron microscopy and cytochemistry and cultured *in vitro* with serial studies of morphology and metabolism. Segments removed from humans are cultured in CMRL 1066 containing insulin and hydrocortisone with or without 5% inactivated fetal calf serum and with or without addition of vitamin A. Segments have been stored at $0 - 4^{o}C$ in L-15 medium for up to 2 days prior to successful culture. Cultures are carried out in plastic Petri dishes on rocking platforms in chambers gassed with 45% oxygen, 50% nitrogen, and 5% CO_2. The epithelial preservation can be seen by both light and electron microscopy and cultured tissues show normal areas of metaplasia and dysplasia. Specimens have so far been maintained for as long as 4 months with good maintenance of ultrastructure.

The ultrastructure of cultured epithelia is similar to epithelia fixed before culture with some modifications of cell type; in many instances the morphology appears better, presumably due to reversible changes induced at the time of surgery, prior to removal. Observations on the cultured bronchi include the demonstration of active incorporation of tritiated leucine, uridine, and thymidine into cellular macromolecules. At the cut edges cells growing around the margin show especially active thymidine incorporation.

Cytochemical studies emphasizing characteristics of Golgi, lysosomes, and cell surface are being carried out on both normal and preneoplastic lesions. This system is very promising as a model for chemical carcinogenesis in human tissue. The present studies represent an initial step in studies to define, in subcellular terms, the events leading from the normal bronchus to invasive carcinoma.

A. Introduction

It is important to know much more about the cellular characteristics of the normal human bronchus and the cellular changes that occur during malignant transformation in response to carcinogenic agents. In particular, it is assumed that these changes will be expressed at the

---

*Supported in part by Contract 4-3237 from the N.C.I.

This is contribution No. 163 from the Cellular Pathobiology Laboratory

organelle and macromolecular levels where they can be visualized by various electron microscopic techniques - especially with cytochemical study of Golgi apparatus and cell surface alterations. Through the use of cultured human tissue, it should also be possible to directly study the subcellular effects of carcinogens.

Specific goals of this project are: 1. to characterize the morphology of normal epithelium and premalignant lesions of the human bronchus at the light- and electron-microscopic levels, and to study the cyto-chemical characteristics of the normal and abnormal epithelium empha-sizing the Golgi apparatus, lysosomes, and cell surface membranes; 2. to culture human bronchial epithelium, both normal and premalignant, and to establish appropriate culture conditions for long term *in vitro* survival; and 3. to determine the effects of benzo(a)pyrene and other suspected respiratory carcinogens on human epithelium in organ culture with the hope of studying the long-term effects of such carcinogens by transplantation of human bronchi into athymic mice.

The ultrastructure of normal and some abnormal epithelium is presented here and compared with the ultrastructure of epithelium maintained in organ culture. The results so far indicate that organ culture of human bronchus is indeed feasible and that good preservation at ultrastruc-tural and metabolic levels can be obtained *in vitro*.

B. Materials and Methods

I. Collection

Human bronchi were obtained at the time of "immediate autopsy" (TRUMP et al., 1974b) within minutes of somatic death or at surgery for ma-lignant or non-malignant disease. To date, 26 samples have been col-lected. Immediateley after removal, different regions of bronchus are collected and prepared for study.

II. Organ Culture

Human specimens are collected under semi-sterile conditions, rinsed with Krebs Ringer phosphate buffer, and transferred to L-15 medium (LEIBOVlTZ, 1963), maintained at $0 - 4°C$. After washing several times in L-15, 1.5 cm square pieces are placed into 60 ml plastic Petri dishes with enough medium to just reach the surface epithelium. Dishes are placed inside a controlled-atmosphere chamber on a rocking stage (10 cycles per minute), so that the surface epithelium is submerged about half the time. The gas phase in the chamber consists of 45% oxygen, 50% nitrogen, and 5% CO_2. Culture medium for human and hamster consists of CMRL 1066, containing 5% inactivated fetal calf serum, 2 mM glutamine, 1 μg insulin, o.1 μg hydrocortisone, 100 units of penicillin, and 100 μg streptomycin per ml. In selected experiments, the culture medium was free of serum. Media and atmosphere are changed every other day.

III. Morphologic Study

Tissues are fixed at time of removal (zero-time samples) and at various times during the organ-culture period. For light microscopy (LM), tis-sues are fixed in 4% formaldehyde (F) in 300 mOsm phosphate buffer

(PO₄) at 25°C, embedded in paraffin, and stained with H & E and PAS. Observations by LM are also made on toluidine blue-stained sections of Epon blocks as described below. For electron microscopy (EM), tissues are fixed at 4°C in 4% glutaraldehyde (G) in 0.1 M cacodylate buffer, pH 7.2. After 3 to 4 hours, bronchial epithelium is trimmed from cartilage and washed in sucrose-cacodylate buffer prior to post-fixation in OsO₄. The epithelium is stained en bloc in uranyl acetate (UAC) in veronal buffer, dehydrated in ethanol, and stained with UAC and lead citrate on the grids. Large semi-thin Epon sections are cut and stained with toluidine blue for orientation.

IV. Cytochemistry

1. Acid Phosphatase Activity (APase)

Tissues are fixed at zero-time and at various times during the culture period for 4 hours at 4°C, either in 4% G in 0.1 M cacodylate, or in 2% F - 1% G in 200 mOsm PO₄ at 4°C. APase is demonstrated by a modified Gomori method (MERCER and BIRBECK, 1966). Epithelium is incubated at 37°C for 1 hour, washed in acetate buffer, rinsed in 0.5% (NH₄)₂S in sucrose-cacodylate buffer, post-fixed in OsO₄ and prepared for EM as in section III above.

2. Unbuffered Osmium Staining (OsO₄)

Tissues are intitially fixed at 25°C in unbuffered 1% OsO₄ (pH 6.0 - 6.5). After 1 hour, epithelium is trimmed and fixation continued for 24 hours at 40°C. After a brief wash in distilled H₂O, epithelium is incubated for 16 to 24 hours in fresh unbuffered 1% OsO₄ at 40°C. Tissue is prepared for EM as in III above.

3. Colloidal Iron Staining

Tissues are fixed in 4% F in 300 mOsm PO₄, or in 2% F - 1% G in 200 mOsm PO₄ for 16 to 24 hours at 25°C. After washing in sucrose-cacodylate buffer, tissue is stained overnight in fresh colloidal iron solution (3 parts colloidal iron to 1 part glacial-acetic acid) at pH 1.8 at 25°C (RINEHART and ABUL-HAJ, 1951). After a brief wash in sucrose buffer, tissue is prepared for EM as in III above; however, en bloc UAC staining is omitted.

4. Phosphotungstic Acid Staining (PTA)

Tissues are fixed as for colloidal iron-staining. After washing in sucrose cacodylate buffer, the epithelium is embedded in glycol-methacrylate and polymerized by UV light (LEDUC and BERNHARD, 1967). After selection of appropriate areas, using semi-thin toluidine blue stained sections, thin sections are cut and stained on grids in 3% PTA at pH 1.0 (0.2 N HCl). After a brief rinse in water, the sections are examined.

To date, only limited observations have been made on the distribution of colloidal iron and PTA and the results represent only preliminary findings.

V. Autoradiography

After 1 week in culture, bronchial pieces are incubated for 6 hours with either: (1) ^{3}H-uridine (15 µCi/ml; sp. act. 27.8 Ci/mM; New England Nuclear; (2) ^{3}H-leucine (15 µCi/ml; sp. act. 58.2 Ci/mM; New England Nuclear; or (3) ^{3}H-thymidine (50 µCi/ml; sp. act. 20 Ci/mM; New England Nuclear). Following fixation in 1.33% OsO$_4$ buffered by 0.1 M s-collidine, pH 7.4, and embedding in Epon, 1.0 µ sections are coated with NTB-2, exposed in the dark for 2 weeks, and autoradiograms are prepared as previously described (BOREN et al., 1974).

C. Results

I. Epithelium Studied Immediately after Removal from Patients

In this material, epithelium ranging from presumably unaltered to that showing various premalignant stages, is seen. Here we will concentrate on more normal areas, with comments on abnormalities of particular interest. Since all epithelium was not from patients with cancer, there is also the opportunity to compare alterations in these two situations.

In this epithelium, we have to date recognized five cell types. The transition between normal and abnormal epithelial structure is extremely difficult to discern, and we are in the process of defining these subtle transitions. We are considering the normal epithelium to be composed of ciliated, mucous, dark non-ciliated, basal, and small granule cells.

1. Ciliated Cells

The tall, columnar cells are joined apically by junctional complexes. From their lateral surfaces, a few small cell processes interdigitate with neighboring cells. Cilia are regularly arranged, and interspersed with microvilli; basal bodies are seen at the cell apex (Figs 1 and 6).

The cytoplasmic density is usually lower than that of adjacent mucous or dark non-ciliated cells. Mitochondria are numerous and often are elongate; orientation is rather random. Endoplasmic reticulum (ER), both RER and SER, tends to be poorly-developed, although in some cells a few long chains of RER are present. Staining with unbuffered OsO$_4$ reveals impregnation of ER, especially in the cell apex and also in the nuclear envelope (Fig. 7). Only rarely is the forming face of the Golgi apparatus stained. The staining reaction is capricious, in that one cell may be heavily stained while neighboring cells show no stain (McDOWELL, 1974).

The Golgi apparatus lies apical to the nucleus, usually oriented so that the concave maturing face of the stack is pointing toward the cell base. Below the concave face of the Golgi apparatus, lysosomes tend to be clustered as a cap at the nuclear pole. The lysosomes are single-membrane-bound, and often contain dense homogeneous contents; they may be round, or elongate and dumb-cell shaped. A few lysosomes contain layered inclusions and debris. APase activity is demonstrated in these lysosomes (Fig. 9) and very rarely activity is also seen in the Golgi apparatus (Fig. 5). Cell filaments, sometimes in clusters, and microtubules are seen. The nuclei are ellipsoidal or rounded and possess one or more nucleoli.

2. Mucous Cells

These tall and columnar cells are joined apically by junctional complexes. From their lateral surfaces, a few cell processes protrude and interdigitate with neighboring cells. The cytoplasmic density usually exceeds that of ciliated cells. The appearance of the apical cell membrane varies according to the amount of mucus in the cell. If only a few mucus droplets are present, microvilli, a few of which are branched, protrude regularly from the apical cell membrane. When the cells are filled with mucus droplets, the cell apex appears distended and domed, and the apical membrane is attenuated. Microvilli are absent from the membrane at the distended pole but may persist at the lateral margins (Fig. 6).

The mucus droplets form large clusters in the apical cytoplasm. Often the droplets are discrete, bound by a single membrane; however, they may fuse into a confluent mass. Some droplets appear structureless, while others contain an arabesque of flocculent material (Fig. 6). They may have an electron-dense core. The RER is well-developed as a collar of long isternae around the nucleus and filling the basal portion of the cells; polysome groups are present. The nucleus lies towards the base of the cell beneath a well-developed Golgi apparatus, consisting of numerous elongate lamellae. Few lysosomes are present.

In OsO₄ stained preparations, the ER appears less stained than in ciliated cells. The nuclear envelope, and occasionally the forming face of the Golgi apparatus, is stained. Mucus droplets are never stained. APase activity is demonstrated in the small lysosomes and is very rarely seen in the maturing Golgi lamellae. Some cells have been seen that bear cilia and also possess apparent mucus granules (Fig. 8).

All electron micrographs presented are of human bronchial epithelium.

Fig. 1. Low power micrograph of normal epithelium (zero-time specimen). Three cell types are shown; basal cells with dense cytoplasm (*B*) which rest on the basal lamina (*Bl*), tall ciliated cells (*Ci*) with pale cytoplasm and dark non-ciliated cells (*Dnc*). Small mucus granules (*m*) are seen in the latter near the well developed Golgi apparatus (*G*). (x 5.950)

Fig. 2. Mucous cell "atrophy" in zero-time specimen. Parts of two cuboidal surface cells are shown. Small microvilli project into the lumen; small membrane-bound bodies lie close to them, yet appear unattached to the microvilli or apical cell membrane (arrows). The Golgi apparatus (*G*) is well developed. A zone of tight-packed microfilaments (*mf*) is present in the cell apices. (x 28.000)

Fig. 3. Compound cilium in zero-time specimen from a non-cancer patient. Note the multiple axial microtubular complexes contained within a single membrane-bound cytoplasmic projection. Invaginations of the cell surface are present at the base, between individual axial complexes (arrows). (x 16.100)

Fig. 4. Fibrogranular material or "filosomes" in the apical cytoplasm of a ciliated cell (zero-time specimen). At the periphery of the area the fibers appear to be organized into patterns resembling microtubular doublets (arrow). Ciliary basal bodies (*bb*). (x 47.000)

Fig. 5. Acid phosphatase activity in the Golgi apparatus of a ciliated cell (zero-time specimen). (x 26.000)

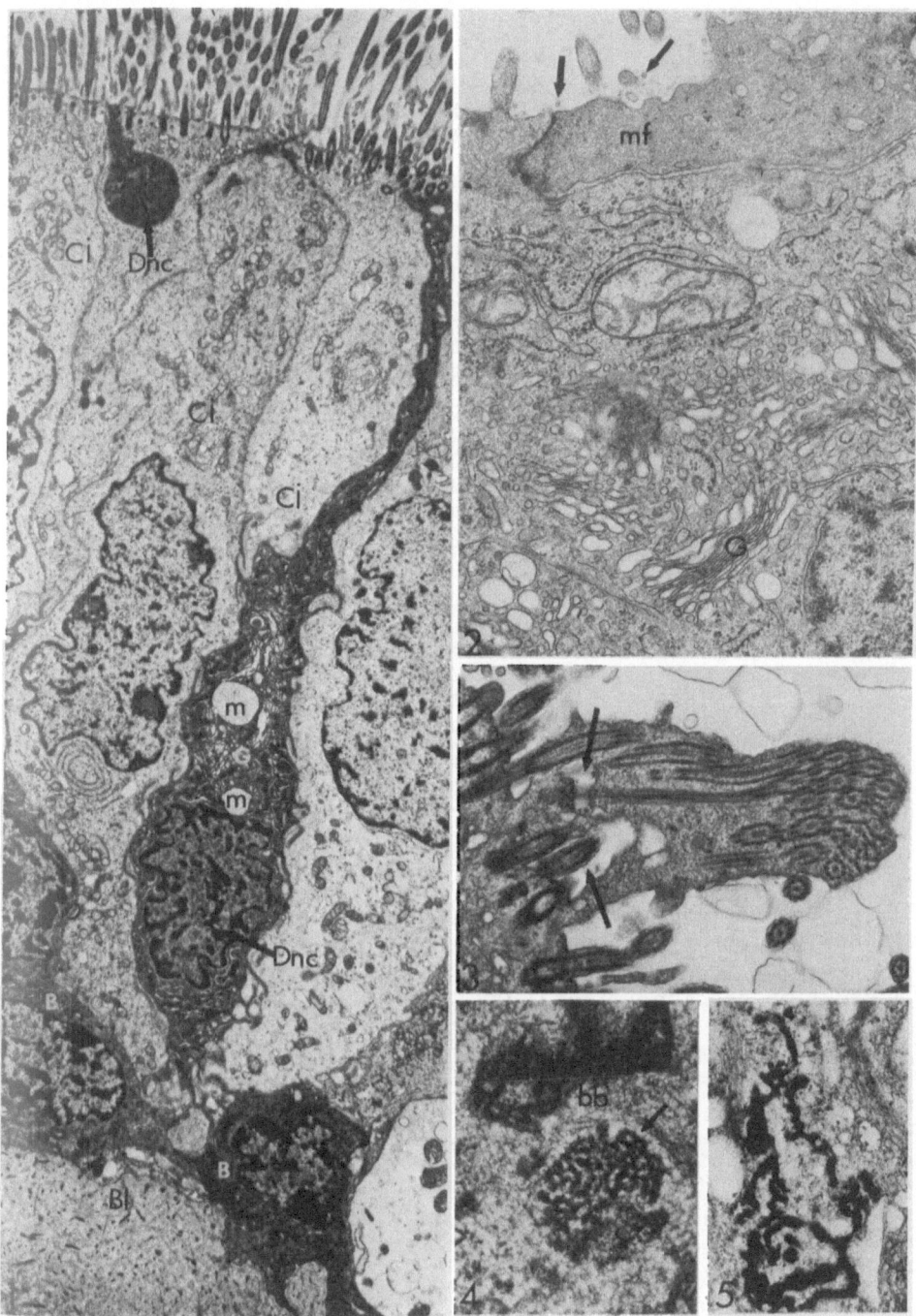

Legends see opposite page

3. Dark Non-ciliated Cells

Some of these cells are thought to represent mucous cells which have discharged their secretion product; such cells have many of the features of mucous cells. Typical "brush cells" (RHODIN and DALHAMN, 1956) have not been seen. The cytoplasm is often particularly dense; microvilli protrude from the cell apex (Fig. 1). The number of these cells varies greatly with different specimens. Cell apices may protrude above, may be level with, or may be below the level of adjacent ciliated cells.When the apical membrane is invaginated, forming a crypt, long microvilli extend into the depression. Usually a few small mucus droplets are seen near the well-developed Golgi apparatus (Fig. 1). Lysosomes tend to be small and sparse. Other cells in this group may represent immature cells undergoing differentiation, and still others a type of sensory receptor (SOROKIN, 1973). These cells demand further investigation and classification.

4. Basal Cells

These polygonal or elongate cells have dense attachment zones where the membrane lies adjacent to the basal lamina. Microvilli vary in number, according to the size of the extracellular space. If the space is large, microvilli appear to be more numerous and intertwine with those of adjacent cells, whereas if the extracellular space is small, the cell membranes seem to be more simple and lie closely parallel with those of adjacent cells. The cells are attached to one another by desmosomes, but these are not numerous.

Fig. 6. A mucous cell (*M*) and a ciliated cell (*Ci*) (zero-time specimen). Note that the discrete mucus granules (*m*) are beginning to fuse to form a confluent mass. An arabesque of flocculent material is seen in the mucus granules. The cell membrane is attenuated at the domed cell apex but microvilli persist at the lateral margins of the mucous cell (arrows). (x 5.600)

Fig. 7. Unbuffered OsO_4 staining in ciliated (*Ci*) and mucous cells (*M*), (zero-time specimen). Note stained ER at apex of ciliated cell and stained nuclear envelope at base (arrow). (x 4.550)

Fig. 8. Apparent mucus granules (*m*) are seen in the apex of a ciliated cell (zero-time specimen). (x 21.000)

Fig. 9. Acid phosphatase activity in a ciliated cell is demonstrated in lysosomes which are clustered as a cap at the nuclear pole, ventral to the Golgi apparatus (*G*) (zero-time specimen). (x 16.100)

Fig. 10. Autoradiograph of 1-week cultured epithelium labelled with ^{3}H-uridine. Note grains over nucleus and cytoplasm. Basal cells (*B*), mucous cells (*M*), ciliated cells (*Ci*) and a dark non-ciliated cell (arrow) are shown. (x 613)

Fig. 11. Autoradiograph showing edge of 1-week cultured explant after ^{3}H-thymidine labelling. Note cells extending around the margin with grains over the nuclei. (x 189)

Fig. 12. Phosphotungstic acid staining of Golgi apparatus in a surface cuboidal cell in 10-day cultured epithelium. Note heavy staining at periphery of some Golgi cisternae (small arrows) while center is free of stain (large arrows). (x 22.400)

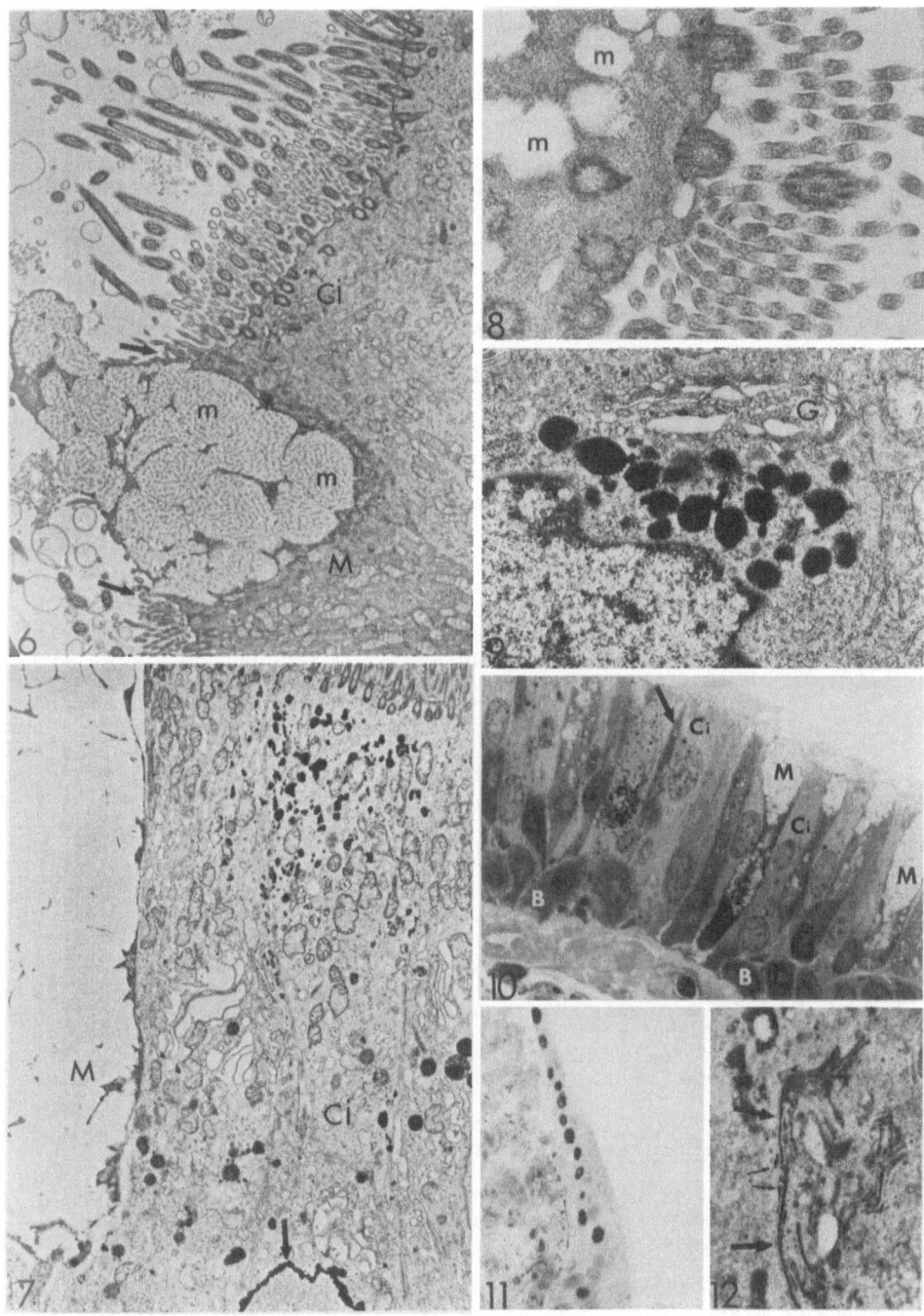

Legends see opposite page

The nucleus is large and oval. ER is present but poorly developed. In OsO₄ stained tissues often both ER and nuclear envelope may be stained in some cells, while in others no stain occurs. A few small lysosomes and, occasionally, maturing Golgi lamellae have APase activity.

Mitochondria are small and not numerous. Tonofilaments in bundles are seen in some cells, especially in those adjacent to the basement membrane.

5. Small Granule Cells

These cells are rare in most specimens and the few observations made to date agree with descriptions of the literature (BENSCH et al., 1965; HAGE, 1973). Occasionally, cells resembling small granule cells apparently reach the surface of the epithelium. The significance of this is presently unknown.

II. Abnormal Epithelium

1. Compound Cilia

Compound cilia have been observed in epithelium from 10 of the 15 patients examined. They have been seen in non-cancerous areas from patients with squamous cell carcinoma, adenocarcinoma, and alveolar cell carcinoma, as well as in epithelium from non-cancerous patients with multiple abscess and fibrosis (Fig. 3). Although this is a commonly observed change, the number of compound cilia seen in any one patient was few. These cilia have been described previously in a human case of bronchial carcinoma (AILSBY and GHADIALLY, 1973), in the tracheobronchial epithelium of hamsters during induction of squamous cell carcinoma with benzo(a)pyrene-Fe_2O_3 (HARRIS et al., 1974), and in the nasal epithelium of the guinea pig infected with Bordetella brochiseptica (DUNCAN and RAMSEY, 1965).

In general, compound cilia contain multiple axial microtubular complexes, and up to 17 complexes have been seen in a cross-section of one compound cilium. In some, microtubules appear randomly arrayed; sometimes, labyrinths consisting of invagination of the cell surface are present between individual axial complexes (Fig. 3). Sometimes the compound cilia are very large and bizarre in shape. Another variant of this abnormality consists of cilia otherwise normal, except that they contain a few additional microtubular components. Occasionally, cilia have been seen within deep recesses of the cell surface.

2. Filosomes or Fibrogranular Areas

"Filosomes" (FRASCA et al., 1967) or fibrogranular areas (SOROKIN, 1968) have been seen in a few of the ciliated cells in epithelium of 6 of the 15 patients examined (Fig. 4). The specimens include epithelium from cases of squamous cell carcinoma, alveolar cell carcinoma, adenocarcinoma, and chronic abscesses. At the periphery of the area, these tangled masses sometimes appear to organize into patterns resembling microtubular doublets (Fig. 4).

3. Mucous Cell Atrophy

This change appears to represent a transformation of normally columnar
cells into cuboidal surface cells that share many features of the normal mucous cells, such as a prominent surface "fuzz", a dark cytoplasm,
and a prominent Golgi apparatus (Fig. 2). They have sparse microvilli
and only occasionally-observed mucus granules. They may also possess
numerous autophagic vacuoles and APase-positive residual bodies.

III. Organ Culture

1. General

Our studies so far indicate that either human bronchi or hamster trachea can be maintained for many weeks in organ culture. Human bronchus
has been maintained for 4 months thus far. As a generalization, the
ultrastructural features of the cells after prolonged culture include
increased numbers of autophagic vacuoles and decreased numbers of mucous cells, whereas cells at the margin of the explant proliferate.
Cultures also show incorporation of uridine, leucine, and thymidine
(Figs 10 and 11). We are here reporting our total experience to date;
differences in characteristics in culture of epithelium from cancer
vs. non-cancer patients are not presently known.

2. Storage

Studies on storage of both human bronchi and hamster trachea indicate
that they can be stored prior to culture. Human bronchus can be stored
for at least 1 day in cold L-15 medium prior to culture and still maintain good morphological appearance after several weeks in culture.
Human bronchus stored for 2 days also shows good preservation, but in
this case a few necrotic cells are seen. At present, the maximum duration of storage of human bronchus at $4^{\circ}C$ is unknown. Observations
concerning storage of hamster trachea are similar to those described
in the human. After storage for 24 hours at $0 - 4^{\circ}C$, epithelial cells
in hamster trachea show condensed mitochondria, dilated ER, and swollen cell sap. As previously suggested (TRUMP et al., 1971), these
changes appear to be reversible in the sense that prolonged culture
reveals no evidence of irreversible cell damage.

3. Changes in Morphology during Culture of Human Bronchus

Changes such as mitochondrial swelling and dilatation of ER, seen to
varying extents in surgical specimens fixed at time of resection
(zero-time), are not seen in cultured specimens, indicating that these
changes are due to anoxia and that they are reversible.

Normal ciliated epithelium has been maintained in organ culture for
8 weeks with good ultrastructural preservation (Fig. 13). Goblet
cells, on the other hand, appear to decrease, possibly through the
discharge of mucus. After several weeks in culture, cells containing
large amounts of mucus are rarely seen, while the culture media contains mucus for approximately 1 month after the cultures have been
started. As tissues are maintained for longer periods of time in
culture, there is a tendency toward change from normal epithelium,
containing ciliated and mucous cells, to an epithelium containing one
or more layers of basal cells and a surface epithelium of cuboidal
cells which have sparse microvilli (Fig. 18). These cuboidal cells

commonly have a few mucus granules, a well-developed "fuzz" coat on the surface membrane (Fig. 16), a prominent Golgi apparatus, and multiple residual bodies containing APase (Fig. 15). They appear similar to those described under mucous cell "atrophy" in II 3 above. Immediately beneath these cells, basal-type cells often contain prominent, long, meandering cisternae of ER (Fig. 18). In addition, other cuboidal shaped cells have cilia and sometimes occasional mucus granules as well, as reported in zero-time samples. Basal cells are prominent in long-term cultures and often have prominent tonofilaments and desmosomes (Fig. 14). They appear to migrate around the edges of the cultures forming a one cell-thick layer. Labelling with ^{3}H-thymidine is seen in this area (Fig. 11).

The connective tissue fibroblasts and smooth muscle cells remain in excellent condition even after several months in culture, despite lack of direct contact with the medium. Gland cells begin to undergo necrosis at 2 months, whereas some fibroblasts and muscle cells exhibit good morphological structure at 3 months and longer.

4. Cytochemistry of Organ-cultured Epithelium

Preliminary observations have been made on the distribution of APase activity, and on staining with colloidal iron, PTA, and OsO$_4$ after short-term culture, i.e., up to 2 weeks. APase activity is present in autophagic vacuoles which seem to be particularly numerous in the surface cuboidal cells with small microvilli; often the maturing Golgi lamella is stained (Fig. 15).

The free surfaces of mucous, ciliated, and cuboidal surface cells are stained with colloidal iron. In ciliated cells, both cilia and microvilli are stained but the iron deposits appear to be less heavy

---

Fig. 13. Ciliated cells in epithelium maintained in organ culture for 6 weeks. Normal ultrastructural morphology is preserved. (x 11.200)

Fig. 14. Portion of a basal cell maintained in organ culture for 8 weeks. Clusters of tonofilaments (T) are present around the nucleus. Basal lamina (Bl). (x 11.200)

Fig. 15. Acid phosphatase activity in a surface cell from 10-day cultured epithelium. Enzyme activity is present in lysosomes (L). One of these (center) contains layered material. Activity is also present in one cisterna of the Golgi apparatus (G). (x. 11.200)

Fig. 16. Portion of a cuboidal surface cell maintained in organ culture for 11 weeks. The microvilli bear a well developed glycocalyx (arrows). Mucus granules (m) are seen, the upper one has an electron dense core. (x 63.000)

Fig. 17. Colloidal iron staining on surface cells maintained 10 days in organ culture. Note that iron deposition on the microvilli and cilia of the ciliated cell (center) is less than that on the microvilli of the non specialized cells at right and left. Cell junctions are present at arrows. (x 12.600)

Fig. 18. Epithelium after 15 weeks in organ culture. The surface cells are very thin and have occasional small microvilli (arrows). The cell adjacent to the basal lamina (Bl) contains long chains of endoplasmic reticulum (ER). (x. 11.200)

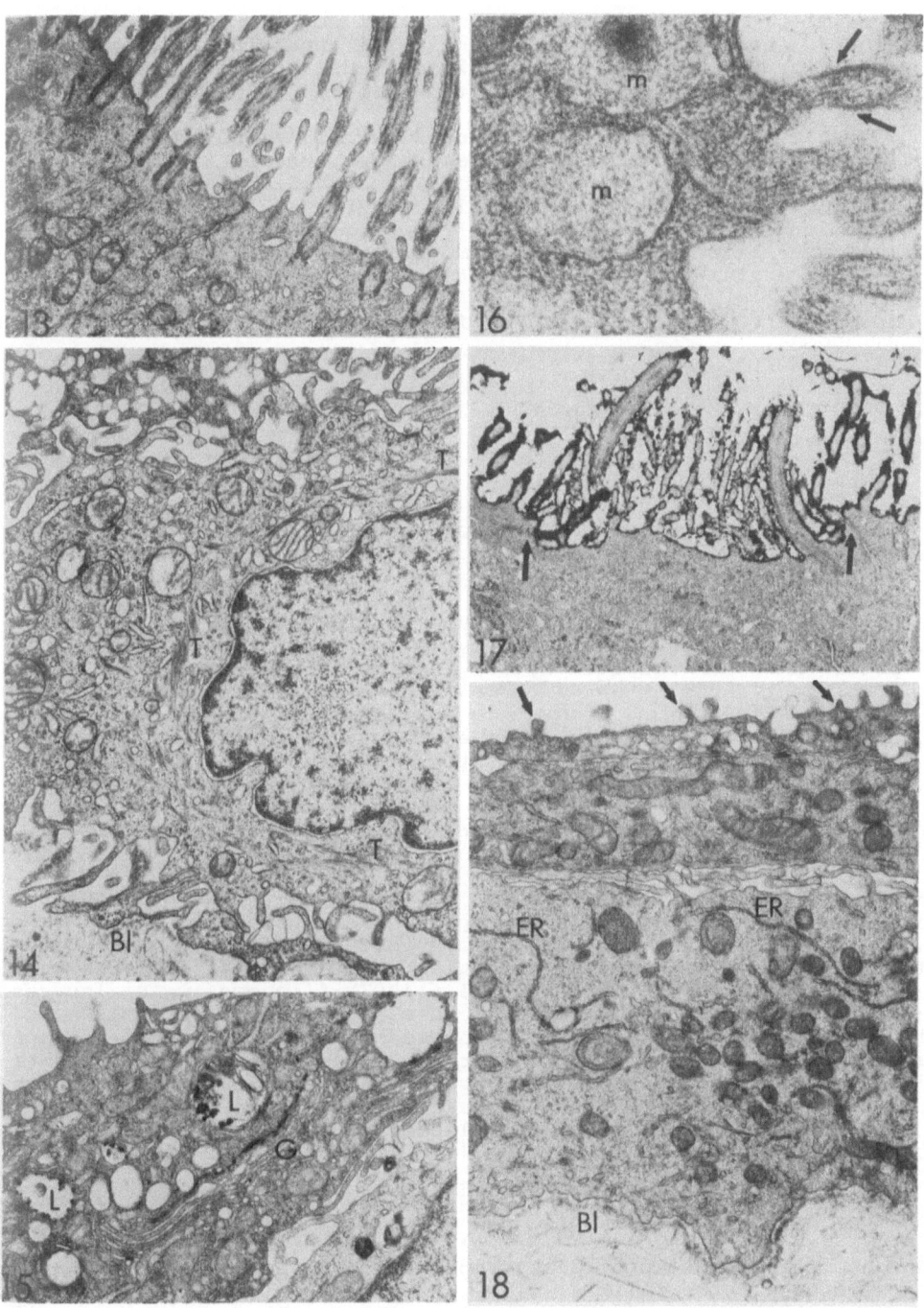

Legends see opposite page

than on microvilli of the surface cuboidal cells which have a well-developed "fuzz" coat (Fig. 17). The Golgi apparatus is not stained, probably due to poor penetration of colloidal iron. In formalin-fixed tissues, mucus droplets are also stained.

In PTA-stained epithelium, the glycocalyx and lateral cell membranes are stained, except at junctional complexes, where stain is absent. Lysosomes, including autophagic vacuoles and multivesicular bodies, are stained in all cells. The Golgi apparatus is also stained, with a gradation of staining occurring from forming (weak stain) to maturing faces (strong stain). In some Golgi saccules, the extremities show greater stain than in the centers (Fig. 12).

Unbuffered OsO₄ stains ER and Golgi-associated vesicles in a few cells of all types.

D. Discussion

These observations indicate that human bronchial epithelium removed at "immediate autopsy" or at time of surgery can be effectively studied by LM, EM, and cytochemistry.

Some of the cell types observed in zero-time samples can only be in part explained on the basis of previous reports. The status of the cells with few microvilli, dense cytoplasm, and occasional mucus droplets (dark non-ciliated cells) remains to be established. They may represent an important intermediate in differentiation.

Abnormal cilia are commonly observed in patients with and without pulmonary neoplasms. These apparently can result from experimental exposure to carcinogens (HARRIS et al., 1974) but they may also represent a sub-lethal, non-specific change. These atypical cilia may be functionally deficient and alter the mucus-ciliary transport system.

Filosomes, or fibrogranular areas, are seldom seen. We have observed them in a few ciliated cells in approximately one-third of all cases examined, including cases of squamous cell carcinoma, adenocarcinoma, alveolar cell carcinoma, and in patients with chronic abscesses. In the extensive study by FRASCA et al. (1967) filosomes were also seen in approximately one-third of all cases examined. Unlike FRASCA et al. (1967), we have not observed any association with annulate lamellae. The latter have not been observed in our material. The significance of fibrogranular areas is obscure. SOROKIN (1968) suggests that they represent the precursors of basal bodies in ciliating cells, whereas FRASCA et al. (1967) postulate that they may represent ciliary breakdown products.

It is striking that bronchi from both human and hamster can be stored for many hours at 0 - 4°C prior to successful culture. During this period, the ultrastructural morphology is altered. The alterations that occur are those previously reported in other stored systems such as rat kidney cortex slices (TRUMP et al., 1974a). The changes that occur, such as condensed mitochondria, dilated ER, and swollen cell sap, have previously been suspected to be reversible (TRUMP et al., 1971). Following culture, these changes did reverse and good ultrastructural morphology and metabolism, including incorporation of leucine, uridine, and thymidine, occurred.

Maintenance of human bronchial organ cultures for as long as 4 months offers an opportunity for a variety of studies on carcinogenic effects and even for long-term studies of histogenesis by subsequent implantation of tissue fragments into immune-deficient animals. The present studies extend the results of O'DONNELL et al. (1973) who were able to maintain human bronchial explants for up to 15 days, using the plasma clot technique.

Mucous cells are difficult to maintain in culture and degranulation of these cells gives rise to one of the more striking changes in culture, i.e., the apparent transformation of mucous cells to non-specialized cuboidal cells with microvilli on their free surfaces. These cells fall into a poorly-characterized category. An increase in autophagic vacuoles and residual bodies was noted in these cells, a change that has been noted earlier in other *in vitro* systems (TRUMP and BULGER, 1967). The fate of ciliated cells is uncertain, but after a time in culture their numbers also decrease. The changes in cell population may reflect the absence of a yet undetermined nutritional factor and/or hormone. The significance of some ciliated cells with apparent mucus granules is unknown.

Preliminary cytochemical studies on epithelium maintained in organ culture are also described. We are directing our cytochemical studies at characterization of the Golgi apparatus and cell surface in normal and abnormal epithelia because changes in cell membranes are considered to play a significant role in the behavioral changes as cells become malignant, such changes being manifest as decreased adhesiveness, decreased contact inhibition, and changes in morphology and antigenic specificity. Emphasis on "outside" cellular markers has directed attention to the Golgi apparatus, which is thought to play a role in determining certain characteristics of the cell surface by its ability to enzymatically link carbohydrate groups to proteins to form informationally-rich macromolecules (WHALEY et al., 1972). The Golgi zone is also intimately related to the formation of lysosomes.

In epithelia removed at time of resection, secondary lysosomes are most common in ciliated cells, although they also occur in basal and mucous cells. APase-staining of Golgi saccules is inconsistent in the samples so far studied. The Golgi apparatus is especially well-developed in the surface cuboidal cells. Unbuffered OsO_4-staining is capricious but potentially stains ER, some Golgi cisternae, and the nuclear envelope in all cell types.

RAMBOURG (1967) has shown that at low pH, PTA staining provides a reliable and simple procedure for staining extracellular cell coats and the maturing Golgi lamellae. The mechanism of the stain is controversial and the true histochemical significance is unknown, but DERMER (1973a), based on controlled studies, proposes that much of the staining is due to the presence of sialic acid in surface-coat glycoproteins, and he has demonstrated changes in PTA staining in malignant breast and bladder tumors (DERMER, 1973b; DERMER and KERN, 1974). PTA staining may provide interesting comparative information in future studies on normal, premalignant, and malignant bronchial lesions fixed at time of resection and also in organ-culture studies where malignant changes are induced. The use of colloidal iron-staining for surface acidic groups also offers promise as a method for studying changes in cell membranes.

E. Summary

Studies of human bronchial epithelium by LM, EM, and cytochemistry
reveal several cell types with uncertainties regarding the role and
function of some of them. Various subtle changes from normal to premalignant change need to be studied. It is possible to culture human
bronchial epithelium *in vitro* for many weeks. These cultures show
little evidence of injury, either at the ultrastructural level, or
in their metabolism as evidenced by uridine, leucine, and thymidine
incorporation. In culture, the number of mucous cells decreases while
the number of non-specialized surface cuboidal cells increases. Cytochemistry reveals secondary lysosomes in all cell types, but at zero-
time they are especially prominent in the ciliated cells. Staining
with APase of maturing Golgi lamellae is capricious. Studies are in
progress to explore the significance of altered staining reactions of
lysosomes, Golgi, and cell surfaces in premalignant and malignant
cells. Human bronchial epithelium can be stored for up to 2 days at
0 - 4°C prior to successful culture. During the storage period, reversible alterations similar to those seen in other systems can be
observed.

These studies represent the first stage of efforts to redefine, in
subcellular terms, the sequence of events leading from the normal
bronchial epithelium to invasive cancer. The type or approach described
should lead to substantive refinement of our current knowledge of histogenesis in this tissue. Methods are described to acquire, store,
transport, and culture human bronchial tissue, as well as to study
cellular effects with various methods including cell kinetics, LM, EM,
and cytochemistry. The primary purpose of our research program is to
examine the cellular effects of carcinogenic compounds in the human,
with the eventual hope of transplanting tissues to appropriate experimental animals where experimental carcinogenesis on human tissues will
then be feasible.

References

AILSBY, R.L., GHADIALLY, F.N.: Atypical cilia in human bronchial mu-
    cosa. J. Path. 109, 75-78 (1973).
BENSCH, K.G., GORDON, G.B., MILLER, L.R.: Studies on the bronchial
    counterpart of the Kultschitzky (argentaffin) cell and innvervation
    of bronchial glands. J. Ultrastruct. Res. 12, 668-686 (1965).
BOREN, H., WRIGHT, E., HARRIS, C.: Methods in Cell Biology (ed. D.
    Prescott), Vol. 8, pp. 277-288. New York: Academic Press 1974.
DERMER, G.B.: Specificity of phosphotungstic acid used as a section
    stain to visualize surface coats of cells. J. Ultrastruct. Res.
    45, 183-191 (1973a).
DERMER, G.B.: Changes in the surface coats of neoplastic human breast
    epithelium. Cancer Res. 33, 999-1002 (1973b).
DERMER, G.B., KERN, W.H.: Surface coats of human transitional epi-
    thelium from normal, low grade and advanced invasive carcinoma of
    the urinary bladder. Amer. J. Path. 74, 18a abstract 49 (1974).
DUNCAN, J.R., RAMSEY, F.K.: Fine structural changes in the porcine
    nasal ciliated epithelial cell produced by *Bordetella bronchiseptica*
    rhinitis. Amer. J. Path. 47, 601-612 (1965).
FRASCA, J.M., AUERBACH, O., PARKS, V.R., STOECKENIUS, W.: Electron
    microscopic observations of bronchial epithelium. II. Filosomes.
    Exp. molec. Path. 7, 92-104 (1967).

HAGE, E.: Electron microscopic identification of several types of endocrine cells in the bronchial epithelium of human foetuses. Z. Zellforsch. 141, 401-412 (1973).

HARRIS, C.C., KAUFMAN, D.G., JACKSON, F., SMITH, J.M., DEDICK, P., SPORN, M.B., SAFFIOTTI, U.: Atypical cilia in the tracheobronchial epithelium of the hamster during respiratory carcinogenesis. J. Path. (1974) in press.

LEDUC, E.H., BERNHARD, W.: Recent modifications of the glycol methacrylate embedding procedure. J. Ultrastruct. Res. 19, 196-199 (1967).

LEIBOVITZ, A.: The growth and maintenance of tissue-cell cultures in free gas exchange with the atmosphere. Amer. J. Hyg. 78, 173-180 (1963).

McDOWELL, E.M.: Unbuffered osmium staining in pars recta of the proximal tubule from rat kidney studied by thin and semi-thin section cytochemistry. Histochemistry 39, 335-344 (1974).

MERCER, E.H., BIRBECK, M.S.C.: Electron Microscopy: A Handbook for Biologists, 2nd ed., p. 87. Oxford: Blackwell Scientific Publ. 1966.

O'DONNELL, T.V., CROCKER, T.T., NUNES, L.L.: Maintenance of normal, metaplastic and dysplastic states of adult human bronchial mucosa in organ culture. Cancer Res. 33, 78-87 (1973).

RAMBOURG, A.: Détection des glycoprotéines en microscopie électronique. Coloration de la surface cellulaire et de l'appareil de Golgi par un mélange acide chromique-phosphotungstique. C.R. Acad. Sci. (Paris) Ser. D 265, 1426-1428 (1967).

RHODIN, J., DALHAMN, T.: Electron microscopy of the tracheal ciliated mucosa in rat. Z. Zellforsch. 44, 345-412 (1956).

RINEHART, J.F., ABUL-HAJ, S.K.: An improved method for histologic demonstration of acid mucopolysaccharides in tissues. Arch. Path. 52, 189-194 (1951).

SOROKIN, S.P.: Reconstructions of centriole formation and ciliogenisis in mammalian lungs. J. Cell Sci. 3, 207-230 (1968).

SOROKIN, S.P.: The Respiratory System. In: Histology, 3rd ed. (eds. Greep, R.O., Weiss, L.). New York: McGraw-Hill Book 1973.

TRUMP, B.F., BULGER, R.E.: Studies of cellular injury in isolated flounder tubules. I. Correlation between morphology and function of control tubules and observations of autophagocytosis and mechanical cell damage. Lab. Invest. 16, 453-482 (1967).

TRUMP, B.F., CROKER, B.P., MERGNER, W.J.: The role of energy metabolism, ion and water shifts in the pathogenesis of cell injury. In: Cell Membranes. Biological and Pathological Aspects, pp. 84-128 (eds. Richter, G.W., Scarpelli, D.G.). Baltimore: Williams & Wilkens 1971.

TRUMP, B.F., STRUM, J.M., BULGER, R.E.: Studies on the pathogenesis of ischemic cell injury. I. Relation between ion and water shifts and cell ultrastructure in rat kidney slices during swelling at O - 4°C. Virchows Arch. Abt. B Cell Path. 16, 1-34 (1974a).

TRUMP, B.F., VALIGORSKY, J.M., DEES, J.H., MERGNER, W.J., KIM, K.M., JONES, R.T., PENDERGRASS, R.E., GARBUS, J., COWLEY, R.A.: Cellular change in human disease. A new method of pathological analysis. Human Path. 4, 89-109 (1974b).

WHALEY, W.G., DAUWALDER, M., KEPHART, J.E.: Golgi apparatus: Influence on cell surfaces. Science 175, 596-599 (1972).

Studies on Carcinogen Binding *in vitro* in Isolated Hamster Tracheas

D. G. Kaufman[1], V. M. Genta[2], and C. C. Harris[1]

[1]Lung Cancer Branch, National Cancer Institute, Bethesda, MD 20014, USA
[2]Instituto di Microbiologia, Spedali Civili, Brescia, Italy

Abstract

An *in vitro* short-term hamster tracheal organ culture system has been studied in an effort to develop an assay system capable of identifying *in vivo* states of increased susceptibility to respiratory carcinogens. Tracheas incubated *in vitro* in medium containing tritiated benzo-(a)pyrene (BaP-^{3}H) have BaP-^{3}H bound to the DNA extracted from the tracheal epithelial cells, then purified and banded in CsCl gradients. Prior intratracheal treatment of hamsters with BaP plus Fe_2O_3 *in vivo* resulted in enhanced *in vitro* binding of BaP-^{3}H to tracheal DNA. This enhanced binding is inhibited by incubation in the presence of 7,8-benzoflavone. Incubation at 0° reduced binding to a greater extent than 7,8-benzoflavone; these results suggest that binding may be composed of two components, one inhibitable by 0° temperatures but not by 7,8-benzoflavone, whereas the inducible component appears completely inhibitable by 7,8-benzoflavone. There was increased binding observed in the tracheas of vitamin A-deficient hamsters and in certain inbred hamster strains. Furthermore, there appears to be an inverse relationship between hamster age and inducible binding levels. The question of whether these results are predictive of the states of susceptibility to respiratory carcinogenesis, is being studied by comparable long-term carcinogenesis tests.

A. Introduction

The question basic to our current studies is whether there are means of identifying people who are at specifically high risk to the development of lung cancer. Can specific individuals be distinguished who, because of genetic or other biologic properties, are more likely to develop lung cancer following a given carcinogen exposure? If these highly susceptible people could be identified, then it might be more feasible to protect this specific group, as compared to the entire population, from dangerous carcinogen exposures. If we can reduce the total lung cancer incidence in this high-risk subpopulation, we might have a substantial effect on the total human lung cancer incidence.

The principal problem is to find the appropriate tests to identify increased susceptibility. Our current efforts are directed at evaluating one such test in animals. These studies are being carried out parallel to life-time carcinogenesis experiments designed to distinguish states of increased susceptibility to lung cancer in an experimental model. Substantial concurrence of the results of both life-time carcinogenesis experiments and our short-term *in vitro* tests would be a validation of the utility of our *in vitro* test. If this test is predictive of lung cancer susceptibility in animals then it might be evaluated to determine its value in the human lung cancer problem.

The specific experimental model used in our life-time carcinogenesis studies is that employing intratracheal instillation of a saline suspension of benzo(a)pyrene (BaP) adsorbed to ferric oxide (Fe_2O_3) in Syrian golden hamsters (SAFFIOTTI et al., 1964, 1968). This procedure has been shown to induce respiratory tract tumors, which resemble the majority of human lung cancers (SAFFIOTTI et al., 1968) and it has been shown to produce a tumor response related to carcinogen dose (SAFFIOTTI et al., 1972a, 1972b). BaP is inert chemically, and covalent binding between BaP cellular macromolecules such as DNA, is presumed to require metabolic activation. This activation has been shown to be mediated by microsomal enzymes and it has been demonstrated in many tissues and species (NEBERT and GELBOIN, 1969). The microsomal enzymes, referred to collectively as the aryl hydrocarbon hydroxylase (AHH) system has the property of inducibility (GELBOIN, 1969), and is inhibited by 7,8-benzoflavone (BF) (WIEBEL et al., 1971).

In the present studies, we have examined the binding of tritiated benzo(a)pyrene (BaP-^{3}H) to the DNA of tracheal epithelial cells during *in vitro* incubation of isolated hamster tracheas. The objective was to determine whether binding differed according to the biologic status of the hamsters from which the tracheas were removed.

B.   Materials and Methods

Male random-bred Syrian golden hamsters (Mammalian Genetics and Animal Production, Division of Cancer Therapy, National Cancer Institute) or male inbred hamsters of strains 15.16 or 87.20 (Telaco) were maintained in pairs on San-I-Cell (Paxton Processing Co.) and given water ad libitum. They were fed either Wayne Lab-Blox (Allied Mills, Inc.) or a vitamin A-deficient diet (General Biochemicals). Vitamin A-deficient hamsters and pair-fed controls were prepared as described previously (HARRIS et al., 1972).

Unlabeled BaP (Aldrich Chemical Co.) was hand ground with an equal quantity of Fe_2O_3 dust (Type R3098; Charles Pfizer, Inc.). This mixture of BaP plus Fe_2O_3, or Fe_2O_3 alone was prepared as a uniform suspension in sterile 0.15 M NaCl solution. Sodium methohexital (Eli Lilly and Co.) dissolved in sterile 0.15 M NaCl solution was given by intraperitoneal injection for anesthesia. Either 5 mg BaP plus 5 mg Fe_2O_3, or 5 mg Fe_2O_3 alone, suspended in 0.2 ml of 0.15 M NaCl were administered intratracheally to hamsters 48 hours prior to *in vitro* experiments. Tracheas were isolated from untreated as well as pretreated hamsters. The tracheas were incubated *in vitro* in short-term organ culture under conditions in which both morphology and biochemical function of the tracheal epithelium are maintained (KAUFMAN et al., 1972). Pairs of tracheas from pretreated or untreated hamsters were incubated for 3 hours in L-15 medium containing 2 mM L-glutamine, 8.0 x 10^{-7} M BaP-^{3}H (20 μCi/ml, final concentration), and 0.04% DMSO. The BaP-^{3}H (specific activity 25 Ci/mmole; Amersham-Searle) was repurified by thin layer chromatography prior to use (KAUFMAN et al., 1973). In cases where it was present, the concentration of BF was 8.0 x 10^{-7} M; in these cases, tracheas were preincubated at 37° for 15 min in medium with BF but without BaP-^{3}H. After *in vitro* incubation the epithelium was separated from the rest of the trachea by scraping into 150 µl of a solution of 0.032 M sucrose containing 0.1 mM Na$_3$EDTA and 0.1 mM potassium phosphate, pH 6.8. This cell suspension was transferred to a small Dounce homogenizer, the suspension was adjusted to 5 mM Na$_3$EDTA and 2% SDS, and the mixture was homogenized at 0°. The homogenate was treated at room temperature with an equal volume of water-saturated phenol and the aqueous phase was separated and saved. A second phenol treatment of the aqueous phase was performed, two volumes of ethanol were added to the final aqueous solution, and the mixture was stored at -20° overnight. The resulting precipitate was sedimented by centrifugation at 10,000 x g for 2 min and the supernatant was discarded. The precipitate was then extracted with multiple aliquots of ether until there was no radioactivity present in the extracts. Following extraction, residual solvent was evaporated in a stream of nitrogen, and the precipitate was dissolved by homogenization in 0.1 M Tris-HCl, pH 7.5 containing 0.15 M NaCl in a Dounce homogenizer. The aqueous solution was then sequentially digested with pancreatic RNase (Worthington Biochemicals, Freehold, N.J.; final concentration 100 µg/ml; previously incubated at 90° for 1 hour to inactivate DNase) at 37° for 1 hour, and pronase (Calbiochem, La Jolla, Calif.; final concentrations 100 µg/ml) at 37° for 1 hour. After enzymatic digestion, the samples were dialyzed at 4° during a 3-day interval against multiple changes of 0.1 M Tris-HCl, pH 7.5 containing 0.15 M NaCl. After dialysis, the sample solutions were adjusted to 5 M CsCl and 4.2 mM Na$_3$EDTA and the samples were centrifuged at 35,000 rpm 66 hours at 20° in a Beckman SW 56 rotor. After centrifugation the CsCl gradients were fractioned into 0.2 ml portions while the absorbance of the effluent stream was continously monitored at 254 nm. Radioactivity was determined for each fraction and the absorbance of peak fractions was determined at 260 nm and 280 nm.

C. Results

I. Effect of Treatment *in vivo*

CsCl gradients of DNA isolated from tracheas that have been incubated at 37° in the presence of BaP-^{3}H are illustrated in Fig. 1. In these cases the tracheas were obtained both from untreated hamsters, and from hamsters which had received an intratracheal administration of BaP plus Fe$_2$O$_3$, or Fe$_2$O$_3$ alone, 48 hours prior to sacrifice. It is evident that a sufficient quantity of DNA is obtained from the tracheas of 2 hamsters to produce a sharp, distinguishable peak on these gradients. It is clear in Fig. 1 that a substantially greater quantity of radioactivity bands coincidently with the DNA from the tracheas of hamsters previously treated *in vivo* with BaP plus Fe$_2$O$_3$. Furthermore, the radioactivity present in the gradients bands coincidently with the DNA peak and both background absorbance at 254 nm and background radioactivity are low. A quantitative comparison of the binding levels as they relate to *in vivo* treatment can be obtained from the data in Table 1. These numbers represent the specific activity of binding determined in peak fraction of the gradients from the quantity of radioactivity (DPM), presumably from bound BaP-^{3}H., normalized to DNA content (µg DNA) in the fractions. In contrast to prior treatment with BaP plus Fe$_2$O$_3$, an intratracheal dose of Fe$_2$O$_3$ alone did not induce greater binding of BaP-^{3}H than in untreated animals.

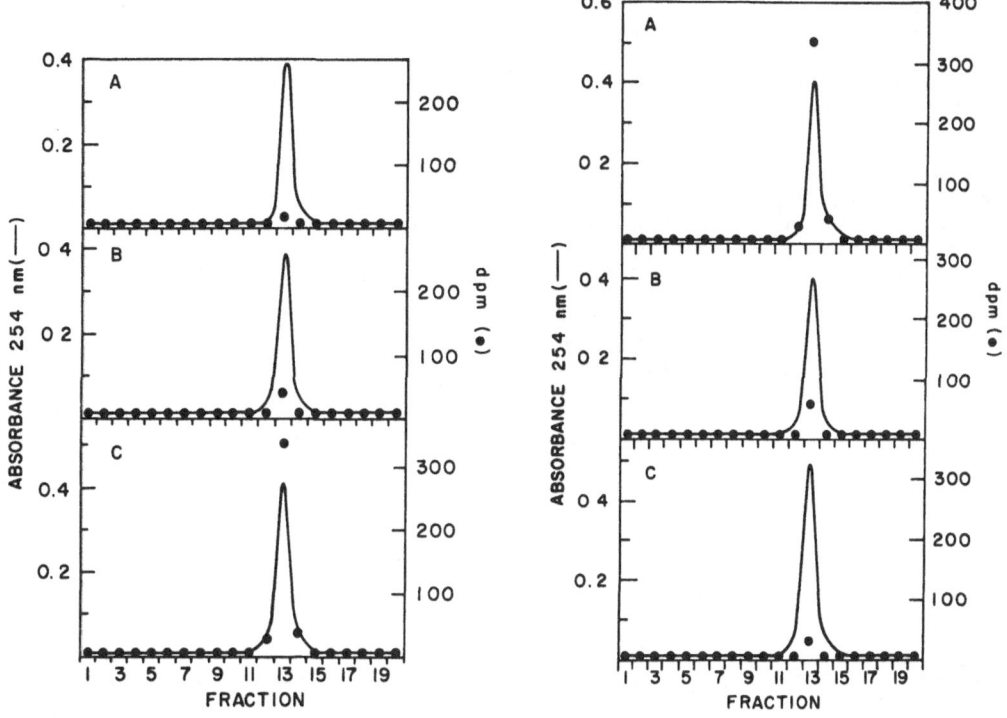

Fig. 1   Fig. 2

Fig. 1 A-C. Effect of prior *in vivo* treatment of hamsters on the subsequent *in vitro* binding of BaP-^{3}H to DNA in isolated tracheas. Tracheas in (A) were isolated from normal animals; in (B) tracheas were isolated from hamsters treated 48 hours previously with a dose of 5 mg of Fe_2O_3 given intratracheally; and in (C) tracheas were isolated from hamsters which had been treated with 5 mg BaP plus 5 mg Fe_2O_3 administered intratracheally 48 hours previously

Fig. 2 A-C. Effect of conditions of *in vitro* incubation on the *in vitro* binding of BaP-^{3}H to DNA in isolated tracheas. Tracheas were isolated from hamsters treated 48 hours previously with 5 mg BaP plus 5 mg Fe_2O_3 administered intratracheally. Isolated tracheas were incubated *in vitro* under (A) standard conditions; (B) with BF added; and (C) with incubation at 0°

II. Inhibition of Binding

In order to rule out the possibility that nonspecific binding is responsible for the preceding findings, the effects of incubation at 0°, and addition of BF (an inhibitor of BaP metabolism) were examined in the *in vitro* incubation system. The CsCl gradients in Fig. 2 compare the effects of standard incubation conditions (Fig. 2A) to those in which BF is added to the incubation medium (Fig. 2B) or in which incubation was carried out at 0° (Fig. 2C). Tracheas were all from animals which had been treated 48 hours previously with an intratracheal dose of BaP plus Fe_2O_3. It is clear from Fig. 2 that both incubation with BF and incubation at 0° result in marked reduction in the amount of BaP-^{3}H binding to DNA. This can be seen quantitatively from the specific activites listed in Table 1. As we have explained previously

(KAUFMAN et al., 1973) the binding observed at $0°$ probably represents the background of nonspecific interaction between BaP-^{3}H and DNA. DNA binding above this background level appears to be distinguishable into two components. In the case where animals were pretreated *in vivo* with BaP plus Fe_2O_3 there appears to be a substantially increased level of binding; this can be reduced by incubation in the presence of BF, to the level seen in untreated and Fe_2O_3-treated animals (under standard conditions at $37°$). There appears to be a small but measurable level of binding above background (i.e. greater than at $0°$) detectable in untreated and Fe_2O_3-treated hamsters and in all tracheas incubated with BF. Thus, this *in vitro* assay may distinguish BaP binding into two components, one induced by BaP, and one not induced. A number of possible reservations to this facile explanation of these results have been offered by us previously (KAUFMAN et al., 1973). These results do not demonstrate that the binding of BaP to DNA is covalent nor that the AHH system is the mediator of this binding.

Table 1. Specific activities of binding of BaP-^{3}H to hamster tracheal DNA: Effects of *in vivo* treatment and *in vitro* incubation conditions

In vitro incubation conditions	*In vivo* treatment[a]		
	Pretreatment with BaP plus Fe_2O_3	Pretreatment with Fe_2O_3	Untreated
BaP-^{3}H, $37°$	12.1 ± 2.5[b,c] (5)[d]	2.4 ± 0.4 (4)	2.7 ± 1.1 (5)
BaP-^{3}H, BF, $37°$	2.4 ± 0.0 (2)	2.4 ± 0.8 (2)	2.6 ± 1.6 (2)
BaP-^{3}H, $0°$	0.8 (1)	1.1 (1)	1.3 ± 1.1 (2)

[a]Hamsters were 12 weeks of age when used in these experiments.

[b]All results are expressed as DPM (BaP-^{3}H)/µg DNA.

[c]Mean ± S.E.

[d]Numbers in parentheses, number of observations.

III. Effects of Vitamin A Deficiency

Vitamin A has been shown to influence the state of differentiation of respiratory tract epithelia (HARRIS et al., 1972; WONG and BUCK, 1971). Furthermore, vitamin A has been shown to affect the process of carcinogenesis in tne respiratory tract. High doses of vitamin A administered following (SAFFIOTTI et al., 1967) or both during and following administration of carcinogen (CONE and NETTESHEIM, 1973) reduce the respiratory tumor incidence in hamsters and rats, respectively. An increased incidence of colon carinomas in rats resulting from aflatoxin was observed in rats maintained in marginal vitamin A status (NEWBERNE and ROGERS, 1973). This evidence led us to suspect that vitamin A deficiency might also represent a state of increased susceptibility to carcinogenesis in tne respiratory tract. Thus, we studied the effect of the vitamin A deficient state on the binding of BaP-^{3}H to the DNA of isolated tracheas during incubation *in vitro*. Vitamin A deficient and pair-fed, vitamin A normal hamsters were prepared as previously described (HARRIS et al., 1972; GENTA et al., 1974), and used in either the weight plateau state or at the first signs of weight loss. Incubation *in vitro* was with BaP-^{3}H alone or with BaP-^{3}H plus BF. There was a substantially greater level of binding in the vitamin A deficient as compared to the vitamin A normal hamsters (Table 2). For both vitamin A normal and deficient hamsters, binding levels were very high without prior induction by treatment with BaP plus Fe_2O_3 *in vivo* (compare with Table 1). Furthermore incubation in the presence of BF reduced binding to very low levels. In previous studies, WATTENBERG (1971, 1972) has shown profound effects on the activity of the AHH system based upon the composition of the diet. We suspect that the differences between the results in Tables 1 and 2 probably relate, at least in part, to the differences between the normal and semi-synthetic diets used in these two experiments.

Table 2. Specific activities of binding of BaP-^{3}H to hamster tracheal DNA: Effects of vitamin A status

In vitro incubation conditions	*In vivo* vitamin A status[a]	
	Vitamin A deficient	Vitamin A normal[b]
BaP-^{3}H, 37°	36.2 ± 10.3[c] (5)[d]	9.7 ± 3.7 (2)
BaP-^{3}H, BF, 37°	1.1 ± 0.2 (4)	1.3 (1)

[a]Hamsters were 8 weeks of age when used in these experiments.

[b]These hamsters were pair-fed vitamin A deficient diet and given vitamin A. They were employed in these studies when the hamsters to which they were pair-fed were symptomatically vitamin A deficient.

[c]All results are expressed as DPM (BaP-^{3}H)μg DNA; mean ± S.E.

[d]Numbers in parentheses, number of observations.

In order to determine whether the increased level of binding detected in the tracheas of vitamin A deficient animals was reversible by vitamin A, experiments were done in which vitamin A was added directly to the incubation medium in which the vitamin A deficient tracheas were maintained. In these experiments, retinyl acetate was present in the incubation medium at concentrations of 5, 10, or 15 μg/ml (1.5-, 3.0-, and 4.5 x 10^{-5} M, respectively) in addition to the BaP-^{3}H. Two separate experiments conducted at each of these concentrations gave binding levels of respectively: 2.8 ± 0.7, 4.1 ± 1.7, and 4.3 ± 0.5 DPM/μg DNA. Thus, the addition of retinyl acetate *in vitro* inhibits the BP binding in vitamin A deficient tracheas, but not to the extent caused by BF. In order to determine whether this inhibition of binding by retinyl acetate was a direct toxic effect, the influence of 5 μg/ml retinyl acetate in the incubation medium was studied in a preliminary experiment on leucine incorporation. The results of this experiment indicate that retinyl acetate does not exert a general toxic effect sufficient to explain the marked inhibition of BaP binding. The three tested levels of retinyl acetate produced comparable levels of inhibition of BaP binding, but since the range of these additions is narrow (1/2 log) it is difficult to establish this as the maximal level of inhibition possible with retinyl acetate. Further studies with both retinyl acetate and with BF will be necessary to determine whether tne effects produced by these two compounds are the results of distinguishable processes.

IV. Effect of Genetic Strain

There is evidence that the inducibility of the AHH system is a genetically determined trait (NEBERT et al., 1972). Variable levels of of inducibility have been observed both in animals and man (BENEDICT et al., 1973; KELLERMANN et al., 1973). Furthermore, there is some evidence that the susceptibility to carcinogenesis in some mouse models relates directly to the inducibility of the AHH system (KOURI et al., 1973).

Life-time carcinogenesis studies demonstrated different susceptibilities of various inbred strains of hamsters to carcinogenesis by either gastric or subcutaneous injection of polynuclear hydrocarbon carcinogens (HOMBURGER et al., 1972). We wished to see whether these strains with different susceptibilities in other organs or tissues showed differences in their ability to bind BaP-^{3}H to their tracheal DNA. Inbred strains 15.16 and 87.20 were selected for their demonstrated susceptibility to subcutaneous or gastrointestinal carcinogenesis (HOMBURGER et al., 1972) and these were compared with random bred Syrian golden hamsters in our *in vitro* assay. The hamsters were either untreated or treated with BaP plus Fe_2O_3 48 hours prior the sacrifice. The data in Table 3 are the results of our single preliminary experiment. Higher levels of *in vitro* binding were found in both inbred strains as compared to the random bred hamsters following an *in vivo* treatment with BaP plus Fe_2O_3. The 15.16 strain showed an elevated level of BaP-^{3}H binding without prior carcinogen treatment in contrast to the results observed with both random bred and the 87.20 strain of hamsters. The effect of BF was studied only in 15.16 strain hamsters and it inhibited both the binding induced by the prior *in vivo* treatment and that which was present without prior induction.

Table 3. Specific activities of binding of BaP-^{3}H to hamster tracheal DNA: Effect of genetic strain of hamsters

	Genetic strain		
In vivo treatment	Random bred	15.16	87.20
None	2.9[b]	6.7 (2.7)[c]	2.8
BaP + Fe_2O_3	8.3	17 (2.5)	18

[a]Hamsters were 14 weeks of age when used in these experiments. *In vivo* treatment with 5 mg BaP plus 5 mg Fe_2O_3 administered intratracheally was carried out 48 hours prior to sacrifice.

[b]All results are expressed as DPM (BaP-^{3}H)/µg DNA.

[c]Numbers in parentheses, the specific activity of binding observed when isolated tracheas were incubated with BF in the incubation medium.

This preliminary data suggests that there are detectable differences in BaP binding in isolated tracheas according to the genetic strain of the hamsters. Interpretation of these differences awaits the results of life-time respiratory carcinogenesis studies with intratracheal instillation of BaP plus Fe_2O_3 in these strains of hamsters. If the level of inducibility of BaP binding reflects the significant factor in carcinogenesis, then an increased susceptibility to respiratory carcinogenesis in both the 15.16 and 87.20 strains would be expected. Conversely, if the level of binding without induction is more closely related to the critical phenomenon, then the present binding data would be consistent with increased susceptibility in the 15.16 strain alone.

V. Effect of Age

In one additional preliminary experiment we examined the effect of
hamster age on the level of BaP binding. Hamsters of 4, 8, or 12 weeks
of age received an intratracheal administration of 5 mg BaP plus 5 mg
Fe_2O_3, and their tracheas were used 48 hours later to determine the
levels of BaP-^{3}H binding *in vitro*. There were substantially higher
levels of binding in the two younger groups of hamsters than in those
12 weeks old (Table 4). BF inhibited binding in the 4 week old hamsters to a level comparable to those previously found in random bred
hamsters (Tables 1 and 3). As in the case with differing binding in
inbred strains, the significance of these binding studies will be
clearer when we known the relationship of respiratory tumor incidence
to the age at which intratracheal instillation is begun.

Table 4. Specific activities of binding of BaP-^{3}H to hamster tracheal
DNA: Effect of age of hamsters

In vitro incubation conditions	Age of hamsters[a]		
	4 weeks	8 weeks	12 weeks
BaP-^{3}H, 37°	41.7[b]	27.3	11.2
BaP-^{3}H, BF, 37°	2.9	–	–

[a]In all cases, hamsters received an intratracheal administration of
5 mg BaP plus 5 mg Fe_2O_3 48 hours prior to sacrifice.
[b]All results are expressed as DPM (BaP-^{3}H)/µg DNA.

D. Discussion

The preceding results demonstrate the binding of BaP-^{3}H to DNA of
tracheal epithelial cells when isolated tracheas are incubated in the
presence of BaP-^{3}H. This binding is enhanced if hamsters receive an
intratracheal instillation of BaP plus Fe_2O_3 48 hours prior to sacrifice. This enhanced binding of BaP-^{3}H is inhibited by incubation with
BF, an inhibitor of BaP metabolism. Incubation at 0° further reduces
the level of binding. These results strongly suggest that the process
resulting in the binding of BaP-^{3}H to tracheal DNA depends, to a great
extent, on metabolic activation of BaP by tracheal epithelial cells,
and also that this activation may be inducible in the tracheal epithelium. In similar studies, HARRIS et al. (1973a) have shown by autoradiography that the binding of BaP-^{3}H to insoluble cellular components is increased in all types of tracheal cells if animals are pretreated with BaP plus Fe_2O_3. As with binding to DNA, autoradiography
reveals an inhibition of binding in all cell types by incubation in
the presence of BF or at 0°. Although induction by *in vivo* treatment
with BaP prior to *in vitro* assay and inhibition by *in vitro* incubation
with BF strongly suggest a role of the AHH system in determining the
results presented here, other factors related to cell function may be
responsible for some part of the binding observed in these cases.
Some of the *in vivo* states studied in this report may have affected the
entry of BaP-^{3}H into tracheal epithelial cells. It is conceivable that
some of these biological states have increased proliferation of tracheal epithelial cells (e.g. HARRIS et al., 1973b) and proliferating
cells may have a greater affinity for the binding of polynuclear hydrocarbon carcinogens to DNA. Direct assays of the AHH activities of

of tracheal epithelium in these various biological states will be necessary to explicitly define the role of this enzyme system.

Our primary aim in these studies was to evaluate a short-term organ culture system for the possibility of relating the extent of binding of BaP-^{3}H to DNA that occurs *in vitro* with the *in vivo* carcinogenic potential of BaP under conditions of altered susceptibility. In vitamin A deficiency the binding of BaP-^{3}H to DNA has been found to be substantially enhanced and this binding appears to be inhibitable by the presence of vitamin A. In addition there was increased inducible binding in inbred hamster strains which previously have been shown to be more susceptible to the development of sarcomas and gastrointestinal carcinomas than random bred hamsters (HOMBURGER et al., 1972). Furthermore, there was a greater level of binding in hamsters of 4 and 8 weeks of age than in older (12 weeks old) hamsters. These results may suggest greater carcinogenic potential due to states of increased susceptibility *in vivo*.

A variety of genetic, nutritional, and physiological states *in vivo* may contribute to the susceptibility of hamsters to carcinogenesis by intratracheal administration of BaP plus Fe_2O_3. Those studied in this report are only a few of the possible *in vivo* susceptibility states which may be investigated. This assay system may, thus, have the ability to predict how *in vivo* states of various types affect susceptibility to carcinogenesis, since presumably the final common pathway in the initiation of carcinogenesis in all of these states is by the binding of BaP to the DNA of the respiratory epithelial cells. This system may be able to provide predictions of carcinogenic susceptibility if the most critical factor in respiratory carcinogenesis is the rate of cell proliferation in the respiratory epithelium just as well as it might if the most critical factor is the rate of polynuclear hydrocarbon metabolism. In contrast, if the most critical facets of the *in vivo* carcinogenesis process occur after the binding of carcinogen to the epithelial cell DNA (e.g. DNA repair, immunological surveillance, etc.) then the results of this assay may be in wide variance to the results of *in vivo* carcinogenesis studies. A clear negative relationship between *in vitro* binding and the results of lifetime carcinogenesis studies would also be a useful result.

It is obvious that a full understanding of the significance of these results will only be available when a suitable number of comparisons between *in vitro* binding studies and *in vivo* carcinogenesis studies are available. At the present time only fragmentary hints of this relationship are available. CONE and NETTESHEIM (1973) have shown that vitamin A administration during periods of administration of methylcholanthrene protects rats from the development of lung tumors. This result would appear to be consistant with our findings of inhibition of BaP binding by vitamin A. Furthermore, preliminary evidence of NETTESHEIM et al. (1973) indicates that vitamin A deficiency makes rats more susceptable to the development of lung cancer.

If the results of this *in vitro* assay concur with a sufficient number of *in vivo* respiratory carcinogenesis studies, then the method may find application in predicting which other *in vivo* states are likely to be states of increased susceptibility to respiratory carcinogenesis. If this assay can consistently predict *in vivo* states of increased susceptibility in hamsters, then a comparable assay might be evaluated for human subjects. Binding of polynuclear hydrocarbon carcinogens to DNA has been demonstrated in organ cultures of human bronchial epithelium obtained from surgical specimens (HARRIS et al., unpublished observation). Cells shed or brushed from the lower respiratory tract or larynx might be evaluated as substitutes for sections of epithelium. An assay of this type in conjunction with one such as that described by KELLERMANN et al. (1973) might be suitable to select the subpopulation of people at greatest risk to the development of lung cancer, since they would determine both risk factors specifically related to the respiratory tract as well as the genetic level of inducible AHH activity (in peripheral blood lymphocytes). Respiratory tract cells may be required to survey the spectrum of influences on the respiratory tract which in summation determine human susceptibility to lung cancer.

Acknowledgements

We thank Mr. REG DAVIES and Miss JEAN GRAF for the preparation of the mixtures of BaP plus Fe_2O_3. We thank Mr. JOSEPH SMITH and Mr. WILLIAM HENDERSON for their help in *in vivo* treatments of the hamsters and in performance of the *in vitro* experiments. We also thank Dr. MICHEL B. SPORN for his continuing advice in the design of these experiments and Mrs. DORIS OVERMAN for her assistance in the preparation of this manuscript.

References

BENEDICT, W.F., CONSIDINE, N., NEBERT, D.W.: Genetic differences in aryl hydrocarbon hydroxylase induction and benzo(a)pyrene-produced tumorigenesis in the mouse. Mol. Pharmacol. 9, 266-277 (1973).

CONE, M.V., NETTESHEIM, P.: Effects of vitamin A on 3-methylcholanthrene-induced squamous metaplasia and early tumors in the respiratory tract of rats. J. nat. Cancer Inst. 50, 1599-1606 (1973).

GELBOIN, H.V.: A microsome-dependent binding of benzo(a)pyrene to DNA. Cancer Res. 29, 1272-1276 (1969).

GENTA, V.M., KAUFMAN, D.G., HARRIS, C.C., SMITH, J.M., SPORN, M.B., SAFFIOTTI, U.: Vitamin A deficiency enhances binding of benzo(a)-pyrene to tracheal epithelial DNA. Nature 247, 48-49 (1974).

HARRIS, C.C., GENTA, V.M., FRANK, A.L., KAUFMAN, D.G., BARRETT, L.A., McDOWELL, E.M., TRUMP, B.F.: Carcinogenic polynuclear hydrocarbons bind to macromolecules in cultured human bronchi. Nature (in press).

HARRIS, C.C., KAUFMAN, D.G., SPORN, M.B., BOREN, H., JACKSON, F., SMITH, J.M., PAULEY, J., DEDICK, P., SAFFIOTTI, U.: Localization of benzo(a)pyrene-^{3}H and alterations in nuclear chromatin caused by benzo(a)pyrene-ferric oxide in the hamster respiratory epithelium. Cancer Res. 33, 2842-2848 (1973a).

HARRIS, C.C., SILVERMAN, T., SMITH, J.M., JACKSON, F., BOREN, H.G.: Proliferation of tracheal epithelial cells in normal and vitamin A-deficient Syrian golden hamsters. J. nat. Cancer Inst. 51, 1059-1062 (1973b).

HARRIS, C.C., SPORN, M.B., KAUFMAN, D.G., SMITH, J.M., JACKSON, F., SAFFIOTTI, U.: Histogenesis of squamous metaplasia in the hamster tracheal epithelium caused by vitamin A deficiency or benzo(a)-pyrene-ferric oxide. J. nat. Cancer Inst. 48, 743-751 (1972).

HOMBURGER, F., HSUEH, S.S., KERR, C.S., RUSSFIELD, A.B.: Inherited susceptibility of inbred strains of Syrian hamsters to induction of subcutaneous sarcomas and mammary and gastrointestinal carcinomas by subcutaneous and gastric administration of polynuclear hydrocarbons. Cancer Res. 32, 360-366 (1972).

574

KAUFMAN, D.G., BAKER, M.S., HARRIS, C.C., SMITH, J.M., BOREN, H., SPORN, M.B., SAFFIOTTI, U.: Coordinated biochemical and morphologic examination of tracheal epithelium. J. nat. Cancer Inst. 49, 783-792 (1972).

KAUFMAN, D.G., GENTA, V.M., HARRIS, C.C., SMITH, J.M., SPORN, M.B., SAFFIOTTI, U.: Binding of ^{3}H-labeled benzo(a)pyrene to DNA in hamster tracheal epithelial cells. Cancer Res. 33, 2837-2841 (1973).

KELLERMANN, G., CANTRELL, E., SHAW, C.R.: Variations in extent of aryl hydrocarbon hydroxylase induction in cultured human lymphocytes. Cancer Res. 33, 1954-1956 (1973).

KELLERMANN, G., SHAW, C.R., LUYTEN-KELLERMANN, M.: Aryl hydrocarbon hydroxylase inducibility and bronchogenic carcinoma. New Engl. J. Med. 289, 934-937 (1973).

KOURI, R.E., SALERNO, R.A., WHITMIRE, C.E.: Relationship between aryl hydrocarbons hydroxylase inducibility and sensitivity to chemically induced subcutaneous sarcomas in various strains of mice. J. nat. Cancer Inst. 50, 363-368 (1973).

NEBERT, D.W., GELBOIN, H.V.: The in vivo and in vitro induction of aryl hydrocarbon hydroxylase in mammalian cells of different species, tissues, strains, and developmental and hormonal states. Arch. Biochem. Biophys. 134, 76-89 (1969).

NEBERT, D., GOUJON, F., GIELEN, J.: Aryl hydrocarbon hydroxylase induction by polycyclic hydrocarbons: Simple autosomal dominant trait in the mouse. Nature New Biol. 236, 107-110 (1972).

NETTESHEIM, P., CONE, M.V., WILLIAMS, M.L.: Effect of vitamin A on induction and growth of squamous cell tumors in the respiratory tract. Proc. Amer. Assoc. Cancer Res. 14, 59 (1973).

NEWBERNE, P.M., ROGERS, A.E.: Rat colon carcinomas associated with aflatoxin and marginal vitamin A. J. nat. Cancer Inst. 50, 439-448 (1973).

SAFFIOTTI, U., CEFIS, F., KOLB, L.H.: A method for the experimental induction of bronchogenic carcinoma. Cancer Res. 28, 104-124 (1968).

SAFFIOTTI, U., CEFIS, F., KOLB, L.H.: Bronchogenic carcinoma induction by particulate carcinogens. Proc. Amer. Assoc. Cancer Res. 5, 55 (1964).

SAFFIOTTI, U., MONTESANO, R., SELLAKUMAR, A.R., BORG, S.A.: Experimental cancer of the lung. Inhibition by vitamin A of the induction of tracheobronchial squamous metaplasia and squamous cell tumors. Cancer 20, 857-864 (1967).

SAFFIOTTI, U., MONTESANO, R., SELLAKUMAR, A.R., CEFIS, F., KAUFMAN, D.G.: Respiratory tract carcinogenesis in hamsters induced by different numbers of administrations of benzo(a)pyrene and ferric oxide. Cancer Res. 32, 1073-1081 (1972a).

SAFFIOTTI, U., MONTESANO, R., SELLAKUMAR, A.R., KAUFMAN, D.G.: Respiratory tract carcinogenesis induced in hamsters by different dose levels of benzo(a)pyrene and ferric oxide. J. nat. Cancer Inst. 49, 1199-1204 (1972b).

WATTENBERG, L.W.: Dietary modification of intestinal and pulmonary aryl hydrocarbon hydroxylase activity. Toxicol. Appl. Pharm. 23, 741-748 (1972).

WATTENBERG, L.W.: Studies of polycyclic hydrocarbon hydroxylases of the intestine possibly related to cancer. Effect of diet on benzo-(a)pyrene hydroxylase activity. Cancer 28, 99-102 (1971).

WIEBEL, F.J., LEUTZ, J.C., DIAMOND, L., GELBOIN, H.V.: Aryl hydrocarbon (benzo(a)pyrene) hydroxylase in microsomes from rat tissues: Differential inhibition and stimulation by benzo-flavones and organic solvents. Arch. Biochem. Biophys. 144, 78-86 (1971).

WONG, Y., BUCK, R.: An electron microscopic study of metaplasia of the rat tracheal epithelium in vitamin A deficiency. Lab. Invest. 24, 55-66 (1971).

The Reversal of Keratinized Squamous Metaplastic Lesions of Vitamin A Deficiency in Tracheobronchial Epithelium by Vitamin A and Vitamin A Analogs in Organ Culture: A Model System for Anti-Carcinogenesis Studies

Michael B. Sporn, Gerald H. Clamon, Joseph M. Smith, Nancy M. Dunlop, Dianne L. Newton, and Umberto Saffiotti

Lung Cancer Branch, Carcinogenesis Program, National Cancer Institute, Bethesda, MD 20014, USA

ABSTRACT

Normal cellular differentiation in tracheobronchial epithelium is dependent on vitamin A. In the absence of vitamin A the normal ciliated and mucus-producing cells of this epithelium are replaced by squamous cells, which are neither ciliated nor mucus-producing, but which do produce keratin. We have developed an *in vitro* system for studying the above process, using organ culture of hamster tracheas in chemically defined, serum-free medium. Keratinized squamous lesions of tracheobronchial epithelium can be induced by absence of vitamin A in the defined medium. Addition of vitamin A or its analogs to the culture (after such lesions have formed) induces reversal of keratinization and growth of a new ciliated and mucus-producing epithelium. A single one-day dose of all-*trans*-retinyl acetate or all-*trans*-retinoic acid is sufficient to effect reversal of keratinization. The hamster tracheobronchial organ culture system is also being used in our laboratory to determine whether vitamin A and its analogs are capable of reversing squamous metaplastic or other preneoplastic lesions that are induced by chemical carcinogens.

Introduction

This paper presents the results of some of our first attempts to develop a model system to study the process of anti-carcinogenesis in respiratory epithelium in organ culture. Two very basic clinical facts about lung cancer in man encourage us to proceed witn this approacn. The first basic fact is that the development of bronchogenic squamous cell carcinoma is a multistage process, with an extremely long latent period in man (AUERBACH et al., 1961, 1962a; SELIKOFF et al., 1967; SACCOMANNO et al., 1971); the latent period for development of clinically manifest disease may be 20 years or more from onset of exposure to the carcinogenic insult. Although many different sets of nomenclature have been used, it is generally accepted tnat during development of bronchogenic squamous cell carcinoma, the respiratory epithelium progresses through a series of stages of metaplasia, with increasing frequency of atypical metaplastic cells, before development of invasive carcinoma. The same process can also be shown to occur during respiratory carcinogenesis in the experimental animal (SAFFIOTTI et al., 1968; HARRIS et al., 1972; SCHREIBER et al., 1974). The second basic fact is that the progression from one stage of metaplasia to the next is not inevitable. Studies with ex-smokers tell us tnat respiratory epithelium has a spontaneous tendency to repair the cellular damage caused by carcinogens (AUERBACH et al., 1962b). It is known that the respiratory epithelium has intrinsic capacity to repair preneoplastic lesions, although obviously this potential is not always adequate to prevent cancer if the carcinogenic insult is excessive. Unfortunately, we do not know now much damage may occur before the preneoplastic lesion becomes irreversible. However, given the fact that the latent period for development of invasive cancer is so long, there exists a unique opportunity to arrest or reverse the progression of malignancy if appropriate anti-carcinogenic measures could be applied at a suitable time during the latent period. Thus, any chemical that is capable of enhancing the intrinsic capacity of the respiratory epithelium to repair preneoplastic lesions offers a potential means to prevent the development of lung cancer.

In our efforts at anti-carcinogenesis, we are thus searching for a means to enhance a natural, physiological process rather than to invent a new biological mechanism. We are seeking a means to heal preneoplastic respiratory epithelium, either to arrest the progression of metaplastic cells or to replace these metaplastic cells with the ciliated and mucus cells which normally line the epithelium. While searching for agents that are capable of modifying the cellular state of tracheobronchial epithelium, one naturally turns to vitamin A, which normally controls the proper physiological differentiation of ciliated and mucus-producing cells in this epithelium (WOLBACH and HOWE, 1925; WONG and BUCK, 1971; HARRIS et al., 1972). It is just these ciliated and mucus cells that disappear from the epithelium during the development of squamous metaplasia induced by carcinogens (AUERBACH et al., 1961; HARRIS et al., 1972). Our efforts in anti-carcinogenesis have been encouraged by the finding, in a number of long-term experimental studies with intact animals, that vitamin A or its analogs has a definite ability to prevent the development of epithelial cancer (BOLLAG, 1970, 1972; CONE and NETTESHEIM, 1973; SAFFIOTTI et al., 1967). The mechanisms whereby vitamin A exerts this protective effect in the intact animal have not yet been fully clarified. Because of the complexity of studying this problem in the intact animal, we have chosen to study it in an organ culture system, as well as continuing with studies on animals.

Although our ultimate goal is the repair of metaplasia induced by carcinogens, to begin with we chose to study the repair of a simpler epithelial lesion, namely keratinized squamous metaplasia induced by vitamin A deficiency. If we could demonstrate healing of this simpler lesion in organ culture, it would increase our confidence in attempting to study healing of metaplasias induced by carcinogens with the same *in vitro* methods. Although our studies on this topic are just beginning, we can report with confidence that in organ culture, vitamin A and its analogs can effectively and rapidly reverse keratinized squamous metaplasia caused by vitamin A deficiency. We have developed an assay that is quick, reproducible, and can be used to measure the biological activity of new synthetic analogs of vitamin A. Biological activity of retinoic acid can be measured at concentrations as low as 10^{-9} molar, which offers a convenient standard for evaluation of any analogs made by the organic chemist.

Materials and Methods

Tne methods that have been used have been described in detail (CLAMON et al., 1974a; SPORN et al., 1974). In brief, we have allowed a tracheal squamous metaplastic lesion to develop in organ culture before

attempting to reverse this lesion with vitamin A or one of its analogs. Tracheas were taken from hamsters that were in very early stages
of vitamin A deficiency and placed in organ culture. At the time of
culture, the animals were still gaining weight; the tracheal epithelium
was generally low columnar or cuboidal, with only occasional patches
of squamous metaplasia. Each trachea was opened from the larynx to
the carina along the membranous dorsal wall and cultured in a serum-
free medium (CMRL-1066; with crystalline bovine insulin, 1.0 µg/ml;
hydrocortisone hemisuccinate, 0.1 µg/ml; glutamine, 2 mM; penicillin,
100 units/ml; and streptomycin, 100 µg/ml, added). Cultures were
gassed with 50% oxygen, 45% nitrogen, and 5% CO_2. The culture dishes
were rocked to allow the tracheas contact with both gas and medium.
All tracheas were grown in medium containing no vitamin A for the
first 4 to 6 days. At the end of 4 to 6 days, some tracheas were harvested, and as can be seen in Tables 1 and 2, almost all of these tracheas had significant squamous metaplasia, and approximately 70% had
keratinized lesions. The tracheas were then divided into different
groups which were treated with either (1) no vitamin A, or (2) vitamin
A acid (β-all-*trans*-retinoic acid), or (3) an analog of retinoic acid.
In typical assays, cultures were treated with retinoic acid or one of
its analogs for a whole week before harvest (Tables 1 and 3), although
in other experiments (Table 2) the treatment with retinoic acid was
for a single day only.

Table 1. Reversal of keratinized squamous metaplastic lesions of vitamin A deficiency in tracheal organ cultures by treatment with retinoic
acid for 7 days[a]

Treatment of cultures	Number of cultures	% of cultures with respective amounts of squamous metaplasia					% of cultures with keratin and keratohya-line granules
		None	Minimal	Mild	Marked	Severe	
No vitamin A, harvested day 4-6	75	7	13	47	29	4	72
No vitamin A, harvested day 11-13	75	3	4	35	40	19	89
β-retinoic acid, 1-week treatment, harvested day 11-13							
10^{-6} M	46	48	41	11	0	0	0
10^{-7} M	22	59	18	18	5	0	0
10^{-8} M	14	14	14	50	7	14	0
10^{-9} M	11	0	18	27	36	18	0
10^{-10} M	12	0	8	42	33	17	75

[a]All tracheas were cultured for the first 4 to 6 days in medium without
vitamin A. At this time some tracheas were harvested, while the rest
were cultured for an additional week in medium containing either:
(1) no vitamin A, or (2) added β-retinoic acid. These tracheas were
harvested on the 11th to 13th day of culture. Cultures were graded as
to percentage of their total epithelium showing squamous metaplasia
on 8 cross sections from the middle of each trachea. If greater than
40% of the total epithelial length was squamous, it was graded as having severe squamous metaplasia; between 10% to 40% was graded as marked;
between 2% to 10% was graded as mild; and less than 2% was graded as
minimal.

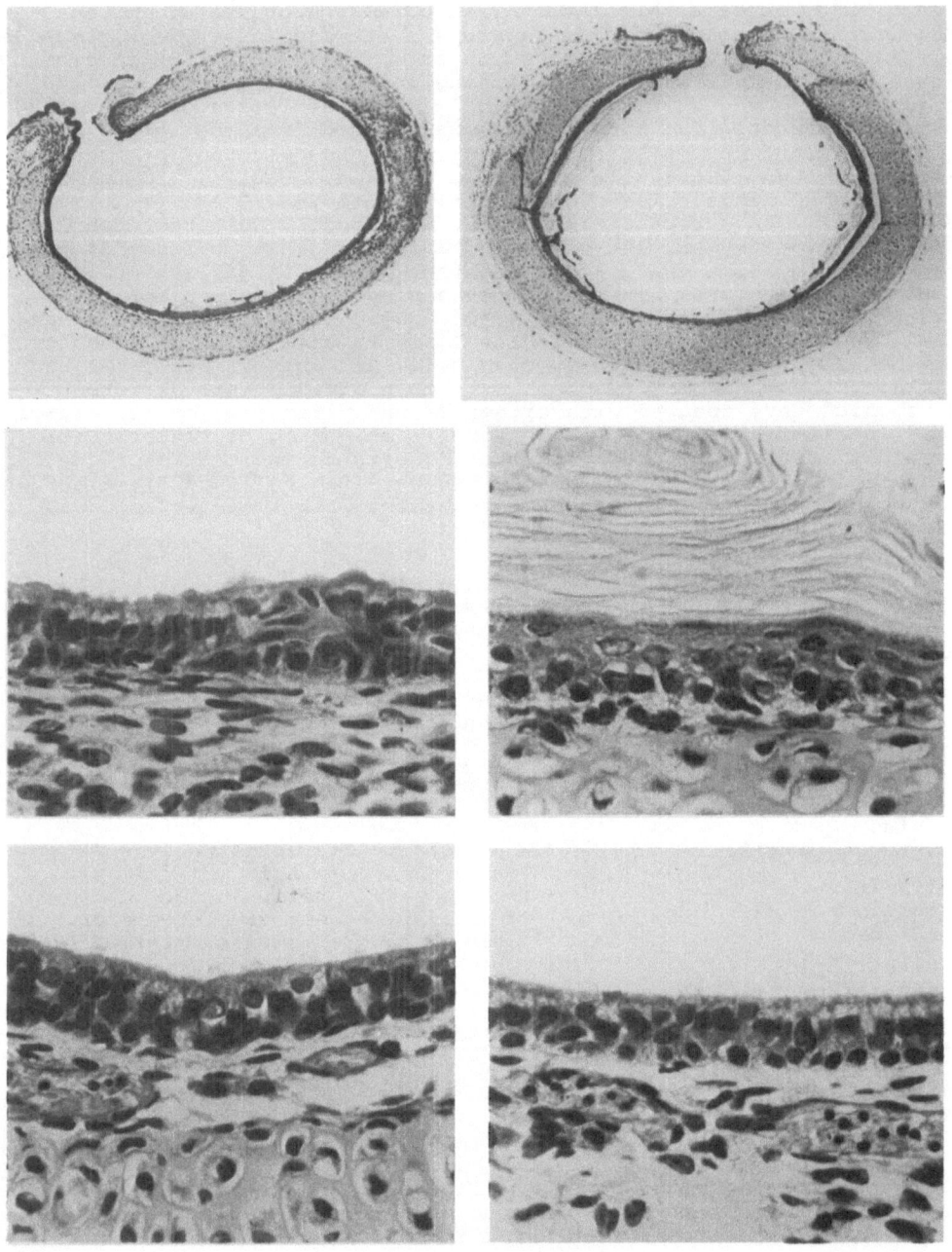

Fig. 1. *Upper left:* Trachea cultured for 10 days without vitamin A, with marked keratinized squamous metaplasia (x 30). *Upper right:* Trachea cultured for 10 days without vitamin A, with severe keratinized squamous metaplasia (x 30). *Middle left:* Minimal squamous metaplastic lesion found in trachea cultured for 4 days without vitamin A (x 375). *Middle right:* Severe squamous metaplastic lesion found in trachea cultured for 10 days without vitamin A. Note presence of keratohyaline

Table 2. Reversal of keratinized squamous metaplastic lesions of vitamin A deficiency in tracheal organ cultures by treatment with retinoic
acid for 1 day[a]

Treatment of cultures	Number of cultures	% of cultures with respective amounts of squamous metaplasia					% of cultures with keratin and keratohya-line granules
		None	Minimal	Mild	Marked	Severe	
No vitamin A, harvested day 6	51	4	8	43	37	8	71
No vitamin A, harvested day 13	52	0	0	10	75	15	100
β-retinoic acid, 1 day only, day 6-7, harvested day 13							
10^{-7} M	6	33	17	50	0	0	0
10^{-8} M	17	6	12	47	29	6	18
10^{-9} M	36	3	14	50	22	11	56
10^{-10} M	6	0	17	33	33	17	86

[a]All tracheas were cultured for the first 6 days in medium without
vitamin A. At this time, some tracheas were harvested. The remainder
were either treated for 1 day with retinoic acid (and then cultured in
medium without vitamin A for the final 6 days), or else were maintained
for the final 7 days in medium without vitamin A. Cultures were graded
as described in Table 1.

Results

Table 1 shows that the squamous metaplastic lesions increase in severity during the period of culture if no vitamin A is added to the
medium during the final 7 days. Conversely, β-retinoic acid can reverse keratinization, if applied for a whole week at concentrations
as low as 10^{-9} molar (0.3 ng/ml). A good dose-response relationship
is also shown in Table 1, in terms of the ability of β-retinoic acid
to reverse squamous metaplasia. It is not necessary to treat cultures
for a full week with β-retinoic acid in order to reverse keratinizing
squamous metaplasia, as shown in Table 2, which shows that a single
day of treatment is adequate. With treatment for a single day only,
the potency of the β-retinoic acid is less by approximately one order
of magnitude, although a good dose response relationship still exists.
Pictures of typical keratinized squamous metaplastic lesions induced
in tracheas in organ culture, and the repair of these lesions by vitamin A *in vitro*, are shown in Fig. 1.

---

granules in surface layer or epithelial cells, as well as heavy keratinization (x 375). *Lower left:* Ciliated, columnar epithelium in trachea
cultured for 4 days without vitamin A, followed by 6 days of culture
with β-retinyl acetate, 0.5 µg/ml (x 375). *Lower right:* Ciliated, columnar epithelium in trachea cultured for 4 days without vitamin A, followed by 6 days of culture with β-retinyl acetate, 0.5 µg/ml (x 375)

580

Table 3. Reversal of keratinized squamous metaplastic lesions of vitamin A deficiency in tracheal organ cultures by treatment with retinoic
acid analogs[a]

Treatment of cultures	Number of cultures	% of cultures with respective amounts of squamous metaplasia					% of cultures with keratin and keratohya-line granules
		None	Minimal	Mild	Marked	Severe	
DACP analog of retinoic acid, 1-week treatment, harvested day 11-13							
10^{-6}M	14	57	0	36	7	0	0
10^{-7}M	19	21	26	32	21	0	0
10^{-8}M	9	11	11	44	33	0	0
TMMP analog of retinoic acid, 1-week treatment, harvested day 11-13							
10^{-6}M	18	39	44	17	0	0	0
10^{-7}M	24	25	8	46	21	0	0
10^{-8}M	6	17	0	67	17	0	17

[a]Control tracheas were cultured without vitamin A, for either 4 to 6
days or for 11 to 13 days, with results of these cultures shown in
Table 1. Other tracheas were cultured for the first 4 to 6 days without vitamin A, and then treated for 1 week with either the dimethyl-
acetylcyclopentenyl (DACP) or trimethylmethoxyphenyl (TMMP) analog of
retinoic acid. Cultures were graded as described in Table 1.

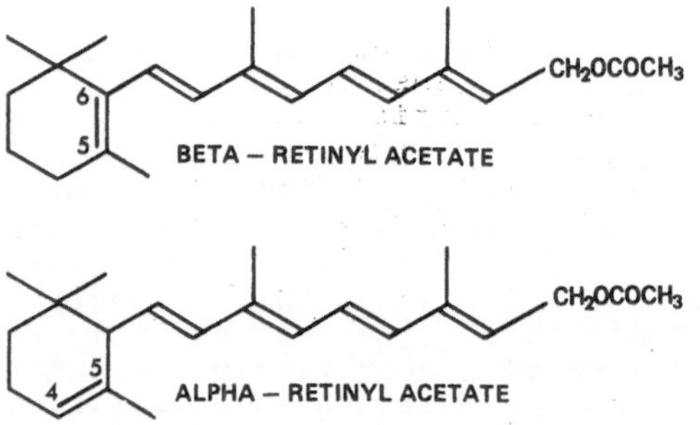

Fig. 2

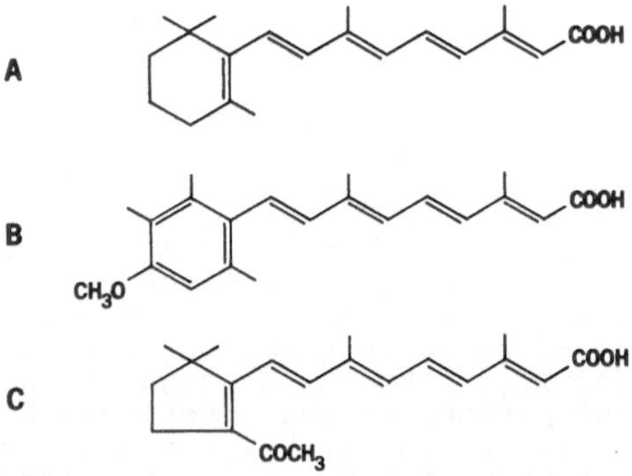

Fig. 3

Fig. 2. Structures of alpha- and beta-retinyl acetate. The naturally
occurring beta isomer has a double bond in the 5-6 position, while
the alpha isomer has a 4-5 double bond

Fig. 3 A-C. Structures of: (A) β-all-*trans*- retinoic acid, (B) its
trimethylmethoxyphenyl (TMMP) analog, and (C) its dimethylacetyl-
cyclopentenyl (DACP) analog

Because the practical usefulness of natural forms of vitamin A in
prevention of cancer and control of preneoplastic cell differentiation
is limited both by inadequate potency and excessive toxicity (BOLLAG,

1972; MOORE, 1967; SAFFIOTTI et al., 1967), we have started an extensive collaboration with Hoffmann-La Roche Inc. to investigate new
synthetic analogs of vitamin A that hopefully will have greater potency and less toxicity. Although it had previously been believed that
the naturally occurring cyclohexene ring (with a 5-6 double bond) was
required for activity of the vitamin A molecule, this concept no longer appears tenable (CLAMON et al., 1974a,b; GOODMAN et al., 1974).
Organ culture studies in our laboratory (CLAMON et al., 1974a) have
shown that α-retinyl acetate, in which the double bond in the cyclohexene ring has been shifted to the 4-5 position (Fig. 2) can reverse
keratinizing squamous metaplasia of tracheobronchial epithelium; and
studies with animals in our laboratory and in Goodman's laboratory
(CLAMON et al., 1974b; GOODMAN et al., 1974) have shown that α-retinyl
acetate can support growth in the hamster or rat. In collaboration
with Hoffmann-La Roche, we have therefore begun to investigate the
activity of a whole series of analogs of retinoic acid (which have
even greater modifications of the ring), in terms of their ability to
reverse keratinized squamous metaplasia of tracheobronchial epithelium.
The assay of two of these analogs (Fig. 3) in organ culture is shown
in Table 3. It can be seen that both the DACP and TMMP analogs have
definite activity at 10^{-8} molar. The data add further confirmation to
the concept that the naturally occurring ring system of the vitamin A
molecule is not essential for all aspects of its physiological activity. We do not yet have any extensive data on the effectiveness of
these anti-carcinogenic agents in respiratory epithelium; however,
in Switzerland, BOLLAG (personal communication) has shown that the
TMMP analog of retinoic acid and its ethyl ester have marked ability
to prevent development of skin papillomas or carcinomas in mice exposed to polycyclic hydrocarbons.

Conclusion

We have developed an *in vitro* system in which one can demonstrate and
analyze the repair or healing of a lesion of respiratory epithelium.
It of course must be realized that our eventual goal, namely the repair of metaplastic lesions induced by carcinogens, may be a much
more complex process than the repair of metaplastic lesions induced
by vitamin A deficiency. However, several known facts make us opti-
mistic that the goal may be achieved. Above all, the important conclusion made by AUERBACH and his colleagues many years ago (1962b),
namely that the respiratory epithelium of man has definite capacity
to repair itself after damage by carcinogens, encourages us to tackle
this difficult problem with organ culture methods. Moreover, the
availability of new synthetic chemical structures with marked ability
to control tne differentiation of respiratory epithelium is another
encouraging development. With the *in vitro* techniques that have been
reported at this symposium, it should now be possible to make a more
complete and sophisticated analysis of the ability of vitamin A and
its analogs to act as effective anti-carcinogenic agents in respiratory epithelium.

Acknowledgments

We thank FRANK E. JACKSON for expert assistance with the photographs,
WILLIAM HENDERSON for feeding of vitamin A-deficient diets, and DORIS
OVERMAN for help in preparation of the manuscript. Vitamin A analogs
were generously provided by Hoffmann-La Roche Inc., insulin by Eli
Lilly and Co., and hydrocortisone hemisuccinate by The Upjohn Company.

582

References

AUERBACH, O., STOUT, A.P., HAMMOND, E.C., GARFINKEL, L.: Changes in
    bronchial epithelium in relation to cigarette smoking and in rela-
    tion to lung cuncer. New Engl. J. Med. 265, 253-267 (1961).
AUERBACH, O., STOUT, A.P., HAMMOND, E.C., GARFINKEL, L.: Changes in
    bronchial epithelium in relation to sex, age, residence, smoking,
    and pneumonia. New Engl. J. Med. 267, 111-119 (1962a).
AUERBACH, O., STOUT, A.P., HAMMOND, E.C., GARFINKEL, L.: Bronchial
    epithelium in former smokers. New Engl. J. Med. 267, 119-125 (1962b).
BOLLAG, W.: Personal communication, 1974.
BOLLAG, W.: Vitamin A and vitamin A acid in the prophylaxis and the-
    rapy of epithelial tumors. Int. J. Vitamin Res. 40, 299-314 (1970).
BOLLAG, W.: Prophylaxis of chemically induced benign and malignant
    epithelial tumors by vitamin A acid (retinoic acid). Europ. J.
    Cancer 8, 689-693 (1972).
CLAMON, G.H., SPORN, M.B., SMITH, J.M., SAFFIOTTI, U.: Alpha- and
    beta-retinyl acetate reverse metaplasias of vitamin A deficiency
    in hamster trachea in organ culture. Nature 250, 64-66 (1974a).
CLAMON, G.H., SPORN, M.B., SMITH, J.M., HENDERSON, W.R.: The effect
    of alpha-retinyl acetate on growth of hamsters maintained on vita-
    min A-deficient diets. Submitted for publication (1974b).
CONE, M.V., NETTESHEIM, P.: Effects of vitamin A on 3-methyl-cholan-
    threne-induced squamous metaplasia and early tumors in the respi-
    ratory tract of rats. J. nat. Cancer Inst. 50, 1599-1606 (1973).
GOODMAN, D.S., SMITH, J.E., HEMBRY, R.M., DINGLE, J.T.: Comparison
    of the effects of vitamin A and its analogs upon rabbit ear car-
    tilage in organ culture and upon growth of the vitamin A-deficient
    rat. J. Lipid Res. 15, 406-414 (1974).
HARRIS, C.C., SPORN, M.B., KAUFMAN, D.G., SMITH, J.M., JACKSON, F.E.,
    SAFFIOTTI, U.: Histogenesis of squamous metaplasia in the hamster
    tracheal epithelium caused by vitamin A deficiency or benzo(a)-
    pyrene-ferric oxide. J. nat. Cancer Inst. 48, 743-761 (1972).
MOORE, T.: Pharmacology and toxicology of vitamin A. In: The vitamins,
    second Ed. (ed. W.H. Sebrell, R.S. Harris). Vol. 1, pp. 280-294.
    New York: Academic Press 1967.
SACCOMANNO, G., ARCHER, V.E., AUERBACH, O.E., KUSCHNER, M., SAUNDERS,
    R.P., KLEIN, M.G.: Histologic types of lung cancer among uranium
    miners. Cancer 27, 515-523 (1971).
SAFFIOTTI, U., CEFIS, F., KOLB, L.H.: A method for the experimental
    induction of bronchogenic carcinoma. Cancer Res. 28, 104-124 (1968).
SAFFIOTTI, U., MONTESANO, R., SELLAKUMAR, A.R., BORG, S.A.: Experi-
    mental cancer of the lung. Inhibition by vitamin A of tne induc-
    tion of tracheobronchial squamous metaplasia and squamous cell
    tumors. Cancer 20, 857-864 (1967).
SCHREIBER, H., SACCOMANNO, G., MARTIN, D.H., BRENNAN, L.: Sequential
    cytological changes during development of respiratory tract tumors
    induced in hamsters by benzo(a)pyrene-ferric oxide. Cancer Res. 34,
    689-693 (1974).
SELIKOFF, I.J., BADER, R.A., BADER, M.E., CHURG, J., HAMMOND, E.C.:
    Asbestos and neoplasia. Amer. J. Med. 42, 487-496 (1967).
SPORN, M.B., CLAMON, G.H., DUNLOP, N.M., NEWTON, D.L., SMITH, J.M.,
    SAFFIOTTI, U.: Activity of vitamin A analogs in cell cultures of
    mouse epidermis and organ cultures of hamster trachea. Submitted
    for publication, 1974.
WOLBACH, S.B., HOWE, P.R.: Tissue changes following deprivation of
    fat-soluble A vitamin. J. exp. Med. 42, 753-777 (1925).
WONG, Y., BUCK, R.: An electron microscopic study of metaplasia of
    the rat tracheal epithelium in vitamin A deficiency. Lab. Invest.
    24, 55-66 (1971).

Transformation of Nonvirus Producing BALB/3T3 Cells by an Environmental Extract*

Margaret A. Sheridan, David A. Axler, Anthony J. Dennis, and
Ralph I. Mitchell

Battelle, Columbus Laboratories, Columbus, OH 43201, USA

ABSTRACT

Nonvirus-producing BALBc/3T3 murine cell cultures were shown to be
susceptible to morphological transformation by a soot extract. This
extract, based on benzo(a)pyrene (BaP) content, was several thousand
times more potent in transforming cells than was pure BaP. The increased activity of the soot extract was not due to induction of an
endogenous 'C' type virus. Chemical analysis identified several polycyclic aromatic hydrocarbon (PAH) carcinogens. Based on their contribution to the total content of the extract, it appears that the increased transforming activity of the soot was due to either synergistic action between the PAHs or the presence of noncarcinogenic promoting agents.

A. Introduction

Since the original claim by PERCIVAL POTT almost two centuries ago
that cancer of the scrotum could be caused by environmental pollutants,
the etiology of a great many other cancers has been linked to environmental chemicals. These cancers can develop from ingestion, inhalation,
or absorption of pollutants through the skin.

The atmospheric carcinogens to which man is exposed are extremely complex. Among those chemicals with which we must be concerned are pollutants caused by the incomplete combustion of hydrocarbon fuels from
industrial sources and from the automobile. Among these are the polycyclic aromatic hydrocarbons.

A variety of polycyclic aromatic hydrocarbons, especially phenanthrene,
induce tumors in several animal species and transform the corresponding cells *in vitro* (BALL and DAWSON, 1969; CHEN and HEIDELBERGER, 1967;
HOMBURGER, 1972). More recently, the carcinogenic activity of extracts
of environmental pollutants have been demonstrated *in vitro*. FREEMAN
et al. (1971) have shown that extracts of city smog are able to morphologically transform virus-infected rat and hamster cells *in vitro*. This
transforming potential was shown to be much greater than could be accounted for by the relatively small percentage of BaP contained in the
sample. GORDON et al. (1972) have reported the transforming potential
of a methanol extract obtained from airborne particulates in high-
passage rat embryo cell cultures and AKR Gross virus-infected NIH
swiss mouse embryo cells.

---

*This work was supported by Battelle Institute grant B1343-0105.

In this paper we report the morphological transforming potential of a methylene chloride extract of carbon black soot on nonvirus-producing BALB/3T3 murine cell cultures. This cell line has been demonstrated to be sensitive to transformation by purified chemical carcinogens (DIPAOLO et al., 1972; TAKANO et al., 1972) and therefore may function as a reliable *in vitro* bioassay for the carcinogenic activity of environmental pollutants.

B. Materials and Methods

BALB/3T3 A31 mouse embryo cells, which demonstrate extreme contact inhibition at confluence, were kindly supplied by Dr. M. LIEBER (Meloy Laboratories, Springfield, Virginia). Cell cultures were maintained according to the strict cultural conditions outlined by TODARO (1969). All cultures were examined for spontaneous release of C-type virus and, although these cells were found to be negative for spontaneous production of virus by the reverse transcriptase assay, they were inducible after pretreatment with BUDR (AARONSON et al., 1971; LIEBER et al., 1973). BaP was obtained as a zone-refined purified solid crystal from Mr. J. HINTON (Columbia, South Carolina). BaP was stored in dark glass containers at -20°C. For subsequent use, BaP was solubilized in Dimethyl Sulfoxide (DMSO) at a concentration of 10 mg BaP per 1.0 ml of DMSO. One ml of this solution was added slowly, with continuous stirring, to 99.0 ml of warm complete Dulbecco's medium to make a working suspension. Soot was obtained by scraping the wall surface of an automobile tunnel located in a large metropolitan area. The solid carbon black soot was extracted in methylene chloride. Using the method of SAWICKI et al. (1970), it was determined that the soot extract contained 0.002% BaP. Stock (1.0 ml) was placed in a sterile, weighed centrifuge tube, allowed to evaporate overnight, and reweighed. The resulting tar layer was resuspended in DMSO at a rate of 1.0 ml DMSO per 1.0 mg of residue. This 1.0 ml solution was then added to 9.0 ml of warm Dulbecco's complete medium to serve as a stock solution. Assays were initiated by planting 500 viable BALB/3T3 cells per 100 mm dish in Dulbecco's complete medium and incubating the cultures for 24 hours at 37°C in a 10% CO_2 - 90% air atmosphere. At 24 hours' postplanting, the medium was removed and replaced with an equal quantity (10.0 ml) of Dulbecco's complete medium containing varying quantities of either soot extract or pure BaP. Following a 48-hour incubation period, the cultures were washed 3 times with Dulbecco's medium (minus calf serum), refed with fresh complete medium, and returned to the incubator. The cultures were fed every 3 days for an additional 12 days and then the cells fixed in methanol, stained with Giemsa, and assayed for transformed colonies. Normal colonies appear flat, thin, evenly stained, and highly contact-inhibited, whereas transformed colonies stain more densely with loss of contact inhibition, as evidenced by the piling up of cells on top of one another. For induction of endogenous 'C' type virus, the reverse transcriptase assay of ROSS et al. (1971) was used. BALB/3T3 cells (1 x 10^5) were seeded onto 60 mm plastic petri plates in Dulbecco's complete media. At 24 hours, the media was removed and the cells treated with BaP or soot extract. Controls consisted of cells treated with growth media only. At 48 hours, all cells were washed. Under these conditions of treatment, the BaP and soot extract are capable of transforming cells *in vitro*. Half of each group was refed with growth media and the other half treated with the halogenated pyrimidine bromodeoxyuridine (BUDR - known to induce endogenous 'C' type virus). At 24 hours, all cells were washed with calf serum-free Dulbecco's medium and refed with complete Dulbecco's media. After 4 days incubation at $37^{\circ}C$ in a 90% air - 10% CO_2 atmosphere, the fluids were collected and assayed for reverse transcriptase activity. Results are expressed as $[^3H]$ TMP incorporated (counts/minute) into poly(dT) product during a 60-minute incubation at $37^{\circ}C$ (minus that incorporated by the same reaction mixture without template). Supernatants from nonproducer cell lines yield between 500 and 2.000 counts/minute in this assay.

C. Results

I. Morphological Transformation by a Soot Extract

Fig. 1 represents the efficiency of cloning (EOC) and the efficiency of transformation (EOT) for both the soot extract and the pure BaP. The dose-response relationship of pure BaP in terms of EOC and EOT follows that reported by others (DIPAOLO et al., 1972).

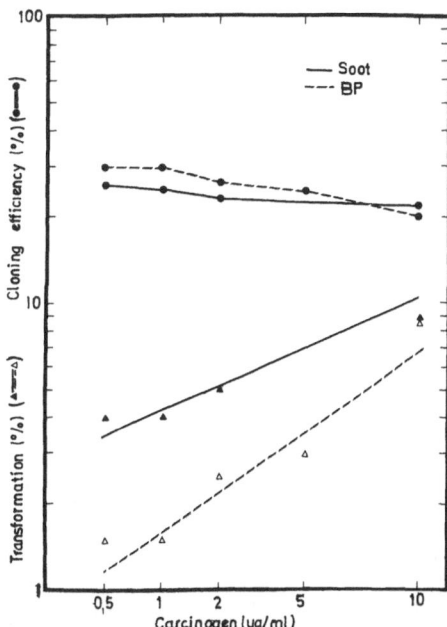

Fig. 1

Neither the pure BaP nor the soot extract was highly cytotoxic at the concentrations employed (note the slow decline in EOC in Fig. 1). However, the soot extract was more potent in inducing morphological transformation than was the purified BaP. Based on the concentration of BaP present in the soot extract (approximately 0.002%), the extract was several thousand times more effective in inducing morphological transformation than was the pure BaP. This observation correlates well with the finding of FREEMAN et al. (1971), that a smog residue containing 0.0007 µg units/ml of BaP transformed rat embryo cultures as efficiently as 0.4 µg/ml of pure BaP.

II. Activation of Endogeneous 'C' Type Virus by a Soot Extract

Among the mechanisms proposed in chemical carcinogenesis is activation of an endogenous oncogenic virus (WHITMIRE et al., 1971). In addition, as indicated earlier, cells that are exogenously infected with non-transforming murine leukemia viruses are more susceptible to transformation by chemical carcinogens (FREEMAN et al., 1971; GORDON et al., 1972). Accordingly, the possibility must be considered that the increased efficiency of transformation by the soot extract may be due to the activation of an endogenous oncogenic virus by a component of the extract. This activation may render the cells more susceptible to the carcinogenic components of the extract. Using the reverse transcriptase assay, virus activation was determined. Table 1 demonstrates the effect of BaP treatment over a wide range of concentrations on the induction of endogenous 'C' type virus. As can be seen, BaP at all concentrations failed to activate virus. From the data presented in Table 2, the soot extract likewise failed to activate endogenous virus from these cells when assayed for reverse transcriptase activity. However, as seen in Tables 1 and 2, the inducibility of endogenous virus is clear from the high level of activation in cells exposed to BUDR with and without BaP or soot.

Table 1. Induction of endogenous 'C' type virus by benzo(a)pyrene

Concentration BaP[a]	BUDR[a]	Supernatant reverse transcriptase activity 10^3 counts/minute)
0.1	--	1.2
0.1	32	150.5
0.5	--	2.0
0.5	32	129.7
5.0	--	1.6
5.0	32	96.4
10.0	--	1.9
10.0	32	113.5
50.0	--	1.5
50.0	32	157.3
--	--	1.3
--	32	118.4

[a]μg/ml.

From this data it appears that activation of endogenous 'C' type virus, based on the reverse transcriptase assay, is not involved in the increased transforming potential of the soot extract.

III. Chemical Evaluation of the Soot Extract

Since BaP is one of the most potent polycyclic aromatic hydrocarbon (PAH) carcinogens, it is used commonly as an index of pollution arising from the combustion of carbonaceous material. It is not, however, the only hydrocarbon found in automobile exhaust which has biological

Table 2. Induction of endogenous 'C' type virus by a soot extract

Concentration soot[a]	BUDR[a]	Supernatant reverse transcriptase activity (10^3 counts/minute)
0.1	--	0.53
0.1	32	13.50
0.5	--	0.37
0.5	32	8.70
5.0	--	0.31
5.0	32	10.10
10.0	--	0.29
10.0	32	13.40
50.0	--	0.41
50.0	32	6.40
--	--	1.10
--	32	11.80

[a] µg/ml.

activity. Accordingly, chemical analysis was performed to identity other PAHs which may be carcinogenic. The same sample of soot extract that was used to perform the transformation and virus induction experiments was analyzed by gas-chromatography-mass spectra techniques. Table 3 lists the PAHs found in the soot extract. Among those identified, the noncarcinogenic compounds are present in highest concentration. Clearly, if one takes into account the total amount of potential carcinogens in the soot extract, the whole extract is still considerably more active than the sum of the individual carcinogenic components.

Table 3. Polycyclic aromatic hydrocarbon analysis of soot extract

Polycyclic aromatic hydrocarbon	Carcinogenic activity[a]	Percent of extract
Anthracene	-	0.01
Methyl anthracene (2 isomers)	+	0.004
Pyrene	-	0.02
Fluoranthene	-	0.02
Methyl pyrenes or fluoranthenes (4 isomers)	+	0.004
Benzanthracene	++	0.002
Benzfluorene (4 isomers)	++	0.01
Benzpyrene or Benzfluoranthene (2 isomers)	+++	0.002
Methyl benzanthracene	+++	0.004
Methyl benzfluorene (4 isomers)	++	0.002
Aceanthrylene	-	0.004

[a] Degree of carcinogenicity from negative (-) to strongly positive (+++). (Data derived from work of others.)

588

D. Discussion

The results reported here demonstrate that nonvirus-producing murine
cell cultures are susceptible to morphological transformation by a
soot extract. The efficiency with which the soot transforms cells is
several thousandfold greater than pure BaP when compared on the basis
of BaP content. These findings are consistent with those reported by
FREEMAN et al. (1971) using a city smog extract and rat and hamster
embryo cells *in vitro* and correlate also with the *in vivo* findings of
KOTIN et al. (1954) using atmospheric extracts in skin-painting experiments on C57 black mice. Since the concentration of BaP in their
preparations could not account for the observed tumor inddence, they
concluded, like FREEMAN et al., that substances other than BaP were
active in promoting or causing the tumors. In many of these systems
referred to previously, the presence of exogenous virus and the possible presence of infectious endogenous virus, perhaps acting as co-
carcinogens or promoters, may make it difficult to interpret the true
role of exogenous chemical promoters. The data presented herein indicates that, at least in the murine BALB/3T3 system, this promoting
action is not due to the chemical activation of endogenous virus.

The possibility remains, therefore, that the low levels of PAH carcinogens in the extract may act synergistically to cause the observed
transformation, or that noncarcinogenic promoters are responsible for
these observations *in vitro*. Ongoing experiments involving the fractionation of the soot extract components and examination of their
synergistic action in various combinations will yield further data
in area.

References

AARONSON, S.A., TODARO, G.J., SCOLNICK, E.M.: Induction of murine
    C-type viruses from clonal lines of virus-free BALB/3T3 cells.
    Science 174, 157-159 (1971).
BALL, J.K., DAWSON, D.A.: Biological effects of the neonatal injec-
    tion of 7,12-Dimethylbenz(α)anthracene. J. nat. Cancer Inst. 42,
    579-591 (1969).
CHEN, T.T., HEIDELBERGER, C.: *In vitro* malignant transformation of
    cells derived from mouse prostate in the presence of 3-methylchol-
    anthrene. J. nat. Cancer Inst. 42, 915-925 (1969).
DIPAOLO, J.A., DONOVAN, P.J.: Properties of Syrian hamster cells
    transformed in the presence of carcinogenic hydrocarbons. Exp.
    Cell Res. 48, 361-377 (1967).
DIPAOLO, J.A., TAKANO, K., POPESCU, N.C.: Quantitation of chemically
    induced neoplastic transformation of BALB/3T3 cloned cell lines.
    Cancer Res. 32, 2686-2695 (1972).
FREEMAN, A.E., PRICE, P.J., BRYAN, R.J., GORDON, R.J., GILDEN, R.V.,
    KELLOFF, G.J., HUEBNER, R.J.: Transformation of rat and hamster
    embryo cells by extracts of city smog. Proc. nat. Acad. Sci. (Wash.)
    68, 445-449 (1971).
GORDON, R.J., BRYAN, R.J., RHINE, J.S., DEMOISE, C., WOLFORD, R.G.,
    FREEMAN, A.D., HUEBNER, R.J.: Transformation of rat and mouse
    embryo cells by a new class of carcinogenic compourds isolated from
    particles of city air. Int. J. Cancer 12, 223-232 (1972).
HOMBURGER, F.: Chemical carcinogenesis in Syrian hamsters. Progr.
    exp. Tumor Res. 16, 152-175 (1972).

KOTIN, P., FALK, H.L., MADER, P., THOMAS, M.: Aromatic hydrocarbons.
  I. Presence in the Los Angeles armosphere and the carcinogenicity
  of atmospheric extracts. Arch. industr. Hyg. 9, 153-163 (1954).
LIEBER, M.M., LIVINGSTON, D.M., TODARO, G.J.: Superinduction of endo-
  genous type-C virus by 5-Bromodeoxyuridine from transformed mouse
  clones. Science 181, 443-444 (1973).
ROSS, J., SCOLNICK, E.M., TODARO, G.J., AARONSON, S.A.: Separation
  of murine cellular and murine leukemia virus DNA polymerases.
  Nature New Biol. 231, 163-167 (1971).
SAWICKI, E., COREY, R.C., DOOLEY, A.E., GISCLARD, J.B., MONKMAN, J.L.,
  NELIGAN, R.E., RIPPERTON, L.A.: Tentative method of microanalysis
  for Benzo(α)pyrene in airborne particulates and source effluents.
  Lab. Hlth. Sci. 7, 56-59 (1970).
TAKANO, K., BALOUGH, L.P., MERKEL, N.S., DIPAOLO, J.A.: Quantitation
  of chemically induced meoplastic transformation of BALB/3T3 cloned
  cell lines. Fed. Proc. 31, 633 (1972).
TODARO, G.J.: Transformation Assay Using Cell Line 3T3 in Fundamental
  Techniques in Virology, pp. 220-228. New York-London: Academic Press
  1969.
WHITMIRE, C.E., SALERNO, R.A., RABSTEIN, L.S., HUEBNER, R.J., TURNER,
  H.C.: RNA tumor-virus antigen expression in chemically induced
  tumors. Virus genome specified common antigens detected by complement fixation in mouse tumors induced by 3-Methylcholanthrene.
  J. nat. Cancer Inst. 47, 1255-1265 (1971).

Concluding Remarks:
Progress in Respiratory Carcinogenesis Bioassays

Michael B. Sporn

Lung Cancer Branch, National Cancer Institute, Bethesda, MD 20014, USA

The one thing that is customary at this time is to try to find some unifying thread or common theme that pertains to the conference as a whole. For this conference that would be most difficult to do, but there is one thing which I am sure the entire audience would agree on, and that is our indebtedness to Dr. KARBE and to Dr. PARK for doing a very outstanding job of organizing this symposium. I don't know of any meeting that I have been to that has been as well planned and as well organized, and where the guests have been as well cared for with excellent hospitality, than as this meeting. So thank you very much Dr. KARBE and Dr. PARK.

Now when it comes to trying to find a central, unifying theme for this entire conference, that is distinctly more difficult; so these very last few remarks may not be entirely agreeable to all of the audience. I would like to suggest that, in terms of what we have been talking about during the last three days, perhaps there is a critical problem which affects the entire field of lung cancer research, particularly as it ultimately pertains to man. It is that we are spending too much time looking at the final product, namely invasive cancer, and not enough on the genesis of the problem. It seems to me that if we are concerned with the problem of progress in respiratory carcinogenesis bioassays, which has been the theme of this conference, basically we come back to the original problem of: What is cancer, and how does it arise? This is a common problem that runs through not only all of lung cancer research but really all of cancer research at this time. I would like to believe that cancer begins not when an invasive tumor is first detectable, but when a carcinogen orignally binds in some biologically meaningful form with a target cell. Now that alone may not be enough to give the final product, namely invasive cancer; but until we do understand the total process of carcinogenesis and understand the mechanism of what cancer really is, we are going to have a difficult time with our eventual goal - namely to prevent or perhaps even to cure this disease.

It thus seems to me that the field of respiratory carcinogenesis bioassays can ultimately be most useful if it enables us to tackle several key problems. First of all: What are the key initiating events in terms of induction of lung cancer? What new assays will enable us to make predictions about the carcinogenicity of various chemicals, and about host factors that modify this carcinogenicity? Secondly, can we develop better assays for studying the process of promotion in order to identify the factors which keep the respiratory epithelium in a state of high cellular turnover so that the initiating events may ultimately lead to invasive cancer? What are the factors that ultimately enable an initiated set of cells to develop into a clone or group of transformed cells that have autonomous growth properties? These are problems, too, for which we need better assays. We have heard during the conference about many factors - whether they be dusts or tobacco smoke or other environmental pollutants - that may be promoting, but mechanistically we still do not have a real understanding of how these promoting agents work. Finally, a third problem would be to develop new bioassays so that we can more adequately define the structural and functional properties of the preneoplastic state. I think that was most strikingly seen this afternoon when we saw four different sets of "preneoplastic cells", but we were unable to give a functional interpretation of what is really meant by this term. We shall certainly need new assays which will help to define this problem.

In the long run, then, if we come to use our assay systems, not just to define <u>what</u> is happening (which is certainly a very needed first step), but <u>if</u> we use our assay systems so that we can understand <u>how</u> it is happening and <u>why</u> it is happening, then I think that we will come closer to our ultimate goal. The types of experimental bioassays that we have heard so much about during the past three days must be used as a foundation for our effort. However, we will need to develop new tools, new techniques, and new methods to answer these very difficult questions so that we can reach the ultimate goal of prevention of lung cancer.

Subject Index

Cells, mesenchymal 519
-, mesothelial 92
-, mucin-secreting 519
-, mucus-producing 575
-, necrobiotic 543
-, neoplastic 495
-, preneoplastic 495
-, proliferation 472
-, - rates 478
-, secretory 529
-, spindle 93
-, spindle-shaped anaplastic 394
Ceramic 431
Cerium hydroxide 409, 411
C3H-10T-1/2 clone 8 498
C3H mouse embryo cells 498
Changes, benign 468
-, carcinogen-induced 507
-, malignant 468
-, metaplastic 465
-, preneoplastic 530
Chemical carcinogen metabolism 26
- carcinogenesis susceptibility 22
- induction 431
Chemicals, environmental 583
Chimney soot 14
Chromate dust 14
Chrome compounds 13
Chromite roast, powdered 93
Chromium oxide, dust of 271
Chrysene 142, 148
Chrysotile 10, 96
Cigarette smoke 2, 48, 320, 454, 485
- - amount of deposition 309
- -, chemical components 486
- - condensate 161, 495, 521, 532
- - condensate, acidic fraction 398
- - condensate, crude 398
- - condensate fractions 48, 293
- - condensate, neutral fraction 398
- -, diluted 369
- - in hamsters 360
- -, inhalation 271, 331
- -, inhalation, in Syrian hamsters 369
- -, labeled 300, 309
- -, mainstream 312
- -, particles of 300
- -, particulate phase 309
- -, tumorigenic effects 147
- smoker 485
- smoking 403
Cigarettes, unlabeled 303
Cilia, lack of 167
Ciliary escalator, mucous 476
Clearance 157, 436, 443
- of BaP 207
-, carcinogen 234
-, lung 423
- mechanism 168
-, particle 159

- of ^{210}Po 476
- rates 69, 146
CO-intoxication 294
Coal tar 13
Cobalt oxide 219
- -, dust of 182
- -, inhaled 360
Cocarcinogenic activity of tobacco smoke 235
- agent 271
- effect 346, 404
- - of dust particles 174
- - of ferric oxide dust 234
- factor 419
Cocarcinogenicity 59, 240, 360
Cocarcinogens 10, 38, 369, 380, 486, 493, 588
-, weak 235
Cofactors 3, 7, 12, 38, 419, 485, 513
- in carcinogenesis 234
Collagen 461
Concentration of particles 346
Condensate application, epicutaneous 293
- of automobile exhaust 140, 146
- of cigarette smoke 142
Connective tissue fibroblasts 558
Copper, retention and distribution 128
Cornification of tracheal epithelium 179
Coronene 148
Crocidolite 14
Cumulative response of lesions 397
Cylindroma, bronchial 200
-, bronchiolo-alveolar 200
Cystadenoma 320
Cytochromes, Co-binding 58
Cytogenetic damage 466
Cytopathological effects 234, 238

Degeneration 509
-, hydropic 167
-, myocardial 328
DEN, subcutaneous inoculations 219
Deposition 428, 443
-, alveolar 423
-, experimental 121
-, fractional 117
-, γ-tagged particle 116
- of the gaseous components 405
- of inhaled aerosols 117
-, intrapleural 93
- of particles 293, 297
- of particulates 94
- of ^{210}Po 476
- profile 121
- of radiopaque tantalum powder aerosols 117
-, regional 117
-, selective 121

List of Contributors

Dr. Ernest C. Anderson
Los Alamos Scientific Laboratory
University of California
P.O. Box 1663
Los Alamos, NM 87544, USA

Dr. David A. Axler
Battelle, Columbus Laboratories
505 King Avenue
Columbus, OH 43201, USA

Lucy A. Barret
Dept. of Pathology
University of Maryland School
of Medicine
31 S. Greene Street
Baltimore, MD 21201, USA

Dr. David W. Baxter
Chicago College of Osteopathic
Medicine
1122 East 53rd Street
Chicago, IL 60637, USA

Prof. Dr. John R. Benfield
University of California (UCLA)
Harbor General Hospital
1000 W. Carson Street
Torrance, CA 90509, USA

Dr. Stephan A. Benjamin
Inhalation Toxicology Research
Institute, Lovelace Foundation
5200 Gibson Boulevard Southheast
Albuquerque, NM 87108, USA

Dr. Peter Bernfeld
Bio-Research Consultants, Inc.
9 Commercial Avenue
Cambridge, MA 02141, USA

Dr. M. Blackstone
College of Medicine
Department of Environmental
Health, Kettering Laboratory
University of Cincinnati
3223 Eden Avenue
Cincinnati, OH 45219, USA

Dr. William H. Blair
Mercy Hospital and Medical Center
Stevenson Expressway at King Drive
Chicago, IL 60616, USA

Dr. Bruce B. Boecker
Inhalation Toxicology Research
Institute, Lovelace Foundation
5200 Gibson Boulevard Southheast
Albuquerque, NM 87108, USA

Dr. P.W. Brown
Carreras Rothmans Ltd.
Nevendon Road
GB - Basildon, Essex SS13 1BT

Dr. Horst Brune
Beratungsforum für Präventiv-
medizin und Umweltschutz GmbH
2000 Hamburg 1
Kattrepelsbrücke 1

Dr. Robert H. Busch
Biology Department, Battelle
Pacific Northwest Laboratories
P.O. Box 999
Richland, WA 99352, USA

Dr. Jean Chameaud
Service Médical, Commissariat
à l'Energie Atomique
B.P. No. 1
F - 87640 Razes

Dr. Ivan Chouroulinkov
Institute of Scientific Research
on Cancer, CNRS
B.P. No. 8
F - 94800 Villejuif

Dr. Gerald H. Clamon
Lung Cancer Branch
National Cancer Institute
Bethesda, MD 20014, USA

Dr. Arthur H. Cohen
Departments of Surgery and
Pathology
Harbor General Hospital
Torrance, CA 90509, USA

Dr. Vicki R. Cohen
Insitute of Environmental
Medicine, New York University
Medical Center
550 First Avenue
New York, NY 10016, USA

Prof. Dr. John E. Craighead
Dept. of Pathology
University of Vermont
College of Medicine
Burlington, VT 05401, USA

Dr. Donald A. Creasia
Biology Division
Oak Ridge National Laboratory
P.O. Box Y
Oak Ridge, TN 37830, USA

Dr. Gerald E. Dagle
Battelle
Pacific Northwest Laboratories
P.O. Box 999
Richland, WA 99352, USA

Dr. G.W. Davis
Department of Veterinary
Pathobiology
Ohio State University
Columbus, OH, USA

Dr. Charles F. Demoise
Department Viral-Chemical Oncology
Microbiological Associates
4733 Bethesda Avenue
Bethesda, MD 20014, USA

Dr. Anthony J. Dennis
Biomedical Sciences Section
Battelle, Columbus Laboratories
505 King Avenue
Columbus, OH 43201, USA

Prof. Dr. Walter Dontenwill
Forschungsinstitut der
Cigarettenindustrie e.V.
2000 Hamburg 54
Gazellenkamp 38

Nancy M. Dunlop
Lung Cancer Branch
National Cancer Institute
9000 Rockville Pike
Bethesda, MD 20014, USA

Prof. Dr. Robert L. Farrell
Department of Veterinary Pathology
University of Georgia
Athens, GA 30602, USA

Dr. Ronald E. Filipy
Battelle
Pacific Northwest Laboratories
P.O. Box 999
Richland, WA 99352, USA

Dr. Arthur L. Frank
Lung Cancer Branch
National Cancer Institute
9000 Rockville Pike
Bethesda, MD 20014, USA

Dr. Arthur Furst
Director
Institute of Chemical Biology
University of San Francisco
San Francisco, CA 94117, USA

Dr. Valerio Genta
Laboratorio di Virologia ed
Analisi Microbiologiche
Spedali Civili
I - 25100 Brescia

Dr. W. Ellis Giddens, Jr.
Regional Primate Research Center
University of Washington
Seattle, WA 98195, USA

Dr. Richard A. Griesemer
Oak Ridge National Laboratory
P.O. Box Y
Oak Ridge, TN 37830, USA

Dr. Laima Griciute
Unit of Environmental
Carcinogens
International Research Center
150, Cours Albert Thomas
F - 69008 Lyon

Dr. P.L. Hackett
Battelle
Pacific Northwest Laboratories
P.O. Box 999
Richland, WA 99352, USA

Dr. Fletcher F. Hahn
Inhalation Toxicology Research
Institute, Lovelace Foundation
5200 Gibson Boulevard Southeast
Albuquerque, NM 87108, USA

Dr. John D. Hardy
University of Southern California
School of Medicine
2025 Zonal Avenue
Los Angeles, CA 90033, USA

Dr. Curtis C. Harris
Lung Cancer Branch
National Cancer Institute
Bethesda, MD 20014, USA

Dr. Mary C. Henry
Life Sciences Division
IIT Research Institute
10 West 35th Street
Chicago, IL 60616, USA

Dr. W.J. Higgins
Carreras Rothmans Ltd.
Nevendon Road
GB - Basildon, Essex SS13 1BT

Dr. William Ho
Institute of Chemical Biology
University of San Francisco
2130 Fulton Street
San Francisco, CA 94117, USA

Dr. Charles H. Hobbs
Inhalation Toxicology Research
Institute, Lovelace Foundation
5200 Gibson Boulevard Southeast
Albuquerque, NM 87108, USA

Dr. Laurence M. Holland
Los Alamos Scientific Laboratory
University of California
P.O. Box 1663
Los Alamos, NM 87544, USA

Prof. Dr. Freddy Homburger
Bio-Research Consultants, Inc.
9 Commercial Avenue
Cambridge, MA 02141, USA

Doras D. Hubert
Health Research Institute
Fairleigh Dickinson University
285 Madison Avenue
Madison, NJ 07940, USA

Dr. R.J. Jones
Carreras Rothmans Ltd.
Nevendon Road
GB - Basildon, Essex SS13 1BT

Dr. Robert K. Jones
Inhalation Toxicology Research
Institute, Lovelace Foundation
P.O. Box 5890
Albuquerque, NM 87115, USA

Dr. Masayoshi Kanisawa
Department of Pathology
Tokyo Metropolitan Institute
of Gerontology
35-2 Sakaecho
Itabashiku Tokyo, 173, Japan

Dr. Phyllis Kaplan
Assistant Professor of Environ-
mental Health
Kettering Laboratory
University of Cincinnati
Medical Center
3223 Eden Avenue
Cincinnati, OH 45219, USA

608

Dr. Eberhard Karbe
Battelle-Institut e.V.
6000 Frankfurt/M. - 90
Am Römerhof 35

Dr. David G. Kaufman
Lung Cancer Branch
National Cancer Institute
Bethesda, MD 20014, USA

Dr. Joseph Kendrick
Oak Ridge National Laboratory
P.O. Box Y
Oak Ridge, TN 37830, USA

Dr. Ann R. Kennedy
Dept. of Physiology, Harvard
School of Public Health
665 Huntington Avenue
Boston, MA 02115, USA

Dr. Norbert Kmoch
Medizinische Hochschule Hannover
Abt. für Exp. Pathologie
3000 Hannover-Kleefeld
Karl-Wiechert-Allee 9

Dr. Kari Köster
Battelle-Institut e.V.
6000 Frankfurt/M. - 90
Am Römerhof 35

Dr. Richard E. Kouri
Co-Project Director
Department of Viral-Chemical
Oncology
Microbiological Associates
4809 Bethesda Avenue
Bethesda, MD 20014, USA

Dr. Jacques LaFuma
Centre d'Etudes Nucléaires
de Fontenay-aux-Roses
Départment de Protection
Commissariat à l'Energie Atomique
B.P. No. 6
F - 92260 Fontenay-aux-Roses

Dr. Bernhard P. Lane
Dept. of Pathology
Health Sciences Center
State University of New York
at Stony Brook
Stony Brook, NY 11794, USA

Dr. Sidney Laskin
New York University Medical Center
Department of Environmental
Medicine
550 First Avenue
New York, NY 10016, USA

Dr. Maxwell Layard
National Institutes of Health
National Cancer Institute
9000 Rockville Pike
Bethesda, MD 20014, USA

Dr. Philippe Lazar
Institut National de la Santé
et de la Recherche Médicale
Unité de Recherches Statistiques
16 Bis,
Avenue Paul-Vaillant-Couturier
F - 94800 Villejuif

Dr. David W. Lindsay
Carreras Rothmans Ltd.
Research Division
Nevendon Road
GB - Basildon, Essex SS13 1BT

Dr. Morton Lippmann
Institute of Environmental Medicine
New York University Medical Center
550 First Avenue
New York, NY 10016, USA

Dr. Hermann Lisco
Dept. of Anatomy
Harvard Medical School
25 Shattuck Street
Boston, MA 02115, USA

Dr. John B. Little
Harvard School of Public Health
665 Huntington Avenue
Boston, MA 02115, USA

Prof. Dr. Clayton G. Loosli
University of Southern California
School of Medicine
2025 Zonal Avenue
Los Angeles, CA 90033, USA

Dr. Russell M. Madison
Microbiological Associates, Inc.
4733 Bethesda Avenue
Bethesda, MD 20014, USA

Dr. R. Masse
Centre d'Etudes Nucléaires
Commissariat à l'Energie Atomique
B.P. No. 6
F - 92260 Fontenay-aux-Roses

Dr. Roger O. McClellan
Inhalation Toxicology Research
Institute, Lovelace Foundation
P.O. Box 5890
Albuquerque, NM 87115, USA

Dr. Elizabeth M. McDowell
Dept. of Pathology
University of Maryland
School of Medicine
31 S. Greene Street
Baltimore, MD 21201, USA

Dr. Robert B. McGandy
Dept. of Physiology
Harvard School of Public Health
665 Huntington Avenue
Boston, MA 02115, USA

Dr. H. Metivier
Centre d'Etudes Nucléaires
Commissariat à l'Energie Atomique
B.P. No. 6
F - 92260 Fontenay-aux-Roses

Dr. M. Michiels
Institute of Scientific Research
on Cancer, CNRS
B.P. No. 8
F - 94800 Villejuif

Eliza Miller
National Institutes of Health
National Cancer Institute
9000 Rockville Pike
Bethesda, MD 20014, USA

Dr. Sandra L. Miller
Dept. of Pathology
State University of New York
at Stony Brook
Stony Brook, NY 11790, USA

Dr. Ralph I. Mitchell
Biomedical Sciences Section
Battelle, Columbus Laboratories
505 King Avenue
Columbus, OH 43201, USA

Prof. Dr. Ulrich Mohr
Medizinische Hochschule Hannover
Abt. für Exp. Pathologie
3000 Hannover-Kleefeld
Karl-Wiechert-Allee 9

Dr. M. Morin
Centre d'Etudes Nucléaires
Commissariat à l'Energie Atomique
B.P. No. 6
F - 92260 Fontenay-aux-Roses

Dr. Brooke T. Mossman
Dept. of Pathology
University of Vermont
College of Medicine
Burlington, VT 05401, USA

Dr. J.C. Nénot
Centre d'Etudes Nucléaires
Commissariat à l'Energie Atomique
B.P. No. 6
F - 92260 Fontenay-aux-Roses

Dr. Paul Nettesheim
Oak Ridge National Laboratory
Biology Division
P.O. Box Y
Oak Ridge, TN 37830, USA

Dianne L. Newton
Lung Cancer Branch
National Cancer Institute
Bethesda, MD 20014, USA

Dr. D. Nobile
Centre d'Etudes Nucléaires
Commissariat à l'Energie Atomique
B.P. No. 6
F - 92260 Fontenay-aux-Roses

Dr. Masahiko Okita
Department of Surgery and
Pathology
Harbor General Hospital
Torrance, CA 90509, USA

Dr. Richard J. Olson
Biology Department, Battelle
Pacific Northwest Laboratories
P.O. Box 999
Richland, WA 99352, USA

Dr. Ray F. Palmer
Battelle
Pacific Northwest Laboratories
P.O. Box 999
Richland, WA 99352, USA

Dr. James Park
Battelle
Pacific Northwest Laboratories
P.O. Box 999
Richland, WA 99352, USA

Dr. Roger Perraud
Service Médical
Commissariat à l'Energie Atomique
B.P. No. 1
F - 87640 Razes

Dr. Curtis D. Port
IIT Research Institute
10 West 35th Street
Chicago, IL 60616, USA

Dr. J. Pradel
Commissariat à l'Energie Atomique
Département de Protection
Sanitaire
B.P. No. 6
F - 92260 Fontenay-aux-Roses

Dr. James R. Prine
Los Alamos Scientific Laboratory
University of California
P.O. Box 1663
Los Alamos, NM 87544, USA

Dr. Harvey A. Ragan
Battelle
Pacific Northwest Laboratories
P.O. Box 999
Richland, WA 99352, USA

Dr. Gerd Reznik
Medizinische Hochschule Hannover
Abt. für Exp. Pathologie
3000 Hannover-Kleefeld
Karl-Wiechert-Allee 9

Dr. N. Richdale
University of Cincinnati
College of Medicine
Department of Environmental Health
Kettering Laboratory
3223 Eden Avenue
Cincinnati, OH 45219, USA

Dr. Chester R. Richmond
Los Alamos Scientific Laboratory
University of California
P.O. Box 1663
Los Alamos, NM 87544, USA

Dr. A.B. Russfield
Pathology Department
St. Vincent Hospital
Worcester, MA 01610, USA

Dr. Umberto Saffiotti
DCCP, National Cancer Institute
Bethesda, MD 20014, USA

Dr. Charles L. Sanders
Battelle
Pacific Northwest Laboratories
P.O. Box 999
Richland, WA 99352, USA

Dr. Richard B. Schlesinger
Institute of Environmental Medicine
New York University Medical Center
550 First Avenue
New York, NY 10016, USA

Prof. Dr. Dietrich Schmähl
Deutsches Krebsforschungszentrum
Institut für Toxikologie
und Chemotherapie
6900 Heidelberg
Im Neuenheimer Feld 280

Dr. Klaus G. Schmidt
Deutsches Krebsforschungszentrum
Institut für Toxikologie
und Chemotherapie
6900 Heidelberg
Im Neuenheimer Feld 280

Dr. Arthur Sellakumar
Department of Environmental
Medicine, School of Medicine
New York University
550 First Avenue
New York, NY 10016, USA

Dr. Margaret A. Sheridan
Battelle
Columbus Laboratories
505 King Avenue
Columbus, OH 43201, USA

Dr. W. Skupinski
Centre d'Etudes Nucléaires
Commissariat à l'Energie Atomique
B.P. No. 6
F - 92260 Fontenay-aux-Roses

Dr. David O. Slauson
Inhalation Toxicology Research
Institute, Lovelace Foundation
5200 Gibson Boulevard Southeast
Albuquerque, NM 87108, USA

Joseph M. Smith
Lung Cancer Branch
National Cancer Institute
Bethesda, MD 20014, USA

Dr. William E. Smith
Health Research Institute
Fairleigh Dickinson University
285 Madison Avenue
Madison, NJ 07940, USA

Dr. Michael B. Sporn
Lung Cancer Branch
Carcinogenesis Program
National Cancer Institute
Bethesda, MD 20014, USA

Dr. Mearl F. Stanton
National Institutes of Health
National Cancer Institute
9000 Rockville Pike
Bethesda, MD 20014, USA

Dr. Frej Stenbäck
Eppley Institute for Research
in Cancer
University of Nebraska
Medical Center
42nd and Dewey Avenue
Omaha, NB 68105, USA

Dr. Sherman F. Stinson
University of Southern California
School of Medicine
2025 Zonal Avenue
Los Angeles, CA 90033, USA

Dr. Bruce O. Stuart
Divison of Biomedical and
Environmental Reasearch, USAEC
Washington, DC 20545, USA

Dr. Margaret Terzaghi
Dept. of Physiology
Harvard School of Public Health
665 Huntington Avenue
Boston, MA 02115, USA

Prof. Dr. Benjamin F. Trump
Dept. of Pathology
University of Maryland
School of Medicine
31 S. Greene Street
Baltimore, MD 21201, USA

Dr. Alfred P. Wehner
Battelle
Pacific Northwest Laboratories
P.O. Box 999
Richland, WA 99352, USA

Dr. Carrie E. Whitmire
Department of Experimental
Oncology
Microbiological Associates
4809 Bethesda Avenue
Bethesda, MD 20014, USA

Dr. Kristina Wilcox
Institute of Chemical Biology
University of San Francisco
San Francisco, CA 94117, USA

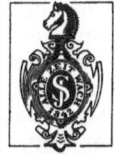

Springer-Verlag
Berlin
Heidelberg
New York

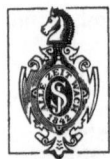

Springer-Verlag
Berlin Heidelberg New York

München Johannesburg London Madrid
New Delhi Paris Rio de Janeiro Sydney
Tokyo Utrecht Wien

Kwa Hong Giok
An Experimental Study of Pituitary Tumours

Genesis, Cytology and Hormone Content
17 figures. IV, 94 pages. 1961
DM 26,—; US $10.70
ISBN 3-540-02714-9

Proceedings of the 9th International Cancer Congress, Tokyo, October 1966

Congress Lectures and Official Speeches.
Editor: R.J.C. Harris
8 figures. VIII, 126 pages. 1967.
(UICC Monograph Series, Vol. 9)
Cloth DM 32,—; US $13.10
ISBN 3-540-04011-0

Complete text of the important lectures
on recent trends in cancer research
delivered by leading authorities at the
Tokyo congress. Among the topics
reviewed are the following: Site variation of the alimentary tract cancer in
man and experimental animals as
indicators of diverse etiology, by
H.L. Stewart; Viral carcinogenesis, by
R. Dulbecco; Cancer immunology by
G. Klein; Chromosomic aberration and
cancer, by J. Lejeune; and The
molecular basis of translation of the
genetic message, by Nobel prizewinner
S. Ochoa.

Proceedings of the International Cancer Congress, Tokyo, October 1966

Panel Discussions. Editor: R.J.C. Harris
111 figures. XII, 288 pages. 1967.
(UICC Monograph Series, Vol. 10)
Cloth DM 75,—; US $30.60
ISBN 3-540-04012-9

Selected panel discussions held at the
Tokyo congress. The following fields
are covered: the epidemiology and
pathogenesis of cancer of the stomach;
an evaluation of techniques of cancer
detection; radiation as a cancer hazard
in man; techniques and results of anti-
smoking campaigns; chemotherapy
as an adjuvant to surgery and radiation therapy; the evaluation of controlled clinical trials; advances in the
management of leukemias and
lymphomas; and the management of
advanced cancer.

Potential Carcinogenetic Hazards from Drugs

Evaluation of Risks
Editor: R. Truhaut
24 figures. X, 249 pages (58 pages
in French). 1967. (UICC Monograph
Series, Vol. 7)
Cloth DM 75,—; US $30.60
ISBN 3-540-04009-9

The proceedings of this UICC Symposium, held in Paris from 3 to 6
November 1965, contain papers on the
qualitative and quantitative evaluation
of the carcinogenic risks of the main
categories of drugs, plastic substances
used in surgery, and radio-isotopes used
for diagnostic purposes.
Information on the potential carcinogenic effects of certain drugs in
scattered throughout the literature;
it appeared desirable to collect and
submit it to the scrutiny of onco-
logists, pharmacologists, and toxico-
logists.

Prices are subject to change without notice